Robotic Assisted Hernia Repair

Karl A. LeBlanc
Editor

Robotic Assisted Hernia Repair

Current Practice

Springer

Editor
Karl A. LeBlanc
Our Lady of the Lake Physician Group
Baton Rouge, LA
USA

ISBN 978-3-030-23024-1 ISBN 978-3-030-23025-8 (eBook)
https://doi.org/10.1007/978-3-030-23025-8

This Springer imprint is published by the registered company Springer Nature Switzerland AG
The registered company address is: Gewerbestrasse 11, 6330 Cham, Switzerland

This textbook is dedicated to my wife, Zinda. Without her support over all these years, I could not have accomplished what I have in my career.

Contents

Part I

General Topics

Robotic Technologies (Past, Present and Future)

1

Brian S. Peters, Priscila R. Armijo, and Dmitry Oleynikov

1.1 Introduction

Surgical robotic technologies and their ancillary systems have been proposed to improve patient outcomes via shorter recoveries and limited scarring while allowing surgeons increased dexterity and visualization [1]. The prototype for discussion of modern robotic systems capable of application in the surgical theater is the *da Vinci*, a well-established platform whose development dates to the turn of the century. Additionally, implementation of and demand for robotic surgical platforms has fueled growth in the sector leading to an increase in the number of products in development as well available for purchase. General surgery trends indicate movement toward minimally invasive procedures when available, many of which are well suited to robotic-assisted surgical platforms [2].

With each new implementation of a robotic-assisted surgical platform, the foothold technology has secured in the operating theater strengthens. Therefore, to understand the general picture and survey the minimally invasive robotic-assisted surgery landscape, a historical review of the origins of these entities is indicated. Here the critical developments, evolutionary phases, adverse events, cost of development and purchase, as well as barriers to care and training will be

B. S. Peters
College of Medicine, University of Nebraska Medical Center, Omaha, NE, USA

P. R. Armijo
Center for Advanced Surgical Technology, University of Nebraska Medical Center, Omaha, NE, USA

D. Oleynikov (✉)
Center for Advanced Surgical Technology, University of Nebraska Medical Center, Omaha, NE, USA

Department of Surgery, University of Nebraska Medical Center, Omaha, NE, USA
e-mail: doleynik@unmc.edu

K. A. LeBlanc (ed.), *Robotic Assisted Hernia Repair*,
https://doi.org/10.1007/978-3-030-23025-8_1

discussed. The historical record on safety and feasibility of robotic assisted surgery platforms throughout their evolution may elucidate the current state of affairs.

1.2 Ancient Past

The journey of understanding the origin of robotic-assisted surgery begins in the centuries leading to the Age of Pericles and the founder of the Hippocratic School of Medicine, Hippocrates of Kos. Greek physicians in the years Before the Common Era (BCE) limited their practice to surgery of bone and muscle while ignoring internal organs as inconsequential causes of disease [3]. The sequence of examination, diagnosis, prognosis and treatment was developed and refined, while magical and religious hypotheses of pathology were ostracized [3]. Historically the evolutionary origin of robotics is rooted in the mythology and scholarship of ancient Greece, China, and Egypt [4].

During the age of Hippocrates, the likeness of a robotic entity was not unknown and could be found in Greek mythology via poetry. For instance, the Greek dactylic hexametric poem the Iliad portrayed Hephaestus as the forefather of modern technological platform designers via his Automata [5]. The Greek god of blacksmiths and craftsmen, Hephaestus was said to have a workshop on Olympus where he engineered items for the gods while delegating executive design oversight to a team of Cyclopes forgers [5]. Hephaestus' automata, self-operating machines capable of autonomous actions of their own free will, are an example of man's predilection for creativity and imagination and a starting point for the discussion of robotic evolution. Each Automaton was said to be mobile, functional, and programmable [6]. These early entities of mechanical operation foreshadow the existence of modern controllable computer programmable devices by millennia and in this text act as the genesis of robotic ideation.

The passage of time from Before Common Era (BCE) to Common Era (CE), is marked by several other written examples of creative manifestations prefiguring robotic technology. For instance, Yan Shi's Chinese automatons who in the Lie Zi text (1000 BCE) were capable of walking, posturing, and performing humanlike mannerisms. These designs of leather and wood were designed by Yan Shi to be compartmentally dependent on hierarchical systems [7]. When a component controlling a specific movement was removed, that movement was lost while unaffected functionality remained [7]. Shi's automaton design incorporating subdivision of process by systematic control is a remarkable example of fiction's harbingering ability and generally parallels modern platforms.

A further example of invention with foundational influence on modern robotic technology is the work of Hero of Alexandria. An Egyptian engineer, Hero wrote several works on his efforts in mathematics and mechanical experimentation. His user-configurable automated systems were described in text as incorporating pneumatic, catoptric, and mechanical components to manipulate objects and light [8]. One such effort, Heron's aeolipile, was a radial steam turbine which created rotational force via propulsive jet expulsion [8]. While the aeolipile had only loose similarities to modern day robotic-assisted surgical technology platforms, it serves as an ancient surrogate for intellectual thought on the input/output computing communication utilized in modern day computer processing. Just as the data input into a processing system is that which is received, the heat added to the aeolipile acted as a signal in the interaction between user and system. Similarly, the steam producing torque was the output corollary.

The connection between ancient tinkerer and today's billion-dollar industry is not direct, rather a chain that has been established over time through the individual links created by each contributor to robotic technology evolution. One such connection was formed by Ismail al-Jazari, the 1206 CE Muslim author of *The Book of Knowledge of Ingenious Mechanical Devices*. The Anatolian artisan contributed automata capable of the first-known feedback control function. The device incorporated mechanical design elements which allowed an operator to fine tune fluid dynamics through a manual interface which regulated operational outputs [9]. Al-jazari's illustrated descriptions clearly delineate progress in input and feedback control system innovation; reservoir volume regulation via valve modulation dependent flow rate in temporal water clock design [9].

Note that technology progressed in a stepwise fashion and successive progressions were made based on principles set forth in preceding scientific efforts. Each generational achievement progressed the ceiling of technology synergistically and various contributions combined to facilitate future achievements. For instance, the mechanical engineering advancements made by the Greeks utilizing air, vacuum, and balance principles profoundly influenced the work of al-Jazari [10].

1.3 Modern Period

In the eighteenth century, Swiss watchmaker Pierre Jaquet-Droz developed automata capable of programmable actions arguably equivalent to computing as it is currently understood [11]. His mechanical devices incorporated elements derivative of his own work on intricate watch complications, or those functions of a timepiece in addition to displaying the hours, minutes, and seconds [11]. One invention, The Writer, was comprised of 6000 individual parts and could systematically interpret a program disk and translate the input into hand written text up to 40 characters [11]. Crank loaded spring power enabled the android's system of interchangeable cams and gears to actuate the read-only program, in addition to various mannerisms, sans outside intervention [11].

Countless others contributed: Philon of Byzantium, Giovanni de la Fontana, Juanelo Turriano, Athanasius Kircher, Heri Maillardet, Leonardo da Vinici, Wolfgang von Kempelen, Salomon de Caus. Attributing the origin of an entire faction of science to a single person, geographical location, or even millennium would be erroneous. The list presented here should not be considered exhaustive and merely represents a fraction of the applicable contributions to the sector.

1.4 Robot

Heretofore the term automaton was described in myth, literature, and historical engineering design as a machine with the capability of actuating movements or functions, complex or otherwise. However, in 1920 Czech author Karel Čapek penned a play entitled *R.U.R. Rossumovia Univerzální Roboti* (Rossum's Universal Robots). In this work, Čapek modified the Slavnoic word for forced-labor servitude (rabota), and the term Robot was coined [12]. The fictional play describes the use of robotic biotechnological workers who were mass produced to complete tasks unappealing to residents of its dystopian central European setting [13]. The etymology of the word robot developed further when, in 1979, The Robot Institute of America bestowed a formal definition: "a reprogrammable, multifunctional manipulator designed to move materials, parts, tools, or specialized devices through various programmed motions for the performance of a variety of tasks" [12].

1.5 Contemporary Period

Born in the United States, though raised and educated in England, William Grey Walter was a neuroscientist known for his contribution to the increased clinical use of electroencephalograms (EEG) [14]. In addition to the use of EEG to treat epilepsy, Walter pioneered the use of EEG to detect localized brain tumors through delta and theta patterns of activity. His work in the 1940s to understand the cerebral rhythm lead to the construction of an apparatus which incorporated electrodes and a camera to visualize and scrutinize the phase and frequency of the EEG. The device contained cathode ray tubes (CRT), like those used in that era's televisions, each connected to an electrode attached to the patient [15]. The collection of 22 individual CRTs was then photographed, resulting in a brain mapping technique that predates neuro-imaging as it is now known [15]. Additionally, Walter's research in neurophysiology eventually led to his involvement in a project with lasting contributions in the field of robotics. During the late years of the 1940s Walter created a series of mechanical inventions designed to mimic human behavior [16]. A pair of successive iterations were named the Electromechanical Robot (Elmer) and the Electro Light Sensitive with Internal and External Stability (Elsie) respectively [14]. The robots were comprised of vacuum tubes, motors, and a photoelectric cell, and were collectively named Machina Speculatrix. This manifestation of robotic ingenuity was separated from preceding automata through its ability to autonomously interact with an environment. The sensory system of M. Speculatrix could identify the presence of physical objects, the intensity of light, and would modulate its motility as a function of those environmental characteristics [16]. While exploring its environment M. Speculatrix could travel towards moderate light, avoid bright light and objects, thus effectively decide on the most favorable conditions in which to exist [16]. A mobile photosensitive tactile robot that displayed complex environmental condition recognition, M. Speculatrix incorporated biological principles in its design which would persist in future robotic development efforts [17].

Joseph F. Engelberger and George C. Devol founded the first proper robotics company Unimation [Danbury, Connecticut] after their initial collaboration in 1956 [18]. As the Korean War waned, Engelberger's position as an engineer of aircraft parts for military contracts became vulnerable. Eventually, after corporate reorganization by his employer, he was able to secure funding and transition his team to a division focused on developing an industrial robot [19]. It was Devol who developed and patented the applicable technology, but Engelberger acted as spokesperson and championed the cause by serving up his visionary promotional showmanship in a calculated manner conducive to securing the interest of investors [18]. During its initial development, the anthropomorphic robot named *Unimate* was built using a polar coordinate design: a two-dimensional system where points on the plane are relative by distance and angle to a central reference point and direction respectively [19]. The platform was capable of 5 degrees of freedom (DOF) via a pair of axes and gears powered by 1000 psi hydraulics [19]. Novel design innovations allowed the incorporation of digital controls, magnetic drum memory, optical positioning feedback, and intrinsic power supplies [19]. The result was a complex programmable system containing technological elements with scope and scale surpassing any previously known robotics platform. The Unimate was utilized by industrial applications such as diecasting, spot welding, and eventually automobile manufacturing and assembly [19]. Engelberger's advocacy for the incorporation of "smart" machines like the Unimate promised safer work site conditions and increased productivity, ultimately leading to licensing agreements with companies including Nokia, Kawasaki, General Motors, BMW, and Mercedes [18, 20].

Once the development and industrial implementation of new technology had been established, the door opened for broader applications of use. Accordingly, the capabilities of the Unimate platform were quickly adapted for use in the medical field. While working at Unimation, Victor Sheinmann adapted a Unimate platform in 1978 into a Programmable Universal Machine for Assembly (PUMA) (Westinghouse Electric, Pittsburgh, PA) [21]. The evolution of PUMA's application from agent of industrial assembly efficiency to one of greater surgical precision sparked a movement and signified a turning point in the origin of robotic-assisted surgery.

1.6 Healthcare Robotics

One of the first implementations of a robot-assisted surgery platform in healthcare was in 1985 by Kwoh et al. [22]. Kowh and his team adapted a PUMA for use in stereotactic brain tumor biopsy, with radioactive implantation and deep brain stimulation theorized as secondary indications for use (Fig. 1.1) [22]. Previously, frame mounted CT-guided stereotactic apparatuses were used to navigate instruments through brain tissue. However, these stereotactic devices were difficult to couple with their CT imaging counterparts; manually adjusting instrument position via graduated positioning scales on the frame according to CT imaging findings was inefficient and limiting. Therefore, improvements in automation and

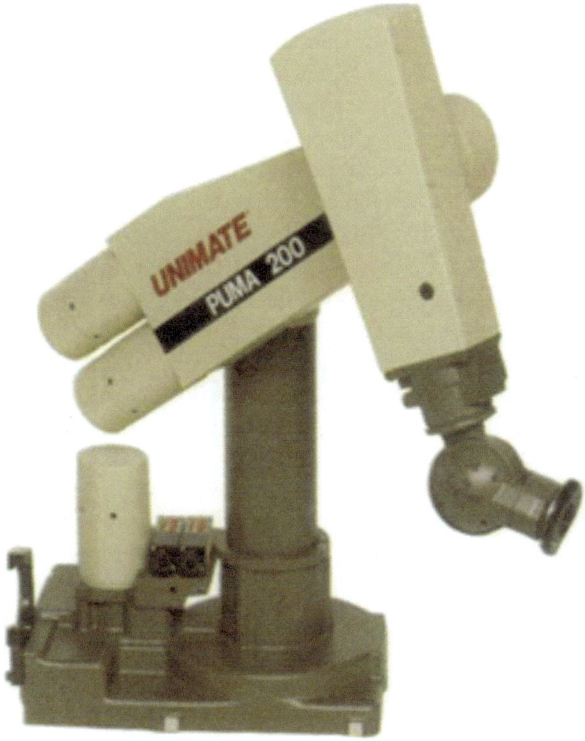

Fig. 1.1 PUMA 200

instrument manipulation capability were desired. Kwoh et al. retrofit the commercially available industrial robot UNIMATION PUMA 200 with a Siemens DRH CT scanner [22]. This combination resulted in a platform that could be programed, controlled by a computer, and allowed instrument manipulation accurate to 0.05 mm. Interfacing a computerized tomographic scanner with contemporary robotic technology resulted in faster procedure times than previously available with stereotactic frames adjusted by hand [22]. Iterations of the PUMA ushered in a new era in medicine, one where the realization of robotic-assisted surgery was no longer fiction but reality.

Another pioneering application of technology was the development of the robotic-assisted surgery platform the Arthrobot [Vancouver BC] for bone mountable hip arthroplasty [23]. Biomedical researchers Dr. James McEwen, Geof Auchinlek, and Dr. Brian Day oversaw the development of the system which assisted an orthopedic surgeon by manipulating the position of the joint by adjusting the limb held in the robotic arm's gripper [23, 24]. Voice recognition capabilities allowed the surgeon to interact with the system using 20 spoken words for command input and speakers emitting closed-loop communication for command confirmation [23]. Like many integrations of technology in medicine, the goal of the Arthrobot was safer procedures and quality improvement in outcomes over existing techniques [24].

Extending previous efforts of orthopedic surgeons to incorporate robotic technology by adapting the foundational principals of the PUMA 560, the Thomas J. Watson Research Center developed ROBODOC (Curexo Technology Corporation). The milling robot was used in 1986 for total hip replacement procedures to core the femoral shaft thereby facilitating femoral-prosthesis integration with 96% precision [25]. This “press fit” preparation of the femoral canal allowed fitting a prosthesis without the use of bone cement [26]. The robotic platform’s accuracy was accomplished through the combination of a high-speed drill and CT imaging [21]. Hip arthroplasty prosthesis sizing via image-directed robotic-assisted femoral preparation was shown to improve on the conventional hand broach femoral coring technique, which was 75% accurate [25]. After a successful clinical trial of 300 patients, ROBODOC earned FDA approval becoming the first robotic-assisted surgery platform to do so (Fig. 1.2) [27]. Preoperative planning and programming of autonomous robotic platforms operating under the supervision of medically trained personnel was thus available for the first time to provide a level of execution beyond that which is capable by the human hand [12].

Temporally paralleling the previously described orthopedic platform was the development of a robotic-assisted surgical platform for use in urology. The PROBOT (Integrated Surgical Supplies Ltd.) was an adaptation of the PUMA 560 system for use in transurethral resection of the prostate (TURP). Its design incorporated a novel circular metal safety frame which maintained the robotic arm and resection instrumentation position within the relatively small prostatic operating window [25, 28]. The platform incorporated on-line imaging and used a 3D model of the prostate to enhance the interface between surgeon and system. The PROBOT was proven successful in clinical trials for robotic-assisted resection of prostatic tissue, although it failed to gain traction necessary for widespread clinical adoption [29].

Foundational advancements in robotic-assisted surgical platforms were necessary for the development of future efforts. The successful demonstration of each

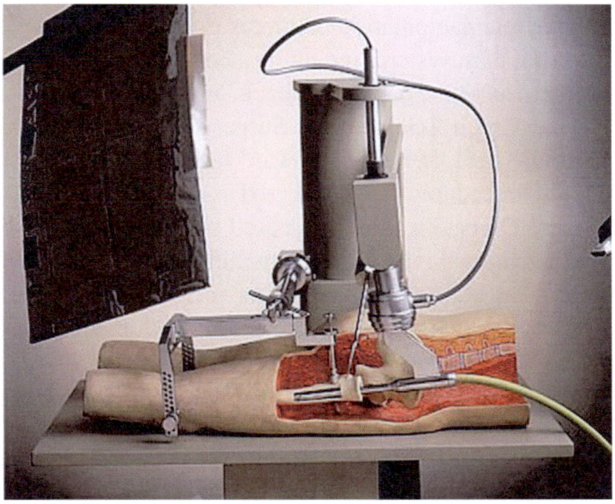

Fig. 1.2 ROBODOC developed by Integrated Surgical Supplies, Inc

subsequent system provided a tangible bastion for continued development and progress. Previously in this historical review of robotic-assisted surgical platforms, developers strove to integrate programmable computer controlled robotic technology into open surgery to positively impact procedures. Modern Robotic Hernia Surgery, however, is founded on the use of laparoscopy. The crux of the transition from the former to latter was the development of a technology for remotely manipulating robotic platform extensions while separated by a distance. This spatial detachment of operator control and mechanical actuation was termed telepresence by the technologist Scott Fisher, PhD [27].

In the mid-1980s the National Air and Space Administration (NASA) Ames Research Center began working on telepresence to provide remote access surgery [30]. To provide an interface environment between a robotic entity controlled by a spatially separated operator, telepresence required the application of a virtual reality [12]. Multidiscipline research cooperation between teams led by Scott Fisher at NASA-Ames and Philip Green at the Stanford Research Institute (SRI) division focused on robotic telemanipulation and resulted in several hardware developments [30]. The team's contributions included the first head-mounted display (HMD), which was developed to display data from NASA's Voyager [25]. Additionally, the efforts of multiple collaborators resulted in the DataGlove, an interactive interface between user and 3D virtual reality environments [25]. Progress in software was necessary to drive the application of these devices and VPL, Inc. led by Jaron Lanier, developed an object-orientated program to that end. Lanier was an early proponent of the vernacular dubbed virtual reality and his visual programming language allowed the creation of computer programs using graphical elements rather than text [31]. The combination of experts with diverse backgrounds in biomechanics, robotics, and virtual reality led to collaboration which proved to be instrumental in the origin of modern robotic-assisted surgery. The late 1980s marked a time which realized crossover between robotics designed for industrial use, telepresence, and robotic telemanipulation technologies applied to medicine signifying the emergence of robotic-assisted surgery [32]. The prototype platform developed by Green for robotic telemanipulation in microsurgery at SRI showcased characteristics found in many modern systems including a control console, telemanipulation of interchangeable instruments, haptic feedback, and HD-3D visualization [32].

The Green Telepresence Surgery System possessed inherent capabilities that naturally lend themselves toward laparoscopic surgery. For instance, early laparoscopic procedures were criticized as inferior to open procedures due to their diminished 3-D visualization, decreased dexterity, and loss of haptic feedback compared to conventional means. These qualities attracted the interest of Richard Satava MD, a surgical endoscopist who was instrumental in the 1992 establishment of the advanced biomedical technologies division at the Defense Advanced Research Projects Agency (DARPA) [25]. The influx of funding provided by the Pentagon supported a nidus for further development of robotic-assisted surgery platforms [25]. The military's mission was to develop The Green Telepresence Surgery System into a platform capable of providing forward battlefield surgical care to soldiers with potentially mortal wounds through robotic telemedicine [25]. The concept was to mount the robotic arms in a Bradley Fighting Vehicle to establish Medical Forward Advanced Surgical Treatment (MEDFAST) with a surgeon operating via telepresence from the safety of a Mobile Advanced Surgical Hospital (MASH) [25]. In 1994, vascular surgeon Jon Bowersox performed an ex vivo porcine intestinal anastomosis from a MASH-to-MEDFAST unit during a combat exercise [21, 32]. The procedure utilized wireless microwave data transfer and marked the first telesurgery demonstration.

DARPA funding was influential in the development of additional systems with a catapulting effect on sector advancement. For instance, the Automated Endoscopic System for Optimal Positioning (AESOP) from Yulun Wang's Computer Motion, Inc. established in 1993, was the first platform specifically designed for abdominal laparoscopic surgery approved by the Food and Drug Administration (Fig. 1.3). The system incorporated voice recognition software to allow control of an endoscopic camera fixed to a robotic arm [30]. The robotic endoscopic camera was capable of 23 voice-controlled commands via 7 degrees of freedom and increased image stability for improved visualization of the surgical field [30]. Following its introduction, systems derivative of AESOP have been used in hundreds of thousands of minimally invasive surgical procedures in a variety of fields [32]. Advantages of AESOP

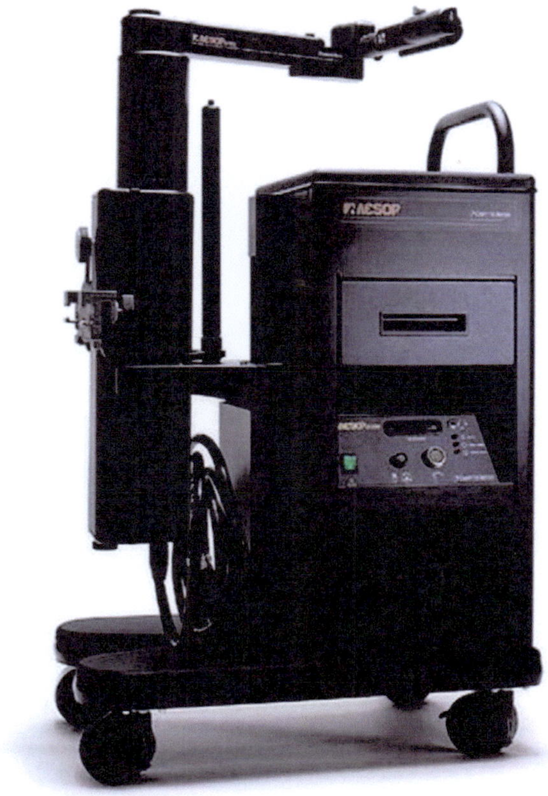

Fig. 1.3 Computer Motion's AESOP (Automatic Endoscopic System for Optimal Positioning)

over conventional hand held camera operation were described in a Johns Hopkins study showing no increase in operating time while using standard laparoscopic port placement in 17 different procedures such as nephrectomy, retroperitoneal lymph node resection, and Burch Bladder suspension [33]. In addition to providing a more stable view, AESOP eliminated the need for a camera controlling assistant, effectively allowing a laparoscopic surgeon to operate solo [21]. This seemingly small contribution brought robotic-assisted surgery platforms one step closer to autonomy by whittling the human component down to one. However, with increased dependence on technology came associated voice control drawbacks such as command to action latency, dialect recognition, integration and adaptation of technique, and potentially distracting talking [21].

Extensive modifications to the AESOP system resulted in Computer Motion's introduction of the ZEUS operating system, the first formal master-slave platform (Fig. 1.4). With this type of system, end effector instrumentation is exclusively actuated by a surgery control center workstation without autonomous programming input from the platform itself [27]. The master portion consists of a video monitor console and 2 surgeon operated handles, left and right, to control the respective robotic arm slaves. With three independent arms and all the functionality of AESOP's voice activated camera system, ZEUS could manipulate 2 instruments with 4 degrees of freedom [12]. Instruments with articulating end-effectors as well as conventional endoscopic instruments with straight shafts were available for use. Special glasses allowed the surgeon 3D visualization provided by a Storz imaging system (Karl Storz Endoscopy, Santa Barbara, CA, USA) [21]. By physically separating the surgeon and patient, ZEUS could reduce operator tremor through its electromechanical interface. Additionally, the computer system could scale operator joystick input up to a factor of 10 thereby allowing precise instrument control

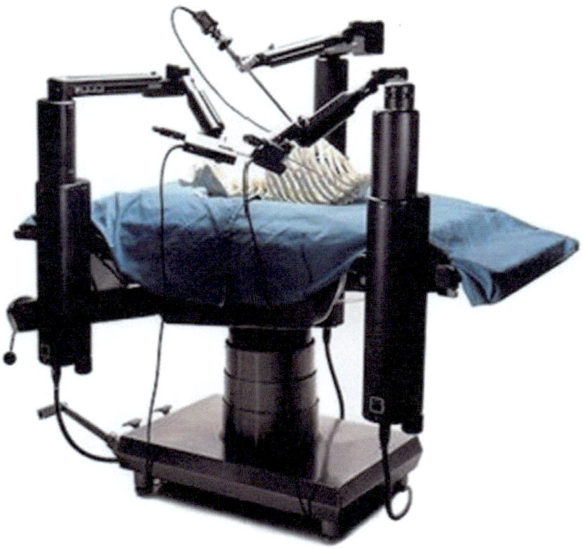

Fig. 1.4 ZEUS robotic system

beyond that which is capable by hand [25]. For instance, scaling handle input from 1 cm to 1 mm allowed end effector actuation with greater accuracy. Future systems would incorporate this technology to achieve precision not otherwise possible.

In 1998, the ZEUS operating system was successfully used by Falcone et al. for laparoscopic uterine tubal reanastomosis microsuturing at the Cleveland Clinic [34]. Additionally, in 1999 Reichenspurner et al. performed the first coronary bypass anastomosis using a robotic-assisted surgical system in porcine and canine models [35]. Numerous other studies contributed to data indicating the safety, feasibility, and increased dexterity provided by the platform in gynecologic and adnexal procedures [30]. ZEUS gained FDA approval in 2001 [12]. In 2001, the French surgeon Jacques Marescaux, successfully demonstrated the capability of a robotic-assisted surgical platform to perform a tele-surgical procedure on a scale previously only theorized. Leading a team of surgeons at the Institute for Research into Cancer of the Digestive System (IRCAD) in New York, Marescaux used the ZEUS surgical robot to perform a minimally invasive cholecystectomy on a patient in Strasbourg, France without any intra-operative complications [36]. The event was named the Lindbergh Operation in homage to Charles Lindberg, the pilot who first flew an airplane across the 3600-mile transatlantic route from New York to Paris, France. The Lindbergh Operation overcame numerous technical challenges including telecommunication delay resulting from bandwidth and digital conversion limitations [36]. Utilizing Computer Motion's SOCRATES telepresence software, the distance spanning patient-side and surgeon-side components of the ZEUS platform was connected via fiber optics allowing data transfer at a rate of 10 megabits per second [12, 36]. This groundbreaking event demonstrated the realization of telesurgery and would fuel future moonshots in the development of robotic-assisted surgery platforms.

Meanwhile, following the Bowersox MEDFAST-to-MASH procedure, Frederick H. Moll MD acquired the license to the SRI Green Telepresence Surgery system and along with Robert Younge and John Freund created Integrated Surgical Systems (now Intuitive Surgical) [21]. While the future directions of long-distance telesurgery were intriguing to Moll, the surgeon entrepreneur began to focus the company's resources on improving conventional civilian minimally invasive surgery, specifically laparoscopy. Using the intellectual property from the SRI acquisition, Intuitive Surgical developed a robotic-assisted surgery prototype in 1997 [32]. Named after Leonardo da Vinci, the fifteenth century inventor known for his study of human anatomy, a lineage of prototypes were refined including Lenny, Leonardo, and MONA [37]. In 1997, MONA was used to telesurgically perform the first robotic-assisted laparoscopic cholecystectomy on a 72-year-old woman in Dendermonde, Belgium [38]. The final prototype of the system was named the da Vinci Surgical System with commercial marketing beginning in 1999. This final iteration marked the first truly integrated robotic surgical system approved by the FDA in 2000 for general laparoscopic surgery [39]. While platforms predating da Vinci utilized endoscopy equipment operated by assistants to the surgeon, the da Vinci allowed a surgeon to work solo, like the AESOP technology utilized in the ZEUS platform. Additionally, da Vinci's arms were considerably smaller in dimeter than the PUMA 560, measuring only 1-cm, and allowed incision walls without leverage which lowered infection risk by minimizing contact of exposed tissue and the robotic arms [39]. As time passed, the da Vinci Surgical system would eventually become the dominate system in the field of robotic-assisted surgery. However, in the beginning the system faced fierce competition from competitors such as Computer Motion's Zeus. Distinguishing capabilities of early da Vinci models included seven degrees of freedom owing to end effector joint articulation, haptic feedback, and 3D vision [32]. Technically, the key was a smaller size, three-dimensional binocular stereoscopic endoscopic imaging system transmitted to a surgeon console [21]. The earliest version of the system had three arms, one for the endoscope, and two for instruments. The 12 mm endoscope contained a pair of 5 mm cameras; left and right aspect perception allowed a 3D visual reproduction of the surgical field [32]. Robotic arms were controlled by the surgeon via left and right hand joysticks mounted to the console as well as foot pedals for additional operational command [32]. End effectors were capable of a variety of actions including insufflation, illumination, and cautery.

1.7 Twenty-First Century

The rush to incorporate new robotic-assisted surgical platforms led to numerous studies collecting data on feasibility, safety, and benefit over conventional techniques. Between 1999 and 2001, Gettman et al. showed data indicating that the da Vinci system could perform laparoscopic Anderson-Hynes pyeloplasty for primary ureteropelvic junction obstruction in less time than necessary for conventional laparoscopy and without open conversion or complications [40]. Additionally, in 2002, Horgan et al. successfully performed ten living donor human laparoscopic nephrectomies at the University of Illinois at Chicago [41].

Furthermore, the first open heart operation exclusively using a robotic-assisted surgery platform was completed in 1998 with the da Vinci for a minimally invasive mitral valve surgery (MIMVS) on a 52-year old woman with an atrial septal defect [42]. Each demonstration expanded the variety of procedures da Vinci was capable of. By 2000 the platform was FDA approved for adult and pediatric urologic, general laparoscopic, gynecologic laparoscopic, general non-cardiovascular thoracoscopic, and cardiothoracic surgical procedures.

Despite its many successes, in the late 1990s and early 2000s the future market domination of Intuitive Surgical's da Vinci was not guaranteed. Early on, a budding rivalry between da Vinci and ZEUS was punctuated by their unique modi operandi. Although both robotic-assisted surgical platforms were similar in their master-slave multi-limbed telepresence controlled surgeon-side console to patient-side instrument layout, each had unique strengths resulting from their varied upbringing. While the ZEUS platform's workstation provided the surgeon a comfortable chair in which to view imaging via a monitor, the inherent perception was one of being separated from the patient. In contrast, da Vinci's workstation incorporated stereoscopic image visualization located directly above the hand-held joysticks. This spatial relationship between hand-held controls and visualization modality provided the sensation that the robotic end effectors were extensions of the joystick and that the patient was directly in front of the surgeon [25]. Moreover, although ZEUS and da Vinci both utilized computer enhanced visualization, the NASA and US Army derived telepresence based da Vinci was shown to outperform ZEUS and conventional laparoscopy in a variety of tasks. For instance, in one study indicating overall usability, suturing and knot-typing times were significantly lower using the da Vinci system compared to ZEUS and conventional laparoscopy [43]. Additionally, da Vinci outperformed the competitors in task errors as well as subjective assessments such as fluidity, efficacy, precision, dexterity, tactile feedback, tremor reduction, and coordination [43]. The da Vinci platform's subjective and objective performance superiority was contributed to its greater range of motion and articulation provided by more degrees of freedom than that of the ZEUS platform. Additionally, its binocular vision, motion scaling, and joystick ergonomics were cited as attributing to its superiority [43]. Although ZEUS allowed independent right and left robotic arm control as well as AESOP voice-operated 2D endoscopic visualization, its limitations in geometric accuracy, stability, tactile feedback were unable to compensate. Ultimately, when compared to the ZEUS system, the da Vinci system's intuitive interaction characteristics were shown to produce shallower user learning curves and shorter times during laparoscopic procedures such as nephrectomy, adrenalectomy, pyeloplasty, and surgical anastomosis [44]. In this case, history was written by the victor and in 2003 Computer motion merged with Intuitive Surgical thus neutralizing the patent war. The ZEUS system was discontinued leaving the da Vinci as the sole robotic-assisted surgical platform available for commercial purchase [12]. Later versions of da Vinci including the 2006 da Vinci S, 2009 da Vinci Si, and the 2011 single-site da Vinci Si each contributed to the development of the modern platform: the da Vinci Xi and X (Figs. 1.5, 1.6, 1.7, and 1.8).

The stepwise development of successive iterations contributed to the current Xi product. For instance, the da Vinci S reduced set-up complications and improved visualization by upgrading camera technology to utilize high-definition 3-dimensional (HD-3D) technology. Additionally, the da Vinci S furthered the ease of interaction between surgeon and platform by incorporating an interactive touch screen display. A few years later, the da Vinci Si offered a dual console for use in training junior team members like a car with 2 steering wheels for driver instruction. The Si also added substantial imaging capabilities to its design. For instance, the da

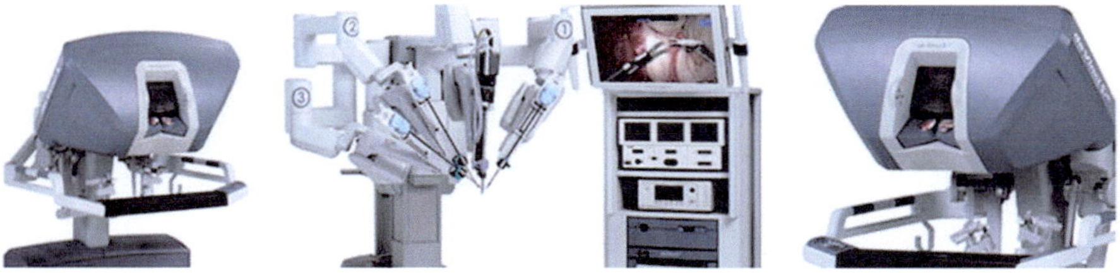

Fig. 1.5 The da Vinci® Surgical System (Intuitive Surgical, Inc., Sunnyvale, CA)

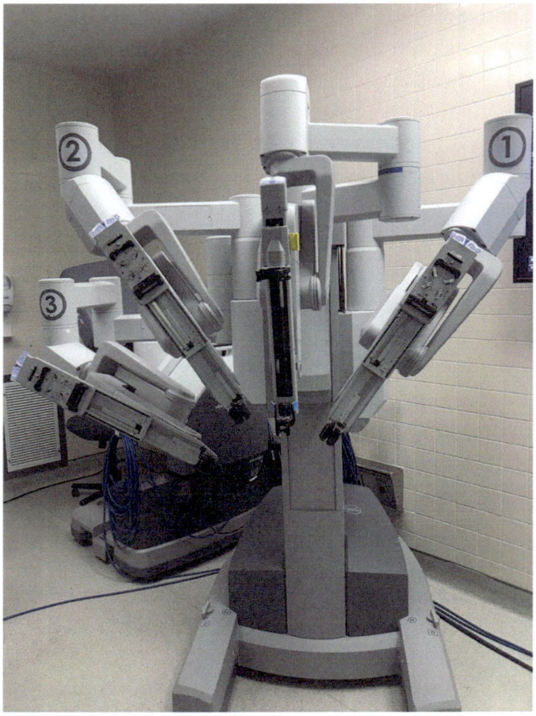

Fig. 1.6 da Vinci Si

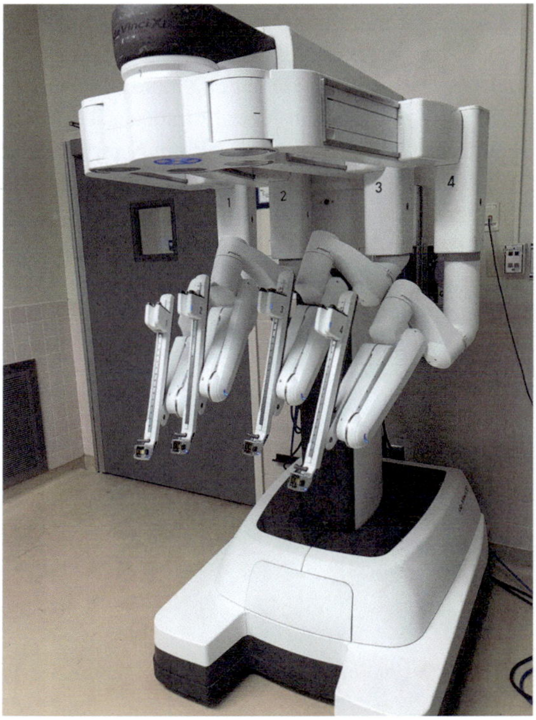

Fig. 1.7 da Vinci Xi

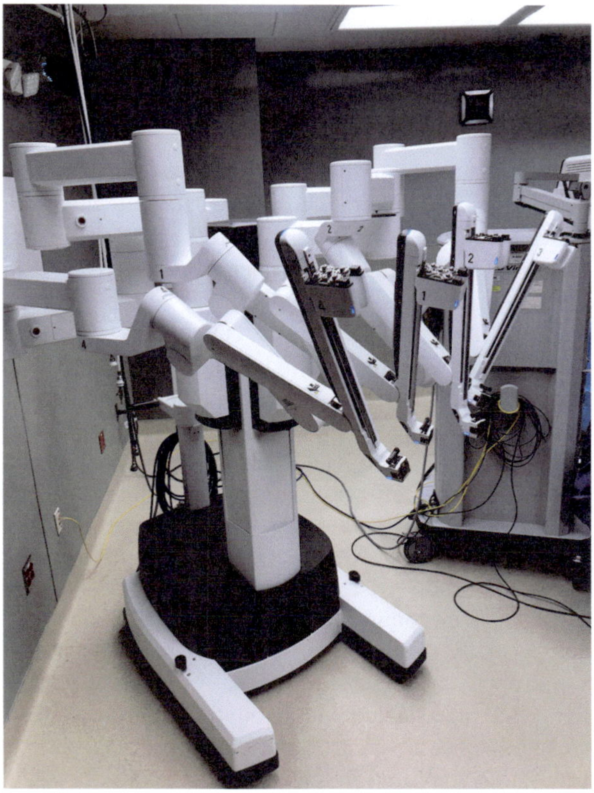

Fig. 1.8 da Vinci X

Vinci Si integrated TilePro, a multi-input function that allowed additional video sources from EKG and ultrasound to be displayed alongside HD-3D video. Additionally, the Si provided near-infrared real-time imaging via the Firefly Fluorescence Imaging Endoscope [12]. The single-site da Vinci Si was released to specifically provide enhanced functionality for single incision laparoscopic surgery (SILS). Single-site specific platform design allowed instrument access via a five-lumen port entered through a 1.5 cm incision [45]. Applications of SILS via the umbilicus include cholecystectomy, hysterectomy, and salpingo-oophorectomy [45]. In 2014, the da Vinci Xi was released. The Xi was unique in that its robotic arms were orientated parallel to each other rather than the previous circular arrangement [12]. The da Vinci Xi compiled the successful characteristics of previous iterations into a single master console and mobile platform with boom-mounted robotic arm. Each of the 4 arms can provide three degrees of freedom, with an additional seven degrees of freedom provided by Intuitive Surgical's EndoWrist technology. The EndoWrist attempts to impersonate the movements of the human wrist, thereby increasing the dexterity and functionality of end effector instrumentation [46]. Visualization in the Xi is handled by HD-3D visualization via a pair of cameras while instruments are controlled through telemanipulators with adjustable finger-cuff style ergonomic loops [47]. User comfort is maximized with intraocular distance adjustment, head-rest padding, and arm rests [47]. Motion of instruments is driven by cable joints distal to the robotic arm and tremor filtration with motion scaling achieve precise movements [46].

As a result of generations of refinement, historical competitive success, and current widespread clinical application, the da Vinci Surgical System is the modern-day workhorse in the field of robotic-assisted procedures. Most current applicable discussions in the literature include data generated from procedures utilizing the da Vinci Surgical System. As a result, the platform is rightly held as the prototypical example for conversion from open surgery and conventional laparoscopy to robotic-assisted procedures.

As in any competitive arena, challengers to the throne will come in droves. The success earned by the da Vinci Surgical System, the most commonly used robotic assisted surgical system, has given impetus to a growing sector of developers. One such platform, the Senhance was derived from a system previously known as the ALF-X Robotic Surgical System from TransEnterix, Morrisville, NC [48, 49]. Controlled remotely with three manipulator arms like that of the da Vinci, laparoscopic handles translate the surgeon's movements to actuators with multiple degrees of freedom. Although its end effector instruments do not articulate like the da Vinci's EndoWrist, the Senhance robotic system improves on the da Vinci's feedback shortcomings by integrating true haptic feedback. Whereas the da Vinci uses visually displayed cues to provide feedback to the operator concerning the force opposing the distal end of instruments while interacting with tissue, the Senhance offers actual tactile haptic force feedback. Tactile feedback provides an elevated sense of control and connectedness between physician and patient by translating sensation to the surgeon's hand [48, 49]. The tactile haptic force feedback incorporated by the Senhance works in tandem with a novel eye-tracking technology which uses the surgeon's point of visual foveation to center the camera image. This contrasts with the da Vinci system in which the surgeon controls the camera with a foot switch. The Senhance has been shown in clinical surgeries to be safe. For instance, in a 45-patient study of inflammatory bowel disease, colorectal cancer, adenoma, or diverticular disease with complications requiring surgery, the Senhance was used with three procedures converted to standard laparoscopy [50]. A champion for newcomers, the Senhance has become the first major robotic-assisted surgical platform other than the da Vinci implemented in a major hospital, being available for use at The Florida Hospital Institute for Surgical Advancement in November, 2017 [51].

The rising tide lifts all boats, and that aphorism rings true in the momentum observed in the robotic-assisted surgical platform sector. All new technologies possess inherent shortcomings that provide an angle of attack for prospective startups. For instance, console based robotic surgical systems are large, and the equipment requires a considerable amount of space and a disruptive choreography in the operating room. To reduce the impact of that footprint in the operative theater, Cambridge Medical Robotics Ltd., Cambridge, UK has developed the Versius Robotic System. The Versius Robotic System is modular, and more lightweight

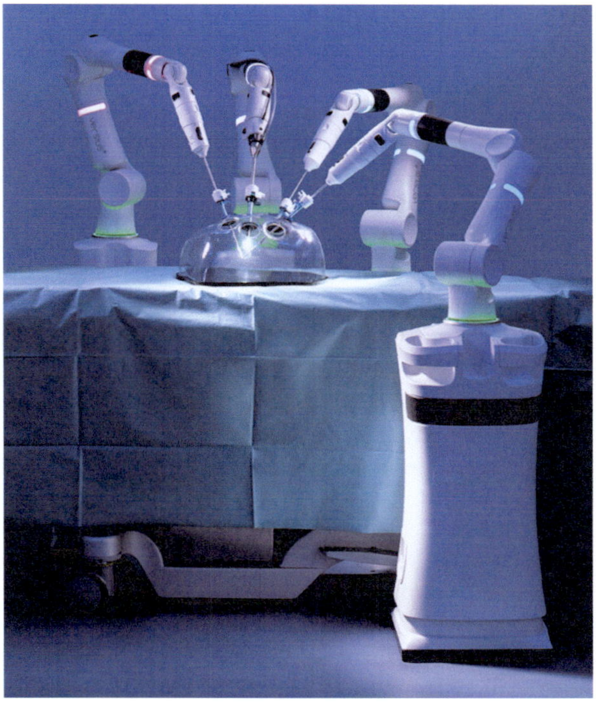

Fig. 1.9 Versius Robotic System

than the aforementioned platforms (Fig. 1.9). Its design provides increased flexibility compared to the established competitors, while allowing more versatile positioning relative to the patient [52]. Functionality comparable to its contemporaries includes multiple modular wristed robotic arms with haptic force feedback and HD-3D display designed for laparoscopic renal, gynecological, upper GI, and colorectal surgeries. Estimates for FDA approval have targeted a 2018 date, with proof of success in electro-surgery, needle driving, tissue manipulation and suturing shown at The Evelyn Cambridge Surgical Training Centre in cadaveric trials [52].

General surgery has been trending toward less invasive procedures when available, with robotic-assisted laparoscopy leading the way. Laparoscopy has been shown to benefit outcomes through shorted hospitalization time and reduced scarring [53]. The rising use of robotic platforms in minimally invasive procedures has been supported by their ability to address limitations conventional laparoscopic places on a surgeon's dexterity, visualization, and sensory feedback [54, 55]. The da Vinci Surgical System has been commonly used in robotic-assisted laparoscopic surgery since 2000, with 3400 systems in use worldwide in 2015 [47, 56]. At the time of publication of this textbook, there will probably exist newer robotic platforms available to the surgical community, other than the ones previously cited. The use of robotic-assisted surgical platforms for current use in hernia repair thus indicates a retrospective view of the procedure's origin.

1.8 Hernia Repair

Surgical repair of groin hernias increases with age with one study reporting that 4.2% of patients 75–80 years old receive treatment [57]. The abnormal tissue movement through its normal wall of containment most commonly involves the inguinal and femoral type, with hiatal, incisional, and umbilical hernias among other prevalent types [58]. Throughout an adult's life, the risk of developing a groin hernia is 27% and 3% for men and women respectively [59]. When asymptomatic watchful waiting is considered prudent. However, acute incarceration and strangulation of herniated tissue indicate emergency surgery. Additionally, data shows that pain symptoms will result in surgical referral within 10 years [58]. The largest risk factors are male sex, advanced age, and family history. However, additional conditions associated with risk include chronic obstructive pulmonary disease, lower body-mass index, and smoking [58]. Counterintuitively, the risk of developing a hernia from heavy lifting was shown to be inconclusive by systematic review [60].

Because untreated hernias can become large and noticeable, the groin hernia in adults has been recorded in history as far back as ancient Greece [61]. The Greek origin of the word Hernia indicates the pathophysiology through its translation from bud or sprout [62].

Earthenware statuettes from ancient eastern Mediterranean civilizations depict female umbilical hernias dating to the fifth century BCE. Additionally, in the smooth-sided Pyramid of Teti in Saqqara Egypt a funeral complex housed a 2500 BCE solid sculpture depicting the reduction of an inguinal hernia [61]. Further evidence of ancient hernias includes the mummified inguinal hernia of the fourth pharaoh of Egypt's Twentieth dynasty [61]. The Egyptian Ebers Papyrus, which dates to 1550 BCE, includes the first medical evidence of written hernia documentation. The 20-meter-long scroll was presumably less wieldy than today's electronic medical records systems. Centuries of advances in hernia surgery included the work of Gabriel Fallopius, Fabricius Aquapendente, Lorenz Heister as well as a litany of contributors to medical science understanding, some of whom are mentioned here [61]. Heister, a German surgeon was the first to report a direct inguinal hernia. The Dutch physician Petrus Camper studied inguinal hernias in the 1750s, leading to the eponymous anterior abdominal wall fascia. Franz Kaspar Hesselbach, a German surgeon, is best known for his description of the cribriform (Hesselbach's) fascia, the interfoveolar (Hesselbach's) ligament, and the inguinal (Hesselbach's) triangle. His 1806 medical text regarding the 3 anatomical structures was highly contributory to the practice of Hernia surgery [63]. The Spanish surgeon Antonio de Gimbernaty Arbós first divided the lacunar ligament to expand the femoral ring for incarcerated femoral hernia treatment [64].

Continuing advancements in the twentieth century allowed various surgical treatments for patients experiencing the chronic pain and obstruction caused by hernias. Harvard Medical School graduate Henry O. Marcy and his 1881 text on the inguinal region and related surgical repair were foundational for the surgical curing of hernias [65]. Marcy's techniques included high ligation of the hernia sac, transplantation of the cord, and reconstructive closure of the inguinal ring [65]. However, it was Italy's Edoardo Bassini who is generally recognized as the father of modern hernia surgery. In 1884, Bassini published a method for inguinal canal repair following hernia sac displacement. It was his herniorrhaphy technique that gained lasting notoriety due to its exclusive use of sutures for the reconstruction of the inguinal canal's posterior wall [66]. Bassini's technique was shown to lower hernia recurrence from 100% to 10% compared to the conventional anterior wall repair [62]. In 1939, Chester B. McVay MD published "A fundamental Error in the Bassini Operation for Direct Inguinal Hernia", the title of which leaves little requirement for elucidation and provides an example of the stepwise progression toward modern standard operating procedures [67]. McVay, a surgeon from South Dakota, advocated the use of the pectineal ligament for its stability in holding sutures [67]. Further contributions from the French surgeon Henri Fruchaud include two texts: "Surgical anatomy of the groin region", and "Surgical treatment of groin hernias" [68]. Each of Fruchaud's books provided detailed figures regarding the anatomic surgical treatment of groin hernias via reconstruction. His research attacked the conventional dichotomy of inguinal and femoral regions in the abdominocrural area [68]. Furthermore, Fruchaud pioneered abdominal access to the thigh and first identified the peritoneal piriform fossa while advocating for a deep reconstruction of the abdominal wall in place of simply closing the inguinal canal or femoral ring [68]. Tensionless repair using Marlex mesh, a synthetic polymer material to strengthen the inguinal canal, was described by Lichtenstein in 1990 [69]. Lichtenstein incorporated the monofilament polypropylene mesh to prevent tension of suture lines while providing a physical barrier to tissue protrusion [69].

The first laparoscopic hernia repair was reported by Ralph Ger and described the closure of patent vaginal processes in beagle dogs using staples applied laparoscopically [70]. That study identified advantages of using laparoscopic technique to manage indirect inguinal hernias including: smaller incisions, elimination of dissection, decreased risk to adjacent anatomy, and reduction of recurrence [70]. The Ger technique included a peritoneal incision that allowed a polypropylene mesh to eliminate the pathologic space followed by re-approximation of the peritoneum. Methods of mesh based repair inspired advancements in techniques to secure the synthetic material such as tacking and transfascial suture fixation. Further refinements of the procedure saw the implementation of polypropylene plugs and patches. For instance, in 1991 Corbitt compared laparoscopic and conventional herniorrhaphy using a Mersilene plug and patch graft for tension free closure [71].

Eventually, advancements in technology that ead to robotic-assisted procedures such as prostatectomy resulted in the crossover of platform use to hernia repair. The first robotic-assisted inguinal hernia repairs were published by urologists who performed intraperitoneal inguinal herniorrhaphy concomitantly to robotic-assisted laparoscopic radical prostatectomies [72, 73]. Later, the feasibility of independent robotic-assisted inguinal hernia repair was shown by Cadière et al. in 2001[74]. In that study, the world premiere of an independent inguinal hernioplasty utilizing the da Vinci surgical platform was demonstrated. A cohort of 146 patients underwent a variety of procedures with no morbidity related to the system reported. In that feasibility study, the successful use of a robotic-assisted surgical platform in the anatomical confinement inherent to hernia repair displayed the benefits of computer enhanced tasks [74]. Furthermore, the da Vinci was noted to excel in intra-abdominal tasks in a small space owing to its mobility and ergonomic instrument end effectors. Several characteristics of the robotic-assisted surgical platform used were reported to improve surgical task quality, including: intra-abdominal articulation of instruments, 3-dimensional visualization, and scaling and stabilization of instrument motion [74].

Current techniques for laparoscopic hernia repair include the transabdominal pre-peritoneal (TAPP) repair, and the totally extra-peritoneal (TEP) repair. In one study, decreased recovery room time and lower average pain was found with robotic-assisted when compared to conventional laparoscopic TAPP [75]. In that study by Waite et al., the robotic-assisted approach was determined to be feasible, although robotic-assisted suturing of the peritoneal flap attributed to longer overall operative time vs. conventional laparoscopy. Additionally, that study found that the direct cost and contribution margin, the product's price less associated variable costs, was roughly equal between the two techniques [75]. In a prospective cohort study by Iraniha et al., outcomes and longitudinal life quality of patients who underwent robotic assisted TAPP inguinal hernia repair were found to be positive. In that study, 82 patients underwent robotic-assisted TAPP, with low recurrence, low pain, and high post procedural quality of life [76].

One metric with which to compare conventional and robotic-assisted incisional hernia repair techniques is hospital length of stay (LOS). In one study of intraperitoneal mesh placement, 454 patients received conventional laparoscopic treatment, with 177 patients receiving robotic-assisted treatment. It was found that the conventional group required a longer LOS of one day vs. the robotic-assisted median LOS of zero days [77]. The shorter LOS came without increases in readmission and postoperative complication. Additionally, a decreased risk was reported of wound morbidities such as surgical site infection and surgical site occurrence including cellulitis, non-healing incision, fascial disruption, ischemia, and necrosis [77]. For instance, robotic-assisted intraperitoneal mesh replacement was shown to have a 9% decreased risk of surgical site occurrence when compared to conventional laparoscopic procedures [77]. However, in that study the operative times of robotic-assisted repairs were 16% more likely to last longer than 2 h compared to conventional laparoscopy [77].

Additional studies have assessed patient outcomes while comparing conventional laparoscopic techniques their robotic-assisted brethren. For instance, in a study of 21,565 patients in New York, outcome measurements were recorded between those two techniques for ventral hernia repair. Among the measures were complications, hospital length of stay (LOS), readmission within 30 days, as well as emergency department visit within 30 days [78]. It was reported, after analysis accounting for variables to estimate treatment effect, that patients who underwent robotic-assisted ventral hernia repair has shorter LOS and lower complication rates [78].

1.9 Robotic-Assisted Surgery Logistics

The use of robotic-assisted surgical platforms in procedures such as inguinal hernia repair has been steadily increasing. A report from Data of the American College of Surgeons National Surgical Quality Improvement Program showed that 13.8% of 510 patients undergoing unilateral inguinal hernia repair from 2012 to 2016 had robotic-assisted procedures vs. 48.1% and 38.1% having laparoscopic and open approaches respectively [79].

Another multi-institutional case series reporting on robotic-assisted laparoscopic ventral and incisional hernia repair described teaching and community hospital outcomes [80]. The study of 368 patients demonstrated the safety of intra-corporeal hernia defect closure by robotic-assisted platform, with intraoperative bowel injury occurring in 0.5% of cases [80]. In that study, conversion to open procedure occurred in 3 patients for reasons of defect size unamenable to closure, adhesion density, and intraoperative bowel injury [80].

While an increase in the number of surgeons implementing robotic-assisted platforms in their practice has been shown, there are barriers to that growth. For instance, the learning curve experienced by surgeons while training on a new system may inhibit the rate at which new patients are exposed to robotic-assisted hernia surgery. One representation of the challenge to surgeons in becoming proficient at robotic-assisted hernia repair included the experience threshold of 50 cases [81]. Additionally, parameters such as operating room size, previous experience with other robotic platforms, existing routines and procedural layout contribute to the integration timeline [82].

Research organizations have forecasted that surgical robot annual revenues more than $20 billion will be realized by 2021 [83]. This growing presence increases the options of surgeons and indicates the increasing representation of robotics in the field of hernia surgery. The cost per procedure is a known barrier to the use of robotic-assisted platforms in the operating suite. One study reported that the use of the da Vinci surgical system increased the cost up to $1500.00 [84]. Further studies are indicated to determine the long-term economics of their use.

1.10 Future Directions

Meaningful predictions require a realistic assessment of current capabilities to accurately map progress. Given the explosive changes and advancements observed in robotic development, speculation on future clinical use is difficult. Machine learning, artificial intelligence, and robotics will likely become increasingly utilized in most aspects of medicine. International Data Corp (IDC), a research firm producing manufacturing forecasts for commercial robotics, predicts developments in a variety of technologies applicable to robotic-assisted surgical platforms used in hernia repair [85]. For instance, improved capability and performance may be facilitated by innovation in computer vision, navigation, and semiconductor technologies. Additionally, the cost of use will likely decrease as more vendors enter the marketplace. Increased competition leading to products in multiple price points seem likely in the face of an information and communications technology landscape estimated to breach $80 billion by 2020. The scope of that sector should provide adequate resources to support the continued research and development of robotic platforms [86]. It was reported that robotic technologies in 2006, which had considerably more capabilities than those of the 1970s, could be purchased for 80% less than those available 30 years prior [87]. Industrial robots with historical prices of hundreds of thousands of dollars can be purchased today for around $20,000. The impact of less expensive options will likely increase with healthcare companies systematically reviewing return on investment before purchasing a robotic system.

The transition of applications and resources from on premise to cloud based software hosting may also improve the capabilities of future systems [85]. For instance, cloud based software will allow robotic platforms to become part of a network of information shared by multiple systems working collectively to improve efficiency and productivity. The deployment of highly automated platforms working collaboratively in the same workspace may provide opportunities for tomorrow's surgeon to take on additional thought processes and challenges [86].

References

1. Peters BS, Armijo PR, Krause C, Choudhury SA, Oleynikov D. Review of emerging surgical robotic technology. Surg Endosc. 2018;32:1636–55. https://doi.org/10.1007/s00464-018-6079-2.
2. Armijo PR, Pagkratis S, Boilesen E, Tanner T, Oleynikov D. Growth in robotic-assisted procedures is from conversion of laparoscopic procedures and not from open surgeons' conversion: a study of trends and costs. Surg Endosc. 2018;32:2106–13. https://doi.org/10.1007/s00464-017-5908-z.
3. Suvajdzic L, Dendic A, Sakac V, Canak G, Dankuc D. Hippocrates—the father of modern medicine. Vojnosanit Pregl. 2016;73:1181–6. https://doi.org/10.2298/VSP150212131S.
4. Smith, WD. (2019) Hippocrates. Encyclopedia Britannica. Retrieved from https://www.britannica.com/biography/Hippocrates. Access date 28 Aug 2019.
5. Asthma AJ. (2019) The Theoi Project: Greek Mythology. Retrieved from https://www.theoi.com/. Access date 28 August 2019.
6. Graziosi B, Haubold J. (Eds.). (2010). Homer: Iliad. Cambridge UK: Cambridge University Press.
7. Ronan CA. The shorter science and civilisation in China. Cambridge: Cambridge University Press; 1985.
8. O'Connor J, Robertson E. (1999) Heron of Alexandria. The MacTutor History of Mathematics Archive. Retrieved from http://www-history.mcs.st-and.ac.uk/Biographies/Heron.html. Access date 28 Aug 2019.
9. Hill DR. Mechanical engineering in the medieval near east. Sci Am. 1991;264:100–5.
10. Valery JP. (2017) Fathers of Robotics: Ismail Al-Jazari. Robot Shop Community. Retrieved from https://www.robotshop.com/community/blog/show/fathers-of-robotics-ismail-al-jazari. Access date 28 Aug 2019.
11. Freed L, Ishida S. (1995) History of Computers. Hightstown, NJ USA: Ziff-Davis Publishing.
12. Marino MV, Shabat G, Gulotta G, Komorowski AL. From illusion to reality: a brief history of robotic surgery. Surg Innov. 2018;25:291–6. https://doi.org/10.1177/1553350618771417.

13. Flatow, I. (2011) Science Diction: The origin of the word 'robot'. National Public Radio. Retrieved from https://www.npr.org/2011/04/22/135634400/science-diction-the-origin-of-the-word-robot. Access date 28 August 2019.
14. Bladin PF. W. Grey Walter, pioneer in the electroencephalogram, robotics, cybernetics, artificial intelligence. J Clin Neurosci. 2006;13:170–7.
15. Sabbatini RME (1997) The History of the Electroencephalogram. Brain & Mind Magazine. Retrieved from http://www.cerebromente.org.br/n03/tecnologia/historia.htm. Access date 28 August 2019.
16. Walter WG. A machine that learns. Sci Am. 1951;185:60–4.
17. Porter B. (2015). What the tortoise taught us: the story of philosophy. Lanham, Maryland USA. Rowman & Littlefield Publishers.
18. Feder BJ, Danbury C. He brought the robot to life. New York Times 21; 1982.
19. Munson GE. THE RISE AND FALL OF UNIMATION INC.-A story of robotics innovation & triumph that changed the world. Robot-Congers:36; 2010.
20. Anandan TM (2017) The Robotmakers-Yesterday, Today and Tomorrow. Robotic Industries Association. Retrieved from https://www.robotics.org/content-detail.cfm/Industrial-Robotics-Industry-Insights/The-Robotmakers-Yesterday-Today-and-Tomorrow/content_id/6513. Access date 28 August 2019.
21. Kalan S, Chauhan S, Coelho RF, Orvieto MA, Camacho IR, Palmer KJ, Patel VR. History of robotic surgery. J Robot Surg. 2010;4:141–7.
22. Kwoh YS, Hou J, Jonckheere EA, Hayati S. A robot with improved absolute positioning accuracy for CT guided stereotactic brain surgery. IEEE Trans Biomed Eng. 1988;35:153–60.
23. Lechky O. Worlds first surgical robot in BC. Med Post. 1985;21:92–3.
24. Mohammad S. Robotic surgery. J Oral Biol Craniofac Res. 2013;3:2. https://doi.org/10.1016/j.jobcr.2013.03.002.
25. Satava RM. Surgical robotics: the early chronicles: a personal historical perspective. Surg Laparosc Endosc Percutan Tech. 2002;12:6–16.
26. Spencer EH. The ROBODOC clinical trial: a robotic assistant for total hip arthroplasty. Orthop Nurs. 1996;15:9–14.
27. Lane T. (2018) A short history of robotic surgery. Ann R Coll Surg Engl. 100(6 sup):5–7. https://doi.org/10.1308/rcsann.supp1.5.
28. Davies B, Hibberd R, Ng W, Timoney A, Wickham J. The development of a surgeon robot for prostatectomies. Proc Inst Mech Eng H. 1991;205:35–8.
29. Harris S, Arambula-Cosio F, Mei Q, Hibberd R, Davies B, Wickham J, Nathan M, Kundu B. The Probot—an active robot for prostate resection. Proc Inst Mech Eng H. 1997;211:317–25.
30. Lanfranco AR, Castellanos AE, Desai JP, Meyers WC. Robotic surgery: a current perspective. Ann Surg. 2004;239:14–21. https://doi.org/10.1097/01.sla.0000103020.19595.7d.
31. Jost B, Ketterl M, Budde R, Leimbach T. Graphical programming environments for educational robots: open roberta-yet another one? 2014. p. 381–6.
32. Pugin F, Bucher P, Morel P. History of robotic surgery: from AESOP and Zeus® to Da Vinci®. J Visc Surg. 2011;148:S3.
33. Partin AW, Adams JB, Moore RG, Kavoussi LR. Complete robot-assisted laparoscopic urologic surgery: a preliminary report. J Am Coll Surg. 1995;181:552–7.
34. Falcone T, Goldberg J, Garcia-Ruiz A, Margossian H, Stevens L. Full robotic assistance for laparoscopic tubal anastomosis: a case report. J Laparoendosc Adv Surg Tech A. 1999;9:107–13.
35. Reichenspurner H, Damiano RJ, Mack M, Boehm DH, Gulbins H, Detter C, Meiser B, Ellgass R, Reichart B. Use of the voice-controlled and computer-assisted surgical system ZEUS for endoscopic coronary artery bypass grafting. J Thorac Cardiovasc Surg. 1999;118:11–6.
36. Marescaux J, Leroy J, Gagner M, Rubino F, Mutter D, Vix M, Butner SE, Smith MK. Transatlantic robot-assisted telesurgery. Nature. 2001;413:379.
37. Hoznek A. History of robotic surgery in urology. In: Anonymous Robotic UrologySpringer; 2008. p. 1–9.
38. Himpens J. Telesurgical laparoscopic cholecystectomy. Surg Endosc. 1998;12:1091.
39. Samadi D. History and the future of Robotic Surgery. 2018.

40. Gettman MT, Peschel R, Neururer R, Bartsch G. A comparison of laparoscopic pyeloplasty performed with the daVinci robotic system versus standard laparoscopic techniques: initial clinical results. Eur Urol. 2002;42:453–8.
41. Horgan S, Vanuno D, Benedetti E. Early experience with robotically assisted laparoscopic donor nephrectomy. Surg Laparosc Endosc Percutan Tech. 2002;12:64–70.
42. Carpentier A, Loulmet D, Aupecle B, Kieffer JP, Tournay D, Guibourt P, Fiemeyer A, Meleard D, Richomme P, Cardon C. Computer assisted open heart surgery. First case operated on with success. C R Acad Sci III. 1998;321:437–42.
43. Nguan C, Girvan A, Luke PP. Robotic surgery versus laparoscopy; a comparison between two robotic systems and laparoscopy. J Robot Surg. 2008;1:263–8.
44. Sung GT, Gill IS. Robotic laparoscopic surgery: a comparison of the da Vinci and Zeus systems. Urology. 2001;58:893–8.
45. IntuitiveSurgical (2018) da Vinci Xi Single-Site Instruments and Accessories. Retrieved from https://www.intuitive.com/en-us/-/media/Project/Intuitive-surgical/files/pdf/1025290ra-isi-brochure-single-site-digital-low-res-394110.pdf?la=en&hash=F24EC0B5DB9C62BDD688F77409A3CA50. Access date 28 August 2019.
46. Hanly EJ, Talamini MA. Robotic abdominal surgery. Am J Surg. 2004;188:19–26.
47. Simorov A, Otte RS, Kopietz CM, Oleynikov D. Review of surgical robotics user interface: what is the best way to control robotic surgery? Surg Endosc. 2012;26:2117–25.
48. Fanfani F, Monterossi G, Fagotti A, Rossitto C, Gueli Alletti S, Costantini B, Gallotta V, Selvaggi L, Restaino S, Scambia G. The new robotic TELELAP ALF-X in gynecological surgery: single-center experience. Surg Endosc. 2016;30:215–21. https://doi.org/10.1007/s00464-015-4187-9.
49. Fanfani F, Restaino S, Rossitto C, Gueli Alletti S, Costantini B, Monterossi G, Cappuccio S, Perrone E, Scambia G. Total laparoscopic (S-LPS) versus TELELAP ALF-X robotic-assisted hysterectomy: a case-control study. J Minim Invasive Gynecol. 2016;23:933–8. https://doi.org/10.1016/j.jmig.2016.05.008.
50. Spinelli A, David G, Gidaro S, Carvello M, Sacchi M, Montorsi M, Montroni I. First experience in colorectal surgery with a new robotic platform with haptic feedback. Color Dis. 2017; https://doi.org/10.1111/codi.13882.
51. Haskins O. (2015) TransEnterix completes SurgiBot pre-clinical FDA work Bariatric News. http://www.bariatricnews.net/?q=node/1856. Access date 28 August 2019.
52. Thibault M. Finally details on Medtronic's Robotics Platform. 2016.
53. Kumar A, Yadav N, Singh S, Chauhan N. Minimally invasive (endoscopic-computer assisted) surgery: technique and review. Ann Maxillofac Surg. 2016;6:159–64. https://doi.org/10.4103/2231-0746.200348.
54. Oleynikov D. Robotic surgery. Surg Clin North Am. 2008;88:1121–30.
55. Walker AS, Steele SR. The future of robotic instruments in colon and rectal surgery. Semin Colon Rectal Surg. 2016;27:144–9.
56. DACH Medical Group (2019) Retrieved from https://www.dach-medical-group.com/en/. Access date 28 August 2019.
57. Burcharth J, Pedersen M, Bisgaard T, Pedersen C, Rosenberg J. Nationwide prevalence of groin hernia repair. PLoS One. 2013;8:e54367.
58. Fitzgibbons RJ Jr, Forse RA. Groin hernias in adults. N Engl J Med. 2015;372:756–63.
59. Primatesta P, Goldacre MJ. Inguinal hernia repair: incidence of elective and emergency surgery, readmission and mortality. Int J Epidemiol. 1996;25:835–9.
60. Svendsen SW, Frost P, Vad MV, Andersen JH. Risk and prognosis of inguinal hernia in relation to occupational mechanical exposures—a systematic review of the epidemiologic evidence. Scand J Work Environ Health. 2013;39:5–26.
61. Hernia Specialists (2019) Hernia History. Retrieved from https://herniaspecialists.com/hernia-history/. Access date 28 Aug 2019.
62. Basile F, Biondi A, Donati M. Surgical approach to abdominal wall defects: history and new trends. Int J Surg. 2013;11:S20–3.
63. Tubbs RS, Gribben WB, Loukas M, Shoja MM, Tubbs KO, Oakes WJ. Franz Kaspar Hesselbach (1759–1816): anatomist and Surgeon. World J Surg. 2008;32:2527–9.
64. Puig–La Calle J, Marti-Pujol R. Antonio de Gimbernat (1734–1816): anatomist and Surgeon. Arch Surg. 1995;130:1017–20.

65. Zimmerman LM. Henry O. Marcy, pioneer of hernial surgery. Q Bull Northwest Univ Med Sch. 1949;23:501.
66. Negro P, Gossetti F, Ceci F, D'Amore L. Made in Italy for hernia: the Italian history of groin hernia repair. Ann Ital Chir. 2016;87:118–28.
67. Herzog BF. Chester B. McVay: small-town surgeon, world-famous herniologist. Surgery. 2007;141:119–20.
68. Stoppa R, Wantz G. Henri Fruchaud (1894–1960): a man of bravery, an anatomist a surgeon. Hernia. 1998;2:45–7.
69. Lichtenstein IL, Shulman AG, Amid PK. Use of mesh to prevent recurrence of hernias. Postgrad Med. 1990;87:155–60.
70. Ger R, Monroe K, Duvivier R, Mishrick A. Management of indirect inguinal hernias by laparoscopic closure of the neck of the sac. Am J Surg. 1990;159:370–3.
71. Corbitt JD Jr. Laparoscopic herniorrhaphy. Surg Laparosc Endosc. 1991;1:23–5.
72. Finley DS, Rodriguez E Jr, Ahlering TE. Combined inguinal hernia repair with prosthetic mesh during transperitoneal robot assisted laparoscopic radical prostatectomy: a 4-year experience. J Urol. 2007;178:1296–300.
73. Joshi AR, Spivak J, Rubach E, Goldberg G, DeNoto G. Concurrent robotic trans-abdominal pre-peritoneal (TAP) herniorrhaphy during robotic-assisted radical prostatectomy. Int J Med Robot. 2010;6:311–4.
74. Cadiere G, Himpens J, Germay O, Izizaw R, Degueldre M, Vandromme J, Capelluto E, Bruyns J. Feasibility of robotic laparoscopic surgery: 146 cases. World J Surg. 2001;25:1467–77.
75. Waite KE, Herman MA, Doyle PJ. Comparison of robotic versus laparoscopic transabdominal preperitoneal (TAPP) inguinal hernia repair. J Robot Surg. 2016;10:239–44.
76. Iraniha A, Peloquin J. Long-term quality of life and outcomes following robotic assisted TAPP inguinal hernia repair. J Robot Surg. 2018;12:261–9.
77. Prabhu AS, Dickens EO, Copper CM, Mann JW, Yunis JP, Phillips S, Huang L, Poulose BK, Rosen MJ. Laparoscopic vs robotic intraperitoneal mesh repair for incisional hernia: an Americas hernia society quality collaborative analysis. J Am Coll Surg. 2017;225:285–93.
78. Altieri MS, Yang J, Xu J, Talamini M, Pryor A, Telem DA. Outcomes after robotic ventral hernia repair: a study of 21,565 patients in the state of New York. Am Surg. 2018;84:902–8.
79. Charles EJ, Mehaffey JH, Tache-Leon CA, Hallowell PT, Sawyer RG, Yang Z. Inguinal hernia repair: is there a benefit to using the robot? Surg Endosc. 2018;32:2131–6.
80. Gonzalez A, Escobar E, Romero R, Walker G, Mejias J, Gallas M, Dickens E, Johnson CJ, Rabaza J, Kudsi OY. Robotic-assisted ventral hernia repair: a multicenter evaluation of clinical outcomes. Surg Endosc. 2017;31:1342–9.
81. LeBlanc KA, Kingsnorth A, Sanders DL. Management of abdominal hernias. London: Springer; 2018.
82. Randell R, Honey S, Hindmarsh J, Alvarado N, Greenhalgh J, Pearman A, Long A, Cope A, Gill A, Gardner P. A realist process evaluation of robot-assisted surgery: integration into routine practice and impacts on communication, collaboration and decision-making. Health Services and Delivery Research 5; 2017.
83. Feussner H, Ostler D, Kranzfelder M, Kohn N, Koller S, Wilhelm D, Thuemmler C, Schneider A. Surgery 4.0. In: Anonymous Health 4.0: how Virtualization and Big Data are Revolutionizing HealthcareSpringer; 2017. p. 91–107.
84. Barbash GI, Glied SA. (2010). New technology and health care costs—the case of robot-assisted surgery. New England Journal of Medicine, 363(8), 701–4.
85. Violino B. (2016) The future of robotics: 10 predictions for 2017 and beyond. ZDNet. Retrieved from https://www.zdnet.com/article/the-future-of-robotics/. Access date 28 August 2019.
86. Violino B. (2016) Meet your robot colleague: The advance of collaborative robotics. ZDNet. Retrieved from https://www.zdnet.com/article/the-advance-of-collaborative-robotics/. Access date 28 August 2019.
87. Huse B. (2006) The Perfect Swarm: Robots Past, Present and Future. Robotic Industries Association. Retrieved from https://www.robotics.org/content-detail.cfm/Industrial-Robotics-Industry-Insights/The-Perfect-Swarm-Robots-Past-Present-and-Future/content_id/1040. Access date 28 August 2019.

Adoption of Robotic Technology in Surgical Practice

2

Ekatarina Elliott, John J. Hall, Erik B. Wilson, Shinil K. Shah, and Melissa M. Felinski

2.1 Introduction

Technological innovations continue to help advance surgical technique as well as aid in the development of new less invasive procedures. Robotic-assisted laparoscopic (RAL) surgery is increasingly utilized by surgeons for minimally invasive surgery and as a way to potentially overcome limitations of traditional laparoscopy. Although RAL surgery was initially utilized by surgical subspecialties such as urology as a preferred tool for performing minimally invasive surgery (prostatectomy), it has gained momentum among general surgeons due to its broad-based application for complex procedures, including hernia repair.

In this chapter, we review the general advantages and disadvantages of RAL surgery, facilitators and barriers to adopting robotic technology, as well as the training requirements necessary to incorporate RAL surgery into practice. There is a lack of literature regarding adoption of robotics in practice, which makes an evidence based review of this topic difficult. We will aim to note the evidence, where available, to support our discussion.

E. Elliott · J. J. Hall · E. B. Wilson · M. M. Felinski (✉)
Division of Minimally Invasive and Elective General Surgery, Department of Surgery, McGovern Medical School, University of Texas Health Science Center at Houston, Houston, TX, USA
e-mail: melissa.felinski@uth.tmc.edu

S. K. Shah
Division of Minimally Invasive and Elective General Surgery, Department of Surgery, McGovern Medical School, University of Texas Health Science Center at Houston, Houston, TX, USA

Michael E. DeBakey Institute for Comparative Cardiovascular Science and Biomedical Devices, Texas A&M University, College Station, TX, USA

K. A. LeBlanc (ed.), *Robotic Assisted Hernia Repair*,
https://doi.org/10.1007/978-3-030-23025-8_2

2.2 Advantages

Since 2003, when then first RAL ventral hernia repair was performed [1], multiple series have been published highlighting the feasibility and potential advantages of this technique [2–8]. The majority of the data are limited to retrospective studies as well as large database reviews. RAL techniques have been reported in the repair of all types of abdominal wall hernias, including diaphragmatic hernias [9, 10]. Additionally, robotic hernia surgery has facilitated novel approaches to extraperitoneal mesh placement, including transabdominal preperitoneal, total extraperitoneal, as well as minimally invasive retrorectus approaches [3, 6, 11–13]. RAL surgery differs from traditional laparoscopy by placing a user interface between the surgeon and patient. The use of RAL techniques continues to increase. Although it is frequently thought of as a method to convert open operations to their minimally invasive counterpart, this is not always the case [14].

Features provided by RAL platforms include a surgeon console, stereoscopic vision, intuitive movements, tremor filtration, motion scaling, and wristed instruments. Purported benefits of these features include potential ergonomic advantages (not always uniformly reported, however) [15], improved visualization, camera stability, depth perception, dexterity, and precision and accuracy of movements that allows ease of the performance of complicated technical maneuvers, including intracorporeal suturing. Specific advantages in hernia surgery may include the enhanced ability to remove the hernia sac, perform primary fascial closure, suture (as opposed to tacking) mesh in place and easier performance of the retrorectus and posterior component separation (transversus abdominis release) in a minimally invasive manner [16]. In certain cases, it allows surgeons to forgo the need for a bedside assistant. These features are thought, in part, to help facilitate the more widespread dispersion and adoption of RAL surgery. In general, in abdominal wall surgery, outcomes of robotics are superior that of open operations, and are generally equivalent to their laparoscopic counterpart [16].

It is important to note that specifically with ventral/incisional hernias, there is certainly room for improvement in surgical technique. Minimally invasive ventral hernia repair does not necessarily decrease recurrence rates, but has been noted to decrease surgical site infection rates [17]. However, adoption of laparoscopic ventral hernia techniques by surgeons continues to be low. Recent estimates from large database reviews demonstrate that although the use of laparoscopic ventral hernia repair techniques is increasing, only 23% of ventral hernia repairs are performed laparoscopically. Additionally, only 6% of patients with complex incisional hernias undergo laparoscopic surgery [18, 19]. With newer platforms and technologies, robotics may finally start to fulfill the promise of being able to increase the number of minimally invasive hernia repairs performed, not by conversion of laparoscopic to robotic cases, but by converting traditionally open to minimally invasive cases.

2.3 Disadvantages/Barriers

Robotic technology potentially aids in the ability to overcome some important challenges that have prevented the more widespread dissemination of minimally invasive hernia surgery. However, there are some important disadvantages to note. The loss of tactile feedback/haptics is a major limitation and can affect how surgeons apply, develop, and master their skill set with the current generation of robotic platforms. Haptic feedback is integrated into some of the newer RAL platforms (TransEnterix, Morrisville, NC).

The physical space required for current robotic platforms can pose challenges to operating room setup. Newer robotic platforms have overcome some of these limitations by allowing for flexibility of the robotic patient side cart position. Lengthy set-up and docking times can be overcome with proper training, communication, and practice. Although decreased operative times tends to come with increasing experience [20], potential areas for rapid time savings, even early in the learning curve, include decreasing the time from incision to docking and sitting on the console, as well as efficiency with instrument exchange and undocking of the robotic platform. The anticipated development of other robotic platforms could advance these areas of improvement further.

In a value based society, and important in the discussion of actual cost is the debate regarding cost effectiveness of RAL surgery. For example, the actual cost difference of a robotic ventral hernia repair may be as high as 25% more [21]. In a recent retrospective analysis of 3665 cases from the National Inpatient Sample, the average cost of the robotic group was $13,441 versus $10,739 when performed laparoscopically. Zhamak et al. did conclude that additional costs are lower in high volume robotic centers [21]. There are multiple ways surgeons can reduce procedure costs, including minimizing the number of disposable instruments used, elimination of tackers/staplers, transition of traditionally open operations to their minimally invasive equivalent (such as with open abdominal wall reconstruction), and reduction of operating time with increased experience.

Increased costs associated with RAL technology, without a consistent improvement in outcomes, are frequently noted as one of the most pressing limitations for more widespread adoption. Initial (capital) purchase costs, annual maintenance expenses, as well as the cost of disposable instruments all contribute to the increased costs associated with RAL surgery. Historically dominated by a single company, Intuitive Surgical, Inc. (Sunnyvale, CA), over a dozen RAL surgical platforms are anticipated to enter the market over the next several years [22]. The introduction of new, competing platforms, some with specialty specific indications, will hopefully drive competition and potentially decrease cost. Additionally, pilot programs to determine the cost-effectiveness of RAL platforms in cost-constrained environments are underway, including a unique program from Intuitive Surgical, Inc. that has resulted in donation of RAL platforms to five county hospitals across the United States.

2.4 Training Requirements

Professional standards as well as institutional requirements must be met in order for a surgeon new to robotic-assisted surgery to safely incorporate this technology into clinical practice. Adoption of robotic technology in resident education is discussed in detail in the previous chapter. Though we recognize that no standardization for robotic procedures exists currently, there are several resources for surgeons considering the adoption of RAL techniques into their practice that are available.

Similar to Fundamentals of Laparoscopic Surgery and Fundamentals of Endoscopic Surgery, required now for current graduates of general surgery residency programs for eligibility for board certification by the American Board of Surgery, a Fundamentals of Robotic Surgery curriculum has been developed and is currently undergoing validation studies (www.frssurgery.org). Structured robotic surgery training programs for fellows are offered through multiple specialty groups including the Association of Program Directors for Colon and Rectal Surgery (APDCRS) as well as the Society of American Gastrointestinal and Endoscopic Surgeons (SAGES) [23, 24]. The majority of recently surveyed general surgery residency programs have formal structured curriculums for resident robotic surgery training [25]. Many surgical residents/surgeons who want to pursue further structured training in robotic surgery elect to do minimally invasive surgery and related fellowships accredited by The Fellowship Council (Los Angeles, CA), some of which offer robust robotic surgery training experiences.

The training of surgeons who are already in practice deserves discussion. There are a multitude of training resources available. Intuitive Surgical, Inc. (Sunnyvale, CA) has created training programs to help assist surgeons who wish to perform RAL surgery. These pathways are generally designed to help meet the requirements for hospital credentialing, however, one will have to refer to their own hospital for additional specific institutional requirements. A company representative must first observe the surgeon's current laparoscopic or open technique in a live case. The surgeon is then introduced to robotic surgery through the use of the robotic simulator platform. Basic tasks such as trocar placement, docking and undocking of the robot, camera and instrument control, and suturing with wristed instruments is emphasized. The surgeon must attend a case observation hosted by an epicenter surgeon. An epicenter surgeon has performed at least 500 robotic cases. This is a time where the two surgeons discuss the value of robotics in relation to their practice and how the learning curve can be best managed. The epicenter surgeon will often also serve as the post-training proctor. The surgeon selects a training date and two days of post training. The surgeon will attend several practice sessions consisting of skill drills on the simulator and must complete a series of online modules and assessments. The online module certificate is submitted to the training lab prior to the training date. On training day, the surgeon will perform various skills on a cadaver led by a proctoring surgeon and Intuitive trainer. Upon completion, the surgeon will be awarded a training certificate from Intuitive Surgical, Inc. The surgeon will then submit this certificate to their hospital, in addition to any specific institutional requirements, to begin the approval process. A proctor is selected to attend the surgeon's first 3–5 robotic cases (this varies with individual hospital bylaws). The proctor will complete an evaluation of the surgeon's robotic skills after each case and submit them to the hospital. After the proctored case series is completed and the surgeon is granted robotic privileges by the hospital, the surgeon may perform robotic-assisted cases independently.

As surgeons introduce RAL techniques into practice, there are several important considerations in regards to continued development of operative skills. In addition to personal case volume, advanced company sponsored specialty specific robotic surgery training courses are offered. Case observations and mini-fellowships may serve to help hasten the learning curve. Multiple societies offer mentored training experiences, including new programs via the International Hernia Collaboration (IHC), which started as a closed discussion board on Facebook (Menlo Park, CA) for discussion of topics related to hernia surgery [26]. SAGES now offers a MASTERS program, which is designed to offer structured post surgical training in a variety of surgical specialties, including hernia and robotic surgery [27]. Various other social medial platforms, including the Robotic Surgery Collaboration [28], and discussion boards sponsored by SAGES, allow for dispersion of advice to surgeon initiated questions as well as an informal platform to discuss technique, share operative videos, and offer and receive technique related feedback. Additionally, there are now a number of texts focusing specifically on RAL techniques for a variety of operations [29–32].

There are also online services for skill improvement where you can upload your case to a secure site for review by a panel of experts. The panel of experts will then asses various skills including depth perceptions, dexterity, efficiency, force sensitivity, and robotic control and provide scoring and feedback [C-SATS, www.csats.com]. Operative surgical videos are an additional educational resource for learning a specific technique. Numerous surgical societies, associations (including the Clinical Robotic Surgery Association), as well as industry post surgical videos on their websites for surgeons to review and learn from.

2.5 Adoption of Robotics into Practice

Regardless of the number of procedures performed to achieve independent status, the key to being safe, proficient, and efficient with RAL techniques is appropriate case selection and repetition. Avoid initiation of this experience with the most complicated cases. An ideal case for the novice robotic surgeon to begin with may be an inguinal hernia. This procedure provides a confined area with anatomical landmarks that aid in operative consistency. The preperitoneal dissection and suturing technique with peritoneal flap closure performed during robotic-assisted laparoscopic inguinal hernia repair are invaluable skills which can then be translated to more complex procedures. It is also a procedure that can be performed, even during the learning curve, with a similar cost profile to the traditional laparoscopic equivalent (by elimination of the use of dissecting balloons and tackers, for example) [33].

It is imperative that these robotic cases are performed with regular frequency. As the old adage says, practice makes perfect. This is also important for optimization of operating room staff training and efficiency of set-up, including patient and patient cart positioning, sterile coverage of robotic arms, and docking of the robot, all of which can be time consuming when robotic platforms are new to an institution. We also recommend, as mentioned above, the continuation of skill development with the robotic simulator modules, participation in additional case observations, industry courses, and/or mini-fellowships, in addition to having the assistance of an experienced colleague. When performing more complicated procedures, robotic technology should be introduced in a staged or hybrid approach. In gastric bypass, one may consider during the initial cases doing a single portion of the case robotically (i.e., the gastrojejunostomy) and doing the rest laparoscopically. For inguinal hernias, one may start with known direct inguinal hernias and primary, non-recurrent hernias. For ventral hernias, experience with intra-peritoneal techniques is necessary prior to attempting more complex preperitoneal and retrorectus approaches. If mesh fixation takes a prolonged amount of time, consideration of the performance of half of the fixation with robotic suturing, and half with tacks until suturing becomes more efficient. There is a tradeoff between operative time and equipment costs that is sometimes difficult to balance. We emphasize the value of video recording and review of these videos of your own cases.

Once robotic technique for a specific case is optimized, learn to work efficiently and then aim to reduce costs. A robotic surgeon should be knowledgeable of the technological options available to him or her. The key to cost reduction in RAL surgery, specific to hernia surgery, is minimization of the use of disposable instruments. Graspers, for example, can double as a second needle driver. Monopolar shears can often take the place of more expensive energy devices. Industry provided data, to compare individual surgeon costs to the national average may help expose unnecessary increased disposable equipment costs [34]. Use of enhanced recovery protocols in RAL cases may help decrease post procedure hospital length of stay secondary to pain and delayed return of bowel function.

2.6 Conclusion

RAL assisted surgery is growing in popularity, with a pace that often is faster than the data published to support its use. Newer, specialty specific robotic platforms may help to increase efficiency, decrease cost, and improve outcomes, however this remains to be seen. Increased peri-operative times and costs with RAL techniques may still prove advantageous in certain cases, if RAL techniques allow for traditionally open procedures to be performed in a minimally invasive manner. Safe and effective adoption of RAL techniques should be encouraged, but this requires particular attention to appropriate training, initial case selection and experienced proctorship. Additionally, continued learning after initial training through the use of the many resources available to practicing surgeons will provide continuous improvement.

References

1. Ballantyne GH, Hourmont K, Wasielewski A. Telerobotic laparoscopic repair of incisional ventral hernias using intraperitoneal prosthetic mesh. JSLS. 2003;7(1):7–14.
2. Kirkpatrick T, Zimmerman B, LeBlanc K. Initial experience with robotic hernia repairs: a review of 150 cases. Surg Technol Int. 2018;33:139–47.
3. Belyansky I, Reza Zahiri H, Sanford Z, Weltz AS, Park A. Early operative outcomes of endoscopic (eTEP access) robotic-assisted retromuscular abdominal wall hernia repair. Hernia. 2018;22(5):837–47. https://doi.org/10.1007/s10029-018-1795-z.
4. Altieri MS, Yang J, Xu J, Talamini M, Pryor A, Telem DA. Outcomes after robotic ventral hernia repair: a study of 21,565 patients in the state of New York. Am Surg. 2018;84(6):902–8.
5. Walker PA, May AC, Mo J, Cherla DV, Santillan MR, Kim S, Ryan H, Shah SK, Wilson EB, Tsuda S. Multicenter review of robotic versus laparoscopic ventral hernia repair: is there a role for robotics? Surg Endosc. 2018;32(4):1901–5. https://doi.org/10.1007/s00464-017-5882-5.
6. Carbonell AM, Warren JA, Prabhu AS, Ballecer CD, Janczyk RJ, Herrera J, Huang LC, Phillips S, Rosen MJ, Poulose BK. Reducing length of stay using a robotic-assisted approach for retromuscular ventral hernia repair: a comparative analysis from the Americas hernia society quality collaborative. Ann Surg. 2018;267(2):210–7. https://doi.org/10.1097/SLA.0000000000002244.
7. Gonzalez A, Escobar E, Romero R, Walker G, Mejias J, Gallas M, Dickens E, Johnson CJ, Rabaza J, Kudsi OY. Robotic-assisted ventral hernia repair: a multicenter evaluation of clinical outcomes. Surg Endosc. 2017;31(3):1342–9. https://doi.org/10.1007/s00464-016-5118-0.
8. Allison N, Tieu K, Snyder B, Pigazzi A, Wilson E. Technical feasibility of robot-assisted ventral hernia repair. World J Surg. 2012;36(2):447–52. https://doi.org/10.1007/s00268-011-1389-8.
9. Mertens AC, Tolboom RC, Zavrtanik H, Draaisma WA, Broeders I. Morbidity and mortality in complex robot-assisted hiatal hernia surgery: 7-year experience in a high-volume center. Surg Endosc. 2018; https://doi.org/10.1007/s00464-018-6494-4.
10. Galvani CA, Loebl H, Osuchukwu O, Samame J, Apel ME, Ghaderi I. Robotic-assisted paraesophageal hernia repair: initial experience at a single institution. J Laparoendosc Adv Surg Tech A. 2016;26(4):290–5. https://doi.org/10.1089/lap.2016.0096.
11. Orthopoulos G, Kudsi OY. Feasibility of robotic-assisted transabdominal preperitoneal ventral hernia repair. J Laparoendosc Adv Surg Tech A. 2018;28(4):434–8. https://doi.org/10.1089/lap.2017.0595.
12. Maciel V, Mata W, Arevalo G, Zeichen M, Glass T. Robotic retro-rectus repair of parastomal hernias. J Robot Surg. 2018; https://doi.org/10.1007/s11701-018-0874-6.
13. Sugiyama G, Chivukula S, Chung PJ, Alfonso A. Robot-assisted transabdominal preperitoneal ventral hernia repair. JSLS. 2015;19(4) https://doi.org/10.4293/JSLS.2015.00092.
14. Armijo PR, Pagkratis S, Boilesen E, Tanner T, Oleynikov D. Growth in robotic-assisted procedures is from conversion of laparoscopic procedures and not from open surgeons' conversion: a study of trends and costs. Surg Endosc. 2018;32(4):2106–13. https://doi.org/10.1007/s00464-017-5908-z.
15. Armijo PR, Huang CK, High R, Leon M, Siu KC, Oleynikov D. Ergonomics of minimally invasive surgery: an analysis of muscle effort and fatigue in the operating room between laparoscopic and robotic surgery. Surg Endosc. 2018; https://doi.org/10.1007/s00464-018-6515-3.
16. Henriksen NA, Jensen KK, Muysoms F. Robot-assisted abdominal wall surgery: a systematic review of the literature and meta-analysis. Hernia. 2018; https://doi.org/10.1007/s10029-018-1872-3.
17. Holihan JL, Alawadi Z, Martindale RG, Roth JS, Wray CJ, Ko TC, Kao LS, Liang MK. Adverse events after ventral hernia repair: the vicious cycle of complications. J Am Coll Surg. 2015;221(2):478–85. https://doi.org/10.1016/j.jamcollsurg.2015.04.026.
18. Mason RJ, Moazzez A, Sohn HJ, Berne TV, Katkhouda N. Laparoscopic versus open anterior abdominal wall hernia repair: 30-day morbidity and mortality using the ACS-NSQIP database. Ann Surg. 2011;254(4):641–52. https://doi.org/10.1097/SLA.0b013e31823009e6.

19. Savitch SL, Shah PC. Closing the gap between the laparoscopic and open approaches to abdominal wall hernia repair: a trend and outcomes analysis of the ACS-NSQIP database. Surg Endosc. 2016;30(8):3267–78. https://doi.org/10.1007/s00464-015-4650-7.
20. Muysoms F, Van Cleven S, Kyle-Leinhase I, Ballecer C, Ramaswamy A. Robotic-assisted laparoscopic groin hernia repair: observational case-control study on the operative time during the learning curve. Surg Endosc. 2018; https://doi.org/10.1007/s00464-018-6236-7.
21. Khorgami Z, Li WT, Jackson TN, Howard CA, Sclabas GM. The cost of robotics: an analysis of the added costs of robotic-assisted versus laparoscopic surgery using the National Inpatient Sample. Surg Endosc. 2018; https://doi.org/10.1007/s00464-018-6507-3.
22. Peters BS, Armijo PR, Krause C, Choudhury SA, Oleynikov D. Review of emerging surgical robotic technology. Surg Endosc. 2018;32(4):1636–55. https://doi.org/10.1007/s00464-018-6079-2.
23. APDCRS. Robotic colorectal surgery training program. http://www.apdcrs.org/wp/member-resources/robotic-colorectal-surgery-training-program/.
24. SAGES. SAGES robotics fellows course. https://www.sages.org/robotics-fellows-course/.
25. George LC, O'Neill R, Merchant AM. Residency training in robotic general surgery: a survey of program directors. Minim Invasive Surg. 2018;2018:8464298. https://doi.org/10.1155/2018/8464298.
26. Ghanem O, Logghe HJ, Tran BV, Huynh D, Jacob B. Closed Facebook groups and CME credit: a new format for continuing medical education. Surg Endosc. 2018; https://doi.org/10.1007/s00464-018-6376-9.
27. SAGES. Masters program. https://www.sages.org/masters-program/.
28. Myers CG, Kudsi OY, Ghaferi AA. Social media as a platform for surgical learning: use and engagement patterns among robotic surgeons. Ann Surg. 2018;267(2):233–5. https://doi.org/10.1097/SLA.0000000000002479.
29. Kudsi OY, Jones DB, Carbonell AM, Yiengpruksawan A. Atlas of robotic surgery. 1st ed: Cine-Med, Inc; 2018.
30. Robotic-assisted minimally invasive surgery: a comprehensive textbook: Springer; 2019. https://doi.org/10.1007/978-3-319-96866-7.
31. LeBlanc KA. Laparoscopic and robotic incisional hernia repair: Springer; 2018.
32. The SAGES manual of robotic surgery. 1st ed: Springer; 2018. https://doi.org/10.1007/978-3-319-51362-1.
33. Waite KE, Herman MA, Doyle PJ. Comparison of robotic versus laparoscopic transabdominal preperitoneal (TAPP) inguinal hernia repair. J Robot Surg. 2016;10(3):239–44. https://doi.org/10.1007/s11701-016-0580-1.
34. Intuitive Surgical I. https://www.dvexeceducation.com/index.php.

Enhanced Recovery After Hernia Repair

3

Frederik Berrevoet

3.1 Introduction

Enhanced recovery after surgery (ERAS) protocols have gained more and more attention over the last decade. These protocols were initially developed by a group of academic surgeons in Europe in 2001 [1]. The concept focused on several components: a multidisciplinary team working together around the patient, a multimodal approach to resolve issues that delay recovery and cause complications, a scientific, evidence-based approach to protocols and a change in management using interactive and continuous feedback.

The initial ideas focused on enhancing recovery and reducing complications by modifying the metabolic response to surgical insult rather than just limiting length of stay. Later on, ERAS was implemented as a fundamental challenge in the care of the surgical patient during their peri-operative contacts: outpatient clinic, preoperative unit, the operating room, postoperative recovery unit, and the ward. Each unit has its own focus, personnel, and specialists to improve patient care.

There are 24 core elements of ERAS care that have scientific support for their use (Table 3.1). These components are distributed along the patient pathway and delivered by different departments and professionals within the hospital, which explains why the surgeon, as the clinician with overall responsibility for the patient, has the best opportunity for a comprehensive view to guide the process. As the underlying process in enhancing the patient recovery is minimizing and mitigating the effects of surgical stress, pain management and acceleration of intestinal recovery are probably key factors in ERAS protocols. However, surgical stress is also influenced by many other factors, such as catabolism, immune dysfunction, impaired pulmonary function, increased cardiac demands, coagulation-fibrinolytic dysfunction, cerebral

F. Berrevoet (✉)
Department of General and HPB Surgery and Liver Transplantation, Ghent University Hospital, Ghent, Belgium
e-mail: frederik.berrevoet@ugent.be

K. A. LeBlanc (ed.), *Robotic Assisted Hernia Repair*,
https://doi.org/10.1007/978-3-030-23025-8_3

Table 3.1 Perioperative factors to enhance surgical recovery

Preoperative
Medical optimization of chronic disease
Cessation of smoking and excessive intake of alcohol
Prehabilitation
Preoperative nutritional screening and, as needed, assessment and nutritional support
Diabetes management and preoperative HgbA1c < 7.0
Structured preoperative information and engagement of the patient and relatives or caretakers
Preoperative carbohydrate treatment
Prophylaxis against nausea and vomiting
Preoperative prophylaxis against thrombosis
Antibiotic prophylaxis, first generation cephalosporin for most; vancomycin in high-risk groups
Alcohol-containing skin preparation
Intraoperative
Standardized anesthesia, avoiding long-acting opioids
Maintaining fluid balance to avoid over- or underhydration, administer vasopressors to support blood pressure control
Control of body temperature using warm air flow blankets and warmed intravenous infusions
Minimal invasive surgical techniques
Epidural anesthesia for open surgery
Restrictive use of surgical site drains
Removal of nasogastric tubes before reversal of anesthesia
Postoperative
Postoperative blood sugar 120–160 mg/dL
Early removal of urinary catheters and intravenous fluids (morning after surgery)
Multimodal approach to control of nausea and vomiting
Multimodal approach to opioid-sparing pain control
Early mobilization (day of surgery)
Early intake of oral fluids and solids (offered the day of surgery)
Use of chewing gums and laxatives and peripheral opioid-blocking agents (when using opioids)
Intake of protein and energy-rich nutritional supplements
Prepare for early discharge

dysfunction, alterations in fluid homeostasis, sleep disturbances, and fatigue. These factors can be managed through a variety of approaches, including alterations in surgical technique, preoperative and postoperative practices, and pharmacologic interventions. In this chapter we will discuss several of these factors in order to facilitate patient recovery.

There are multiple factors that influence a successful hernia repair, including surgical technique, tissue plane dissection, and choice of mesh prosthetic implanted. In addition to these surgeon-entrusted factors, there are multiple elements of preoperative and postoperative care that greatly affect outcomes. Of these elements, many are patient-specific factors that are modifiable. Thus, there is great potential to improve outcomes by ameliorating detrimental patient factors before an elective hernia repair.

Wound complications such as surgical-site infections (SSIs) are the most common postoperative complication in patients undergoing ventral hernia repair. Such complications can lead to increased emergency room visits, hospital readmissions, greater time in clinic, or reoperations to manage wound complications. Additionally, perioperative surgical-site occurrences, including SSI, seroma, wound ischemia, and dehiscence, can greatly increase the risk of hernia recurrence. In an effort to support and promote optimal wound healing, reduce infection, and enhance early postoperative recovery, enhanced recovery pathways have been developed for hernia repair.

Secondly, as care of the hernia patient is complex and many issues that might contribute to the recovery of the patient are not yet fully understood, ERAS protocols should not only be attentive to short-term goals, such as reduction of length of stay, but should also investigate the impact on the larger recovery of the patient. Improvement in any area without regard to the overall process may lead to sub-optimization and unintended consequences are likely to follow.

3.2 Pre-Operative Measurements

3.2.1 Smoking Cessation

Smoking is probably the best modifiable patient risk factor and relatively well studied [2–6]. The deleterious effect of smoking on wound healing is well known and has several mechanisms. Smoking leads to elevated blood levels of carbon monoxide, which binds hemoglobin, shifts the oxygen-hemoglobin dissociation curve to the left, and decreases oxygen tissue delivery by as much as 15%. Smokers therefore have a clear disadvantage in regard to wound healing and their ability to overcome wound morbidity, particularly surgical site infections (SSI).

The evidence to support the negative effect of smoking on postoperative wound morbidity can be shown by a meta-analysis, including nearly 480,000 subjects in different surgical areas, which associated smoking with an increased rate of wound necrosis, dehiscence and SSI [7]. Specifically in the context of abdominal wall repair, smoking has been routinely associated with wound morbidity. Because hernia repair relies intensely on proper wound healing, any reduction of blood and tissue oxygenation and impairment in collagen deposition within fresh wounds can greatly affect the outcome of a hernia repair [2, 8, 9]. Additionally, abdominal wall repairs frequently require the use of mesh and various tissue plane dissections, and thus reinforce the need for smoking cessation before repair. An important study by Sorensen et al. demonstrated that smoking cessation for 30 days is adequate to show alleviation of many deleterious effects of cigarettes [10]. Given this high-quality literature demonstrating a clear correlation between active cigarette use and impaired wound healing, it should now be mandatory for patients to cease all smoking activity for a minimum of 30 days preoperatively for those undergoing elective hernia repair. Although laparoscopic and other minimally invasive techniques benefit patients with reduced wound complications, active tobacco use still adds impairments to wound healing.

In a Cochrane review of 13 randomized controlled trials recruiting smokers before elective surgery, seven trials looked at the association of preoperative abstinence with postoperative complications [11]. For the two trials that compared intensive interventions at least 4 weeks before surgery, a reduction in all complications and wound morbidity was found. Interventions less than 4 weeks from surgery were not able to demonstrate a significant impact on morbidity, and were less likely to lead to long-term smoking cessation.

When patients report 100% abstinence, urine can be tested for the tobacco plant alkaloid anabasine, an insecticide found in cigarettes that has been suggested to evaluate smoking cessation. Although non-smokers will almost always test negative (100% specificity), smokers can still test negative (sensitivity 41%). Patients who sincerely report complete cessation and test negative for urine anabasine can considered abstinent. If urine anabasine is negative, surgery should then best be scheduled at least 4 weeks after smoking cessation [12, 13].

3.2.2 Weight Loss

Obesity also has a well-documented impact on complications following abdominal wall repair, including wound necrosis, SSI, reoperation, and hernia recurrence. Regardless of the surgical technique employed for VHR, hernia recurrence increases linearly as body mass index (BMI) increases [14, 15]. Regarding wound morbidity in hernia repair subjects, Fischer and colleagues reported a graded relationship with obesity: OR 1.25, 1.42, and 1.66 for a BMI of 30 to 35, 35 to 40, and greater than 40, respectively [16].

Obese patients in need of a repair of their hernia should be counseled preoperatively on the importance of weight loss. The surgeon should bring the patients to realize they can have a positive impact on their surgical outcome. Medical and surgical weight loss are certainly options, but evidence that these interventions have an impact on outcomes of a subsequent hernia repair is currently unavailable. Therefore, there is currently no consensus on the best approach to achieve weight loss goals or what BMI goal is optimal.

For selective patients who have associated medical comorbidities and whose abdominal wall is not so complex, bariatric surgery is also an option. However, definitive hernia repair at the time of their bariatric procedure is not recommended unless there is significant risk of incarceration and strangulation.

Finally, seeing patients at 3-month intervals to monitor success increases compliance, demonstrates the surgeon's commitment to the patient, and will motivate patients to achieve their goals.

3.2.3 Diabetes Optimization

Although not studied in a dedicated fashion relative to abdominal wall reconstruction, glucose management is important for all stages of patient care related to hernia repair. Preoperative glycemic control is essential for optimal outcomes. This is routinely measured in the preoperative setting with glycosylated hemoglobin (HbA1c). Considerable data exist regarding the negative impact of poorly controlled diabetes in regard to wound morbidity after general, orthopedic, and cardiothoracic surgery [17]. Given the dramatic association with wound morbidity and poorly controlled diabetes, it can be generally recommended for patients to have an HbA1c less than 8. Those with poorly controlled diabetes should be managed similarly to obese patients in that they are not scheduled for surgery. Instead they should be instructed to set a goal for their HbA1c, and scheduled to visit an endocrinologist for close monitoring.

Peri- and postoperative glucose control is another essential component to reduce wound complications in both diabetic and non-diabetic patients. Therefore, appropriate glycemic control is vital within the first 24 h of the postoperative period to optimize outcome and reduce wound complications. Guidelines recommend a range of 110–150 mg/dL [18].

3.2.4 Nutritional Optimization

Numerous randomized controlled trials and reviews demonstrated the role that nutritional therapy plays in the ability of patients to heal and recover following surgery. Although most hernia patients are not severely malnourished, patients suffering from an enterocutaneous or enteroprosthetic fistula can be relatively catabolic or nutritionally depleted. Importantly, for patients identified as severely malnourished, good data have shown that preoperative total parenteral nutrition reduces non-infectious postoperative complications [19].

Ideally, the combination of an increasing prealbumin level and slightly elevated or normal CRP level gives assurance that the patient's nutritional status is improving. The Mini Nutritional Assessment (MNA) can also help in assessing patients' nutritional status. For hospital inpatients, low MNA scores are associated with mortality, prolonged length of stay, and greater likelihood of discharge to nursing homes [20, 21].

Brief preoperative fasting is among the ERAS recommendations. During earlier times a long preoperative fasting period was mandatory, but it was shown that 150 ml of water can improve gastric emptying and was safe 2–3 h before surgery [22]. Another area of metabolic manipulation is preoperative carbohydrate loading. This metabolic strategy uses an isotonic carbohydrate solution given 3 h preoperatively to alter stress metabolism and decrease insulin resistance. In most Western surgical settings, the "routine", however, is for the patient to fast after midnight before surgery in the morning.

3.2.5 Prehabilitation

One of the newer areas of interest is the concept of prehabilitation, which takes measures to improve a patient's functional status in preparation for surgery. A recent meta-analysis of randomized controlled trials that included subjects undergoing abdominal surgery and who were randomized to prehabilitation techniques or not, found that inspiratory muscle training, aerobic exercise, and/or resistance training can decrease postoperative complications. Most dramatic was the reduction in pulmonary complications. This might be of interest in patients suffering from large incisional hernias with loss of domain. Currently, there are many ongoing trials to evaluate the effectiveness of prehabilitation techniques in regard to abdominal surgery.

3.3 Intra-operative Measures

3.3.1 Skin Preparation and Decolonization Protocols

The need for appropriate surgical field disinfection is well known. Iodine and chlorhexidine-based skin preparations are equally effective, provided that alcohol is a primary ingredient within the preparation solution [23–25]. The use of preoperative showers with antiseptic soaps or antiseptic agents to decrease SSIs has been rather inconclusive [26]. It may even change the normal protective skin flora and even increase the risk of SSI [27].

3.3.2 Perioperative Antibiotics

Perioperative antibiotic prophylaxis has been routinely established for surgical procedures, especially when using mesh. According to existing guidelines, patients undergoing routine ventral hernias repair should be given prophylaxis using a first-generation cephalosporin [28]. During the procedure, antibiotics should be redosed based on duration of surgery and antibiotic half-life. Regarding the use of postoperative antibiotics, no benefit of dosing antibiotics after the skin has been closed in clean cases has been shown [28, 29].

3.3.3 Surgical-Site Infections (SSI)

Compared with other clean non-hernia surgeries, SSI rates are noted to be higher for ventral abdominal wall surgery. These complications can be quite severe and expose the patient to significant morbidity, mortality and cost of care. Another aspect of infections and hernia repair is the use of synthetic meshes, which are necessary for successful outcomes in the majority of this type of surgery. The macroporous (light/medium weight) polypropylene has the best chance of salvage [30, 31]. Although decolonization is no doubt effective, its implementation is work-intensive. Obesity, mesh repair, immunosuppression, and operative time are known to be more associated with wound morbidity.

3.3.4 Improving Postoperative Intestinal Function

Postoperative ileus and nausea or vomiting are important complaints after surgery, especially when extensive adhesiolysis might be necessary during ventral hernia repair. Alvimopan is an opioid antagonist, mainly affecting peripheral receptors.

After oral administration, it specifically antagonizes the opioid receptors in the gastrointestinal (GI) tract responsible for postoperative ileus (POI) and postoperative nausea/vomiting. The sequelae of bloating, pain, nausea, and vomiting can delay the tolerance of PO intake, prolong hospital stay, and impede the tolerance of enteral pain medications. Thus, POI can be a primary determinant of hospital stay and may potentially be quelled by alvimopan.

The evidence regarding the use of alvimopan most clearly supports its usage after open bowel resections or total abdominal hysterectomy [32]. Although not labeled for large open ventral hernia repair, alvimopan might be incorporated into an ERAS pathway for larger incisional hernia repair.

3.4 Post-operative Measures

3.4.1 Use of Abdominal Binders and Early Mobilization

An abdominal binder can be applied, mainly as an additional tool to increase patients' comfort, not because of a strict medical reason. The evidence is extremely low [33]. It is best applied while the patient is still in the operating theater, and patients are instructed to wear the binder until clinical follow-up 3–4 weeks postoperatively. There is no evidence that abdominal binders influence neither the seroma rate nor seroma severity. Patients should be mobilized postoperatively as soon as possible, even shortly after leaving the recovery ward. Both respiratory and rehabilitation physiotherapy should be recommended, especially after repair of larger ventral hernias.

3.4.2 Multimodal Pain Control

One of the biggest challenges in ERAS for ventral hernia repair is adequate pain control. Regardless of the repair type, almost all hernia repairs require fascial re-approximation and some degree of mesh fixation, all of which induce pain. Although multiple protocols exist, the principal components of postoperative multimodal pain regimen include an immediate acting narcotic, acetaminophen, gabapentin, and possibly non-steroidal anti-inflammatory drugs (NSAIDs).

Intravenous paracetamol (acetaminophen) has a central analgesic effect and has a more rapid/predictable onset than opioids. Furthermore, it is not restricted by the return of bowel function and the ability to tolerate an oral diet. It does not induce the side effects of opioids, such as sedation, respiratory depression, and ileus. There is also no concern of bleeding or impaired renal function as with nonsteroidal anti-inflammatory drugs (NSAIDs). Its use, however, should still be cautioned in patients with hepatic insufficiency. Overall, paracetamol seems to improve postoperative pain and potentially limits narcotic consumption. Acetaminophen is routinely given around the clock because it carries a high-safety profile and therefore, when dosed appropriately, patients will routinely be discharged with acetaminophen as a primary analgesic. NSAIDs represent another class of non-opiates but should be cautiously used with elderly patients given the risk of kidney injury. Therefore, NSAIDs are reserved for non-elderly patients for only a short duration.

Gabapentin remains another useful analgesic following hernia repair. Some RCTs have demonstrated the benefits of pain control and reduced opioid use without the side-effect profile of opiates [34]. Although some patients experience sedative effects from gabapentin, this effect is less frequent than with opiates. Because of the extensive myofascial dissection, muscle spasms can be common. Although typically thought of as an anxiolytic, diazepam can be an effective muscle relaxant in the postoperative setting. Diazepam is typically started on postoperative day 1 or 2, allowing for evaluation of sedation. Because of these sedative effects and greater addictive profile of benzodiazepines, diazepam might be routinely excluded at discharge.

Local and regional blocks are also a useful adjunct for analgesia. Transversus abdominis plane (TAP) blocks have gained popularity given its blockade of intercostal, subcostal, ilioinguinal, and iliohypogastric nerves [35, 36]. The TAP block is a regional anesthetic technique that is inserted in the triangle of Petit, with the needle penetrating the abdominal wall until it reaches the TAP that is between internal oblique and transversus abdominis muscles. For midline abdominal procedures, the block is performed under direct visualization bilaterally to provide a better midline anesthesia. Several studies have demonstrated the benefit of TAP block during abdominal surgery in regard to reduction of postoperative pain, narcotic consumption, and hospital LOS [37]. With regard to epidural anesthesia, there is a lack of evidence for the efficacy of adequate pain relief in AWR patients. This lack of benefit, difficulty with placement in obese patients, along with other side effects (e.g. hypotension, urinary retention, etc.), along with increased length of stay, has led to abstinence from this type of analgesia in the majority of patients undergoing AWR.

So, the aim of a multimodal pain regimen should be: decreased postoperative pain, while significantly reducing opioid consumption. Although opiates are still an important aspect of adequate pain relief at this time, a reduction in narcotic use is favored (Table 3.2).

Table 3.2 Multimodal pain control perioperatively

Multimodal pain control
Intraoperative TAP block with Exparel 20 mL diluted to 120 mL
Patient-controlled analgesia until taking PO
Paracetamol 1 g IV per 6 h for 48 h
Transition to 1000 mg PO per 6 h scheduled
Oxycodone 5–10 mg PO 4 times/day when needed
Gabapentin 300 mg PO three times a day until discharge
Valium 5 mg IV 4 times daily for 48 h
Hold in case of obstructive sleep apnea or sedation
Half dose for patients over 65 years
NSAIDs added when needed
Start 48 h postoperatively
Hold for any renal dysfunction

3.4.3 Early Enteral Feeding

Keeping patients "nil per os" has been the rule, at least until return of bowel function. However, multiple studies have demonstrated success with early enteral feeding [38, 39]. Early nourishment to the patient leads to multiple metabolic benefits, as well as reducing postoperative ileus and decreasing length of hospitalization, without added risk. Most patients tolerate early feeding without the need for nasogastric tube placement.

3.5 Discussion

3.5.1 Measuring Quality in Hernia Surgery

Measuring, reporting, and comparing outcomes, are important steps toward rapidly improving outcomes and making reasonable choices about reducing costs. Within hernia surgery, there is a need for the full assessment of quality throughout lifetime of that patient when measuring outcomes. ERAS implementation might favor short term outcomes, but might be less effective in changing long-term benefits for the patient. With the use of mesh, the long-term outcomes, of intraperitoneal meshes and mesh devices in particular, might result in significant patient harm with reoperations, chronic pain, fistula formation or other mesh-related complications. However, it is very difficult to obtain this kind of data collection. A recent example of how this can be done is provided through the American Hernia Society Qualitative Collaboration [40]. They prospectively collect demographic patient risk factors, perioperative details, and long-term follow-up using validated patient-reported outcome measures, including the PROMIS pain scale, the Ventral Hernia Recurrence Inventory, and the Hernia-Related Quality of Life Survey (HERQLES) abdominal wall functional scores [41, 42]. From this data evidence-based guidelines were published to improve quality outcomes, including elimination of routine preoperative outpatient chlorhexidine scrubs, elimination of routine bowel preparation before elective hernia repair, the potential downside of epidural utilization in ventral hernia repairs, and methods to reduce readmissions after ventral hernia repair [27, 43, 44]. Establishment of clinical quality improvement programs is an excellent way to develop means to track and improve outcomes. This tool allows individual programs to interpret interventions in all patients and apply those interventions only to those who will receive the greatest benefit.

3.5.2 Patient Selection for ERAS After Surgery Protocols

Hernias of the abdominal wall might present in different ways, various width, and multiple locations, while ERAS protocols in hernia surgery mainly will focus on surgical repairs associated with longer length of hospital stay. This then includes primary and recurrent ventral, incisional, and parastomal hernias. There is not that much literature to support the identification of appropriate patient populations for enrollment in ERAS hernia protocols. It is not yet well studied, nor is it entirely clear which patient populations are appropriate for enrollment into ERAS pathways. Although certain protocols demonstrated benefits from ERAS, individual patients might have to be excluded based on placement of biologic mesh due to contaminated fields, and other potential sequelae requiring prolonged hospital stay [45].

Patients undergoing abdominal wall reconstruction may not meet the enrollment criteria set forth in studies from other areas in surgery. Future studies would indeed benefit from inclusion of all subjects followed by subgroup analyses to determine appropriate patients for inclusion in hernia-specific ERAS protocols moving forward.

3.5.3 Implementation of ERAS

Evidence suggests that change in clinical practice occurs 15 years after clear evidence is available [46]. A growing amount of literature on barriers to implementation reports that factors that enable the successful implementation of ERAS include not only a willingness to change to ERAS, formation of multidisciplinary teams and thereby improved communication and collaboration, and support by hospital management, but also standardization of order sets and care processes and the use of audits. Barriers to implementation are a general resistance to change, lack of time and staff, and poor communication, collaboration, and coordination between departments [47, 48].

3.5.4 Outcomes with the ERAS Protocol

There are many stakeholders in surgical care, i.e. professionals from various disciplines as well as managers, politicians, payers, and the general public are involved, as are the medical device and pharmaceutical industries. The early studies reporting on outcomes after ERAS were often met with disbelief, and some thought (incorrectly) that it was careful selection of patients that resulted in a shortened hospital stay. Now diverse groups publishing on consecutive series and using ERAS principles show consistent results [49, 50].

A meta-analysis of randomized trials of the ERAS protocol in patients undergoing colorectal surgery showed that complication rates were reduced by up to 50%, when ERAS principles were used [51]. These studies revealed that not only overall complications were reduced with better compliance, but the most severe complications, which resulted in reoperations or admission to the intensive care unit, decreased as mortality improved.

There are only few studies that directly investigate ERAS protocols when applied to the hernia population. ERAS protocols are mostly targeted at patients undergoing open abdominal wall reconstruction, because these patients are hospitalized postoperatively.

Macedo et al. published a systematic review on ERAS protocols in ventral hernias in 2016; they demonstrated a mean reduction in length of stay of 2.07 days and a trend toward decreased readmission rates in the ERAS group [52]. Jensen et al. examined 32 consecutive subjects undergoing giant ventral hernia repair. ERAS protocols were implemented and compared retrospectively to a standard care control group. The main emphasis in the ERAS protocol included preoperative high-dose glucocorticoid administration (methylprednisolone 125 mg intravenous in an effort to attenuate the inflammatory response) and led to low scores of pain, fatigue, and nausea. Other elements differing from the standard pathway included preoperative education on the pathway and expectations of discharge, twice daily discharge assessments, and more aggressive bowel regimens, including gum chewing and scheduled enemas. The primary endpoint of length of stay was decreased after implementation (median 3.0 vs 5.5 days, $p = 0.003$). There were no statistically significant differences between the two groups with respect to rates of readmission, postoperative complications or reoperation [50].

Majumder et al. published a series of ERAS after VHR [45]. This ERAS pathway was broader, including both perioperative care and preoperative patient optimization. Preoperatively, obese patients underwent weight loss counseling, though no specific BMI cut-off was used, and the effect of this counseling on actual preoperative weight loss was not reported. Additionally, patients with diabetes were required to reach a hemoglobin A1c (HbA1c) of <8. Smoking cessation for at least 1 month prior to surgery was mandatory. Intraoperatively, a transversus abdominis plane (TAP) block was performed using liposomal bupivacaine. Postoperatively, patients received hydromorphone PCA, oral oxycodone, oral acetaminophen, diazepam, gabapentin, and non-steroidal anti-inflammatories (NSAIDs). Using this comprehensive ERAS pathway, 100 patients were compared to 100 historical controls. A decreased LOS was observed from 6.1 to 4 days, as well as a reduction in readmission rate. An earlier resumption of regular diet, earlier return of bowel function, and earlier progression to oral narcotic analgesia were also seen in the ERAS group. Recently, Jensen and colleagues published on 94 patients of a larger cohort undergoing ventral hernia repair with their enhanced recovery after surgery pathway. Length of stay was significantly reduced after the introduction of enhanced recovery after surgery (median 4, interquartile range 3–6 days vs. control 5, 4–7 days, $P < 0.001$). There was no difference between the cohorts in the incidence of postoperative complications requiring operative intervention (enhanced recovery after surgery 10.6% vs control 10.4%, $P = 1.0$) or the rate of readmissions (enhanced recovery after surgery 16.0% vs control 12.5%, $P = 0.635$) [53].

3.5.5 Long-Term Benefits of ERAS

The longer-term benefits of rapid, uncomplicated recovery using ERAS principles are less well known. Medium-term outcomes have been sparsely studied [54] and long-term data on outcomes are now only beginning to appear. Patients with higher compliance might have fewer complications, which may affect the observed outcomes. Perioperative complications have been shown to be strongly associated with poor long-term outcomes in very large surgical series [55]. However, whether the ventral hernia patient will also benefit long-term from ERAS measurements has to be studied in the coming years.

References

1. Fearon KC, Ljungqvist O, Von Meyenfeldt M, Revhaug A, Dejong CH, Lassen K, Nygren J, Hausel J, Soop M, Andersen J, Kehlet H. Enhanced recovery after surgery: a consensus review of clinical care for patients undergoing colonic resection. Clin Nutr. 2005;24(3):466–77.
2. Sørensen LT, Toft BG, Rygaard J, Ladelund S, Paddon M, James T, Taylor R, Gottrup F. Effect of smoking, smoking cessation, and nicotine patch on wound dimension, vitamin C, and systemic markers of collagen metabolism. Surgery. 2010;148(5):982–90. https://doi.org/10.1016/j.surg.2010.02.005.
3. Sørensen LT, Hemmingsen UB, Kirkeby LT, Kallehave F, Jørgensen LN. Smoking is a risk factor for incisional hernia. Arch Surg. 2005;140(2):119–23.
4. Sørensen LT, Hemmingsen U, Jørgensen T. Strategies of smoking cessation intervention before hernia surgery--effect on perioperative smoking behavior. Hernia. 2007;11(4):327–33.
5. Yang GP, Longaker MT. Abstinence from smoking reduces incisional wound infection: a randomized, controlled trial. Ann Surg. 2003;238(1):6–8.
6. Petro CC, Haskins IN, Tastaldi L, Tu C, Krpata DM, Rosen MJ, Prabhu AS. Does active smoking really matter before ventral hernia repair? An AHSQC analysis. Surgery. 2018. pii: S0039-6060(18)30499-9. https://doi.org/10.1016/j.surg.2018.07.039. [Epub ahead of print].
7. Sørensen LT. Wound healing and infection in surgery. The clinical impact of smoking and smoking cessation: a systematic review and meta-analysis. Arch Surg. 2012;147(4):373–83. https://doi.org/10.1001/archsurg.2012.5.
8. Jensen JA, Goodson WH, Hopf HW, Hunt TK. Cigarette smoking decreases tissue oxygen. Arch Surg. 1991;126(9):1131–4.
9. Knuutinen A, Kokkonen N, Risteli J, Vähäkangas K, Kallioinen M, Salo T, Sorsa T, Oikarinen A. Smoking affects collagen synthesis and extracellular matrix turnover in human skin. Br J Dermatol. 2002;146(4):588–94.
10. Sorensen LT, Karlsmark T, Gottrup F. Abstinence from smoking reduces incisional wound infection: a randomized controlled trial. Ann Surg. 2003;238(1):1–5.
11. Thomsen T, Villebro N, Møller AM. Interventions for preoperative smoking cessation. Cochrane Database Syst Rev. 2014;3:CD002294. https://doi.org/10.1002/14651858.CD002294.pub4.
12. Moyer TP, Charlson JR, Enger RJ, Dale LC, Ebbert JO, Schroeder DR, Hurt RD. Simultaneous analysis of nicotine, nicotine metabolites, and tobacco alkaloids in serum or urine by tandem mass spectrometry, with clinically relevant metabolic profiles. Clin Chem. 2002;48(9):1460–71.
13. Feldhammer M, Ritchie JC. Anabasine is a poor marker for determining smoking status of transplant patients. Clin Chem. 2017;63(2):604–6. https://doi.org/10.1373/clinchem.2016.265546.
14. Sauerland S, Korenkov M, Kleinen T, Arndt M, Paul A. Obesity is a risk factor for recurrence after incisional hernia repair. Hernia. 2004;8(1):42–6.
15. Desai KA, Razavi SA, Hart AM, Thompson PW, Losken A. The effect of BMI on outcomes following complex abdominal wall reconstructions. Ann Plast Surg. 2016;76(Suppl 4):S295–7. https://doi.org/10.1097/SAP.0000000000000673.
16. Fischer JP, Wink JD, Tuggle CT, Nelson JA, Kovach SJ. Wound risk assessment in ventral hernia repair: generation and internal validation of a risk stratification system using the ACS-NSQIP. Hernia. 2015;19(1):103–11. https://doi.org/10.1007/s10029-014-1318-5.
17. Liang MK, Holihan JL, Itani K, Alawadi ZM, Gonzalez JR, Askenasy EP, Ballecer C, Chong HS, Goldblatt MI, Greenberg JA, Harvin JA, Keith JN, Martindale RG, Orenstein S, Richmond B, Roth JS, Szotek P, Towfigh S, Tsuda S, Vaziri K, Berger DH. Ventral hernia management:

expert consensus guided by systematic review. Ann Surg. 2017;265(1):80–9. https://doi.org/10.1097/SLA.0000000000001701.
18. Ban KA, Minei JP, Laronga C, Harbrecht BG, Jensen EH, Fry DE, Itani KM, Dellinger EP, Ko CY, Duane TM. American College of Surgeons and Surgical Infection Society: Surgical Site Infection Guidelines, 2016 update. J Am Coll Surg. 2017;224(1):59–74. https://doi.org/10.1016/j.jamcollsurg.2016.10.029.
19. Veterans Affairs Total Parenteral Nutrition Cooperative Study Group. Perioperative total parenteral nutrition in surgical patients. N Engl J Med. 1991;325(8):525–32.
20. Cereda E. Mini nutritional assessment. Curr Opin Clin Nutr Metab Care. 2012;15(1):29–41. https://doi.org/10.1097/MCO.0b013e32834d7647.
21. Guigoz Y. The Mini Nutritional Assessment (MNA) review of the literature--What does it tell us? J Nutr Health Aging. 2006;10(6):466–85; discussion 485–7.
22. Maltby JR, Sutherland AD, Sale JP, Shaffer EA. Preoperative oral fluids: is a five-hour fast justified prior to elective surgery? Anesth Analg. 1986;65(11):1112–6.
23. Swenson BR, Hedrick TL, Metzger R, Bonatti H, Pruett TL, Sawyer RG. Effects of preoperative skin preparation on postoperative wound infection rates: a prospective study of 3 skin preparation protocols. Infect Control Hosp Epidemiol. 2009;30(10):964–71. https://doi.org/10.1086/605926.
24. Darouiche RO, Wall MJ Jr, Itani KM, Otterson MF, Webb AL, Carrick MM, Miller HJ, Awad SS, Crosby CT, Mosier MC, Alsharif A, Berger DH. Chlorhexidine-alcohol versus povidone-iodine for surgical-site antisepsis. N Engl J Med. 2010;362(1):18–26. https://doi.org/10.1056/NEJMoa0810988.
25. Berríos-Torres SI, Umscheid CA, Bratzler DW, Leas B, Stone EC, Kelz RR, Reinke CE, Morgan S, Solomkin JS, Mazuski JE, Dellinger EP, Itani KMF, Berbari EF, Segreti J, Parvizi J, Blanchard J, Allen G, Kluytmans JAJW, Donlan R, Schecter WP. Healthcare infection control practices advisory committee. centers for disease control and prevention guideline for the prevention of surgical site infection, 2017. JAMA Surg. 2017;152(8):784–91. https://doi.org/10.1001/jamasurg.2017.0904.
26. Chlebicki MP, Safdar N, O'Horo JC, Maki DG. Preoperative chlorhexidine shower or bath for prevention of surgical site infection: a meta-analysis. Am J Infect Control. 2013;41(2):167–73. https://doi.org/10.1016/j.ajic.2012.02.014.
27. Prabhu AS, Krpata DM, Phillips S, Huang LC, Haskins IN, Rosenblatt S, Poulose BK, Rosen MJ. Preoperative chlorhexidine gluconate use can increase risk for surgical site infections after ventral hernia repair. J Am Coll Surg. 2017;224(3):334–40. https://doi.org/10.1016/j.jamcollsurg.2016.12.013.
28. Bratzler DW, Dellinger EP, Olsen KM, Perl TM, Auwaerter PG, Bolon MK, Fish DN, Napolitano LM, Sawyer RG, Slain D, Steinberg JP, Weinstein RA. American Society of Health-System Pharmacists; Infectious Disease Society of America; Surgical Infection Society; Society for Healthcare Epidemiology of America. Clinical practice guidelines for antimicrobial prophylaxis in surgery. Am J Health Syst Pharm. 2013;70(3):195–283. https://doi.org/10.2146/ajhp120568.
29. Fonseca SN, Kunzle SR, Junqueira MJ, Nascimento RT, de Andrade JI, Levin AS. Implementing 1-dose antibiotic prophylaxis for prevention of surgical site infection. Arch Surg. 2006;141(11):1109–13; discussion 1114.
30. Berrevoet F, Vanlander A, Sainz-Barriga M, Rogiers X, Troisi R. Infected large pore meshes may be salvaged by topical negative pressure therapy. Hernia. 2013;17(1):67–73. https://doi.org/10.1007/s10029-012-0969-3.
31. Le D, Deveney CW, Reaven NL, Funk SE, McGaughey KJ, Martindale RG. Mesh choice in ventral hernia repair: so many choices, so little time. Am J Surg. 2013;205(5):602–7; discussion 607.
32. Tan EK, Cornish J, Darzi AW, Tekkis PP. Meta-analysis: Alvimopan vs. placebo in the treatment of post-operative ileus. Aliment Pharmacol Ther. 2007;25(1):47–57.
33. Christoffersen MW, Olsen BH, Rosenberg J, Bisgaard T. Randomized clinical trial on the post-operative use of an abdominal binder after laparoscopic umbilical and epigastric hernia repair. Hernia. 2015;19(1):147–53. https://doi.org/10.1007/s10029-014-1289-6.

34. Hurley RW, Cohen SP, Williams KA, Rowlingson AJ, Wu CL. The analgesic effects of perioperative gabapentin on postoperative pain: a meta-analysis. Reg Anesth Pain Med. 2006;31(3):237–47.
35. Petersen PL, Hilsted KL, Dahl JB, Mathiesen O. Bilateral transversus abdominis plane (TAP) block with 24 hours ropivacaine infusion via TAP catheters: a randomized trial in healthy volunteers. BMC Anesthesiol. 2013;13(1):30. https://doi.org/10.1186/1471-2253-13-30.
36. Cohen SM. Extended pain relief trial utilizing infiltration of Exparel(®), a long-acting multivesicular liposome formulation of bupivacaine: a Phase IV health economic trial in adult patients undergoing open colectomy. J Pain Res. 2012;5:567–72. https://doi.org/10.2147/JPR.S38621.
37. Petersen PL, Mathiesen O, Torup H, Dahl JB. The transversus abdominis plane block: a valuable option for postoperative analgesia? A topical review. Acta Anaesthesiol Scand. 2010;54(5):529–35. https://doi.org/10.1111/j.1399-6576.2010.02215.x.
38. Barlow R, Price P, Reid TD, Hunt S, Clark GW, Havard TJ, Puntis MC, Lewis WG. Prospective multicentre randomised controlled trial of early enteral nutrition for patients undergoing major upper gastrointestinal surgical resection. Clin Nutr. 2011;30(5):560–6. https://doi.org/10.1016/j.clnu.2011.02.006.
39. McClave SA, Codner P, Patel J, Hurt RT, Allen K, Martindale RG. Should we aim for full enteral feeding in the first week of critical illness? Nutr Clin Pract. 2016;31(4):425–31. https://doi.org/10.1177/0884533616653809.
40. Poulose BK, Roll S, Murphy JW, Matthews BD, Todd Heniford B, Voeller G, Hope WW, Goldblatt MI, Adrales GL, Rosen MJ. Design and implementation of the Americas Hernia Society Quality Collaborative (AHSQC): improving value in hernia care. Hernia. 2016;20(2):177–89. https://doi.org/10.1007/s10029-016-1477-7.
41. Krpata DM, Schmotzer BJ, Flocke S, Jin J, Blatnik JA, Ermlich B, Novitsky YW, Rosen MJ. Design and initial implementation of HerQLes: a hernia-related quality-of-life survey to assess abdominal wall function. J Am Coll Surg. 2012;215(5):635–42. https://doi.org/10.1016/j.jamcollsurg.2012.06.412.
42. Muysoms FE, Deerenberg EB, Peeters E, Agresta F, Berrevoet F, Campanelli G, Ceelen W, Champault GG, Corcione F, Cuccurullo D, DeBeaux AC, Dietz UA, Fitzgibbons RJ Jr, Gillion JF, Hilgers RD, Jeekel J, Kyle-Leinhase I, Köckerling F, Mandala V, Montgomery A, Morales-Conde S, Simmermacher RK, Schumpelick V, Smietański M, Walgenbach M, Miserez M. Recommendations for reporting outcome results in abdominal wall repair: results of a Consensus meeting in Palermo, Italy, 28-30 June 2012. Hernia. 2013;17(4):423–33. https://doi.org/10.1007/s10029-013-1108-5.
43. Krpata DM, Haskins IN, Phillips S, Prabhu AS, Rosenblatt S, Poulose BK, Rosen MJ. Does preoperative bowel preparation reduce surgical site infections during elective ventral hernia repair? J Am Coll Surg. 2017;224(2):204–11. https://doi.org/10.1016/j.jamcollsurg.2016.10.049.
44. Prabhu AS, Krpata DM, Perez A, Phillips S, Huang LC, Haskins IN, Rosenblatt S, Poulose BK, Rosen MJ. Is it time to reconsider postoperative epidural analgesia in patients undergoing elective ventral hernia repair?: an AHSQC analysis. Ann Surg. 2018;267(5):971–6. https://doi.org/10.1097/SLA.0000000000002214.
45. Majumder A, Fayezizadeh M, Neupane R, Elliott HL, Novitsky YW. Benefits of multimodal enhanced recovery pathway in patients undergoing open ventral hernia repair. J Am Coll Surg. 2016;222(6):1106–15. https://doi.org/10.1016/j.jamcollsurg.2016.02.015.
46. Lassen K, Hannemann P, Ljungqvist O, Fearon K, Dejong CH, von Meyenfeldt MF, Hausel J, Nygren J, Andersen J, Revhaug A. Enhanced Recovery After Surgery Group Patterns in current perioperative practice: survey of colorectal surgeons in five northern European countries. BMJ. 2005;330(7505):1420–1.
47. Pearsall EA, Meghji Z, Pitzul KB, Aarts MA, McKenzie M, McLeod RS, Okrainec A. A qualitative study to understand the barriers and enablers in implementing an enhanced recovery after surgery program. Ann Surg. 2015;261(1):92–6. https://doi.org/10.1097/SLA.0000000000000604.

48. Ament SM, Gillissen F, Moser A, Maessen JM, Dirksen CD, von Meyenfeldt MF, van der Weijden T. Identification of promising strategies to sustain improvements in hospital practice: a qualitative case study. BMC Health Serv Res. 2014;14:641. https://doi.org/10.1186/s12913-014-0641-y.
49. Delaney CP, Fazio VW, Senagore AJ, Robinson B, Halverson AL, Remzi FH. 'Fast track' postoperative management protocol for patients with high co-morbidity undergoing complex abdominal and pelvic colorectal surgery. Br J Surg. 2001;88(11):1533–8.
50. Jensen KK, Brondum TL, Harling H, Kehlet H, Jorgensen LN. Enhanced recovery after giant ventral hernia repair. Hernia. 2016;20(2):249–56. https://doi.org/10.1007/s10029-016-1471-0.
51. Varadhan KK, Neal KR, Dejong CH, Fearon KC, Ljungqvist O, Lobo DN. The enhanced recovery after surgery (ERAS) pathway for patients undergoing major elective open colorectal surgery: a meta-analysis of randomized controlled trials. Clin Nutr. 2010;29(4):434–40. https://doi.org/10.1016/j.clnu.2010.01.004.
52. Macedo FIB, Mittal VK. Does enhanced recovery pathways affect outcomes in open ventral hernia repair? Hernia. 2017;21(5):817–8. https://doi.org/10.1007/s10029-016-1553-z.
53. Jensen KK, Dressler J, Baastrup NN, Kehlet H, Jørgensen LN. Enhanced recovery after abdominal wall reconstruction reduces length of postoperative stay: an observational cohort study. Surgery. 2018. pii: S0039-6060(18)30493-8. https://doi.org/10.1016/j.surg.2018.07.035. [Epub ahead of print].
54. Neville A, Lee L, Antonescu I, Mayo NE, Vassiliou MC, Fried GM, Feldman LS. Systematic review of outcomes used to evaluate enhanced recovery after surgery. Br J Surg. 2014;101(3):159–70. https://doi.org/10.1002/bjs.9324.
55. Khuri SF, Henderson WG, DePalma RG, Mosca C, Healey NA, Kumbhani DJ, Participants in the VA National Surgical Quality Improvement Program. Determinants of long-term survival after major surgery and the adverse effect of postoperative complications. Ann Surg. 2005;242(3):326–41; discussion 341–3.

4 Prosthetic Materials for Robot-Assisted Hernia Repair

Karl A. LeBlanc

4.1 Introduction

Incisional hernias will develop in at least 13% and perhaps as many as 20% of laparotomy incisions. The risk of herniation is increased by fivefold if a postoperative wound infection occurs. Other factors that predispose to the development of a fascial defect include smoking, obesity, poor nutritional status, steroid usage, etc. While some of these may be avoided, those patients that are found to have such a hernia can present difficult management problems due to the high potential for recurrence. It has been known for many years that without the use of a prosthetic material, the recurrence rate for ventral hernia repair is as high as 51% [1]. The use of a synthetic material will reduce this rate to at least 10–24% [2]. While these publications are older, they are still relevant in today's management of hernia repair. Recent data still reveals a recurrence rate of 17.1% without the use of mesh, 12.3% with open mesh repair and 10.6% with laparoscopic mesh repair [3].

The laparoscopic repair of incisional and ventral hernias was first performed in 1991 using the Soft Tissue Patch made by W.L. Gore and Associates (Elkhart, DE, USA) [4]. The recurrence rate that has been reported in other recent literature varies from 0–11% but averages approximately 5.5%. A recent publication reported only one recurrence in 368 hernias that were repaired in this multicenter study using the robot technology [5].

The use of prosthetic biomaterials in the repair of hernias of the abdominal wall is a virtual requirement to effectively repair them with robotic technology. As such, it is very important for the surgeon to be as familiar with these materials as they are with the technical aspects of the procedure itself. The "one size fits all" approach to the use of mesh in the repair of hernias is not ideal. The size and location of the hernia that is being repaired, the number of prior repairs and the type(s) of mesh

K. A. LeBlanc (✉)
Our Lady of the Lake Physician Group, Baton Rouge, LA, USA

K. A. LeBlanc (ed.), *Robotic Assisted Hernia Repair*,
https://doi.org/10.1007/978-3-030-23025-8_4

already in place and the co-morbidities of the patient into which this material will be placed should dictate the type of material that will be chosen.

There are several hundred different products that can be used in the repair of the hernias of the abdominal wall. This chapter will identify these goals and the properties of the various biomaterials that are on the market today. In many of the products listed below there is a paucity of published literature that verifies the claims made by the manufacturers. It is very difficult to find Level 1 studies that evaluate the success or failure of the respective materials. It is recommended that the reader is advised to reference the available journals to identify the uses and results of these materials. Finally, a large portion of the information presented was obtained from the respective manufacturer directly but not in all cases. If necessary, the reader should reference the particular manufacturer for in-depth information that cannot be provided in this textbook.

4.2 Indications for Use of Prosthetic Materials

Surgeons recognize that the main purpose in the use of these materials will be the repair of a fascial defect or a weakness in the abdominal wall. This situations will occur in a variety of etiologies (Table 4.1).

Musculofascial tissue strength can be lost in a variety of ways. The most common, of course, would be due to the external etiology of the weakness that develops after a laparotomy or other abdominal incision. Another example would be the loss of tissue with trauma such as gunshot wounds and/or treatment with an open abdomen. The increase of intra-abdominal pressure that results from significant weight gain will result in an internal source of weakening of the abdominal wall fascia. Poor nutrition and/or protein malnutrition are also sources of such problems. Other pre-disposing factors such as emphysema or the chronic bronchitis of individuals that smoke tobacco products results in a constant increase in intra-abdominal pressure because of a frequent cough. Additionally the collagen breakdown that is responsible for emphysema is a systematic effect and not limited to just the pulmonary tissues (i.e. metastatic emphysema). Potentially life-threatening infections such as fasciitis and gangrene will produce large areas of necrosis and resultant tissue loss due to required surgical debridement. More frequently, the development

Table 4.1 Indications for prostheses

Replacement of lost musculofascial tissue caused by:
Trauma
External
Internal
Infection
Reinforcement of native tissue weakness
Aging (laxity of tissues)
Neurological deficit (denervation)

of a postoperative wound infection will increase the risk of herniation by as much a fivefold. It has been known for many decades that nearly 30% of patients that develop a postoperative incisional wound infection will eventually develop an incisional hernia [6]. Modern needs of patients have resulted in the development of products that are not permanent such as biologic meshes or synthetic absorbable products. There are combination materials of these that include permanent components.

The effects of aging and the declining ability of the elderly patients to repair the native tissues will lead to the loss of fascial integrity. This is commonly seen with direct inguinal hernias. It also occurs with the enlargement of the linea alba that is referred to as diastasis recti. These latter defects can enlarge and occasionally become symptomatic, requiring repair.

The most common defect that results from a denervation phenomenon follows the flank incision that is utilized in a nephrectomy, lumbar sympathectomy or an anterior approach to the lumbar interbody fusion for degenerative disc disease. This can occasionally be seen following viral infections such as herpes zoster or even de novo with no predisposing factors. In these entities, there is no defined fascial edge that is seen with the more common anterior abdominal wall hernia defects. This is due to the broad surface of the denervated musculature that has intact fascia but lacks the reinforcement of healthy muscle tissue. Mesh materials are especially necessary for these problems to assure a durable and cosmetically acceptable repair as possible.

4.3 Prosthetic Materials: History

The use of materials for the repairs of hernias can be found in antiquity. It is believed that Heliodorus used cellulose from a cotton or flax plant to effect scarification in the inguinal area to treat herniation in A.D. 25. The use of silver as a synthetic prosthesis was reported in 1900 [7]. Metallic biomaterials have also included the use of tantalum gauze mesh, stainless steel mesh, and silver filigree [8]. None of these materials gained wide acceptance because of the complications that were associated with their usage. These included lack of pliability, seroma development, wound infection, fatigue fractures, herniation through the fracture sites, abnormal scarification, adhesions, loss of structural integrity and allergic reactions. Additionally re-operation on these patients was particularly challenging.

It is interesting that the use of biologic materials was attempted many years ago. The processing and the results varied from the currently available products (Table 4.2).

Table 4.2 Natural prosthetic products

Autogenous dermal grafts	Whole skin grafts
Dermal collagen homografts	Porcine dermal collagen
Autogenous fascial heterografts	Lyophilized aortic homografts
Preserved dural homografts	Bovine pericardium

These materials were used with good results in some cases but scarcity and cost limited their widespread adoption. Real concerns of viral transmission developed following the report of a case of Creutzfeld-Jacobs disease subsequent to the use of a dural homograft in a hernia repair. The development of improved synthetic biomaterials hastened the demise of the use of these products in the past. As we now have seen over the last several years, some of these products have seen resurgence. Updated methods of processing these products have allowed for improved safety and efficacy resulting in an expansion of their use.

A series of nonmetallic synthetic prosthetic biomaterials were used as well (Table 4.3). As with the metal materials, there were significant problems with the outcomes seen with these products. These included infections, sinus tract formation, alteration of the product *in vivo*, and lack of incorporation into the native tissues. The use of the carbon fiber in humans has never been attempted because of concerns of potential carcinogenicity (although it functioned fairly well in the experimental model). As is easily noted, many of these materials are currently in use but with significant modifications that mitigate against the issues noted above.

All of these biomaterials were attempting to address the "ideal characteristics" that were promulgated by Cumberland and Scales [9, 10]. While it is widely felt that the ideal material has yet to be discovered, these criteria are the goals that are sought by the manufacturers (Table 4.4) [11].

While the clinical uses of these prosthetic materials share these considerations, the operating surgeon does, in fact, desire slightly different priorities in the use of the prosthesis within his or her individual patient. Disregarding the obvious need to be non-carcinogenic, the clinical characteristics of the "ideal surgical" material differ from the properties listed above (Table 4.5).

The synthetic prosthetic materials can be divided into the absorbable and nonabsorbable products. The synthetic permanent materials are of many types, sizes, and shapes. The use of these products is commonplace in the repair of virtually all hernias. There has been an increase in the number synthetic absorbable products

Table 4.3 Nonmetallic synthetic products

Fortisan fabric (cellulose)	Polytetrafluoroethylene
Polyvinyl sponge	Polypropylene mesh/gelatin film
Polyvinyl cloth	Polyester-reinforced silicon sheeting
Nylon mesh	Silastic
Carbon fiber	Polyester (as a solid sheet)
Silicon-velvet composite	Carbon fiber

Table 4.4 Ideal properties of synthetic products

No physical modification by tissue fluids	Chemically inert
Does not incite inflammatory or foreign body reaction	Does not produce allergy or hypersensitivity
Noncarcinogenic	Resistant to mechanical strains
Can be fabricated to the form required	Sterilizable

Table 4.5 Ideal *clinical* characteristics of synthetic products

Permanent Repair of the Abdominal Wall (i.e. no recurrences)
In-growth characteristics that result in a normal pattern of tissue repair and healing
No alteration of the compliance of the abdominal wall musculature
Lack of adhesion predisposition
Cuts easily and without fraying
Inexpensive
Lack of long-term complications such as pain or fistula development

over the last several years. There are even hybrid products that include both absorbable and non-absorbable layers. These attempt to capitalize on the attributes of both of these technologies.

The materials that are presented below are given in an arbitrary arrangement and with as accurate information that could be obtained. An effort was made, however, to stratify these products in a classification that grouped similar products together. I have attempted to identify all of the currently available products that are used in most parts of the world at the time of publication. Some of these materials have either no published clinical data or scant information as to the clinical performance characteristics. Therefore, it is certain, that some products and/or details have been overlooked despite my efforts to present all that I could identify. Due to the very large variation in the sizes of the products, little comment regarding the sizes of these products will be given. Similarly, the thicknesses, fiber sizes, weave patterns and pore sizes of most of these products are not discussed at length. The reader is referred to the respective manufacturer for these details.

It should also be noted that not all of these products are available in all countries. Manufacturers may have limited the release of them to only selected areas of the world or have not yet obtained the necessary governmental approvals for clinical distribution at the time of this writing. Additionally, many companies are quite small, are not participants in large nationwide contracts and/or have limited distribution. Therefore, if any of these that are not included it was not because of an intended omission but rather a lack of obtainable information. Finally, it is certain that all of the available products are not included in this compilation or that some of those listed are no longer available due to the lag in this research and actual publication.

4.4 Absorbable Synthetic Biomaterials

The general purpose of these is to act as a bridge of hernia abdominal wall defect or the temporary replacement of absent tissue (Table 4.6). The strength of these materials and the lack of permanency make some of them unsuitable for the permanent repair of any hernia in most cases. However, research has suggested that some of

Table 4.6 Absorbable products

Bio-A, W. L. Gore & Associates, Elkhart, DE
Safil Mesh, B. Braun Surgical, Germany
TIGR mesh, Novus Scientific Pte Ltd., Singapore
Phasix mesh, CR Bard, Providence, RI, USA
Phasix ST mesh, CR Bard, Providence, RI, USA

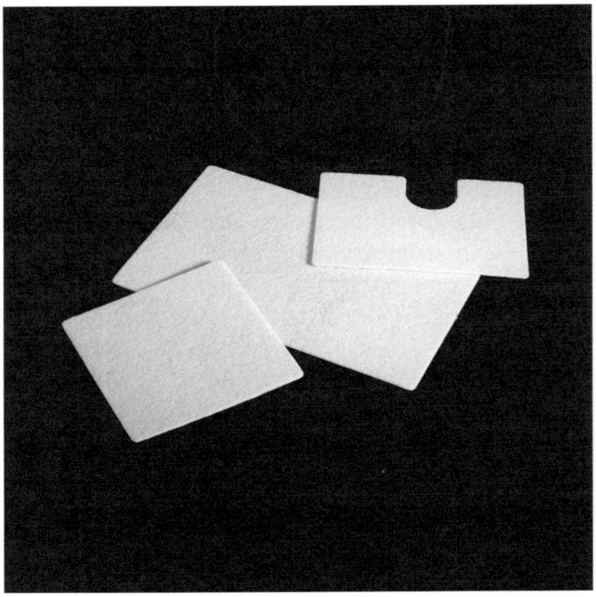

Fig. 4.1 Bio-A

these materials might be preferred in some circumstances rather than a true biologic product. This fact may be due to the fact that biologics require degradation then reconstruction of the collagen of the patient's fascia. These materials do not require the extent of cellular degradation that true biological materials require and seem to progress to reconstructive metabolism more rapidly. This is an area of ongoing research. Clinical usage will be dependent upon the longevity of the material that is sought by the surgeon and the conditional that is being treated.

The *Bio-A* product is made of trimethylene carbonate and polyglycolic acid (Fig. 4.1). It will maintain approximately 70% of its tensile strength for 21 days. It serves as a scaffold to allow for fibroblastic infiltration and replacement by the native collagen of the. Recent studies have shown efficacy for complex situations [12]. *Safil Mesh* is a warp knitted polyglycolic acid material that will retain 50% of its strength at 20 days and is totally resorbed in 60–90 days (Fig. 4.2). It is used to strengthen the closure of the abdominal and chest walls. The above photo also shows the bags into which this material is also shaped for use in splenic preservation.

Phasix is composed of poly-4-hydroxybutyrate (P4HB) that is produced from the byproducts of E. coli metabolism (Fig. 4.3). It is degraded by hydrolytic

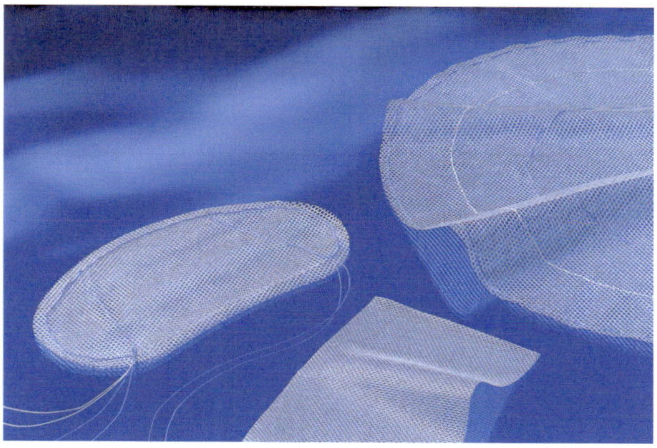

Fig. 4.2 Safil mesh

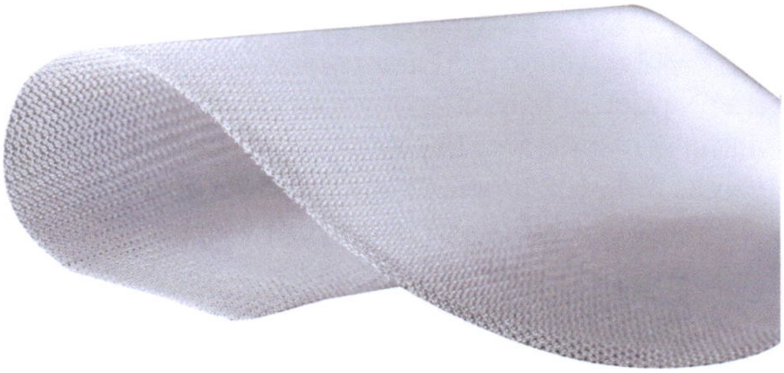

Fig. 4.3 Phasix mesh

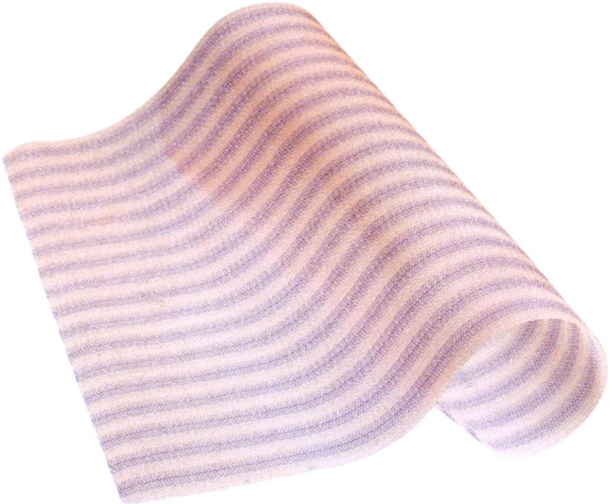

Fig. 4.4 Phasix ST

enzymatic processes. The absorption of the material is minimal until about 26 weeks post-implantation and is essentially complete in about 52 weeks. The mesh is also available with a barrier coating of carboxymethylcellulose and hyaluronic acid as *Phasix ST* (Fig. 4.4). This product can be placed in the intraperitoneal positon against the intestine.

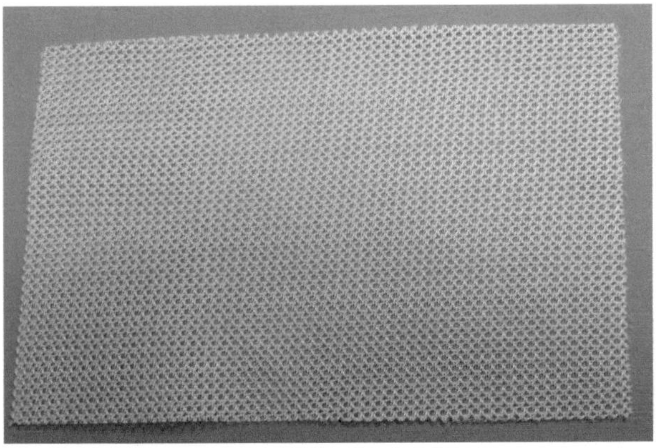

Fig. 4.5 TIGR mesh

TIGR Matrix Surgical Mesh is knitted from two different synthetic resorbable fibers, polyglycolic acid and polylactic acid (Fig. 4.5). The Matrix is warp-knitted in a proprietary way, allowing it to gradually degrade over time. The strength of the Matrix is comparable to conventional permanent implants for the initial six to nine months following implantation. The first fiber (polyglycolic acid) appears to lose its functional capabilities in two weeks while the second fiber (polylactic acid) maintains its strength for approximately nine months. Older products that are still utilized for soft tissue reinforcement including hiatal hernia repair include Vicryl® (Ethicon, Inc. Somerville, NJ, USA) that is either knitted or woven.

4.5 Biologic Products

As noted above, the use of biologic products does not represent a new concept in hernia repair. They are based upon a harvested collagen matrix that is manufactured into sheets of tissue-engineered materials that can be used to repair defects in the abdominal wall. The concept of these materials is that the biologic material will allow the migration of the patient's own fibroblasts onto them so that collagen will be deposited to form a "neo-fascia". For the most part, these are used in open techniques but there has been some usage in laparoscopic methods especially in the repair of hiatal hernias. There is even less usage with robotic assisted hernia repair. These materials are listed for completeness but are not extensively discussed. Further information can be obtained in other publications [13].

There are similarities of all of the biologic products. They are the most expensive of all prosthetic materials that repair or replace the abdominal wall fascia. They are all harvested from an organism that was once alive. The source will dictate the size of the material and in most cases, the thickness of the product. The thickness will be variable in nearly all of them. Some manufacturers have found creative techniques to increase the size of the materials available. All of the products are processed to eliminate all cellular and nuclear material as well as any prions. Following this, another process can be applied to crosslink the collagen at the molecular level. There is only one product that is currently cross-linked as discussed below. The final stage is the sterilization of the prosthesis. It is beyond the scope of this chapter to cover all of these in detail. However, it should be considered, when using any of these materials, that the processing plays a large part into the characteristics and the clinical behavior of them post-implantation.

In general, the biologic products were introduced for use in contaminated fields such as a synthetic mesh infection. While they can be used in this manner, it is recommended that the wound should not possess gross pus as the collagenases of some bacteria and inflammatory cells can degrade these products. These products are sometimes used in the repair of very complex non-infected hernias as well. One concern will be that if the patient possesses an undiagnosed collagen deficiency disorder, the remodeling of these products will not occur properly, leading to a predictable failure of the repair. It has also be learned over the last few years that these products perform best if they have direct contact with some type of vascularized tissue. Intuitively, if the expectation of these biologic scaffolds to become infiltrated by fibroblasts and subsequent collagen deposition, blood supply will deliver these cells more rapidly. Consequently, a higher failure rate will be noted if a biologic prosthesis is used as a "bridge" between fascial edges. It is recommended that if a bridge is unavoidable, then use of the peritoneum of the hernia sac can provide a source of vascular supply.

4.5.1 Bovine Products

The bovine products are from dermis or pericardium (Table 4.7). Only the *SurgiMend* is fetal (dermal) tissue. The associated numbers are the thickness of the four different products in millimeters. *SurgiMend-e* is specifically designed for ventral hernia repair. It is elliptical in shape, perforated and available in 3 mm or 4 mm thicknesses. *Surgimend MP* is similar to the former product in that it is available in four different thicknesses but is also perforated over its entirety. *Tutomesh* and *Tutopatch* are of the same source (pericardium) and are processed in the same manner. The only difference in these two is that the Tutomesh is perforated while Tutopatch is not. *Veritas* is also pericardium and does not require rehydration.

Table 4.7 Bovine biologic prostheses

SurgiMend 1.0,2.0,3.0,4.0, Integra LifeSciences, USA
SurgiMend-e, Integra LifeSciences, USA
SurgiMend MP, Integra LifeSciences, USA
Tutomesh, RTI Biologics, Alachua, FL, USA
Tutopatch, RTI Biologics, Alachua, FL, USA
Veritas, Baxter Healthcare Corporation, Deerfield, IL USA

4.5.2 Cadaveric Products

These are seldom used in the robotic repair of hernias and are listed here for completeness. There is significant variability in the amount of stretch that each of these will undergo either at the time of implantation and subsequent to the procedure (Table 4.8). This stretch varies from product to product and should be accounted for at the time of implantation. These products are not cross-linked and require rehydration. These are also used in the repair of hiatal hernias. *AlloMax* Surgical Graft is 0.8–1.8 mm thick. *Cortiva* and *Cortiva 1 mm* are similar materials that are in two different thicknesses. *Cortiva* is thicker at 1.3 mm (0.8–1.8 mm) and *Cortiva 1 mm* is 1 mm (0.8–1.2 mm). *DermaMatrix* is available in thicknesses of 0.2–0.4 mm, 0.4–0.8 mm, 0.8–1.7 mm, and ≥1.8 mm. *Flex HD Structural* is available in a thick version (0.8 mm–1.7 mm) or an Ultra Thick version (1.8 mm–4 mm).

4.5.3 Porcine Products

There is a significant variation of these materials. Some are laminated, cross-linked, perforated, some require rehydration and others do not (Table 4.9). *BioDesign Hernia Grafts* are three products that are designed for the repair of specific hernias, ventral, inguinal and hiatal. They are all developed from porcine small intestinal submucosa and are the only products with such a source. *Cellis* is porcine dermal collagen and is available in many sizes and different thicknesses. *Fortiva* originates from dermis. *Gentrix Surgical Matrix* is also a laminated product. It is unique in this

Table 4.8 Cadaveric biologic prostheses

AlloMax, Davol, Inc., Warwick, RI, USA
Cortiva, RTI Surgical, Alachua, FL, USA
Cortiva 1 mm, RTI Surgical, Alachua, FL, USA
DermaMatrix, Synthes CMF, West Chester, PA, USA
FlexHD STRUCTURAL, Ethicon, Inc., Somerville, NJ, USA

Table 4.9 Porcine biologic prostheses

Biodesign, Cook Surgical, Inc., Bloomington, IN, USA
Cellis, Meccellis Biotech, La Rochelle, France
Fortiva, RTI Biologics, Alachua, FL, USA
Gentrix Surgical Matrix, ACell, Columbia, MD, USA
Permacol, Medtronic, Minneapolis, MN, USA
Strattice RTM, Acelity, San Antonio, TX, USA
XenMatrix, Davol, Inc., Warwick, RI, USA
XenMatrix AB, Davol, Inc., Warwick, RI, USA
XCM Biologic Tissue Matrix, Ethicon, Somerville, NJ, USA

Fig. 4.6 Strattice laparoscopic

biologic category as it is the only one that is made from the urinary bladder of the pig. *Gentrix* is available as *RS* (two ply), *PSM* (three ply), *PSMX* (six ply), or Plus (8 ply). *Permacol* is a dermal collagen based product that is the only material listed that is cross-linked and is available in thicknesses of 0.5 mm, 1.0 mm, and 1.5 mm.

Strattice Reconstructive Tissue Matrix (RTM) is available in two thicknesses, firm and pliable. It is made from dermis. There are different versions of this product but one is specifically designed for laparoscopic use (Fig. 4.6). *XenMatrix* is also dermal based and is not cross-linked. *XenMatrix AB* contains the antimicrobials, rifampin and minocycline, which are present for over 7 days. *XCM Biologic Tissue Matrix* is also a non-cross-linked porcine dermal product.

4.6 Hybrid Products

This is a relatively new concept in mesh development. There are clear reasons to use a permanent material in the repair of fascial defects. There are real reasons to consider the use of products that are not permanent but seek to increases the levels of collagen deposition to enhance the healing process. These materials seek to capitalize on the benefits of both of these concepts (Table 4.10). These are designed in a fashion for use in robotic assisted repairs.

OviTex, OviTex 1S and 2S is the most recent additions to these class of meshes. They are a combination of ovine gastric submucosal extracellular matrix and embedded polypropylene or polyglycolic acid. There is a four-layer core of this matrix in the *OviTex* version (Fig. 4.7a). *OviTex 1S* has an additional two layers of matrix on one side and the *OviTex 2S* has the core plus two layers on both sides of the product (Fig. 4.7b). Because of these differing designs, the thickness varies from 0.9 mm to 1.1 mm to 1.6 mm. The absorbable component option makes it the only biologic hybrid option with such a concept. The non-biologic portion is constructed with 6 mm pores. These figures are of the permanent component option. The resorbable polymer option is clear and will not be seen. Both *OviTex 1S* and *OviTex 2S* can

Table 4.10 Hybrid products

OviTex, OviTex 1S, Ovitex 2S, Permanent, TelaBio, Malvern, PA, USA
OviTex, OviTex 1S, Ovitex 2S, Resorbable, TelaBio, Malvern, PA, USA
Synecor IP, W. L. Gore & Associates, Elkhart, DE, USA
Synecor PRE, W. L. Gore & Associates, Elkhart, DE, USA

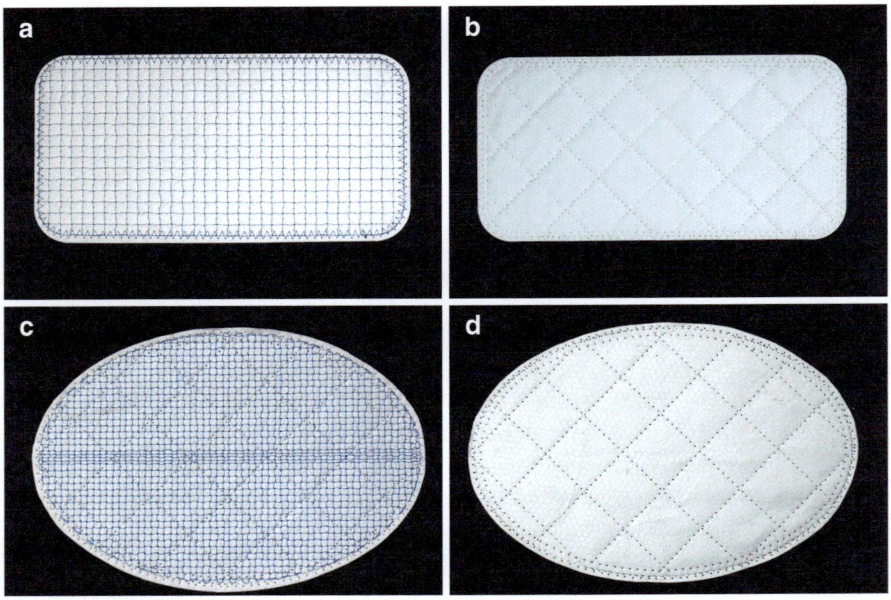

Fig. 4.7 (**a**) Ovitex Core with polypropylene (**b**) Ovitex 1S (Ovitex Core with two additional layers on the shown surface). (**c**, **d**) Ovitex LPR

be placed with visceral contact. There has been a recent addition to the product line that provides a product specific to laparoscopic and robotic usage and placement as an intraperitoneal mesh, the OviTex LPR (Fig. 4.7c, d). The former figure shows the parietal surface while the latter the visceral surface. This contains the polypropylene to provide for permanence in the repair.

Synecor has combined some older materials together. The internal permanent material is polytetrafluoroethylene (PTFE). This is woven into a structure that is similar to other macroporous materials and is not the same are ePTFE. This is sandwiched between two types of polyglycolic acid/trimethylene carbonate (PGA/TMC). The Synecor IP has two different layers. The parietal surface is similar to the Bio-A that is described above (Fig. 4.8, right). The visceral (tissue-separating) side is PGA/TMC is a different structural weave which is quite tight to prevent ingrowth (Fig. 4.8, left). The Synecor PRE has the Bio-A coating on both sides of the PTFE (Fig. 4.9). It is meant to only be used with no visceral contact and must be placed an extraperitoneal plane. These materials can be used either dry or wet.

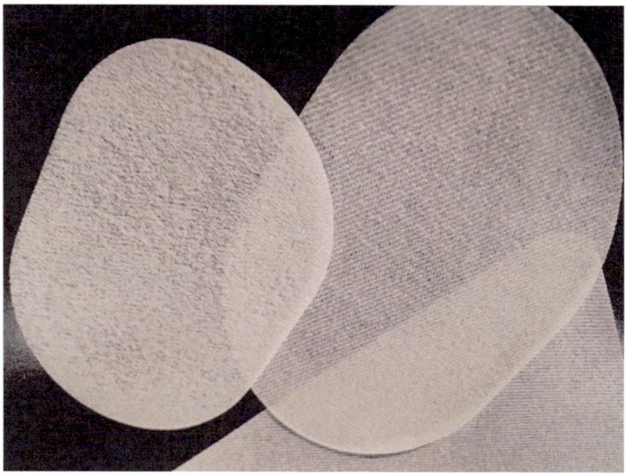

Fig. 4.8 Synecor IP

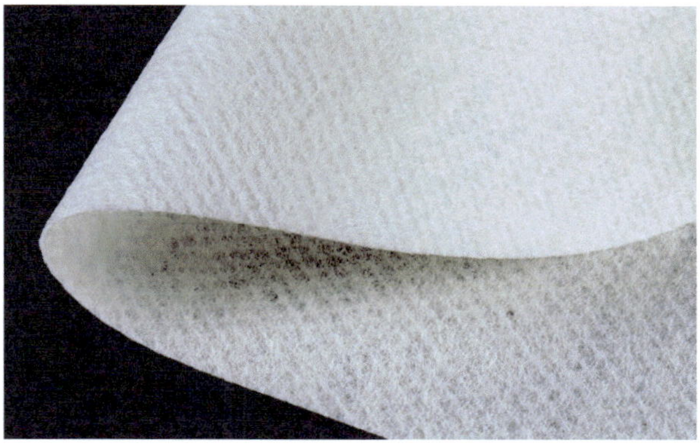

Fig. 4.9 Synecor PRE

4.7 Flat Prosthetic Products

The currently available products in use today are polypropylene (PP), condensed polypropylene (cPP), polyester (POL), polytetrafluoroethylene (PTFE), expanded PTFE (ePTFE) or condensed PTFE (cPTFE). All are available in a variety of sizes and can be cut to conform to the dimensions that are necessary. There are currently so many products on the market today that it is quite difficult to become well versed in all of these materials. The most prominent and commonly used are PP materials (Table 4.11). These can be used either in the open or laparoscopic applications but none are barrier coated and therefore cannot be placed in contact with an intra-abdominal organ. Because of the complexities of pore sizes and the multitude of differing weights and shapes of the PPM within each of these materials, the reader is referred to the manufacturer for further information in the exact densities, weights and pore sizes of these products.

The *2D* products are available in a variety of products and weights. The *2D PPT Std* and the *2D PPT LW* are both knitted and differ in the weight and pore size. The

Table 4.11 Flat polypropylene products

2D PPT Std, Microval, Saint-Just-Malmont, France
2D PPT LW, Microval, Saint-Just-Malmont, France
2D PPNT, Microval, Saint-Just-Malmont, France
Basic mesh, Di.pro Medical Devices, Torino, Italy
Basic Evolution mesh, Di.pro Medical Devices, Torino, Italy
Bard mesh, Davol, Inc., Warwick, RI, USA
Bard Soft mesh, Davol, Inc., Warwick, RI, USA
Biomesh P1, Cousin Biotech, Wervicq-Sud, France
Bulev UL, Di.pro Medical Devices, Torino, Italy
Bulev B5050, Di.pro Medical Devices, Torino, Italy
DynaMesh PP-Standard, FEG Textiltechnik mbH, Aachen, Germany
DynaMesh PP- Light, FEG Textiltechnik mbH, Aachen, Germany
EasyProthes, TransEasy Medical Tech.Co.Ltd., Beijing, China
Hermesh 3,4,5,6,7,8, HerniaMesh, S.R.L., Torino, Italy
Optilene, B. Braun Melsungen AG, Melsungen, Germany
Optilene LP, B. Braun Melsungen AG, Melsungen, Germany
Optilene Mesh Elastic, B. Braun Melsungen AG, Melsungen, Germany
Parietene Flat Sheet, Medtronic, Minneapolis, MN, USA
Parietene Lightweight, Medtronic, Minneapolis, MN, USA
Premilene, B. Braun Melsungen AG, Melsungen, Germany
Premium, Cousin Biotech, Wervicq-Sud, France
Prolene, Ethicon Inc., Somerville, NJ, USA
Prolene Soft Mesh, Ethicon Inc., Somerville, NJ, USA
Prolite, Atrium Medical Corporation, Hudson, NH, USA
Repol Angimesh 0,1,8,9, Angiologica, S. Martino Sicc., Italy
SMX, THT Bio-Science, Montpelier, France
SMH2, THT Bio-Science, Montpelier, France
SMH, THT Bio-Science, Montpelier, France
Surgimesh WN, Aspide Medical, St. Etienne, France
Surgipro Monofilamented, Covidien plc, Dublin, Ireland
Surgipro Multifilamented, Covidien plc, Dublin, Ireland
Surgipro Open Weave, Covidien plc, Dublin, Ireland
TiLENE, GfE Medizintechnik, Nuremburg, Germany
TiLENE Blue, GfE Medizintechnik, Nuremburg, Germany
TiMESH, GfE Medizintechnik, Nuremburg, Germany
TiO_2 Mesh, Bayreuth, Germany
VitaMesh– Getinge Group, Wayne, NJ
VitaMesh Blue – Getinge Group, Wayne, NJ

former is heavy weight while the latter is medium weight and possesses larger pore sizes. The 2D PPNT is a non-woven PP material that is available in three different weights and thicknesses (Fig. 4.10). These meshes are configured in a variety of shapes and sizes as shown.

Basic mesh is a lightweight mesh (Fig. 4.11). Di.pro has developed an ultra lightweight version that is called *Basic Evolution* mesh (Fig. 4.12). *Bard Mesh* is

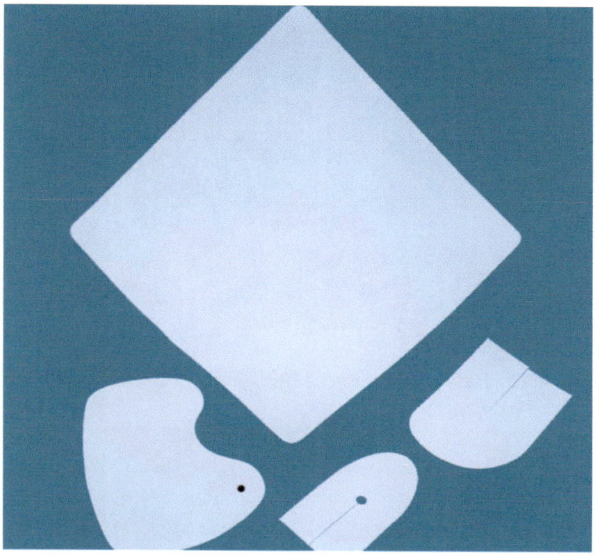

Fig. 4.10 2D PPNT

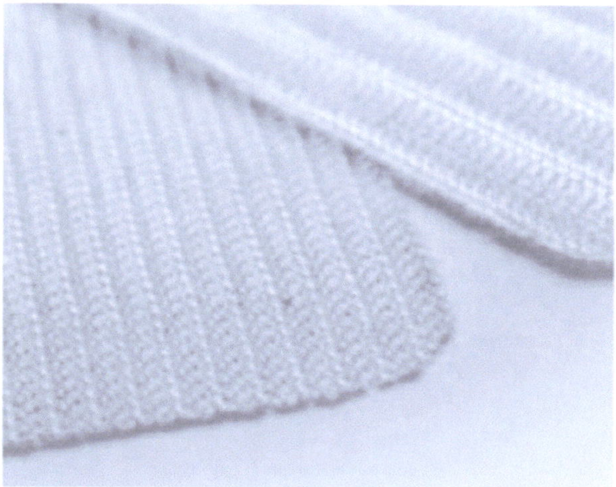

Fig. 4.11 Basic

probably the oldest flat sheet of heavy weight polypropylene in existence, having been brought to market in the early 1960s (Fig. 4.13). It is still in use today and like many of these prostheses, a lightweight and more macroporous version has been developed, the *Bard Soft Mesh* (Fig. 4.14). *Biomesh P1* (Fig. 4.15) is the standard weight material compared to the *Premium* (Fig. 4.16). It is available for extraperitoneal placement in various shapes and sizes for laparoscopic inguinal and ventral hernia repairs. *Bulev B* and *Bulev UL* are somewhat similar to the Basic and Basic Evolution meshes discussed above (Figs. 4.17 and 4.18). The weights of the Bulev products are 48 gm/m^2 and 39 gm/m^2 respectively. They are different in that they possess blue lines to differentiate them from the other meshes and aid in positioning of the product.

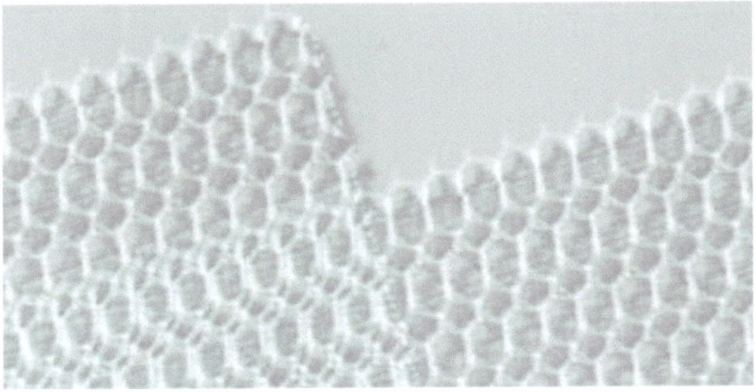

Fig. 4.12 Basic evolution

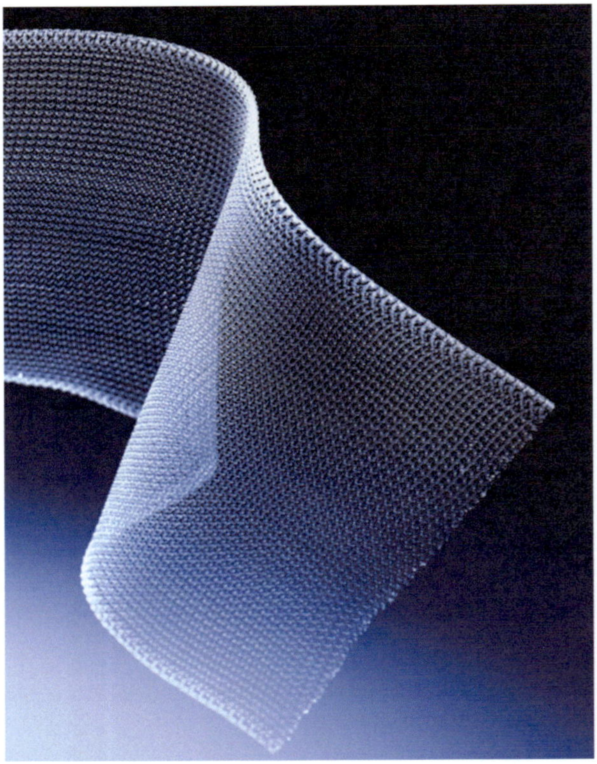

Fig. 4.13 Bard mesh

DynaMesh comes in two weights; *Dynamesh PP—Standard* (Fig. 4.19, right) is twice the weight of the *Dynamesh PP—Light* (Fig. 4.19, left) product. *Easy Prothes* is available as a heavy weight material (90 g/m^2), two medium products (70 g/m^2 and 60 g/m^2), and a lightweight version (40 g/m^2). Figures 4.20 and 4.21 compare the medium and lightweight versions. The *Hermesh 3–8* have a huge variety of sizes and graduated weights from heaviest (3) to lightest (8) and sizes (Fig. 4.22).

Optilene products are all lightweight materials that vary from the heaviest by that name (60 gm/m^2) to the *Elastic* (48 gm/m^2) and the lighter *LP* (36 gm/m^2). The

Fig. 4.14 Bard Soft mesh

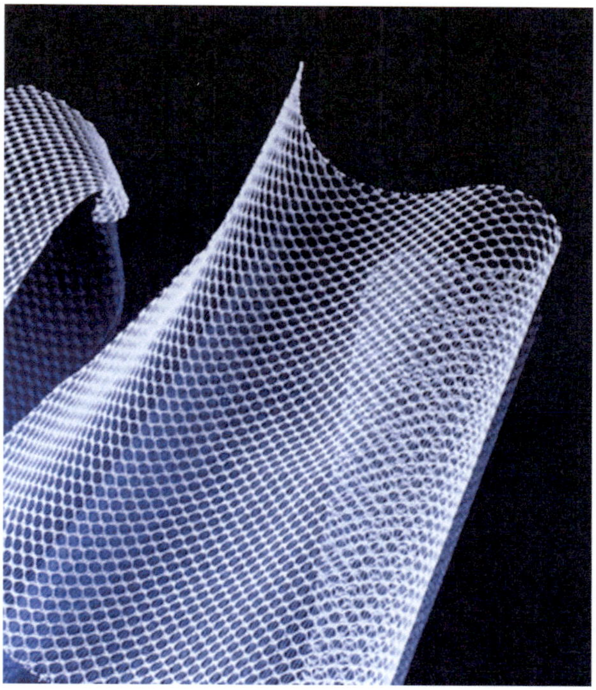

Fig. 4.15 Biomesh P1

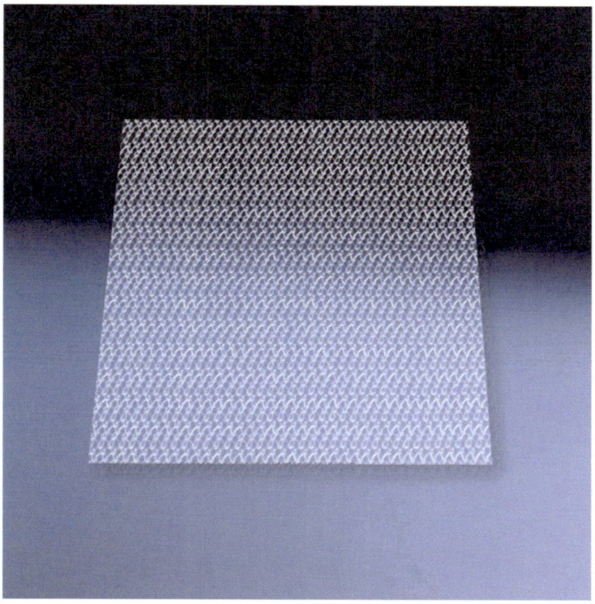

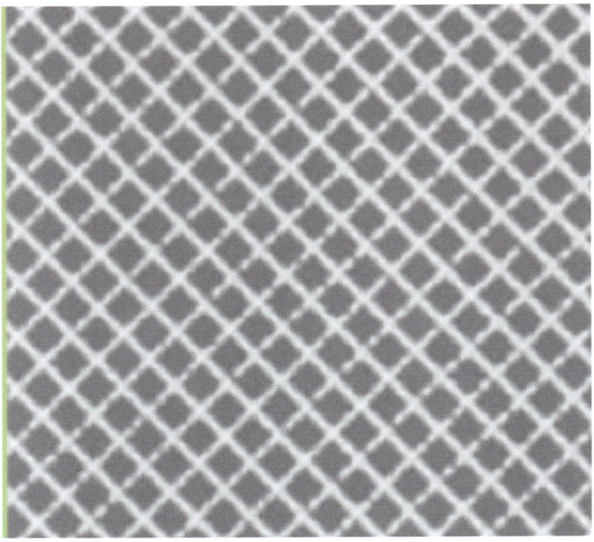

Fig. 4.16 Premium mesh

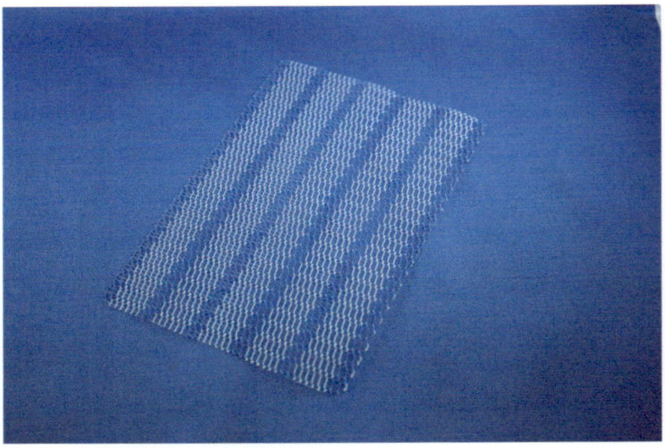

Fig. 4.17 Bulev B

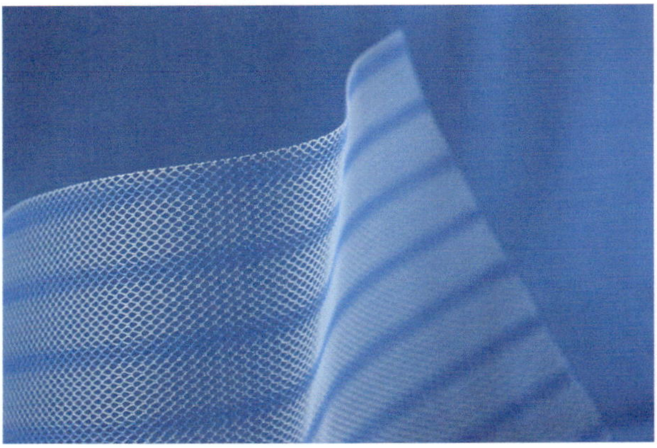

Fig. 4.18 Bulev UL

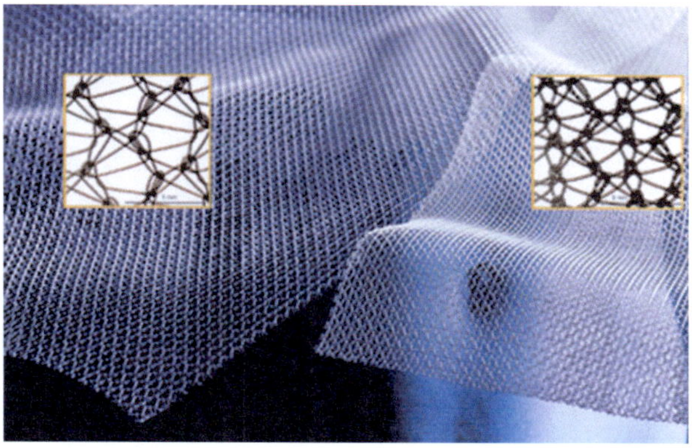

Fig. 4.19 DynaMesh light and standard

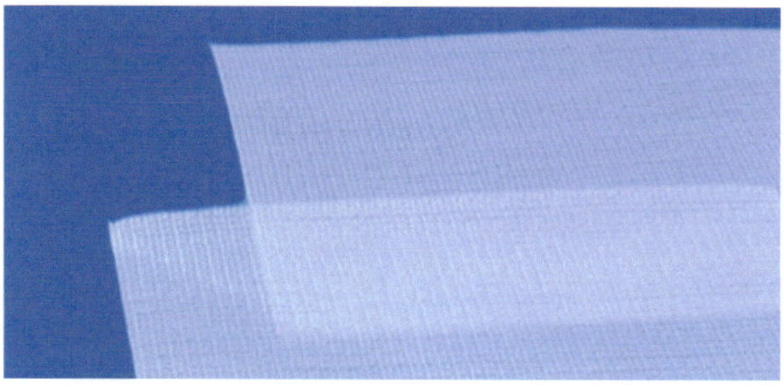

Fig. 4.20 Easy prothes mediumweight

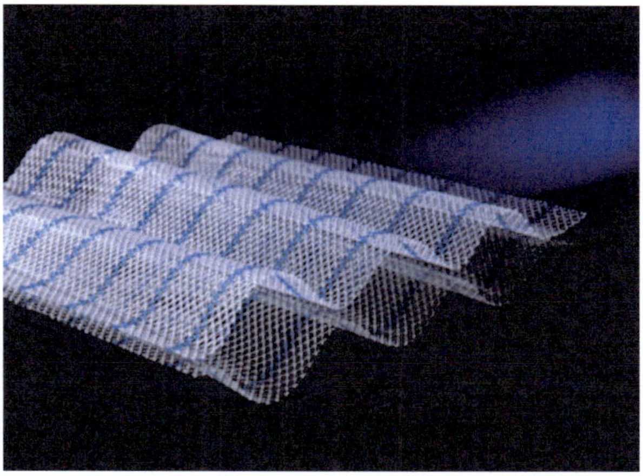

Fig. 4.21 Easy prothes lightweight

Elastic version has unequal pore sizes (3.6 × 2.8 mm) to allow for multidirectional elasticity (Figs. 4.23, 4.24, and 4.25). *Parietene Flat Sheet and Parietene Lightweight* products are monofilament flat sheet products (Fig. 4.26). *Premilene* is the heaviest weight (82 gm/m^2) product in the Braun flat mesh product line (Fig. 4.27). *Premium* mesh is a lightweight product similar to the Biomesh P1 described above (Fig. 4.15) this is configured into various sizes and shapes for use in open or laparoscopic

Fig. 4.22 Hermesh 3-8

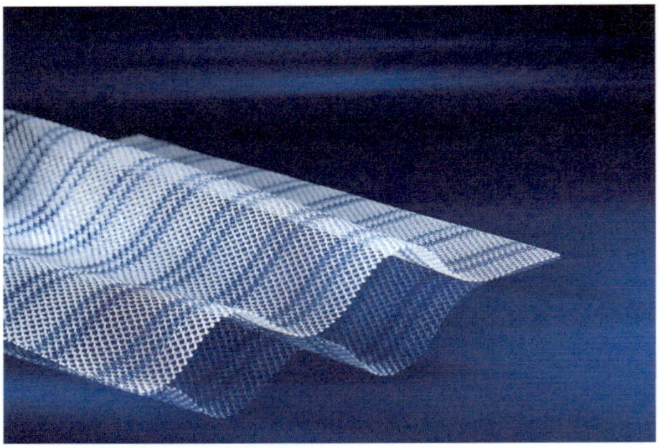

Fig. 4.23 Optilene

inguinal and extraperitoneal ventral hernia repair (Fig. 4.16). *Prolene* is also a heavier weight mesh material and it is one of the older products available (Fig. 4.28). *Prolene Soft Mesh* is the lighter weight version that has larger pores than the original mesh and blue lines through the product (Fig. 4.29). *Prolite* was one of the earliest meshes that were initially introduced as a lighter weight material (Fig. 4.30). Today, it is considered a mid-weight mesh. *Prolite Ultra* possesses even less weight of mesh than Prolite (Fig. 4.31).

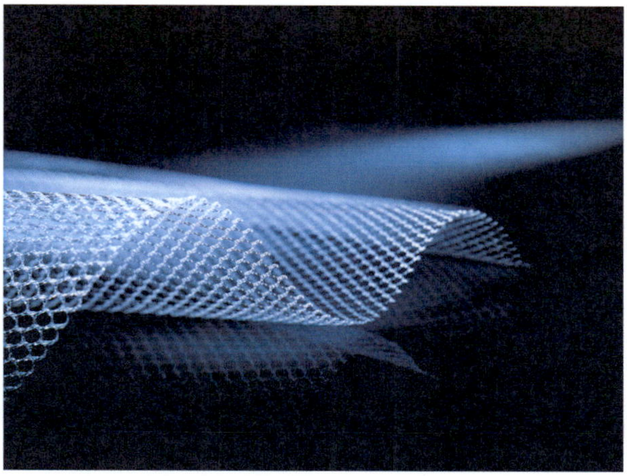

Fig. 4.24 Optilene elastic

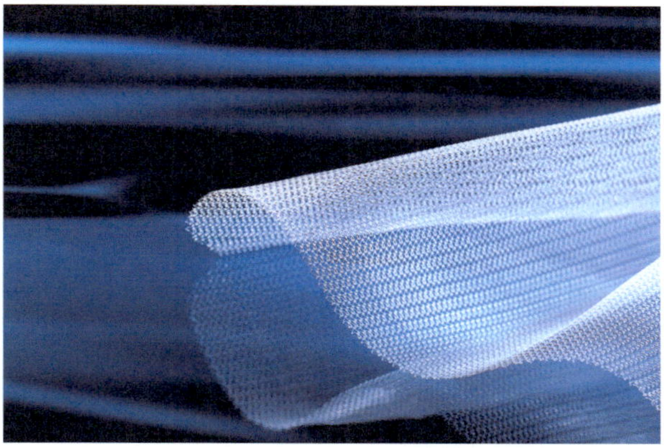

Fig. 4.25 Optilene LP

Fig. 4.26 Parietene flat sheet (All rights reserved; used with permission of Medtronic)

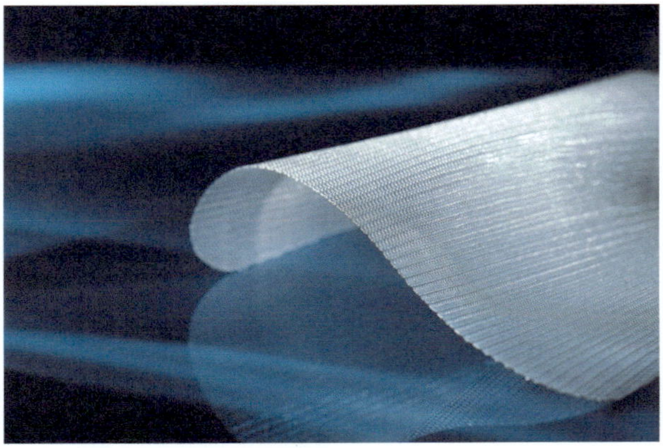

Fig. 4.27 Premilene

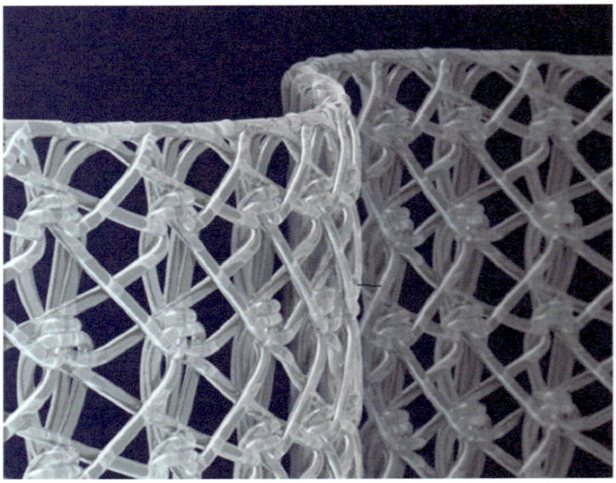

Fig. 4.28 Prolene (Image courtesy of Ethicon, Inc.)

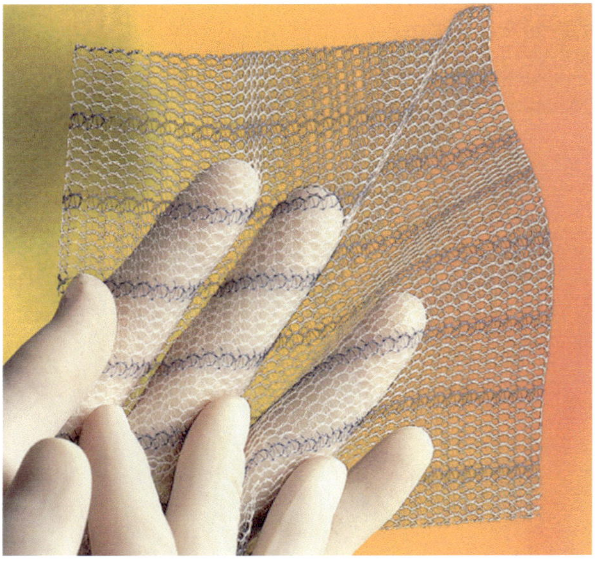

Fig. 4.29 Prolene soft mesh (Image courtesy of Ethicon, Inc.)

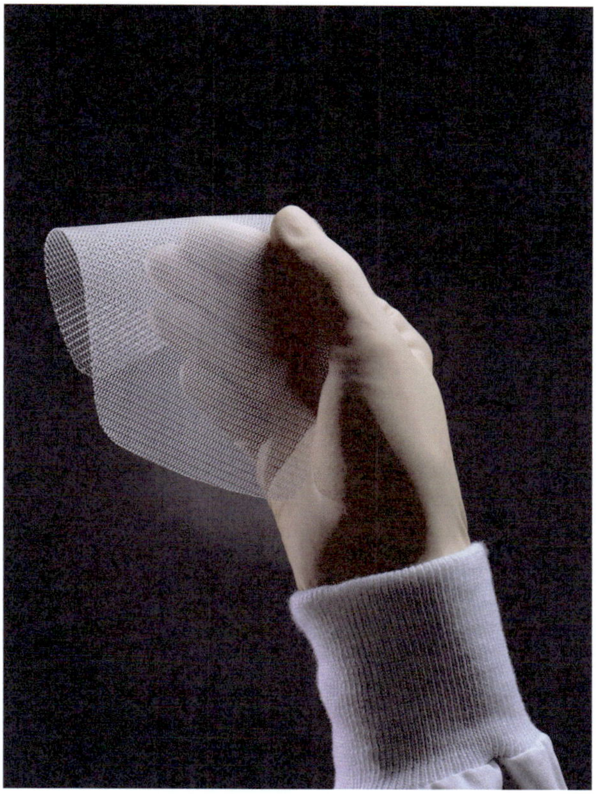

Fig. 4.30 ProLite

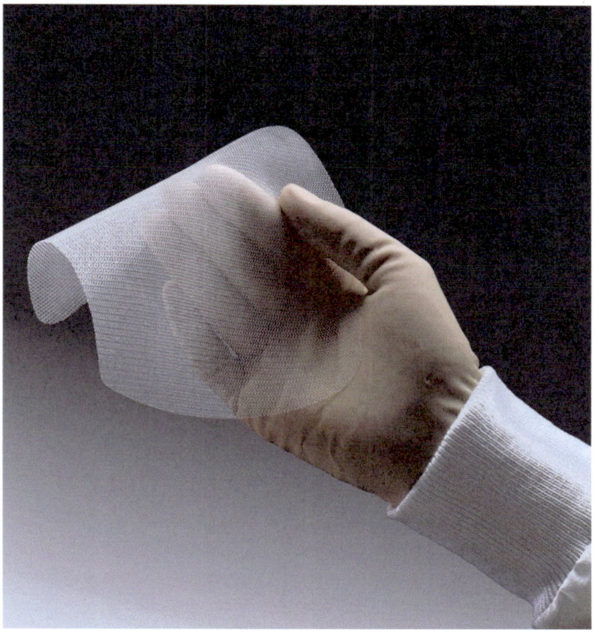

Fig. 4.31 ProLite ultra

Repol Angimesh 0 (lightest), *1, 8, 9* (heaviest) are all similar and differentiated in the weights and weaves from each other. *SurgiMesh WN* is a non-woven microfiber PP product that is extremely lightweight and has a differing microstructure than the other materials listed in this section (Fig. 4.32). It is available in several configurations but cannot be placed against the viscera. *Surgipro* was originally introduced as a multifilament mesh. This product is softer than the monofilament version (Fig. 4.33). The open weave product is called *Surgipro Open Weave* (Fig. 4.34). *SMX* is a heavy product (Fig. 4.35). It is available in a lightweight and ultra light material as *SMH2* and *SMH* respectively (Fig. 4.36). They are part of the "Swingmesh" product line.

TiMESH is a lightweight material that has titanium bonded onto the fibers of the PP using nanotechnology (Figs. 4.37 and 4.38). This coating on the fibers is said to allow ingrowth of collagen in a flexible manner due to the inhibition of the development of a thick scar plate. It is one of the few products in this section that can be used in either the intraperitoneal or extraperitoneal positions. TiLENE Blue has blue lines incorporated into the material to aid in positioning and can also be used in the intra- or extra-peritoneal planes (Fig. 4.39). It is also available without the blue lines as *TiLENE*. *TiO_2 Mesh* is also a titanized PP that is lightweight (47 g/m_2), large pore (2.8 mm) and has blue orientation strips (Fig. 4.40a). It is stated to be hydrophilic so that there is an apparent "stickiness" to the product, which eases intraoperative

Fig. 4.32 SurgiMesh WN

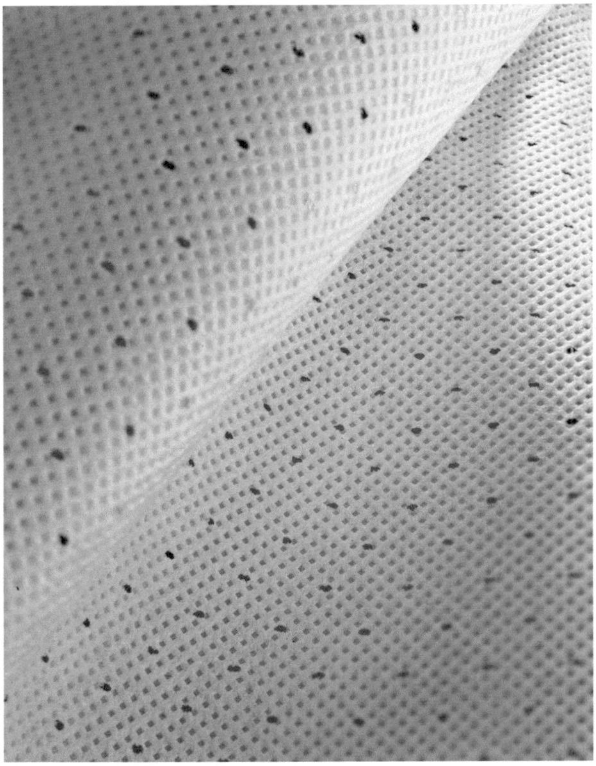

Fig. 4.33 SurgiPro monofilament (All rights reserved; used with permission of Medtronic)

Fig. 4.34 Surgipro open weave (All rights reserved; used with permission of Medtronic)

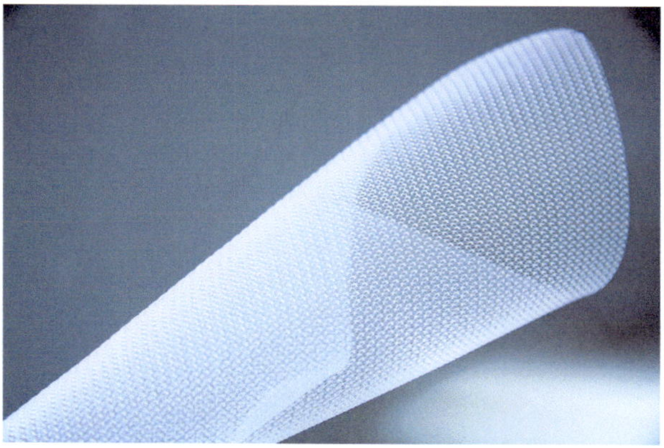

Fig. 4.35 SMX

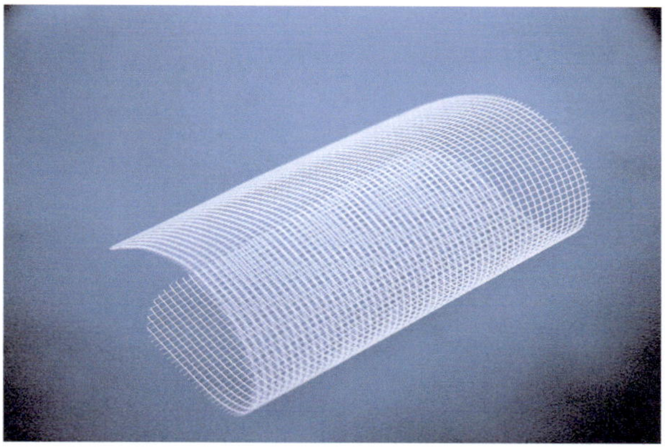

Fig. 4.36 SMH2

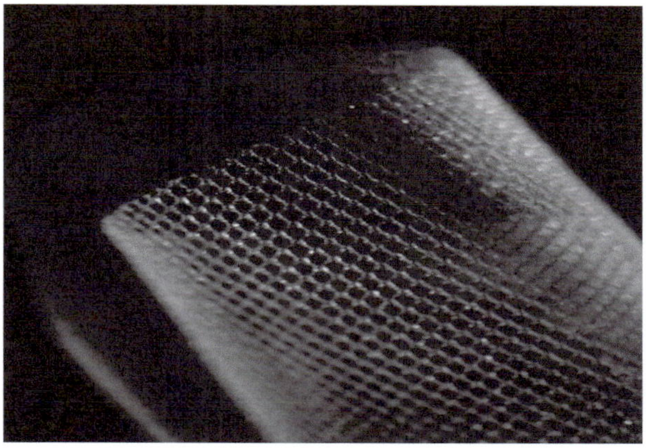

Fig. 4.37 TiMESH

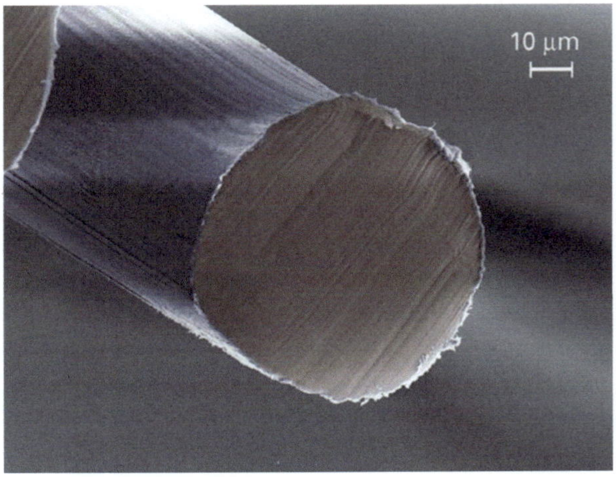

Fig. 4.38 TiMESH SEM

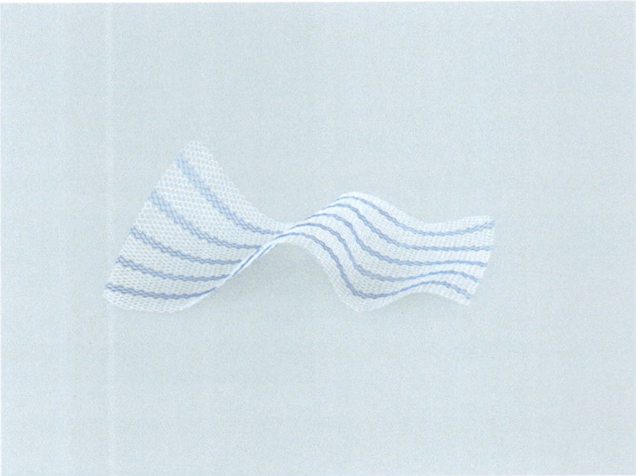

Fig. 4.39 TiLENE blue

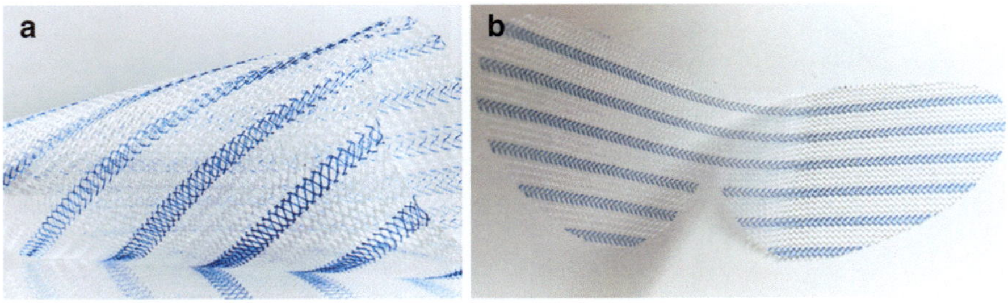

Fig. 4.40 (**a**) TiO2 mesh. (**b**) TiO2—GS

handling. It can be used in either open or laparoscopic inguinal and incisional hernia repairs. It has been configured into the GS-Mesh implant that is 11 × 30 cm and indicated for bilateral inguinal hernia repair (Fig. 4.40b).

VitaMesh is made of condensed PP rather than the traditional PP (Fig. 4.41). These products are singular in that they are made of Regular PP mesh becomes condensed PP mesh through compression during a post-knit heat treatment. This condensing process serves to reduce mesh thickness approximately 70%. This is said to improve deliverability through increased smoothness because fiber crossover points are flattened. Improved recovery of the shape of the mesh is asserted because the knots in the mesh are flattened. This provides greater shape memory than their non-flattened PP. *VitaMesh* is the heavier weight version (50 g/m^2). There is also available as a lighter weight version (28 g/m^2) as *VitaMesh Blue* and is easily differentiated by its blue color (Fig. 4.42).

The differences in the appearance of the prosthetics are easily seen in these photos. The size of the pores of these materials as well as the thickness of the product will have a significant impact on the stiffness. These factors affect the degree of scarring within the tissues. Additionally, the pore sizes vary greatly from each of these products. The lighter weight products have significantly impacted the prosthetic repair of hernias. The current thought is that, for the most part, there is less pain and scar plate with these lightweight, larger pore meshes. They also appear to be easier to treat if they become infected than the heavier weight materials.

Like the polypropylene materials, the polyester flat sheets can be used in inguinal and ventral hernia repair (Table 4.12). The preponderance of the polyester products that are currently available is produced in various configurations and most have some type of coating. These "tissue separating" products are listed later in this

Fig. 4.41 Vitamesh

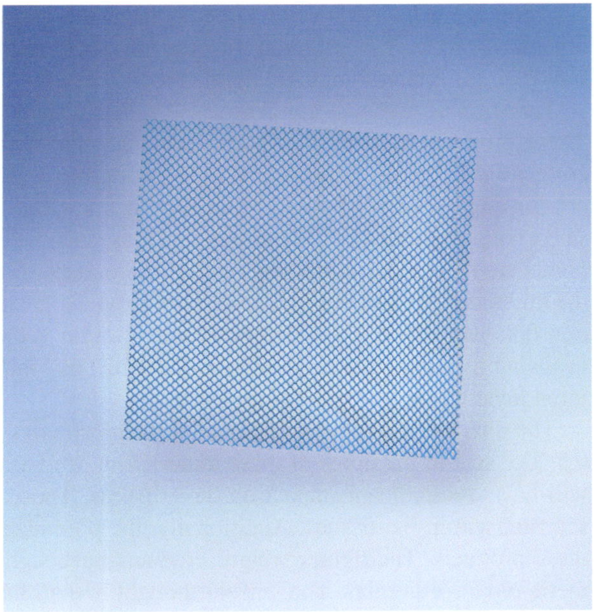

Fig. 4.42 Vitamesh blue

Table 4.12 Flat polyester products

2D PET, Microval, Saint-Just-Malmont, France
Angimesh R2, Angiologica, S. Martino Sicc., Italy
Angimesh R2-1, Angiologica, S. Martino Sicc., Italy
Angimesh R2-9, Angiologica, S. Martino Sicc., Italy
Biomesh A2, Cousin Biotech, Wervicq-Sud, France
Parietex Flat Sheet Mesh, Medtronic, Minneapolis, MN, USA
Parietex Lightweight Mesh, Medtronic, Minneapolis, MN, USA
Parietex Monofilament Macroporous Mesh, Medtronic, Minneapolis, MN, USA
SM2, THT Bio-Science, Montpelier, France
SM3, THT Bio-Science, Montpelier, France
Versatex, Medtronic, Minneapolis, MN, USA

chapter. The ones discussed here are not coated and should not be used in the intraperitoneal space.

The *2D PET, Angimesh R2, R2-1, R2-9* and *Biomesh A2* materials are all fairly similar in appearance. The *2D PET* and *Biomesh A2*, however, has been configured into various shapes and sized to allow use in open or laparoscopic inguinal and open ventral hernia repair (Figs. 4.43 and 4.44). *Angimesh R2* is multifilament polyester (Fig. 4.45). *Angimesh R2-1* and *R2-9* are monofilament materials very similar in appearance and differ only in thicknesses, *R2-1* being thinner than *R2-9* (Figs. 4.46 and 4.47).

The *Parietex Flat Sheet Mesh* is available in two or three-dimensional weaves (Fig. 4.48). The 2D material is more rigid and is touted for robotic repairs due to this

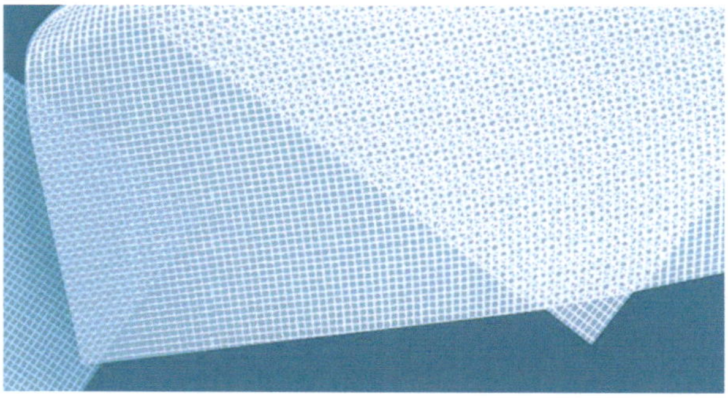

Fig. 4.43 2D PET

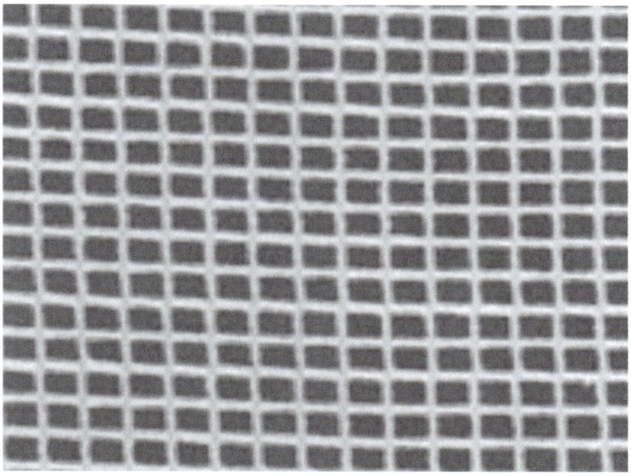

Fig. 4.44 Biomesh A2

fact. The 3D product is more supple and soft. *Parietex Lightweight* product is a monofilament product (Fig. 4.49). *Parietex Monofilament Macroporous* is available in a flat sheet and is a two dimensional construct (Fig. 4.50). *SM2* is a heavyweight bi-dimensional weave material that is indicated for all hernia repairs (Fig. 4.51).

SM3 is a three-dimensional weave of pure polyester that is available in a variety of shapes and sizes and can be used in open or robotic applications (Fig. 4.52). *Versatex* has a 3D construct and is macroporous (Fig. 4.53). It is a medium weight (64 g/m^2) monofilament product and has a central teardrop to be used for positioning.

Expanded polytetrafluoroethylene (ePTFE) prostheses have also been available in a flat sheet configuration for many years (Table 4.13). In fact, the earliest products used in the intraperitoneal space for incisional hernia repair were of ePTFE [4]. Because of their structure, they are solid and white unless an antimicrobial agent has been added.

The current DualMesh products are very similar in construction and are one of the oldest "tissue-separating" products (Fig. 4.54). These all have two distinctly different surfaces. One side (visceral surface) is very smooth and has interstices of

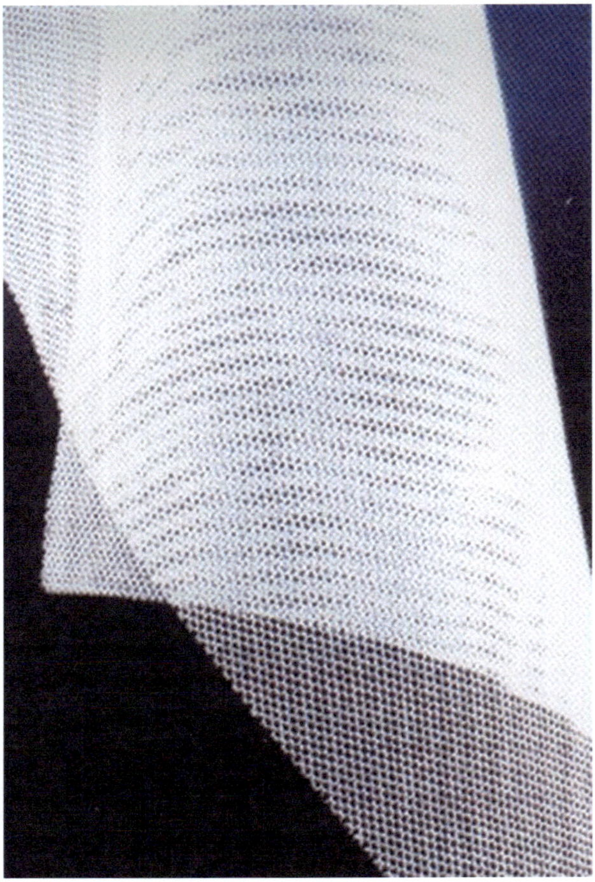

Fig. 4.45 Angimesh R2

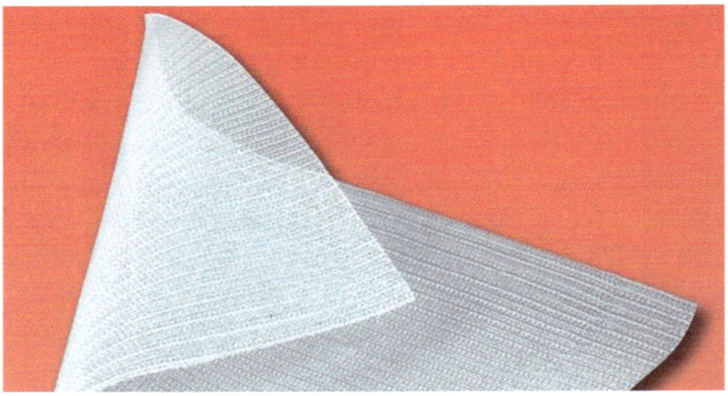

Fig. 4.46 Angimesh R2-1

three microns while the other (parietal surface) has the appearance of corduroy with an approximate "ridge to ridge" distance of 1500 microns. This prosthesis is designed for use in the intraperitoneal space. *DualMesh* is one millimeter in thickness and is available with the impregnation of silver and chlorhexidine as *DualMesh*

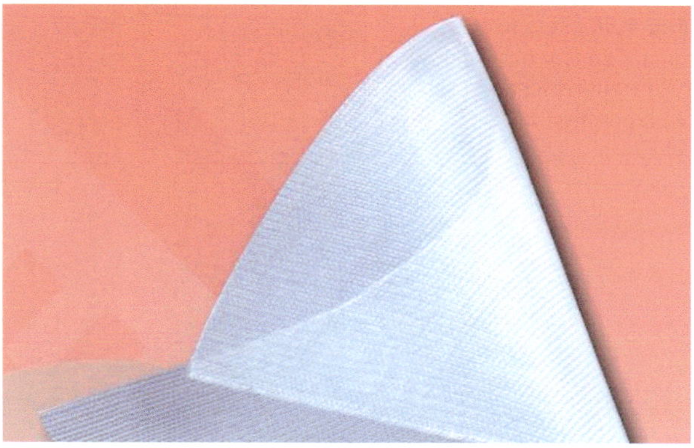

Fig. 4.47 Angimesh R2-9

Fig. 4.48 Parietex flat sheet (All rights reserved; used with permission of Medtronic, Inc.)

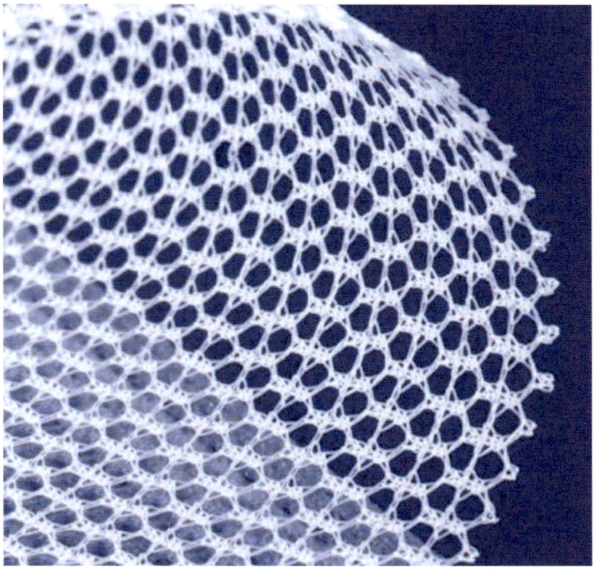

Fig. 4.49 Parietex lightweight mesh (All rights reserved; used with permission of Medtronic, Inc.)

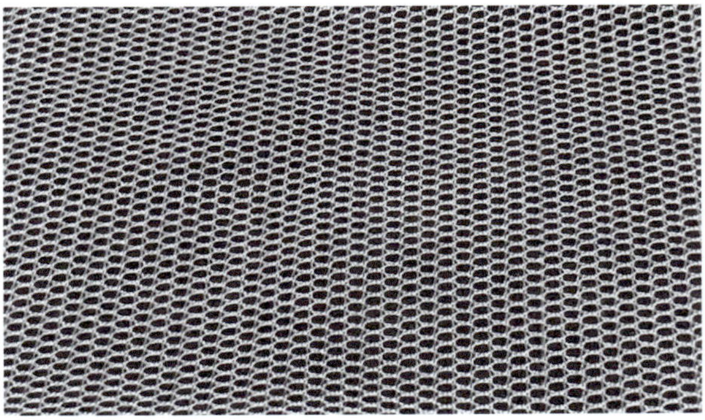

Fig. 4.50 Parietex monofilament macroporous (All rights reserved; used with permission of Medtronic, Inc.)

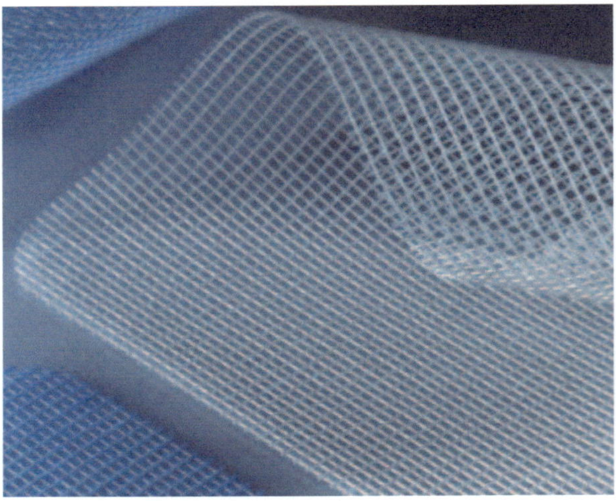

Fig. 4.51 SM2

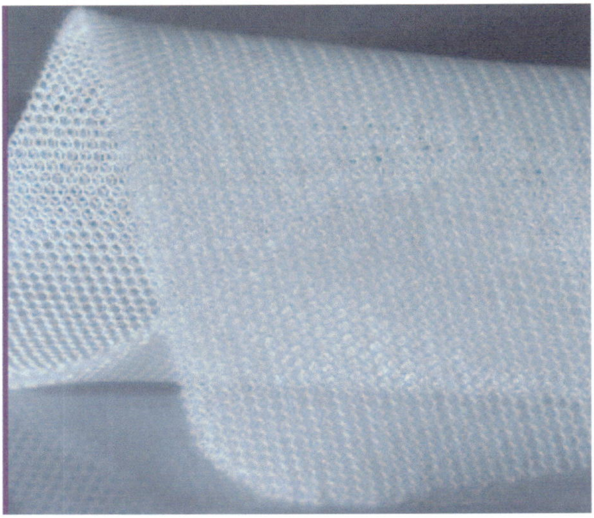

Fig. 4.52 SM3

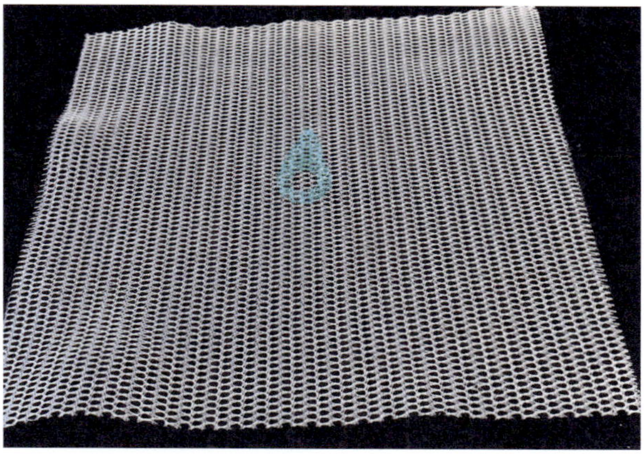

Fig. 4.53 Versatex (All rights reserved; used with permission of Medtronic, Inc.)

Table 4.13 ePTFE products

DualMesh, W. L. Gore & Associates, Elkhart, DE, USA
DualMesh Plus, W. L. Gore &Associates, Elkhart, DE, USA
DualMesh Plus with Holes, W. L. Gore &Associates, Elkhart, DE, USA
Dulex, Davol, Inc., Warwick, RI, USA
MycroMesh, W. L. Gore &Associates, Elkhart, DE, USA
MycroMesh Plus, W. L. Gore &Associates, Elkhart, DE, USA
Soft Tissue Patch, W. L. Gore &Associates, Elkhart, DE, USA

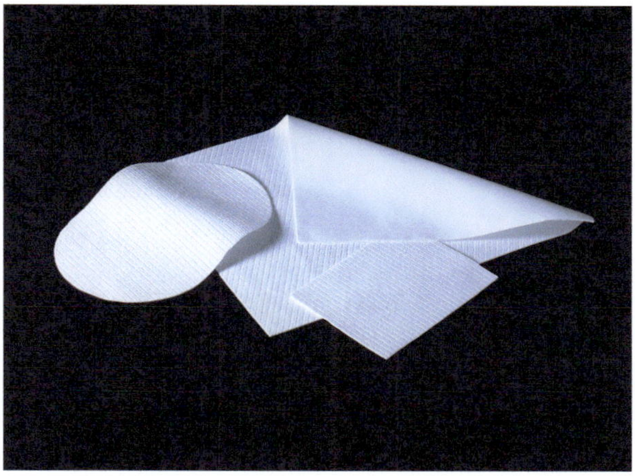

Fig. 4.54 DualMesh

PLUS (Fig. 4.55). The two-millimeter product is only available as DualMesh Plus with the antimicrobial agents within it. These two chemicals are antimicrobial agents that are added to decrease the risk of infection and, because of the silver, impart a brown color to the "PLUS" products. At this time, these products are the only synthetic materials impregnated with any type of any antimicrobial or bactericidal agents. *DualMesh PLUS with Holes* (Fig. 4.56) is of the same construction as

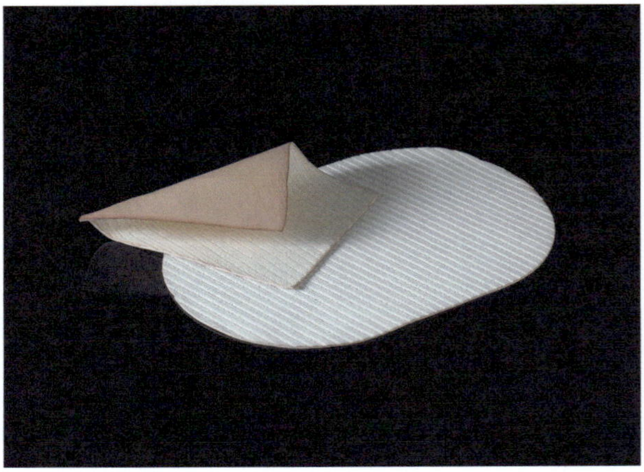

Fig. 4.55 DualMesh PLUS

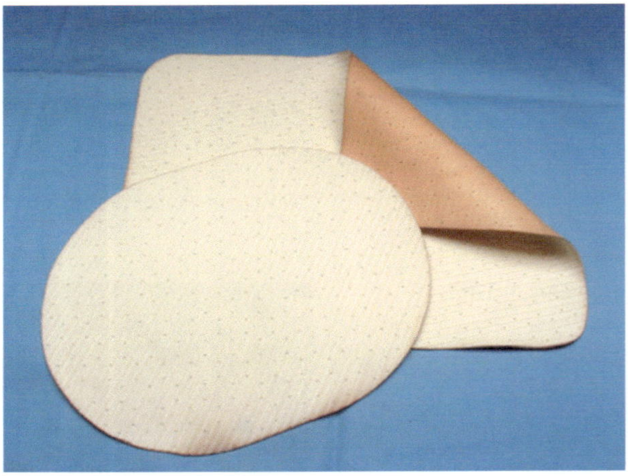

Fig. 4.56 DualMesh PLUS with holes

that of the DualMesh. The penetration of the holes requires that this product be of 1.5 mm in thickness. The concept of the addition of these perforations is that there may be greater penetration of the fibroblasts and other cells across the material and these might reduce the incidence of seroma development.

Dulex is manufactured of laminated ePTFE and is available in 1 mm or 2 mm thicknesses (Fig. 4.57). One surface (parietal) of the material is studded with numerous outcroppings as seen on the scanning electron microscopic view that are approximately 400 microns apart. This gives the product the gross appearance of sandpaper. The intent of this surface is to provide for greater fibroblastic attachment and thereby greater collagen deposition on this parietal surface. The opposite surface (visceral) is smooth and faces the intestine in theintraperitoneal onlay repair.

Fig. 4.57 Dulex

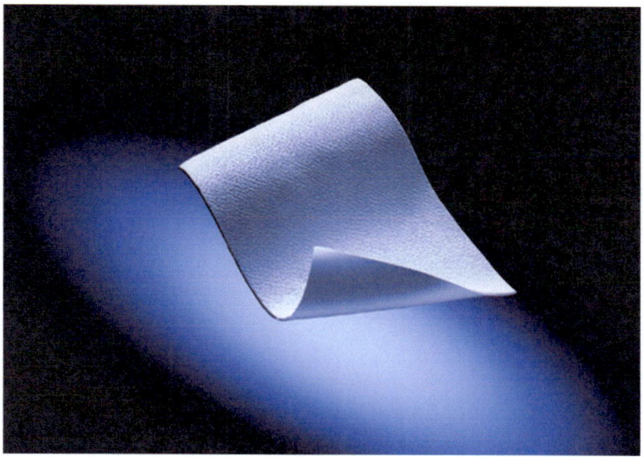

Fig. 4.58 MycroMesh

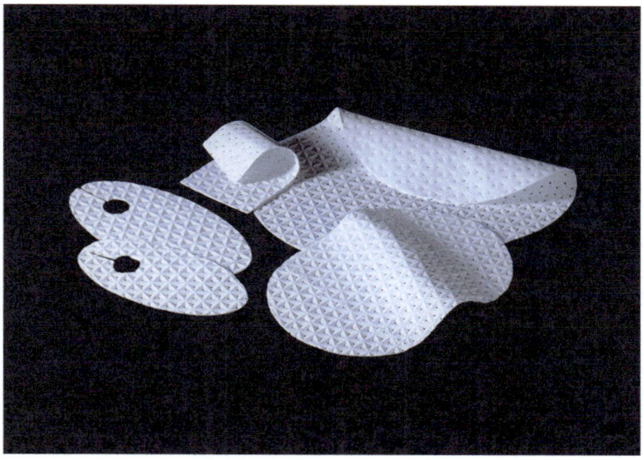

MycroMesh is also a dual-sided perforated prosthetic with one surface of three microns and the other of 17–22 microns (Fig. 4.58). The latter surface is textured. This material is perforated for reasons that are similar to that of the DualMesh Plus with holes. It is only one millimeter thick, however. *Mycromesh PLUS* is impregnated with the antimicrobials silver and chlorhexidine (Fig. 4.59). It is not designed for intraperitoneal usage.

Soft Tissue Patch is the earliest implants of these ePTFE products and was the product utilized in the very first laparoscopic incisional hernia repair (Fig. 4.60) [4]. The variety of available configurations of this product has increased over the last several years. Its use, however, has waned because of the development of the other products that are listed in Table 4.12. Like *MycroMesh*, it should not contact any viscera when used.

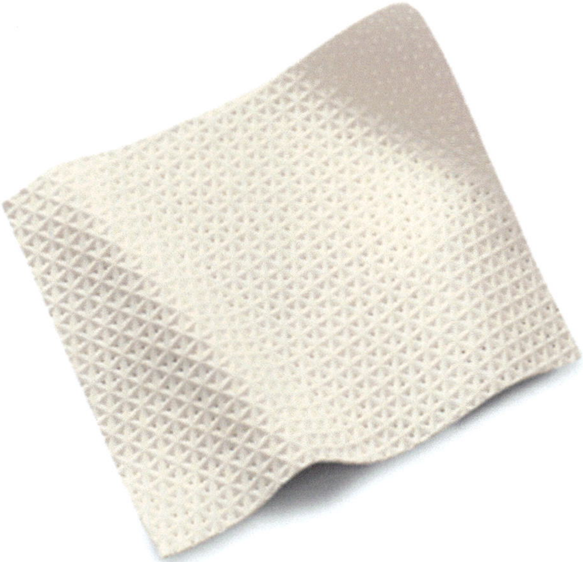

Fig. 4.59 MycroMesh PLUS

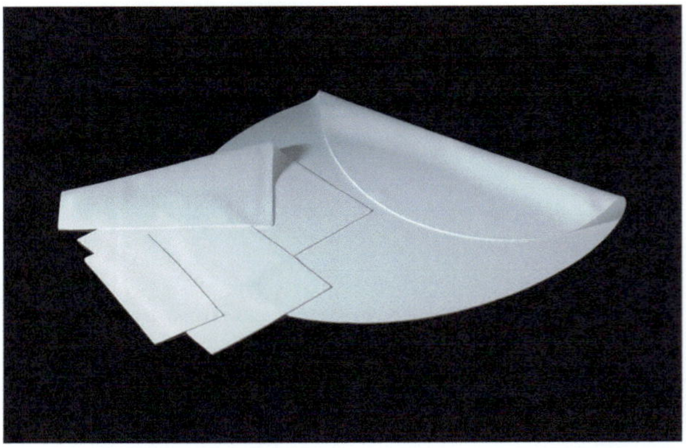

Fig. 4.60 Soft tissue patch

4.8 Miscellaneous Flat Products

There are ranges of materials that do not fit into the exact categories above (Table 4.14). For instance, *Inomesh* is a product made of PVDF and polybutylene adipate with laser cut holes (Fig. 4.61). *MotifMesh* and *Omyra* are identical in design and concept (Figs. 4.62 and 4.63). There are made of condensed PTFE (cPTFE) and designed for use in contact with the intestine. The PTFE is laminated and then condensed with a heated compression process. The nonporous material is then laser micromachined to create the macroporous structure of the final product. They claim to be "a bacterial resistant anti-adhesive mesh."

Table 4.14 Miscellaneous flat mesh products

Inomesh, Medlinx Acacia, Singapore
MotifMESH, Proxy Biomedical Ltd., Galway, Ireland
Omyra, B. Braun Melsungen AG, Melsungen, Germany

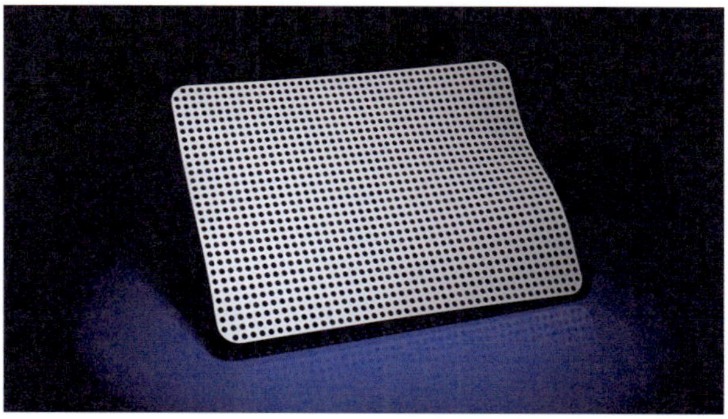

Fig. 4.61 InoMesh

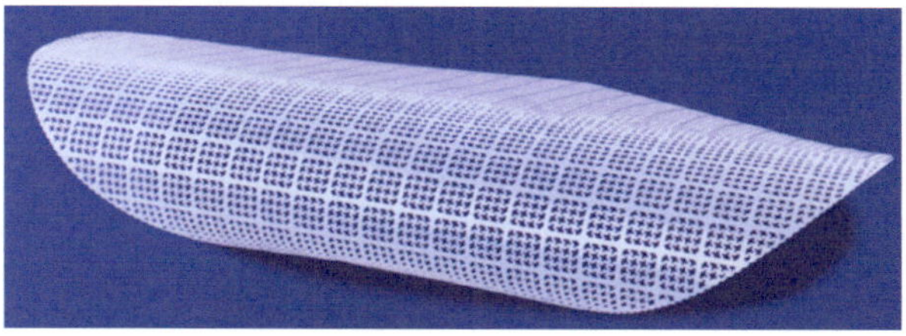

Fig. 4.62 Motifmesh

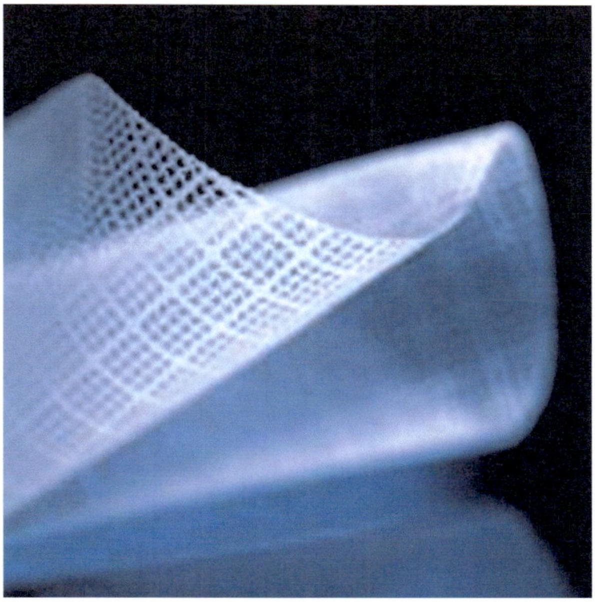

Fig. 4.63 Omyra mesh

4.9 Combination Flat Synthetic Prosthetics

This grouping of these products is made because there is a permanent portion of these materials and an absorbable component to the product. These prostheses are generally not meant to contact any viscera and do not possess a specific shape. (Table 4.15)

Adhesix, Parietene ProGrip, and *Parietex ProGrip* all have self-attaching portions of the prosthesis so that once placed onto the tissue surface, they will fixate themselves (Figs. 4.64 and 4.65). These "gripping portions" are absorbable. The permanent portions of Adhesix and Parietene ProGrip are made of PP while the Parietex ProGrip is POL. *Adhesix* has a coating on one side that is made of polyvinylpyrrolidone and polyethylene glycol. This coating turns into an adhesive gel when it comes into contact with both heat and humidity. *Parietex ProGrip Laparoscopic* is a flat sheet of polyester that has microgrips of polylactic acid that last >18 months (Fig. 4.66). It differs from the other ProGrip products in that it has

Table 4.15 Combination products

Adhesix, Davol, Inc., Warwick, RI, USA
Easy Prothes Partially Absorbable PAF, TransEasy Medical Tech.Co.Ltd., Beijing, China
Easy Prothes Partially Absorbable PAS, TransEasy Medical Tech.Co.Ltd., Beijing, China
4D Laparoscopic Mesh, Cousin Biotech, Wervicq-Sud, France
4D Mesh Ventral, Cousin Biotech, Wervicq-Sud, France
Parietene ProGrip, Medtronic, Minneapolis, MN, USA
Parietex ProGrip, Medtronic, Minneapolis, MN, USA
Parietex ProGrip Laparoscopic, Medtronic, Minneapolis, MN, USA
TiMesh, GfE Medizintechnik, Nuremburg, Germany
Vypro, Ethicon, Inc., Somerville, NJ, USA
Vypro II, Ethicon, Inc., Somerville, NJ, USA
Ultrapro, Ethicon, Inc., Somerville, NJ, USA
Ultrapro Advanced, Ethicon, Inc., Somerville, NJ, USA

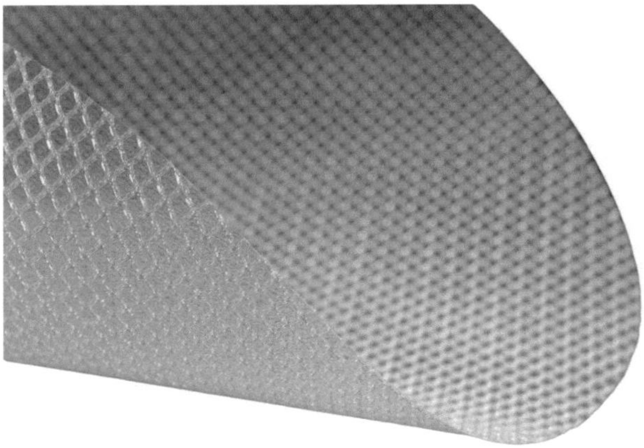

Fig. 4.64 Adhesix

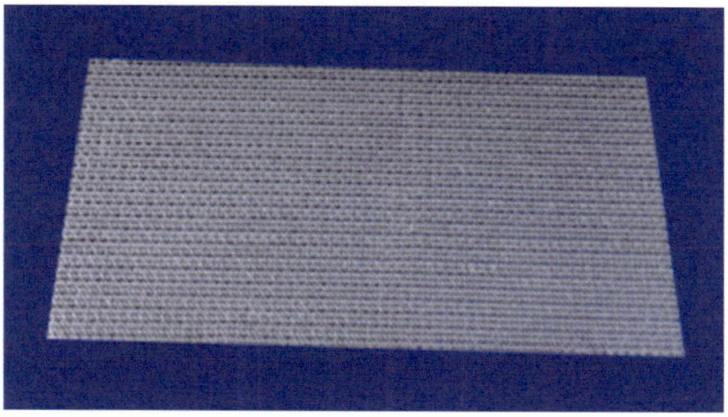

Fig. 4.65 Parietene ProGrip (All rights reserved; used with permission of Medtronic, Inc.)

Fig. 4.66 Parietex ProGrip laparoscopic (All rights reserved; used with permission of Medtronic, Inc.)

a green portion to delineate the medial aspect of the mesh and has a light coating of collagen to make manipulation during robotic use easier.

Easy Prothes Partially Absorbable is a partially absorbable product (Fig. 4.67). It is a combination of PP and poly(glycolide-cocaprolactone) [PGCL] monofilaments. The PGCL portion will be completely absorbed within 90–120 days. It is available in two versions, both of which have a PP weight of 30 g/m^2, which is the final weight of the material after degradation of the absorbable material. The difference lies in the weight of the PGCL, which are 30 g/m^2 in the *PAF* material and 60 g/m^2 in the *PAS* product. *4D Laparoscopic Mesh* is made of a base of a 25% PP base with the remainder of resorbable PLLA (Fig. 4.68). It is approximately 30 gm/m^2 postabsorption. The *4D Ventral* is a flat sheet and differs from the 4D mesh in that it is 40% PP and 60% PLLA (Fig. 4.69).

TiMESH has been described above and is one of the few products in this section that can be placed against the viscera (Fig. 4.37). The materials, *Vypro* (25 gm/m^2) and *Vypro II* (30 gm/m^2) are actually a combination of PP and the absorbable polymer polydioxione (Fig. 4.70). The combination of these materials results in a very pliable and malleable material. Once the polydioxione has been absorbed, the PP that remains has very large interstices (>3 mm) into which the fibroblasts and collagen are deposited. The aim of these types of products is the improvement in the abdominal wall compliance that is more normal

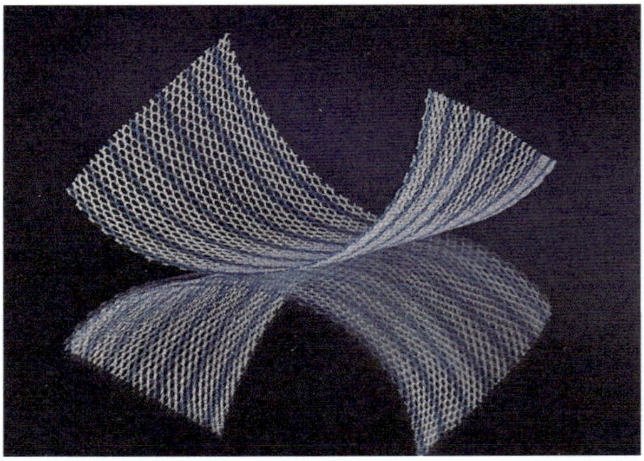

Fig. 4.67 Easy prothes partially absorbable

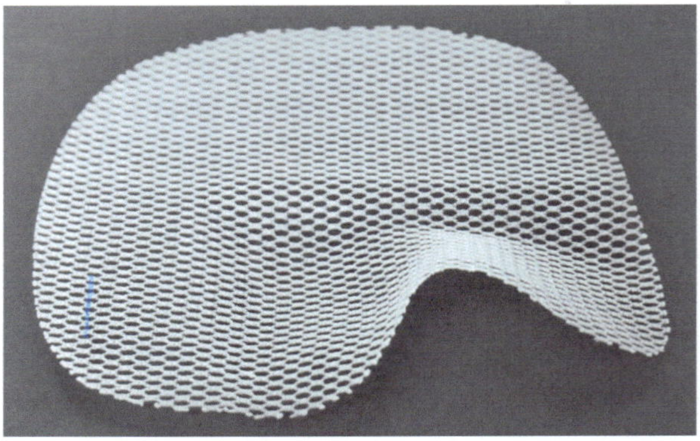

Fig. 4.68 4D laparoscopic

Fig. 4.69 4D ventral

in function because of the very lightweight PP that remains. *Vypro II* is designed for inguinal hernia repair while *Vypro* is made for preperitoneal incisional hernia repair. *Ultrapro* mesh is a similar concept and is manufactured from approximately equal parts of the absorbable poliglecaprone-25 monofilament fiber and the non-absorbable lightweight PP (Fig. 4.71). A portion of the PP is dyed. The

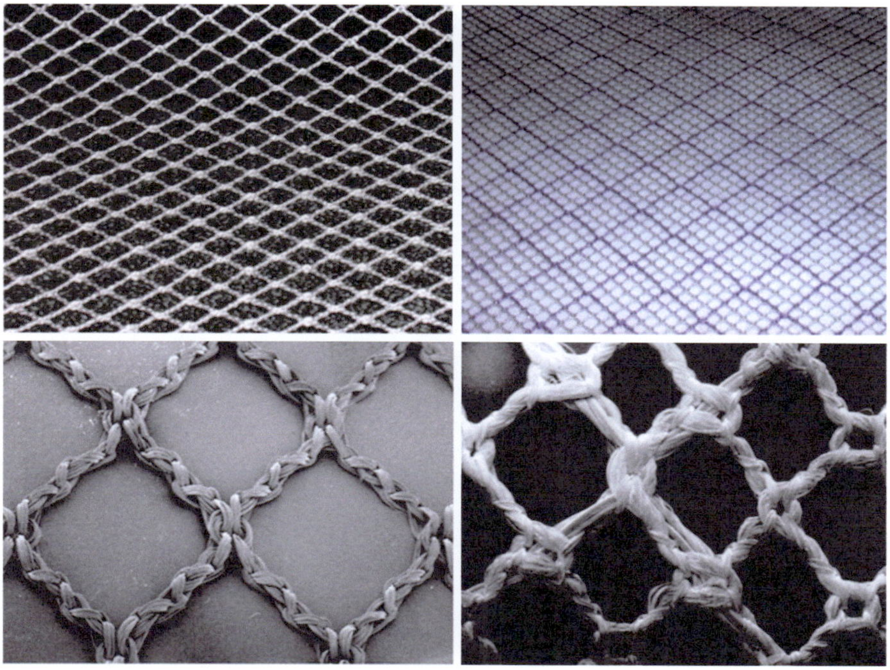

Fig. 4.70 Vypro and Vypro II (Image courtesy of Ethicon, Inc.)

Fig. 4.71 Ultrapro flat mesh (Image courtesy of Ethicon, Inc.)

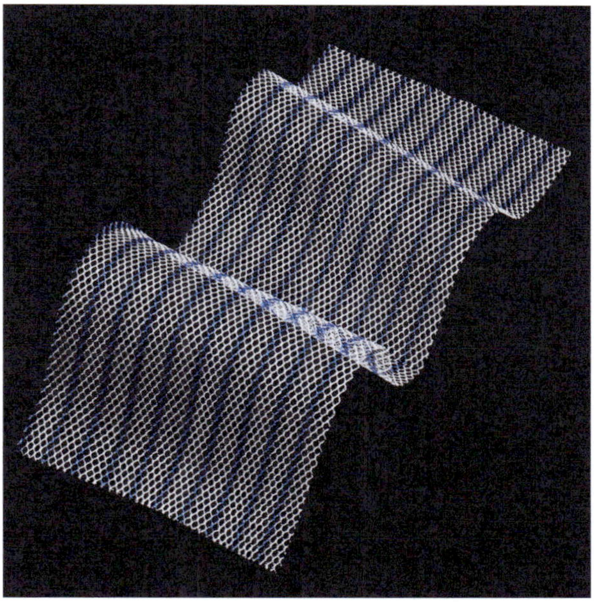

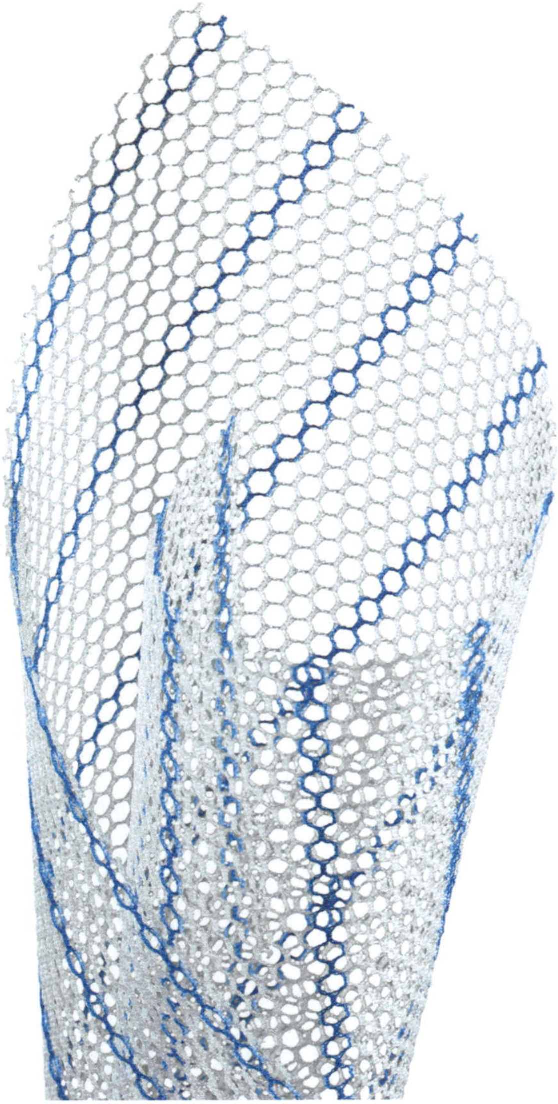

Fig. 4.72 Ultrapro advanced (Image courtesy of Ethicon, Inc.)

absorbable portion is essentially absorbed by 84 days. *Ultrapro Advanced* is similar to the former product but is designed to allow for more stretch of the abdominal wall, allowing a 2:1 stretch (Fig. 4.72). It stretches to the greatest degree perpendicular to the blue stripes.

4.10 Pre-shaped Products for Robotic Inguinal Hernioplasty

Originally the laparoscopic/robotic repair of inguinal hernias involved the use of a flat mesh that was rectangular in shape. This continues to be a frequently used

Table 4.16 Pre-shaped products for robotic inguinal hernia repair

3D Anatomic, Microval, Saint-Just-Malmont, France
3D Max, Davol, Inc., Warwick, RI, USA
3D Max Light, Davol, Inc., Warwick, RI, USA
4D Laparoscopic Mesh, Cousin Biotech, Wervicq-Sud, France
CO3A, THT Bio-Science, Montpelier, France
CO3+, THT Bio-Science, Montpelier, France
C-QUR CentriFX, Getinge Group, Wayne, NJ
Easy Prothes Partially Absorbable 3D Mesh, TransEasy Medical Tech.Co.Ltd., Beijing, China
JG Inguinal, Microval, Saint-Just-Malmont, France
Parietex ProGrip Anatomical, Medtronic, Minneapolis, MN, USA
Parietex Anatomical Mesh, Medtronic, Minneapolis, MN, USA
Parietex Anatomical Mesh with Suture, Medtronic, Minneapolis, MN, USA
Parietex Folding Mesh with Suture, Medtronic, Minneapolis, MN, USA
PS, Microval, Saint-Just-Malmont, France
Premium, Cousin Biotech, Wervicq-Sud, France
SMA, THT Bio-Science, Montpelier, France
SM2+, THT Bio-Science, Montpelier, France
SMH2+, THT Bio-Science, Montpelier, France
SMH2A, THT Bio-Science, Montpelier, France
SM3, THT Bio-Science, Montpelier, France
SM3+, THT Bio-Science, Montpelier, France
SurgiMesh WN, Aspide Medical, St. Etienne, France
Visilex, Davol, Inc., Warwick, RI, USA

material (Tables 4.11 and 4.12). Currently there are a number of pre-shaped products that are designed for this procedure (Table 4.16). These all attempt to ease the placement of the prosthetic over the myopectineal orifice and/or serve to conform to the anatomic configuration at that site of the repair. A few are manufactured so that fixation with any type of fastener is not required.

The *3D Anatomic* implant has very deep curves that are designed to exactly fit the curves of the inguino-pelvic anatomy (Fig. 4.73). There is a mark in the inferior internal edge of the prosthetic to aid in positioning, as there is a right and left product. For the TEP approach, no fixation required. The *3D Max* and *3D Max Light* products are similar in shape and sizes (medium, large and extra large). The difference between these two products is the weight of the PP within each product and pore size. The former is of the heavy weight Bard mesh and the latter is of the lighter Bard Soft Mesh. It is quite apparent in the figure that the lower product is the lighter one (Fig. 4.74). Both have an "M" and an arrow on the medial aspect of the product to indicate the positioning of the prosthesis. These are curved to conform to the shape of the pelvis. Because of this curved shape, there is a right and left product.

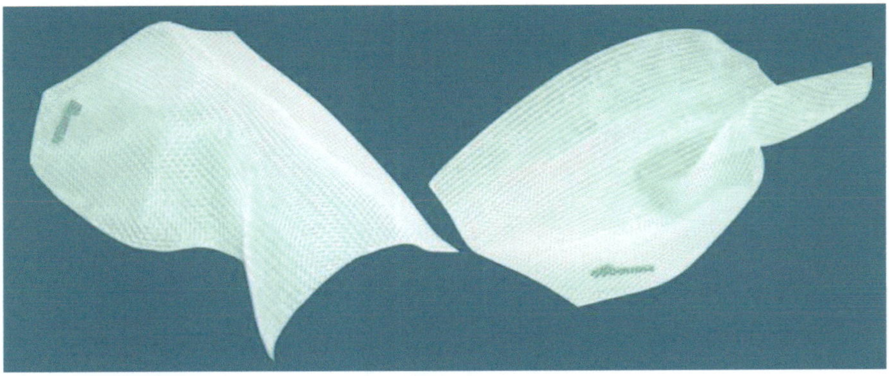

Fig. 4.73 3D anatomic

Fig. 4.74 3D Max regular and light

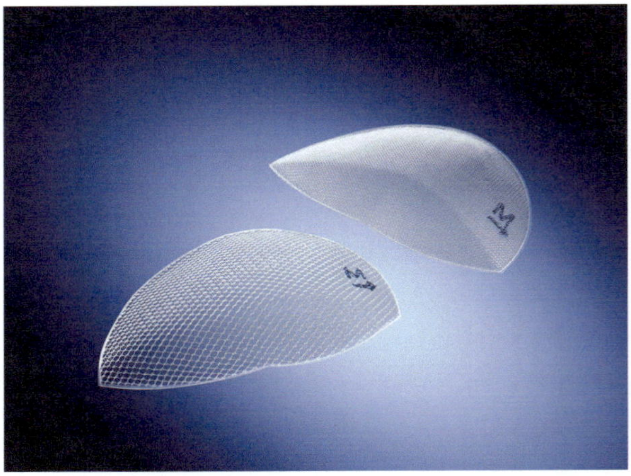

There is also an indentation on the inferior aspect of the product to indicate the location of the iliac vessels. There is no fixation is required with the heavier weight product.

The 4D Mesh product has been described above that is specifically for laparoscopic/robotic repair of these hernias (Fig. 4.68). It is of the same composition as the flat mesh but is shaped for this technique. *CO3A* and *CO3+* are both made of POL with impregnated polyurethane (PUR) and have knitted grips to hold the products in place. These have been configured in many different shapes for laparoscopic/robotic inguinal and ventral hernia repair. *CO3+* is a flat sheet but *CO3A* is specifically designed for laparoscopic/robotic inguinal hernia repair due its configuration (Figs. 4.75 and 4.76).

C-QUR CentriFX is made in a laparoscopic shape (Fig. 4.77). *C-QUR CentriFX* is composed ProLite mesh material coated with Omega 3 Fatty Acid (O3FA) but is shaped for use in either a left or right laparoscopic/robotic repair of inguinal

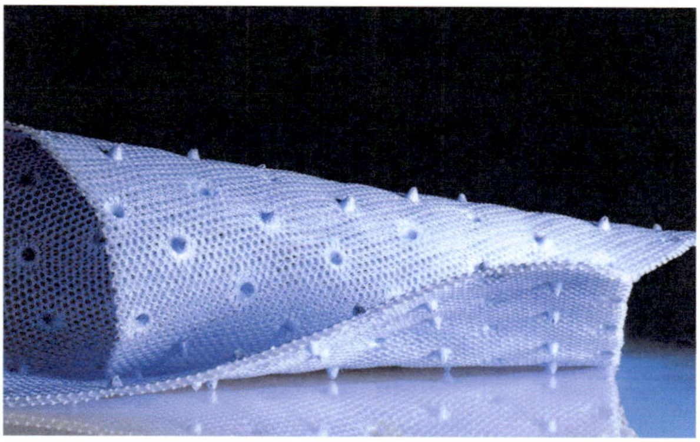

Fig. 4.75 CO3+

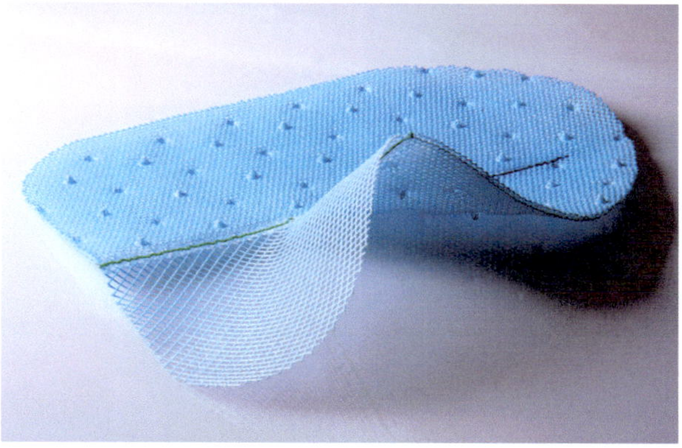

Fig. 4.76 CO3A

hernias. It is one of the few products that can be interchanged in such a fashion. *Easy Prothes Partially Absorbable 3D Mesh* is the only partially absorbable product in this section (Fig. 4.78).

It is made of the same material as the Easy Prothes Partially Absorbable Flat product PAS noted above (Fig. 4.67). The *JG inguinal* implant also has an anatomic shape that includes a raised edge for the cord structures (Fig. 4.79). There is a round black mark to indicate the inferior internal edge, as there is a left and right product. This is available in a standard or lightweight version.

Parietex Lap ProGrip Anatomic is POL with microgrips that has been described above but it is configured as either the left or right for laparoscopic repair specifically (Fig. 4.80). *Parietex Anatomical Mesh* is of the same three-dimensional weave of POL as the other Parietex products on the lower portion of the product making if softer and is designed to lie on the iliac vessels (Fig. 4.81). Its shape is similar to the ProGrip Anatomic but it does not have the microgrips. The portion that is placed on the posterior aspect of the inguinal floor is a more rigid two-dimensional weave to aid in handling. It is generally used with the application of some type of fixation but

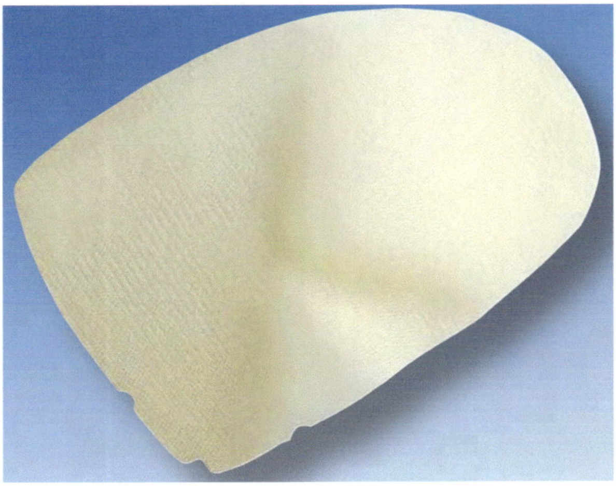

Fig. 4.77 C-QUR CentriFX

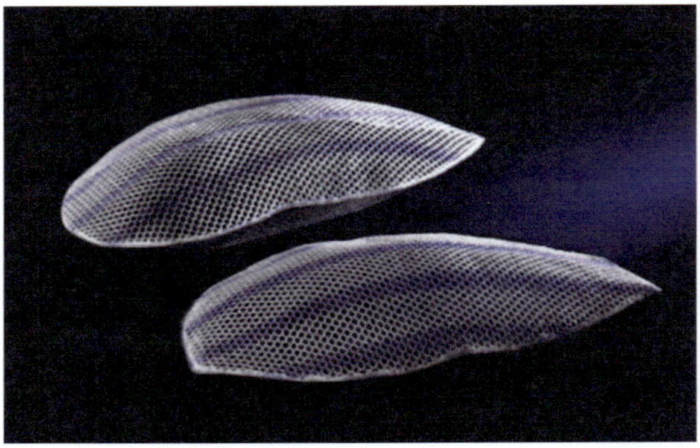

Fig. 4.78 Easy prothes 3D mesh

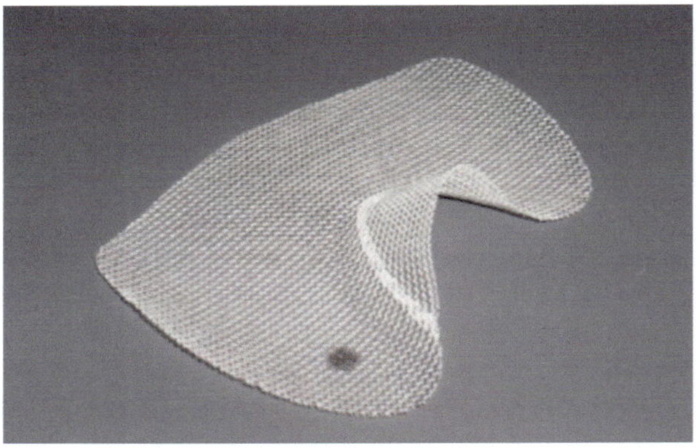

Fig. 4.79 JG inguinal

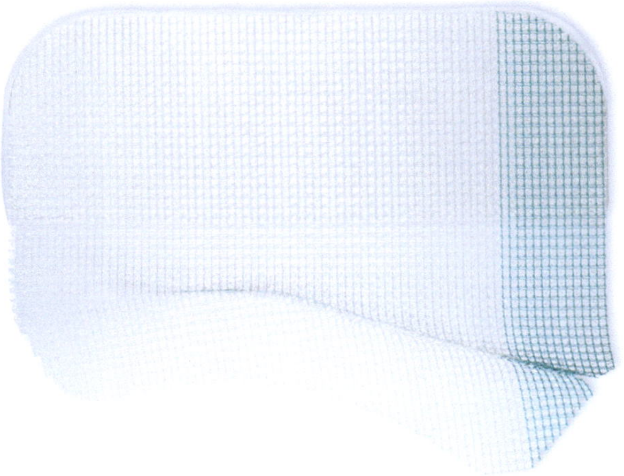

Fig. 4.80 Lap Progrip anatomic (All rights reserved; used with permission of Medtronic, Inc.)

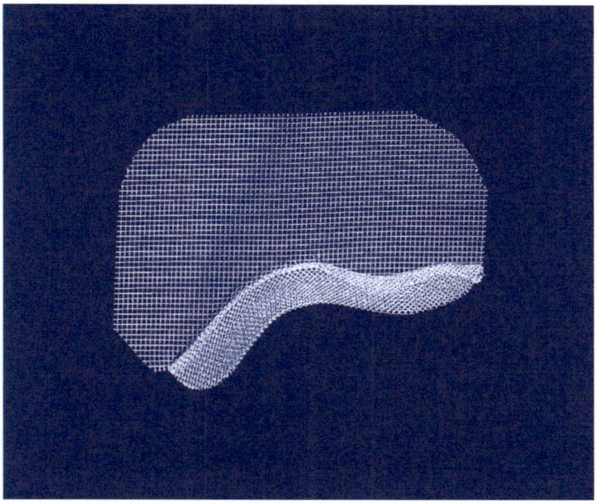

Fig. 4.81 Parietex anatomical mesh (All rights reserved; used with permission of Medtronic, Inc.)

some surgeons do not use fasteners of any kind. It has a left and right design. It is also available with an embedded suture to ease insertion and an included flap to place the cord structures through the product (Fig. 4.82). The *Folding Mesh with Suture* is a flat polyester mesh with rounded edges (Fig. 4.83). As noted in the figure, there is a suture that is woven through the material as an aid in the insertion and deployment of this mesh in the preperitoneal space during the robotic repair. This suture is pulled tight so that the mesh will be drawn into a small somewhat cylindrical shape. It is then placed into the preperitoneal space whereupon the suture is cut, allowing the mesh to resume its original shape. This device is also available with a slit if one desires to place the cord structures through the slit.

PS implant is a nonwoven PP material that is rather ovoid in shape (Fig. 4.84). It can be used for either the left or right inguinal hernia repair and with or without

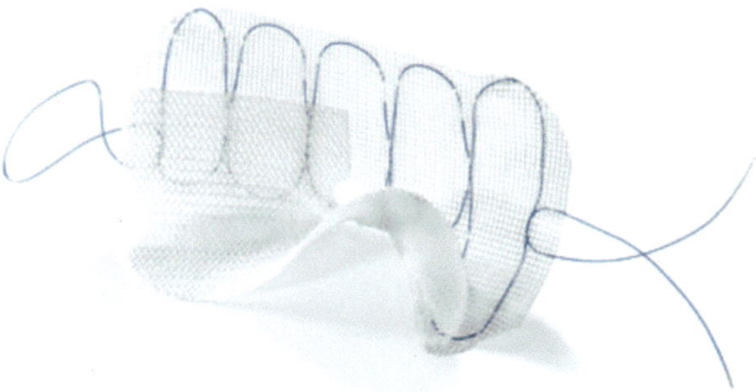

Fig. 4.82 Parietex anatomic with suture (All rights reserved; used with permission of Medtronic, Inc.)

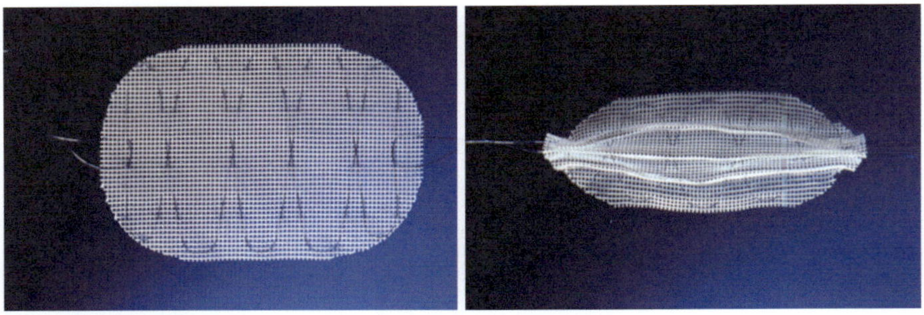

Fig. 4.83 Folding mesh with suture (All rights reserved; used with permission of Medtronic, Inc.)

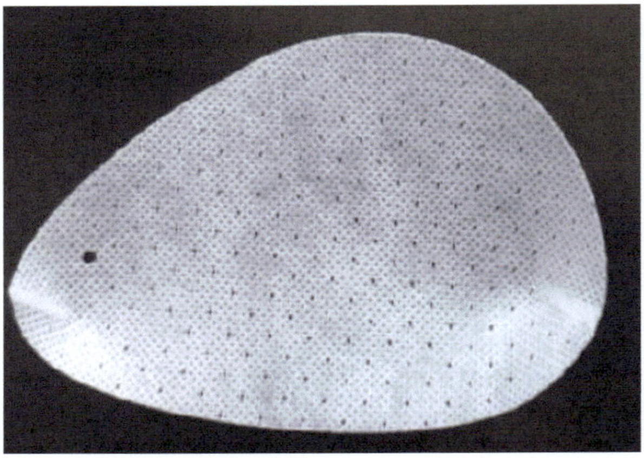

Fig. 4.84 PS implant

fixation. *Premium* mesh is PP that available in various shapes for the laparoscopic repair (Fig. 4.85). There is a blue polypropylene suture to mark the medial side of the product. *SMA* and *SMH2* product are similar products. They are both anatomically shaped but the *SMA* is made of polyester and impregnated PUR (Fig. 4.86). It is preferably used in the TEP repair but could be used in the robotic TAPP as well. *SM2+* is polyester and impregnated PUR and shaped for this repair (Fig. 4.87).

Fig. 4.85 Premium laparoscopic inguinal

Fig. 4.86 SMA

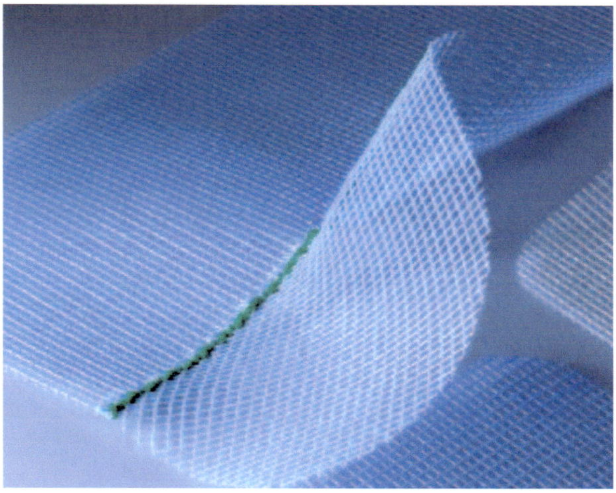

Fig. 4.87 SM2+

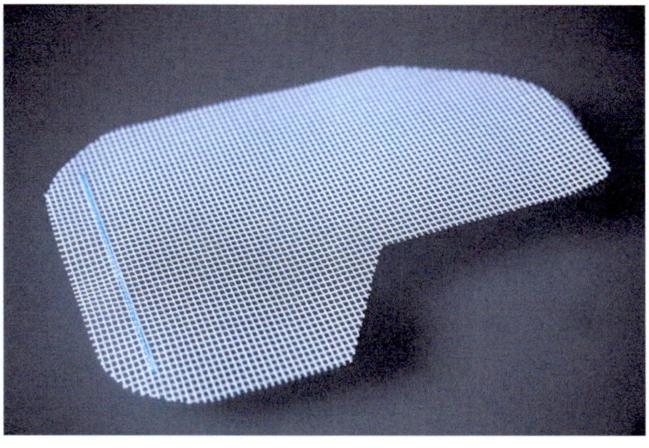

SMH2+ is a product that has a shape similar to the 3D Max and the Easy Prosthes 3D Mesh (Fig. 4.88). It differs in that it is a combination product of permanent material, PP and impregnated polyurethane (PUR). *SMH2A* is also made of PP and PUR but like the *SMA*, it should be used preferably in the TEP approach to inguinal hernia repair due to its shape so for this reason, there has been little use with the robotic approach (Fig. 4.89). *SM3* has been described in the flat mesh section above (Fig. 4.53). This is configured for use in the laparoscopic repair of inguinal hernias.

SurgiMesh WN has the same structure as that of most of the SurgiMesh products listed in the prior tables (Fig. 4.32). There are two laparoscopic products. One is a single flat square sheet with a rounded portion cutout on one corner. This is to be

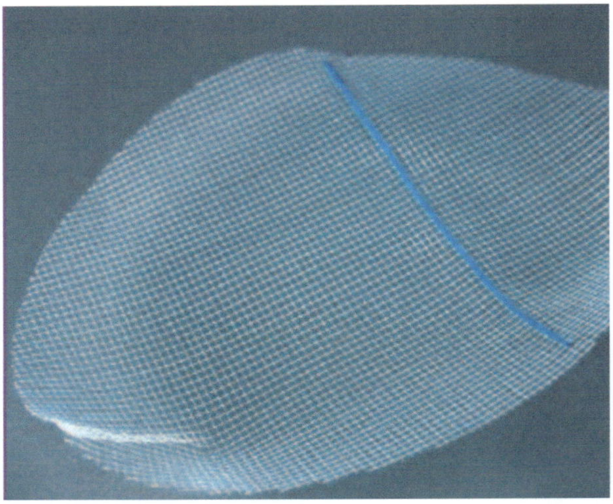

Fig. 4.88 SMH2+

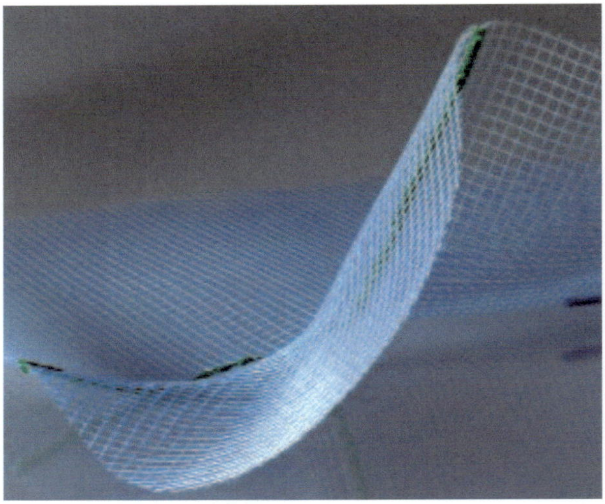

Fig. 4.89 SMH2A

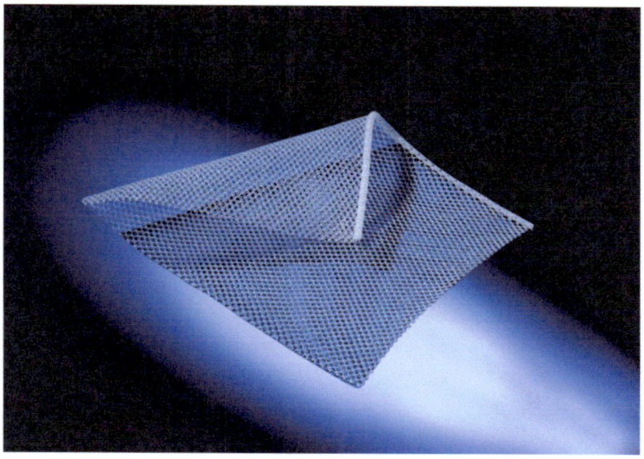

Fig. 4.90 Visilex

placed at Cooper's ligament. The other product has a keyhole and a flap to allow the product to be placed onto the posterior wall of the inguinal canal with the cord structures placed in the keyhole. The flap then covers the slit and keyhole to seal this defect in the mesh. *Visilex* is flat Bard mesh that has a stiffer border designed to ease the manipulation of the product in the preperitoneal space (Fig. 4.90).

4.11 Prostheses for Incisional and Ventral Hernioplasty with an Absorbable Barrier

The original impetus behind the development of these products was the popularity of the laparoscopic methodology. In general, however, all of these prosthetic devices can or have been used in open, laparoscopic and robotic incisional hernioplasties. All of them have the common purpose to repair the hernia and prevent the development of adhesions with the attendant complications associated with this result of the healing process. These are generally referred to as "tissue-separating" meshes as they create an absorbable barrier between the permanent product and the viscera (Table 4.17). They are available in a variety of shapes and sizes, which are too many to enumerate here. The reader is referred to the individual company for further information.

The resorption of that nonpermanent substance leaves a permanent layer of mesh that will incorporate into the tissues of the patient. The controversial part of this idea is the fact that the problems that are related to the development of adhesions following the implantation of a synthetic biomaterial may not become manifest for many years post-implantation. Therefore, the late effects of these products will necessitate many years of follow-up to validate these claims. At the present time, however, these meshes do seem to live up to their expectations.

Adhesix is the same product that was listed in Table 4.15 (Fig. 4.64). It is touted that this can be used in the preperitoneal position, the retrorectus space or as an onlay but it is not designed for use in with contact with the viscera. It is not readily available today.

Table 4.17 Ventral and incisional prostheses with an absorbable barrier

Adhesix, Davol, Inc., Warwick, RI, USA
C-QUR FX, Getinge Group, Wayne, NJ, USA
C-QUR Mosiac, Getinge Group, Wayne, NJ, USA
C-QUR TacShield, Getinge Group, Wayne, NJ USA
C-QUR V-Patch, Getinge Group, Wayne, NJ, USA
Easy Pro Composite Mesh, TransEasy Medical Tech.Co. Ltd., Beijing, China
Parietene Composite, Medtronic, Minneapolis, MN, USA
Parietex Composite Ventral Patch, Medtronic, Minneapolis, MN, USA
Parietex Optimized Composite (PCO_x), Medtronic, Minneapolis, MN, USA
Parietex Optimized Composite (PCO_x) Skirted Mesh, Medtronic, Minneapolis, MN, USA
Parietene DS, Medtronic, Minneapolis, MN, USA
Parietene ProGrip, Medtronic, Minneapolis, MN, USA
Parietex ProGrip, Medtronic, Minneapolis, MN, USA
Physiomesh Open, Ethicon, Inc., Somerville, NJ, USA
Proceed, Ethicon, Inc., Somerville, NJ, USA
Proceed Ventral Patch, Ethicon, Inc., Somerville, NJ, USA
SepraMesh IP, Davol, Inc., Warwick, RI, USA
Symbotex, Medtronic, Minneapolis, MN, USA
Ventralight ST, Davol, Inc., Warwick, RI, USA
Ventralex ST, Davol, Inc., Warwick, RI, USA
Ventrio ST, Davol, Inc., Warwick, RI, USA

C-QUR FX is made of a lightweight Prolite mesh onto which Omega-3 Fatty Acid (O3FA) has been coated onto the product (Fig. 4.91). These fatty acids are in a cross-linked gel that covers both sides of the material and impart a characteristic dark yellow color. O3FA will absorb over a period of 3–6 months. *C-QUR FX* has a lighter coating of the Omega 3 fatty acid that the other C-QUR products possess and therefore, must be placed in the extraperitoneal space. It is also configured for use in open and laparoscopic/robotic inguinal hernia repair. *C-QUR Mosiac* is made of the same materials but has a thicker coating of O3FA (Fig. 4.92). Therefore, it can be used when tissue-separating capabilities are required in the repair of hernias. The *C-QUR V-Patch* is designed for open repair umbilical hernias and trocar site defects but it could be used for smaller incisional hernias as well (Fig. 4.93). It combines the ProLite material such that there is one layer of the C-QUR FX and one layer of the C-QUR mesh itself that are sewn together around an O3FA coated mesh stabilizing ring. The fixation straps would be cut off in the robotic application. *Easy Pro Composite Mesh* is constructed of lightweight PPM with a barrier coating of polylactide-co-carprolactone (Fig. 4.94). It has an "F" on the visceral surface to identify the orientation toward the intestine. It is also available in a precut size for complicated inguinal hernia repair.

Parietene Composite is PP coated with the hydrophilic collagen and other substances that are used in the better-known Parietex Composite discussed below.

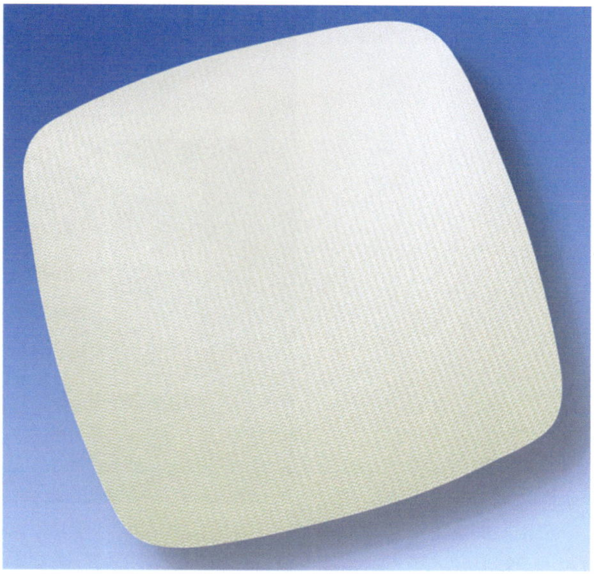

Fig. 4.91 C-QUR FX

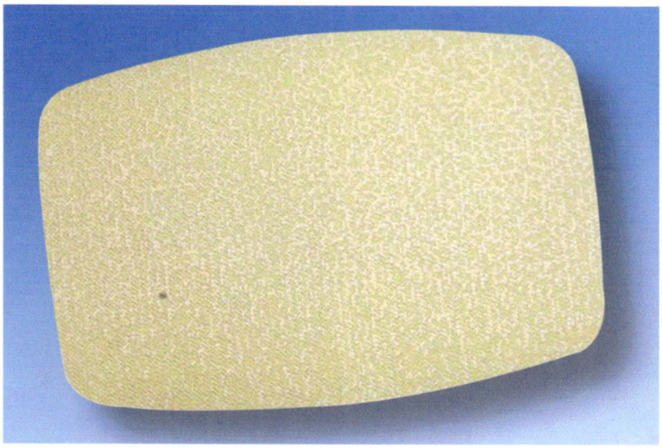

Fig. 4.92 C-Qur Mosiac

Parietex Composite Ventral Patch is designed for the smaller defects in the abdominal wall such as umbilical or epigastric hernias like that of the C-Qur V-Patch (Fig. 4.95). It is supplied with a deployment system that consists of a PGLA structure that is implanted and two nylon suture "positioning" arms that are removed when used in the robotic repair. It has an incorporated hydrophilic layer of a mixture of oxidized Type I atelocollagen, polyethylene glycol and glycerol, which is absorbable. *Parietex Optimized Composite* is the same POL biomaterial that is described earlier in this chapter (Fig. 4.96). It is supplied with or without preplaced sutures. The mesh is available with the attached *AccuMesh Positioning System* that will hold the product in place during fixation (Fig. 4.97). *Parietene DS* is a dual sided product that has Paritene macroporous PP that is coated on one side with glycolide, caprolactone, trimethylene carbonate and lactose (Fig. 4.98). *Parietene ProGrip* and *Parietex ProGrip* also differ in that the former is of PP and the latter is of POL. Both

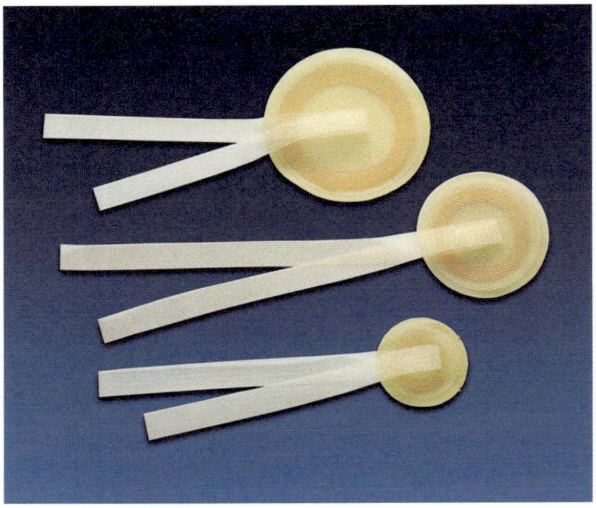

Fig. 4.93 C-QUR V-patch

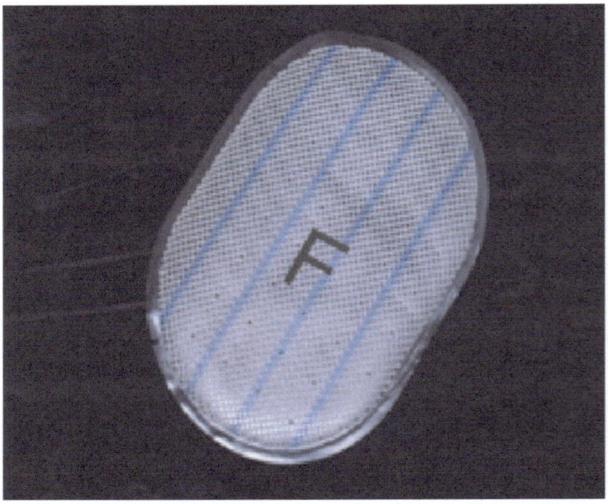

Fig. 4.94 EasyPro composite

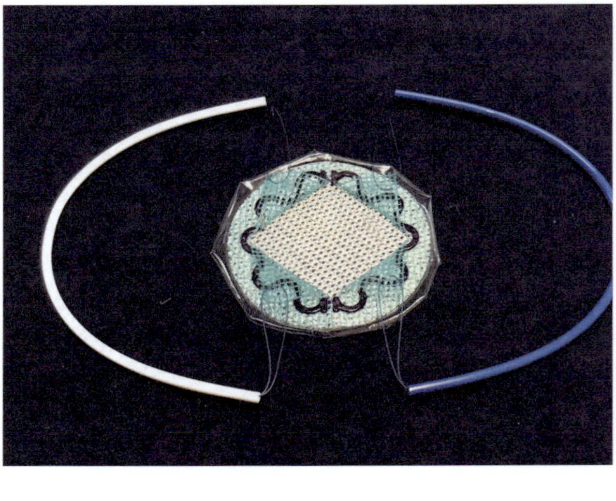

Fig. 4.95 Parietex composite ventral patch (All rights reserved; used with permission of Medtronic, Inc.)

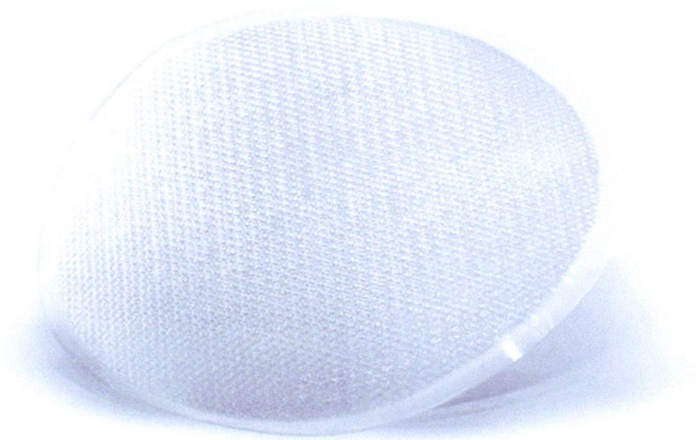

Fig. 4.96 Parietex composite optimized (All rights reserved; used with permission of Medtronic, Inc.)

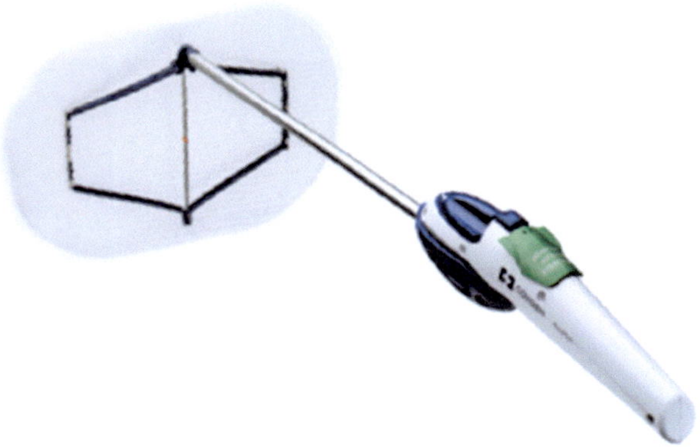

Fig. 4.97 AccuMesh positioning system (All rights reserved; used with permission of Medtronic, Inc.)

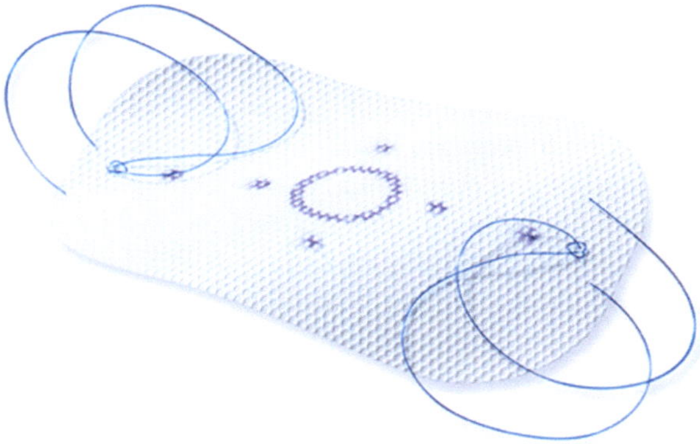

Fig. 4.98 Parietene DS (All rights reserved; used with permission of Medtronic, Inc.)

have the polylactic acid grippers (described earlier in this chapter) so that they potentially do not need fixation. The coating on these products is very minimal so it is not recommended that these products contact the viscera.

Proceed is composed of an oxidized regenerated cellulose (ORC) fabric and Prolene Soft Mesh which is encapsulated by a polydioxanone polymer that holds these materials together (Fig. 4.99). The fabric acts as a barrier to separate the PP from the viscera. The ORC is absorbed within four weeks. It should be noted that

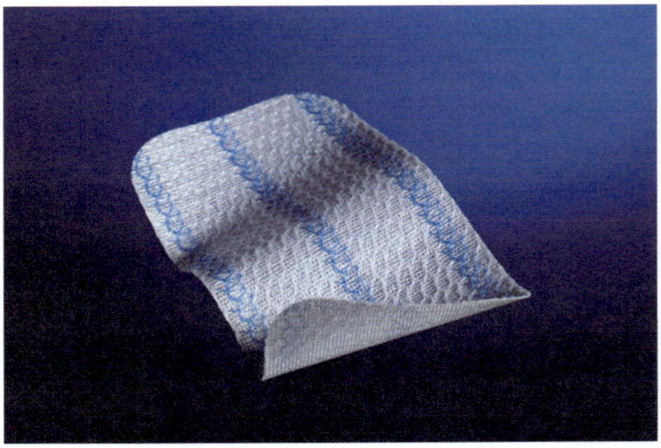

Fig. 4.99 Proceed (Image courtesy of Ethicon, Inc.)

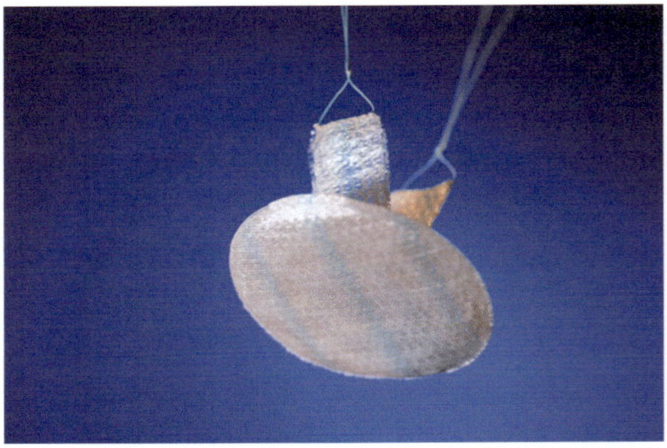

Fig. 4.100 Proceed ventral patch (Image courtesy of Ethicon, Inc.)

the instructions for use state "Proceed Mesh has an ORC component that should not be used in the presence of uncontrolled and/or active bleeding as fibrinous exudates may increase the chance of adhesion formation." The *Proceed Ventral Patch (PVP)* is another version that also has an ORC layer that is placed toward the intestine (Fig. 4.100). In this product, there is an additional layer of polydioxanone polymer and a positioning ring to provide memory. Polyglactin 910 is placed on top of the polydioxanone and is encapsulated with a polydioxanone film. The sutures that are seen in the photo are of polyester. Similar to the other products above, these should be removed in the use for robotic incisional hernia repair.

SepraMesh IP is a single layer of polypropylene is covered by barrier that is a combination of carboxymethylcellulose and hyaluronic acid (Fig. 4.101). It is bound together with polyglycolic acid fibers and has a hydrogel layer on the visceral surface. This product requires brief immersion into saline solution prior to its use to activate the gel, which then causes the hydrogel to swell causing it to swell and cover any fixation devices that are used. This barrier portion of the product is stated to last approximately four weeks. There is a lighter weight version that is Ventralight ST that is the more commonly used product (Fig. 4.102). The "Sepra" technology has been extended to the original Ventralex and Ventrio products (Table 4.18). The

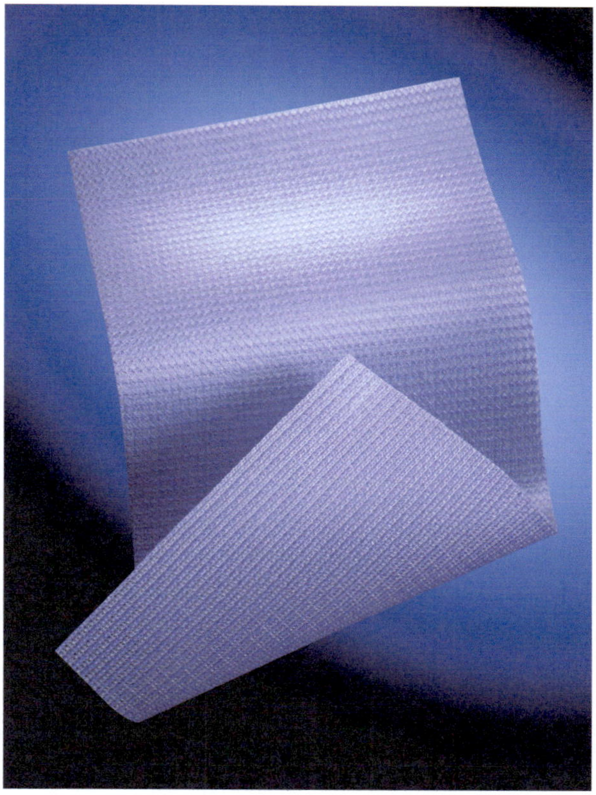

Fig. 4.101 SepraMesh IP

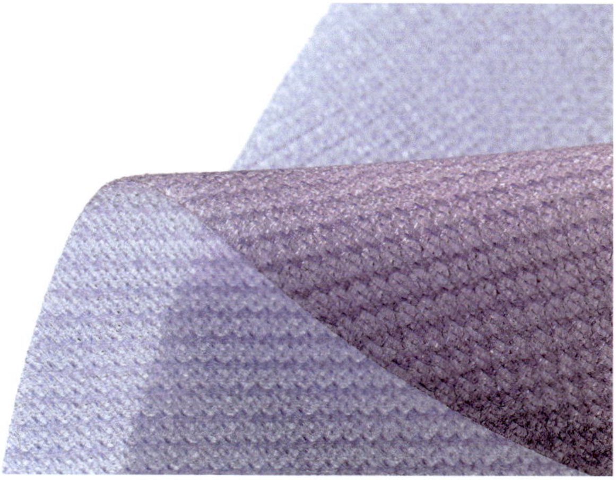

Fig. 4.102 Ventralight ST

Table 4.18 Ventral and incisional products with a permanent barrier

ClearMesh Composite (CMC), Di.pro Medical Devices, Torino, Italy
CO3A, THT-Bio-Science, Montpelier, France
Combi Mesh Plus, Angiologica, S. Martino Sicc., Italy
Composix E/X Mesh, Davol, Inc., Warwick, RI, USA
Composix L/P Mesh, Davol, Inc., Warwick, RI, USA
Composix L/P Mesh with ECHO PS, Davol, Inc., Warwick, RI, USA
DualMesh, W. L. Gore & Associates, Elkhart, DE, USA
DualMesh Plus, W. L. Gore &Associates, Elkhart, DE, USA
DualMesh Plus with Holes, W. L. Gore &Associates, Elkhart, DE, USA
Dulex, Davol, Inc., Warwick, RI, USA
DynaMesh IPOM, FEG Textiltechnik mbH, Aachen, Germany
Intra, Microval, Saint-Just-Malmont, France
IntraMesh T1, Cousin Biotech, Wervicq-Sud, France
IS 180, THT Bio-Science, Montpelier, France
Omyra Mesh, B. Braun Melsungen AG, Melsungen, Germany
MotifMESH, Proxy Biomedical Ltd., Galway, Ireland
MycroMesh, W. L. Gore &Associates, Elkhart, DE, USA
MycroMesh Plus, W. L. Gore &Associates, Elkhart, DE, USA
Prefix, THT Bio-Science, Montpelier, France
Plurimesh (PCMC), Di.pro Medical Devices, Torino, Italy
Rebound HRD V, ARB Medical, Minneapolis, MN, USA
Relimesh, HerniaMesh, Torino, Italy
SMH2+, THT Bio-science, Montpelier, France
SM3+, THT Bio-Science, Montpelier, France
Soft Tissue Patch, W. L. Gore &Associates, Elkhart, DE, USA
SurgiMesh XB, Aspide Medical, St. Etienne, France
TiMesh, GfE Medizintechnik, Nuremburg, Germany
TiO_2 Mesh, Bayreuth, Germany
Umbilical - CMC, Di.pro Medical Devices, Torino, Italy
Ventralex, Davol, Inc., Warwick, RI, USA
Ventrio Hernia Patch, Davol, Inc., Warwick, RI, USA

ePTFE surface of these latter products has been replaced with the tissue-separating material that is used on the SepraMesh IP and Ventralight ST prostheses. These products are called *Ventralex ST* and *Ventrio ST* (Figs. 4.103 and 4.104). *Symbotex* is a polyester material that is lighter in weight than the Parietex PCO (Fig. 4.105). It has the same barrier material as the PCO product described above (i.e. Type I atelo-collagen, polyethylene glycol and glycerol). There is a green marker that is placed as an aid in positioning.

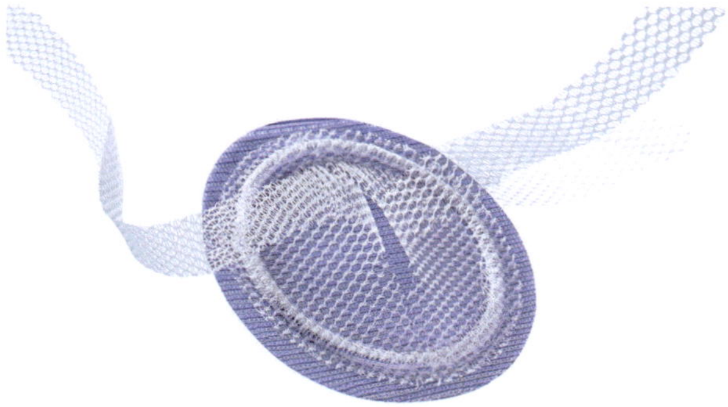

Fig. 4.103 Ventralex ST

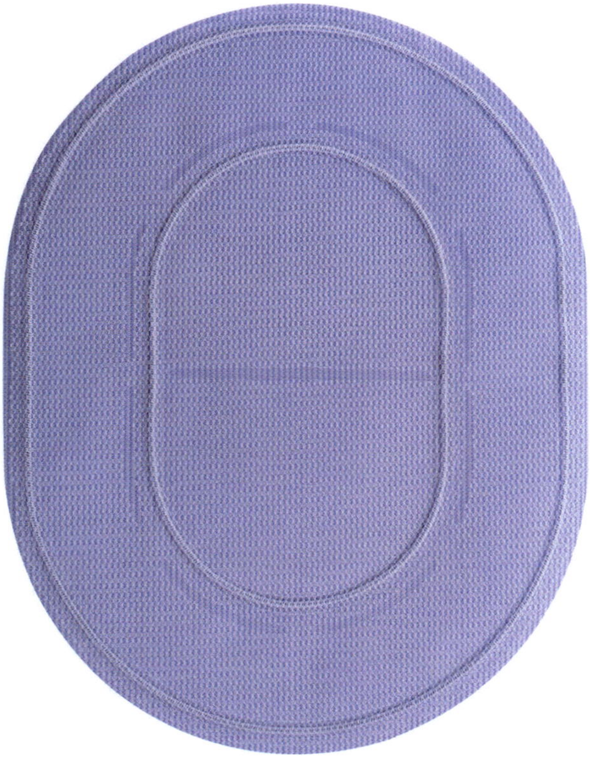

Fig. 4.104 Ventrio ST

4.12 Prostheses for Incisional and Ventral Hernioplasty with a Permanent Barrier

These products are a combination of a single product that is manufactured in two different forms or, more commonly, a combination of two different materials (Table 4.18). The method of fixation of these products to each other differs from each manufacturer. There are some that have been described earlier in this chapter

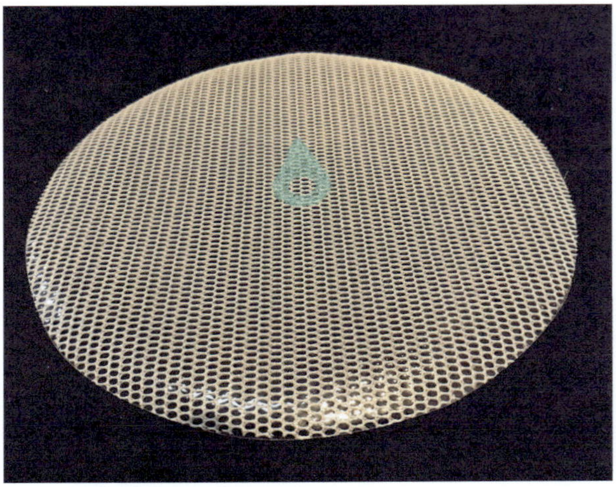

Fig. 4.105 Symbotex ()

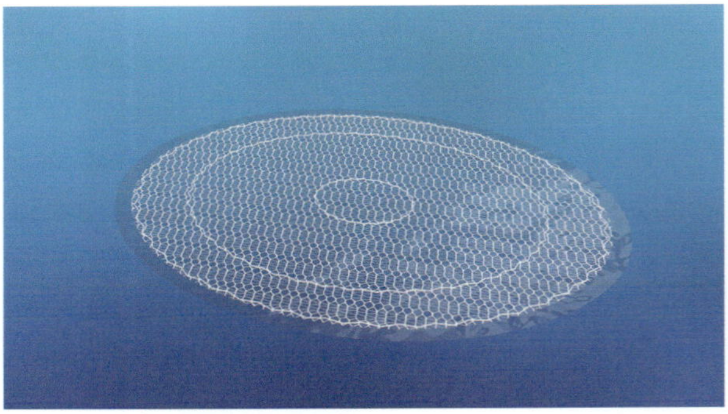

Fig. 4.106 ClearMesh composite

that are single products (ePTFE, cPTFE or PVDF) and are not described again here (Tables 4.13 and 4.14). What is consistent in all of the prostheses is the creation of some type of a barrier to visceral adhesion formation while allowing for parietal ingrowth on the opposite surface of these meshes.

ClearMesh Composite (CMC) is a pure PP mesh (Fig. 4.106). There is a textured side that is composed of a single filament macroporous weave and a non-adhesive side that is composed of a non-porous smooth PP film. It is further designated as *CMC 2P*, which is elliptical in shape and the *CMC 2P-C,* which is round. *CO3A* has been described in the flat mesh section (Fig. 4.76). It is a combination of POL and PUR with grips. *Combi Mesh Plus* is also combination of PP and PUR but also has an attached suture to delineate the parietal surface (Fig. 4.107). The polyurethane layer of all such products faces the viscera. *Composix E/X* mesh is flat Bard mesh on one side (parietal) and ePTFE on the other surface (visceral) (Fig. 4.108). The perimeter edge of the elliptically shaped product is sealed to prevent contact of viscera to the PP. It is a low profile mesh. *Composix L/P* is very similar to the Composix E/X except that the former uses the lighter Bard Soft Mesh rather than the Bard mesh (Fig. 4.109). It is specifically designed for laparoscopic usage and can be used

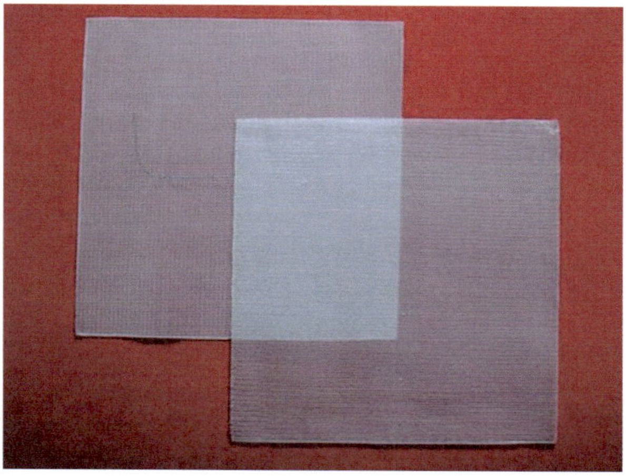

Fig. 4.107 Combi Mesh Plus

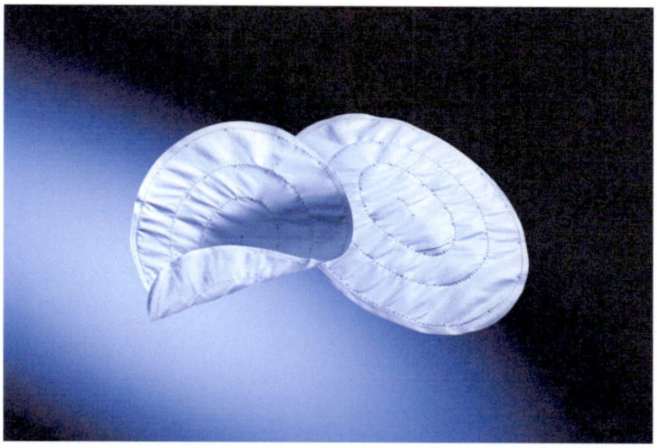

Fig. 4.108 Composix E/X

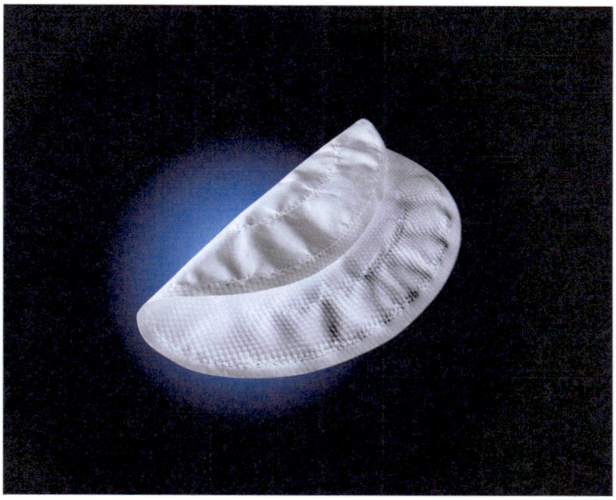

Fig. 4.109 Composix L/P

with a supplied introduction tool. The two mesh layers are sutured together with ePTFE suture. The Composix L/P is also available with the ECHO PS (Fig. 4.110). The green balloon shown in the figure will be inflated to firm up the mesh to allow for accurate positioning and fixation. There is an attached blue tubing on the opposite side (not seen in the figure) that is pulled through the abdominal wall to center the mesh. It is then cut and attached to a syringe that is used to inflate the balloon. Once fixation is completed, the balloon is deflated and removed.

DynaMesh IPOM is a similar PP weave as the DynaMesh described earlier in this chapter (Fig. 4.19) but it is slightly lighter in weight than the latter product (Fig. 4.111). This version is intertwined with a monofilament of polyvinylidene

Fig. 4.110 Composix L/P mesh with Echo PS

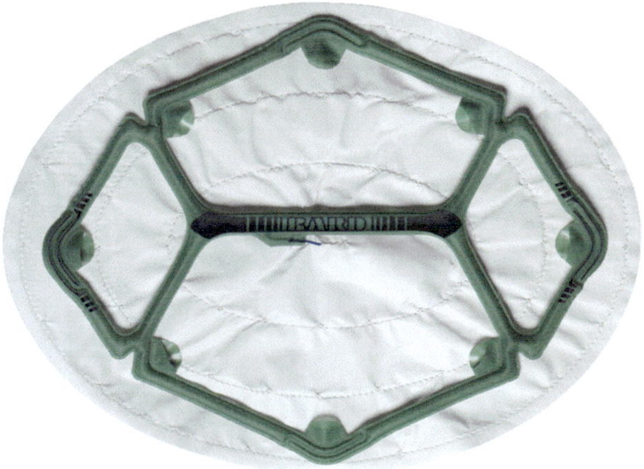

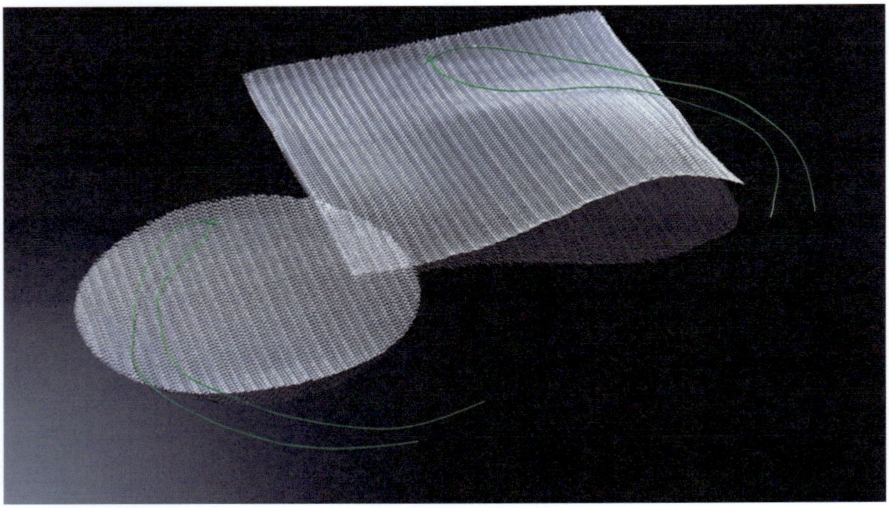

Fig. 4.111 DynaMesh IPOM

fluoride (PVDF). Because of this PVDF tissue-separating component it can be placed onto the viscera. The suture noted in the figure signifies which side should be placed against the abdominal wall, as it is impossible to be certain with the naked eye which side is the parietal surface. *Intra* mesh is a combination of nonwoven PP on one side with a layer of silicone on the other as a tissue separating material (Fig. 4.112). It is one of the few materials available with this silicone barrier. This side is marked with a cross and "intra side" in black silicone ink. *IntraMesh T1* is similar to the Composix product line in that it is composed of one layer of PP and a second layer of ePTFE (Fig. 4.113). It is the only material that possesses lines on the product to delineate the midportions of each side to ease positioning for the laparoscopic/robotic approach. Cousin Biotech also sells a "mesh roller" which is a device to aid in the rolling of these materials to ease insertion into the abdominal cavity through a trocar. *IS 180* is part of the intra-swing composite family, which is a macroperforated three-dimensional POL with a coating of PUR (tissue-separating) on one surface (Fig. 4.114). It is configured in a variety of shapes with or without PP sutures to aid in fixation. The company also has an available *Easy-Catch EC* device to be used for laparoscopic introduction of the material into the abdominal cavity. *Prefix* is similar in concept to the IS 180 but, as shown in the photo, there are

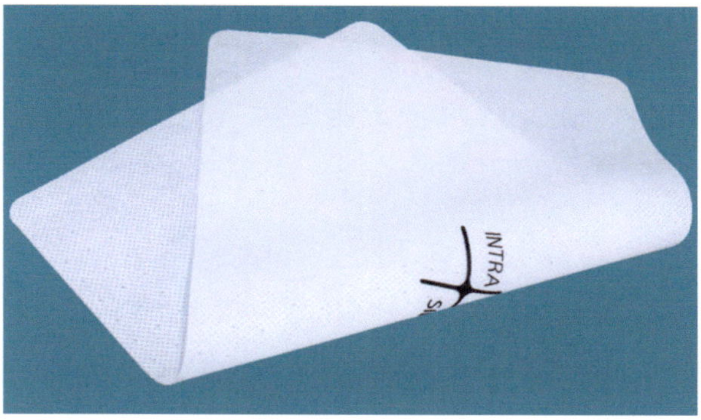

Fig. 4.112 Intra mesh

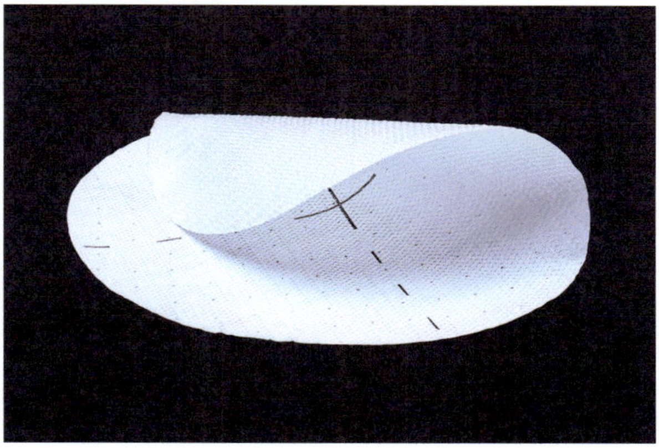

Fig. 4.113 IntraMesh T1

preplaced sutures to allow for positioning of the product (Fig. 4.115). It is one of the few products that include pre-attached sutures with straight needles on them.

Plurimesh (PCMC) is a similar concept as the CMC except that it is designed for incisional or parastomal hernia repair (Fig. 4.116). It has sewn seams that can be

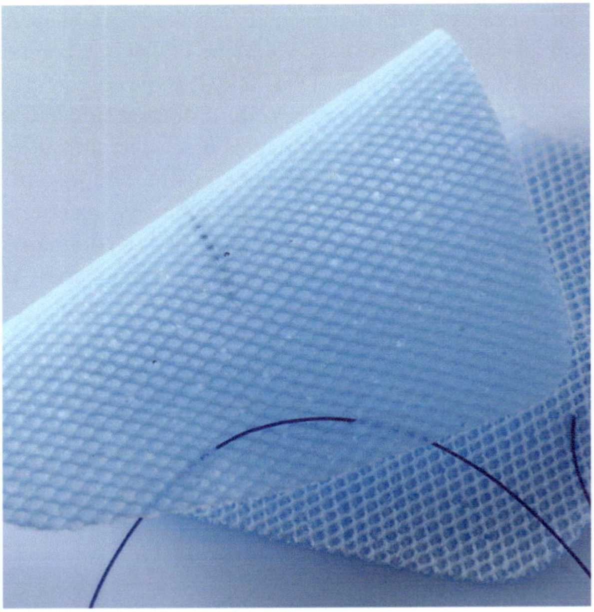

Fig. 4.114 IS 180

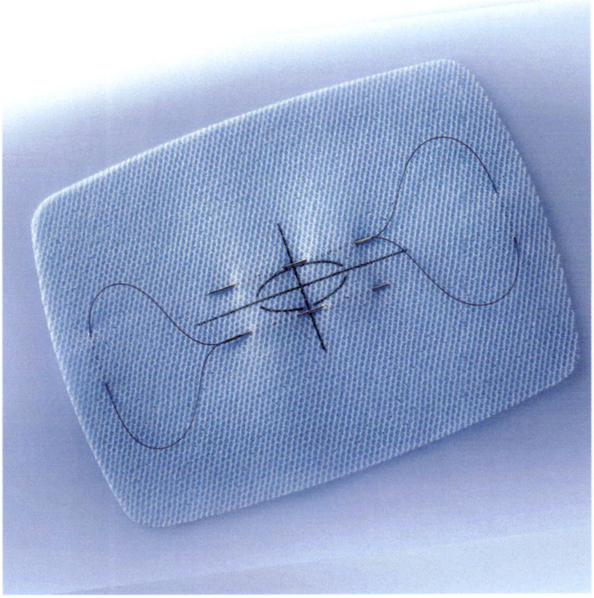

Fig. 4.115 Prefix

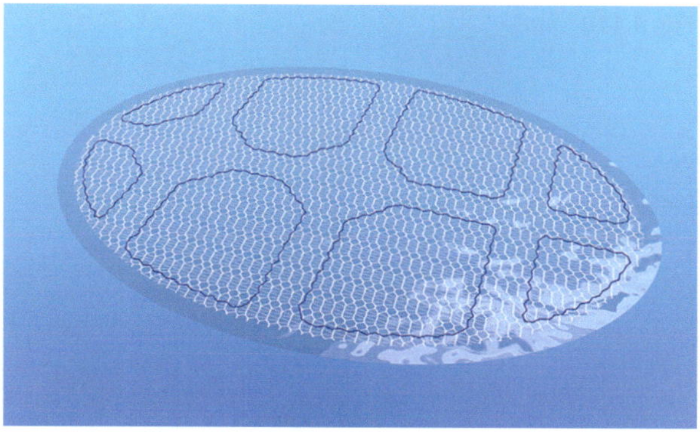

Fig. 4.116 Plurimesh

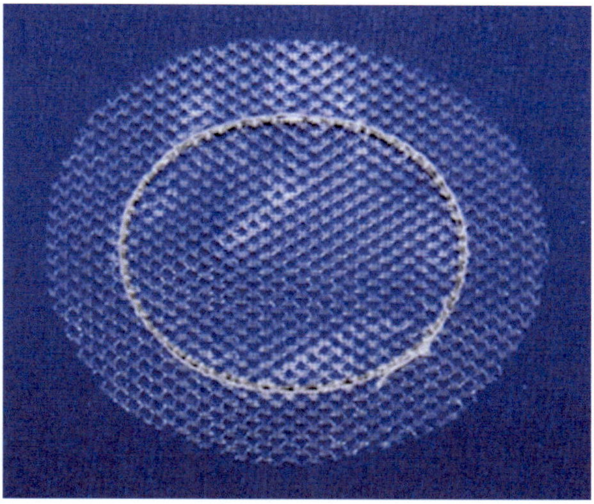

Fig. 4.117 Rebound HRD V

used to cut the mesh to conform to the needs of the hernia treated. *Rebound HRD V* is a unique material in that it is PP that has a ring of nitinol to stiffen the product and is available as an oval shape for umbilical hernia repair (Fig. 4.117). It is designed for use in the preperitoneal space and does not have a separate coating. It is placed in this section due to fact that it has significantly different components. *Relimesh* is another product that incorporates the PP on one surface and ePTFE on the other to allow placement against the viscera. It is a lighter weight product compared to other HerniaMesh products. Because of this, it can be rolled for insertion via a trocar. It is marked to aid in positioning and fixation. *SMH2+* has been previously described in the preformed inguinal hernia mesh section and is PP and PUR. It is also indicated for ventral hernias as well (Fig. 4.88). *SM3+* is polyester with impregnated polyurethane and is a flat mesh but is also configured in anatomical shapes for inguinal or femoral hernia repair (Fig. 4.118).

SurgiMesh XB has a non-woven, non-knitted structure as does the SurgiMesh WN described earlier but it has an additional layer of silicone to allow contact with

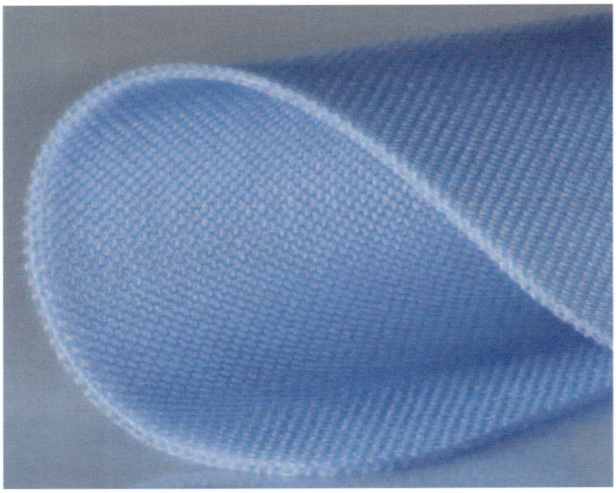

Fig. 4.118 SM3+

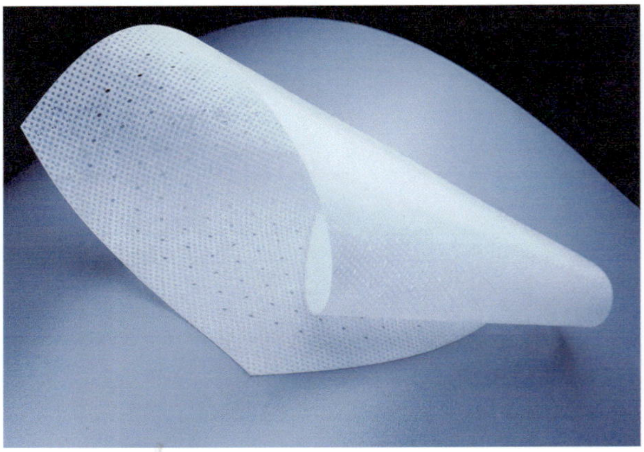

Fig. 4.119 Surgimesh XB

the viscera and is microperforated (Fig. 4.119). This product is available in different shape including a circular one that has an attached suture as a positioning aid (Tintra C). *TiMesh* is the same material that has been described in several locations within this chapter (Fig. 4.37). The titanized PPM can be used in the intraperitoneal location (per the manufacturer). Another titanized PPM is that of *TiO_2Mesh* (Fig. 4.40). This is described in the Miscellaneous Flat Mesh section above. *Umbilical CMC* is round and includes blue stitching and tethers to aid in positioning (Fig. 4.120).

Ventralex is a self-expanding PP device (because of the outer ring of polydioxanone) that has ePTFE on one side to allow placement adjacent to viscera (Fig. 4.121). It is round but smaller than the larger products such as the Composix products described above. It is intended for use in the smaller defects of the abdominal wall such as trocar or umbilical hernias. Two long straps are attached that are very long as this product can be inserted through a laparoscopic trocar to aid in the prevention of trocar hernias. When used during robotic incisional hernia repair, the straps

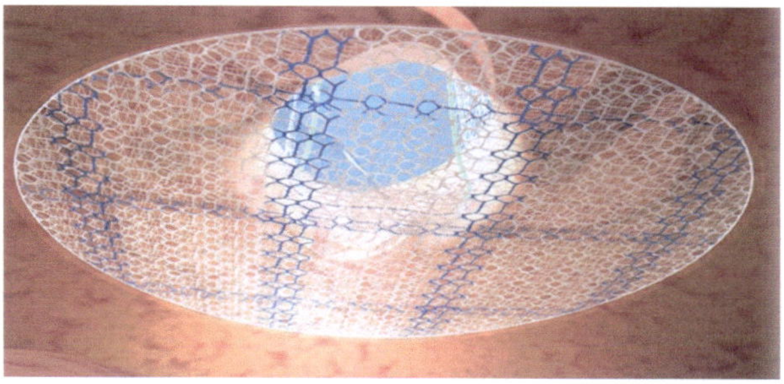

Fig. 4.120 Umbilical CMC

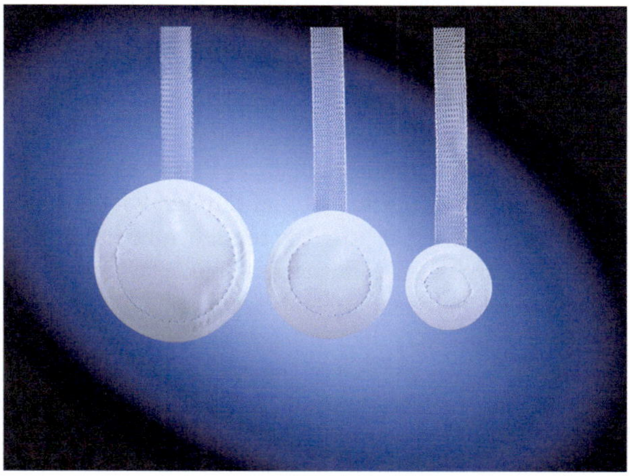

Fig. 4.121 Ventralex

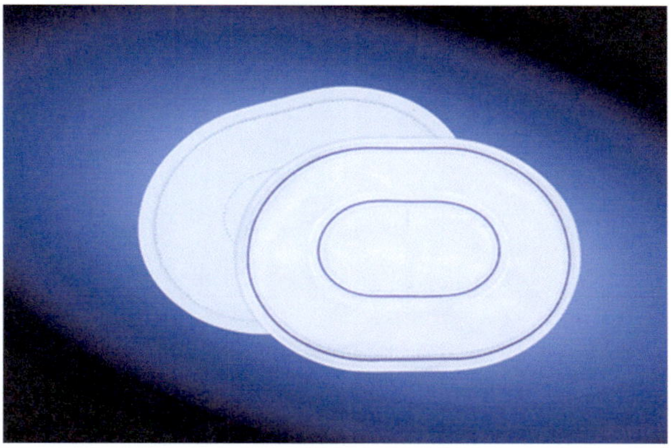

Fig. 4.122 Ventrio hernia patch

should be removed prior to insertion. The *Ventrio Hernia Patch* is comprised of two layers of PP that are stitched to an ePTFE layer as the tissue-separating component (Fig. 4.122). Within the PP surface there are "tubes" that house an absorbable polydioxanone (PDO) monofilament ring(s) to give the mesh rigidity to aid in positioning and fixation. The purple PDO ring is absorbed within 6–8 months.

4.13 Stomal Hernia Prevention and Repair Products

The development of a hernia wherever a stoma is created has been the challenge in the life of all patients with some type of an ostomy. Traditionally, relocation or primary closure was used to repair these hernias but this is now considered a poor choice as this method or repair is fraught with failure in most cases. Consequently, the use of a prosthetic material has become nearly standard to repair these hernias. In fact, recent trends indicate that the use of a mesh of some type when the stoma is created may be the preferred option. Prevention has become the new effort in mesh construction (Table 4.19). Many of these involve the use of one of the biologic, synthetic absorbable or permanent products described earlier in this chapter. As with many of the other products in this chapter, these can generally be used with the open or laparoscopic/robotic techniques. The materials are specific to ostomy hernia repair but other techniques such as the Sugarbaker onlay utilize one of the flat meshes described earlier in this chapter.

Colostomy Mesh is a single layer PP product (Fig. 4.123). It has a five-centimeter hole in the center of the material through which the intestine can be placed during stomal creation. Of course, the mesh can be cut if this product is used in the repair of a parastomal hernia. It is available in a "rigid" and a "semi-rigid" construction. It is not coated and must not be place in the intraperitoneal space.

DynaMesh-IPST, like its parent material, is made of both PVDF and PP (Fig. 4.124). It is preshaped and three-dimensional through which the intestine is placed. This is generally used during the creation of the ostomy rather than during

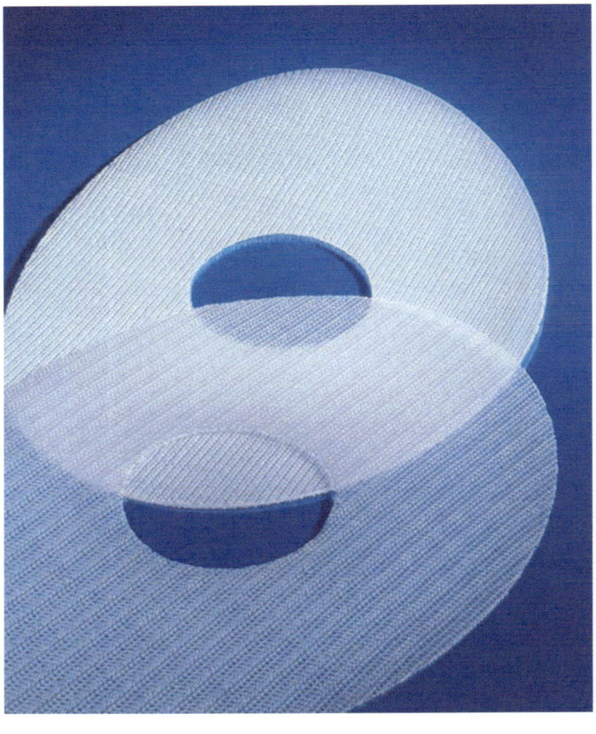

Fig. 4.123 Colostomy mesh

the repair of a parastomal hernia in an effort to prevent the development of a hernia. If used in that fashion it, too, would need to be cut to allow placement around the stomal hernia repair. *Parietex Composite Parastomal Mesh* is of the same material (polyester) as that described previously during descriptions of the Parietex products. This device is supplied in two sizes and is available with a hole or without a hole but with a central band (Figs. 4.125 and 4.126). The available opening of the hole can

Table 4.19 Stomal prostheses

Colostomy Mesh, HerniaMesh, Torino, Italy
DynaMesh-IPST, FEG Textiltechnik mbH, Aachen, Germany
Parietex Composite Parastomal Mesh, Medtronic, Minneapolis, MN
Plurimesh Clear Mesh Composite (PCMC), Di.pro Medical Devices, Torino, Italy
TiLENE Guard, GfE Medizintechnik, Nuremburg, Germany

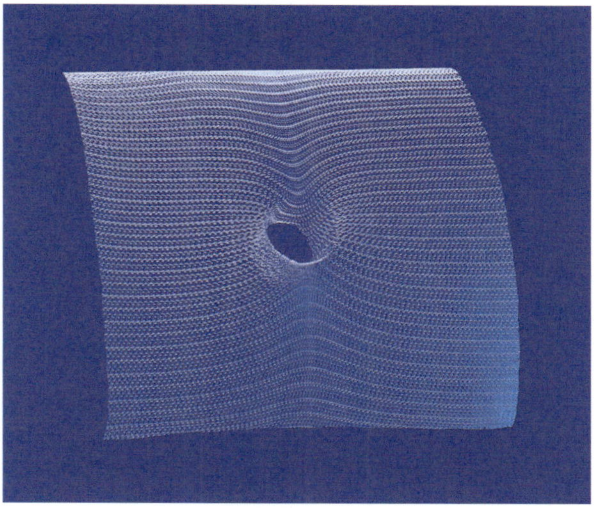

Fig. 4.124 DynaMesh IPST

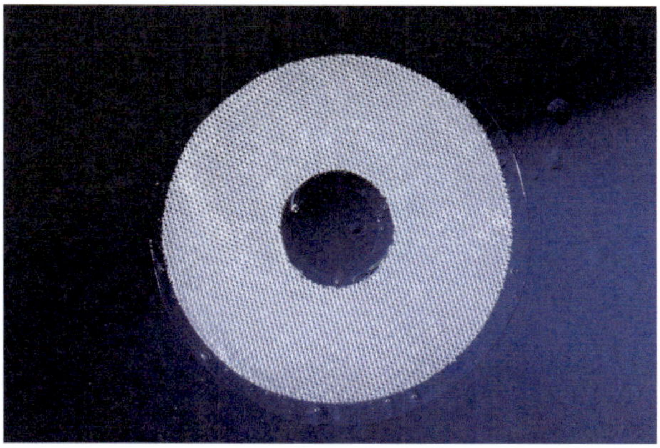

Fig. 4.125 Parietex parastomal with hole (All rights reserved; used with permission of Medtronic, Inc.)

either be 3.5 cm or 5.0 cm. *Plurimesh (PCMC)* has already been described for incisional and ventral hernia repair. It can also be used for parastomal hernia repair (Fig. 4.116). It is supplied in such a manner that it can be cut to confirm to whatever the size the surgeon chooses.

TiLENE Guard is of titanized PP that contains a flap, which is closed after the intestine is placed through the central hole (Fig. 4.127). It is supplied in the light and

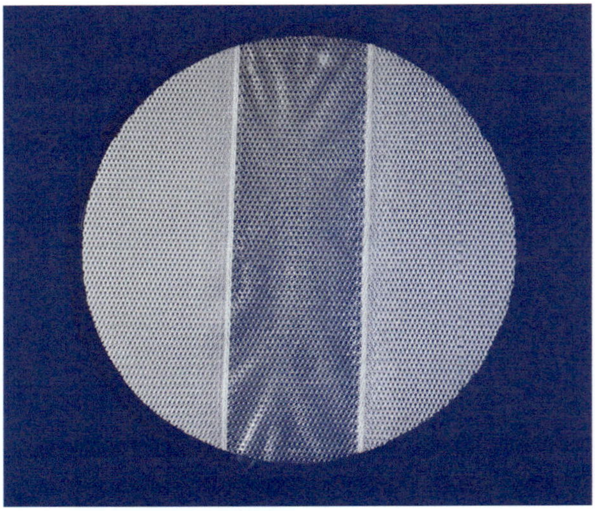

Fig. 4.126 Parietex parastomal without hole (All rights reserved; used with permission of Medtronic, Inc.)

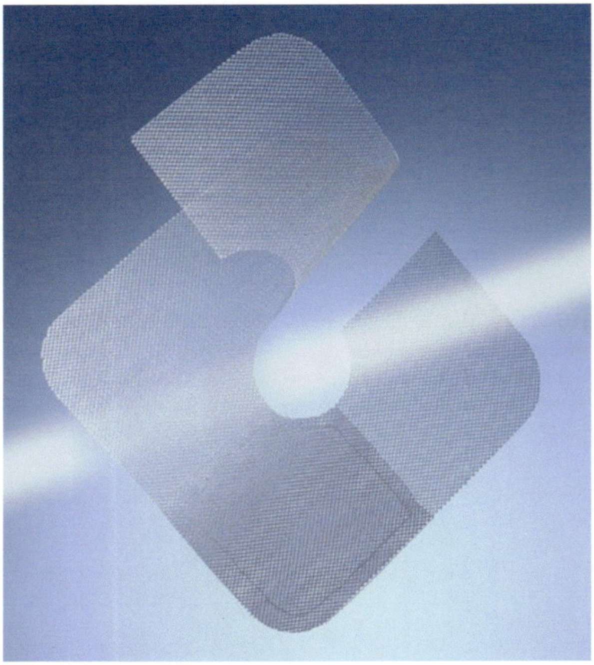

Fig. 4.127 TiLENE guard

dual-weight (light and medium) meshes. There is a set, which contains *TiLENE* mesh that is to be applied as a "sandwich" technique to repair or prevent herniation through the stomal exit location.

4.14 Hiatal Hernia Repair Products

The use of permanent meshes to repair hiatal hernias has been commonplace for many years. The introduction of the biologic products has resulted in a decline in the application of the permanent products at this position. The real concern is of erosion of the product into the esophagus or infection with a permanent prosthesis. While the application of flat meshes such as unprotected PP or POL has been used, these products were designed to mitigate against these concerns (Table 4.20).

Bio-A is the same material discussed at the beginning of this chapter and is not permanent. It is made of the PGA-TMC but is configured into a shape that can be modified by the surgeon if desired (Fig. 4.128). It can be glued or sutured in place. The *Biodesign Hiatal Hernia Graft* is the same family of products described in the biologic section but this has been configured similar to the Bio-A with a "U"-shaped cutout of the material. *RH Implant* is of the similar material of the other products

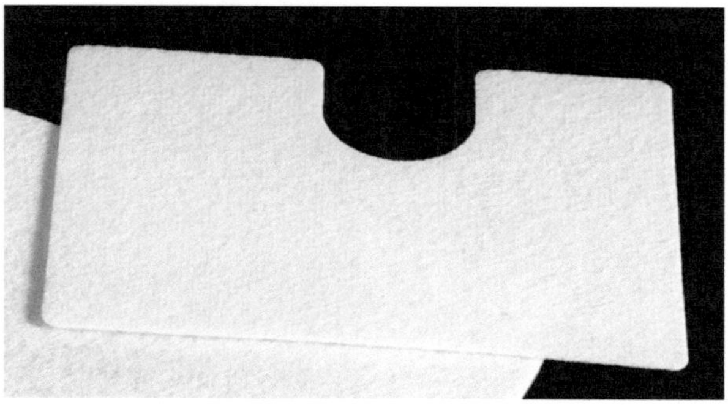

Fig. 4.128 Bio-A hiatal

Table 4.20 Hiatal hernia repair products

Bio-A Hiatal, W.L Gore & Associates, Elkhart, DE, USA
Biodesign Hiatal Hernia Graft, Cook Medical, Bloomington, IL, USA
RH Implant, Microval, Saint-Just-Malmont, France
Parietex Composite (PCO) Hiatal Mesh, Medtronic, Minneapolis, MN, USA
Phasix ST, C.R. Bard, Warwick, RI, USA
TiLENE Hiatus, GfE Medizintechnik, Nuremburg, Germany
TiSURE, GfE Medizintechnik, Nuremburg, Germany

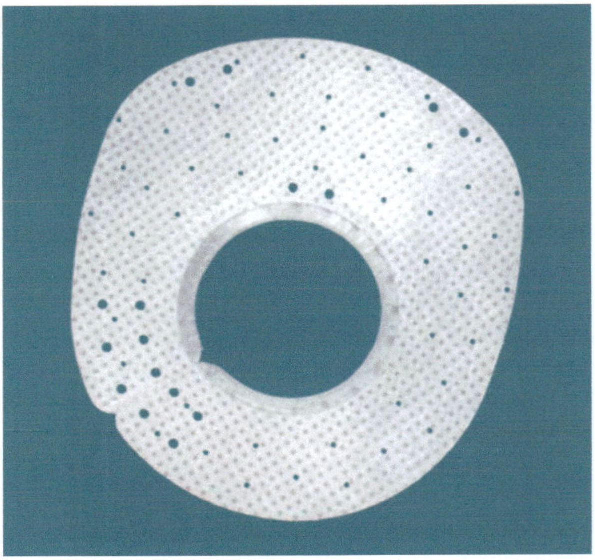

Fig. 4.129 RH Implant

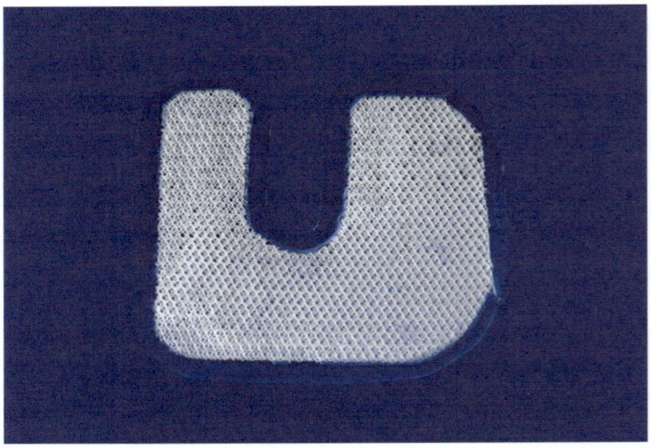

Fig. 4.130 Parietex composite hiatal mesh (All rights reserved; used with permission of Medtronic, Inc.)

from Microval (Fig. 4.129). It is a permanent non-woven PP coated on one side with silicon as the tissue-separating component. The larger perforations are used to suture the mesh in place.

Parietex Composite Hiatal Mesh is made of the same permanent material as the parent PCO product (Fig. 4.130). It possesses a U-shaped defect that is slightly off-center that is to be positioned below the esophagus. The legs of the product will lie on the crura. It is available in two other shapes, a heart shape and a horseshoe shape. *Phasix ST* has recently been approved for use in this application (Fig. 4.4). It does not have a precut design therefore the surgeon must modify a small flat sheet to his or her specifications.

TiLENE Hiatus is made of the titanized PP but in either a rectangle shape with a curve on one side or in an "hour-glass" configuration. *TiSURE* is a rectangular mesh that has a central hole and a flap made from TiMESH (Fig. 4.131). It differs from the other products listed in that it possesses that flap which mandates complete encirclement of the esophagus. It can be fixed with either fibrin glue or sutures. It is not recommended to use metal fixation devices on this product because of the risk of complications from these devices.

4.15 Fixation Devices

Fixation devices became prevalent early in the development of the laparoscopic repair of hernias. They are mostly available as 5 mm versions as these have become the most popular. Most recently, recognition of the fact that these fasteners are only needed on a temporary basis has lead to the introduction of absorbable platforms. Currently, there is a variety of these devices that one may choose to fixate the meshes placed in hernia repair, however, the majority of robotic surgeons sew in the mesh rather than fixate it with one of these devices (Table 4.21). Surgeon preference and mesh selection will dictate the decision. One should consider the total length of these fasteners, as the depth of penetration will be dependent upon the thickness of the mesh used to repair the hernia. For example, a 5 mm fastener will provide no more of tissue penetration than 4 mm when used with 1 mm prosthesis. Additionally, there are significant differences in the types of "heads" these fasteners possess. The reader is referred to the specific manufacturer of these products for more indepth information. Additionally, this is an abbreviated list as many are not available in large areas of the world. Other sources are available that provide a more complete listing of these products [13].

AbsorbaTack is a 5 mm fixation device provides an absorbable synthetic polyester copolymer screw-like fastener derived from PGLA (Fig. 4.132). This device has a 3 cm degree of flex that is allowed to fire the fastener and has a metric scale on the

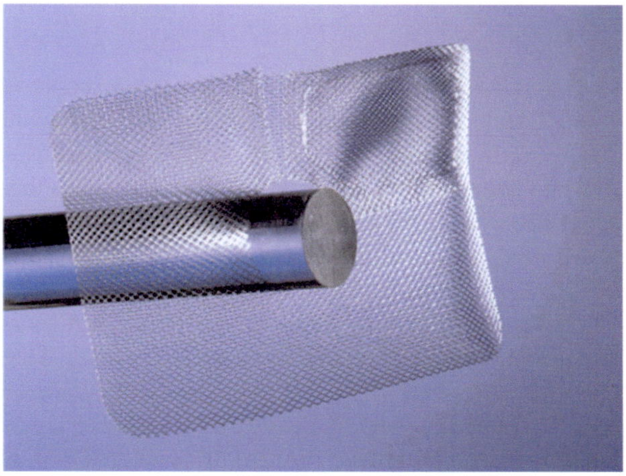

Fig. 4.131 TiSURE

Table 4.21 Fixation devices for hernia repair

AbsorbaTack, Medtronic, Minneapolis, MN, USA
CapSure, Davol, Inc., Warwick, RI, USA
FasTouch, Via Surgical, Tel Aviv, Israel
iMesh Tacker, Corregio (RE), Italy
Optifix, Davol. Inc., Warwick, RI, USA
PermaFix, Davol, Inc., Warwick, RI, USA
ProTack, Medtronic, Minneapolis, MN, USA
ReliaTack, Medtronic, Minneapolis, MN, USA
SecureStrap, Ethicon Inc., Somerville, NJ, USA
SorbaFix, Davol, Inc., Warwick, RI, USA

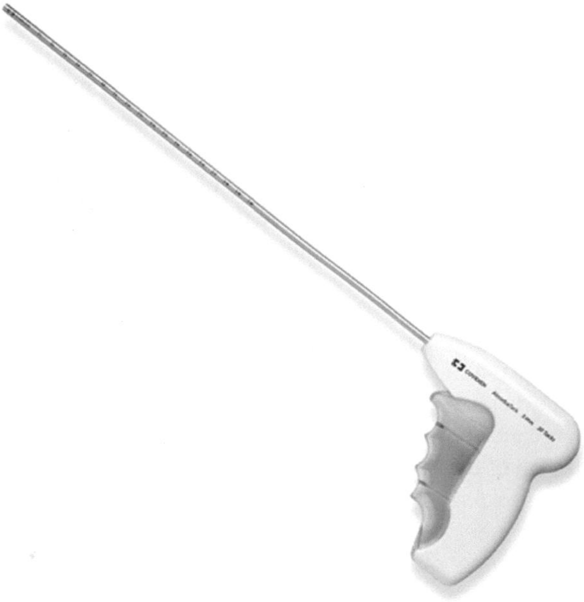

Fig. 4.132 AbsorbaTack (All rights reserved; used with permission of Medtronic, Inc.)

shaft. It measures 5.1 mm in length. The laparoscopic version is available with either 15 or 30 tacks. The tacks are significantly absorbed within 3–5 months with complete absorption within one year. *CapSure* is a permanent product, which has a smooth polyetheretherketone (PEEK) cap and screw theads that are made of 316 L stainless steel. The iMesh tack is also an absorbable PGLA device. It has a depth of purchase of 5.2 mm. Available information states that it has a large variety of loads of 10, 15, 20, 25, 30, or 38 tacks. The tip of the delivery device can articulate up to 60°.

FasTouch is a unique 5 mm device in that it does not employ any of the screw-like fasteners listed in this section (Fig. 4.133). It delivers a suture-like closed "locked" loop (Fig. 4.134). Its shape and size delivers the lowest amount of foreign body to fixate the mesh than any other available product [14]. The permanent fastener is made of poly-carbonate-urethane (PCU). There is also an absorbable

Fig. 4.133 CapSure

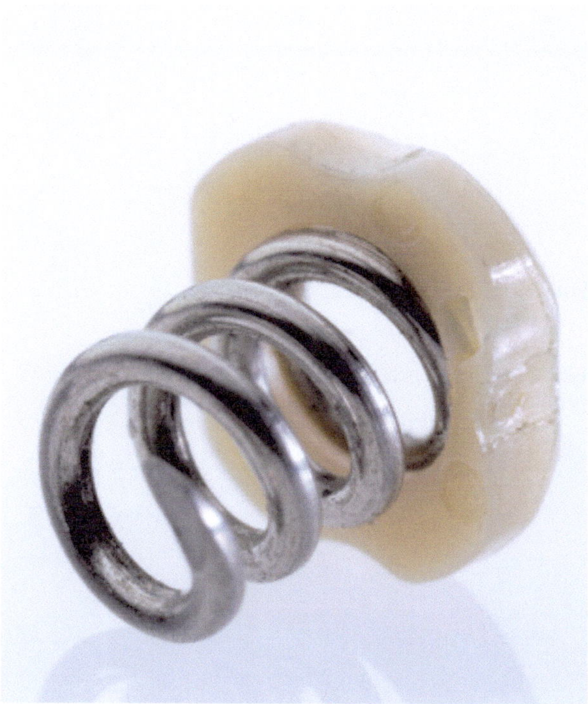

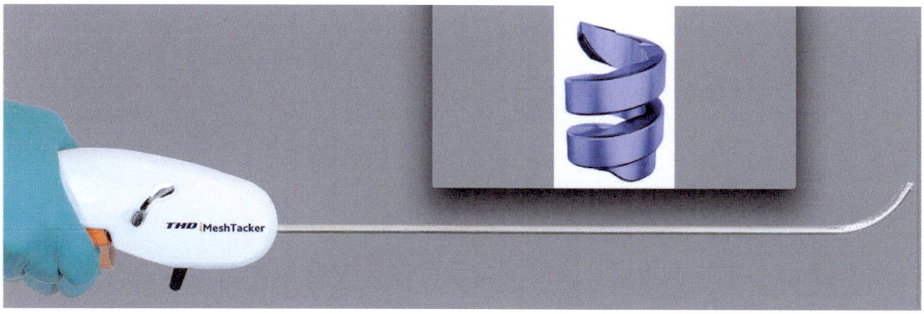

Fig. 4.134 iMesh tacker

version of this device that is made of a co-polymer of L-lactide and glycolide (Fig. 4.135). They can be reloaded with either a 10 or 25 reload.

The *OptiFix* device delivers a poly (D, L)–lactide (PDLLA) fastener that has two barbs on the end of it and two on the shaft (Figs. 4.136 and 4.137). They are delivered over an introducer needle. This product is available in either a 15 or 30 shot shaft. These fasteners are fully absorbed at 16 months. *PermaFix* and *SorbaFix* each deliver the same size (6.7 mm) screw-type fasteners by an identical delivery mechanism with a pilot tip and mandrel (Figs. 4.138 and 4.139). Both of these fasteners are available in either 15 or 30 devices delivered via a 5 mm product. Permafix is

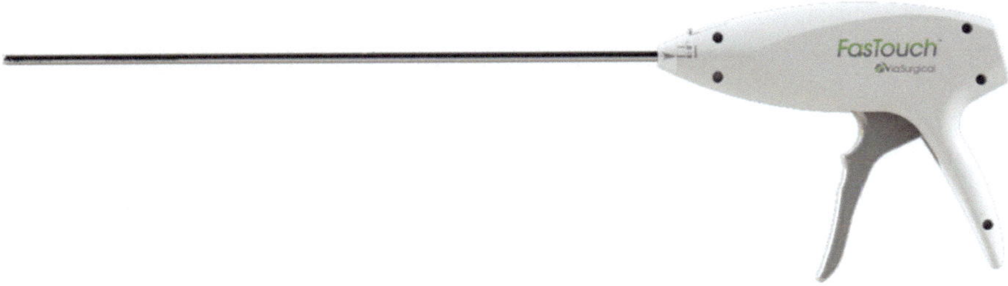

Fig. 4.135 FasTouch

Fig. 4.136 FasTouch permanent

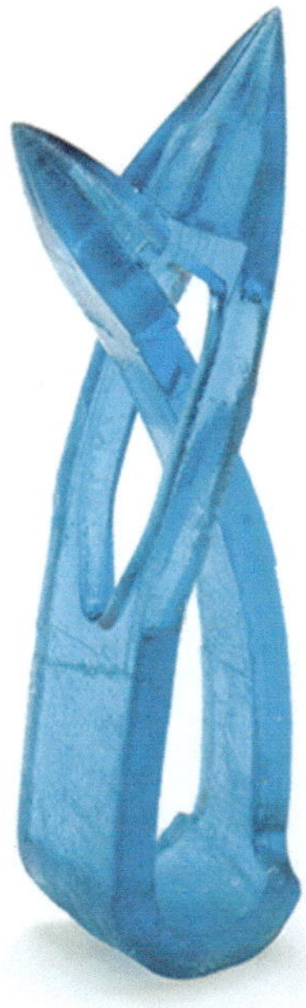

made of a grey molded permanent (nonabsorbable) polymer. SorbaFix is made of the same purple absorbable material as OptiFix.

The *ProTack* is one of the older products that delivers a permanent titanium helical fastener by a 5 mm device that is available with 30 tacks (Fig. 4.140). These are the easiest fixation products to visualize on a plain radiologic study. They are 3.9 mm in total length. *ReliaTack* is an articulating 5 mm device that also delivers a similar screw like absorbable tack (Fig. 4.141). It can be reloaded with a cartridge that contains either 5 or 10 fasteners. It is supplied with either a standard 5.1 mm device or the deep purchase tack that is 7.0 mm in length

Fig. 4.137 FasTouch absorbable

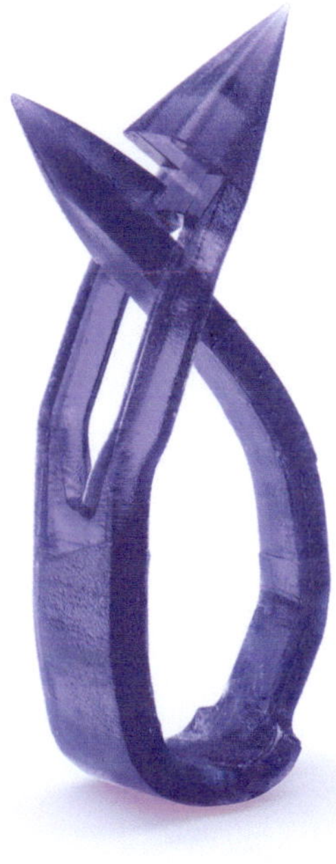

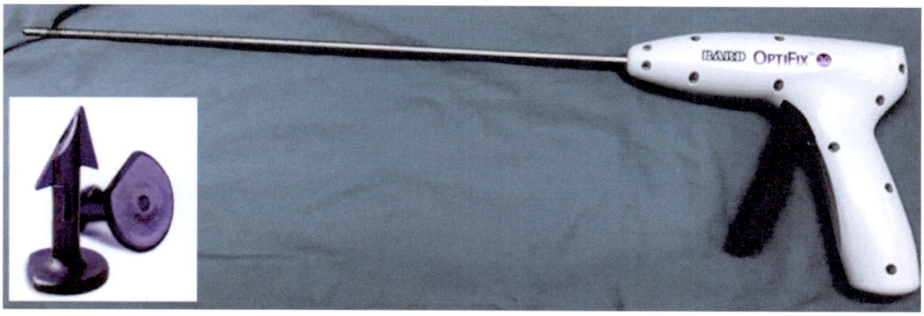

Fig. 4.138 Optifix

(Fig. 4.142). It is the only fastener that is available with two different lengths of tacks from which to choose.

The *SECURESTRAP* is pre-loaded with *25* absorbable straps (Fig. 4.143). The straps are composed of a blend of polydioxanone and L(-)-lactide and glycolide dyed with D&C Violet No. 2. This product does not screw into the tissues and has two legs similar to the staplers. The ends of these straps are barbed to aid in fixation. The width between the points is 3.5 mm. The entire devices length is 6.7 mm but the distance from the inner portion of the strap to the point of fixation of the strap is 4.9 mm (i.e. the “grip”).

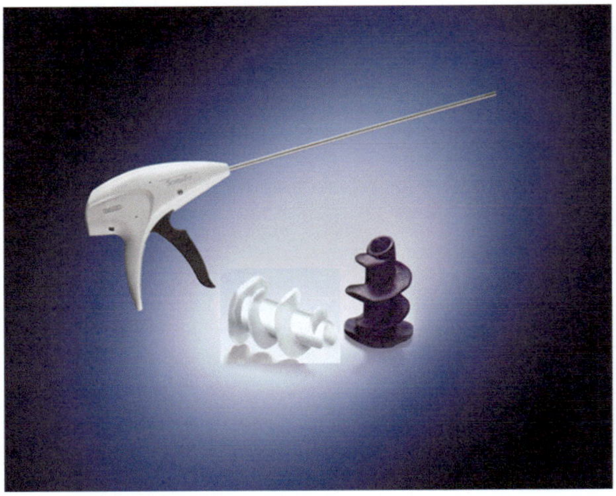

Fig. 4.139 SorbaFix and PermaFix

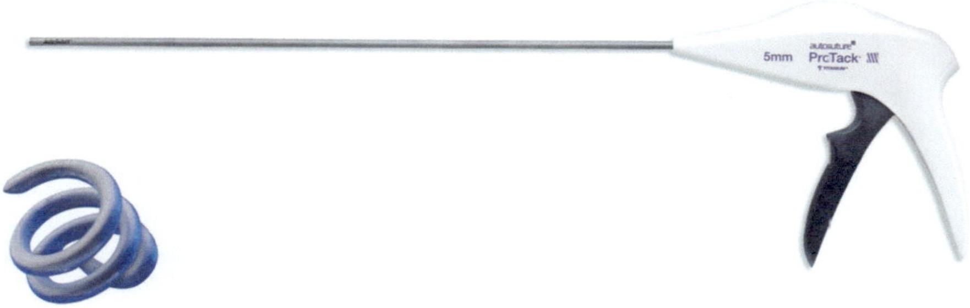

Fig. 4.140 ProTack (All rights reserved; used with permission of Medtronic, Inc.)

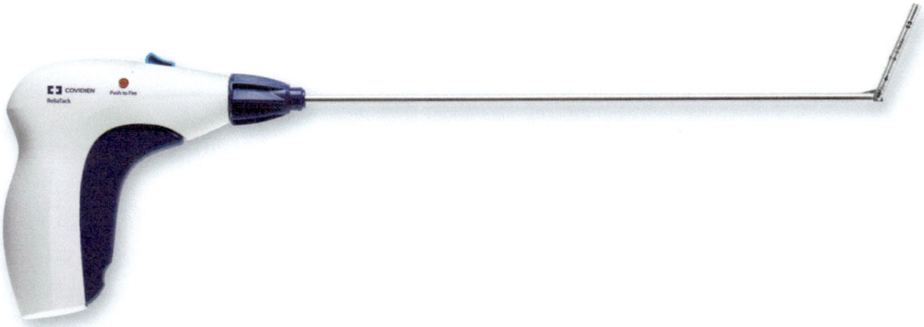

Fig. 4.141 ReliaTack (All rights reserved; used with permission of Medtronic, Inc.)

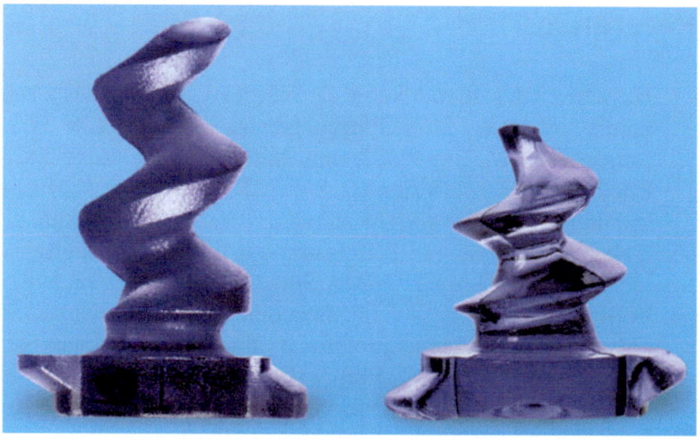

Fig. 4.142 ReliaTack standard and deep purchase (All rights reserved; used 0Medtronic, Inc.)

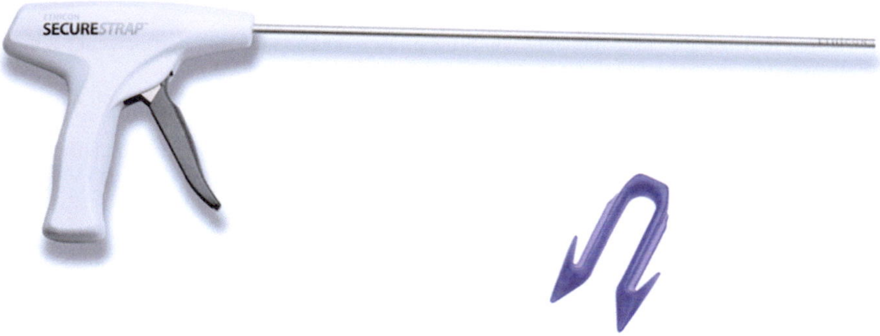

Fig. 4.143 SECURESTRAP (Image courtesy of Ethicon, Inc.)

4.16 Conclusion

The use of a prosthetic material for all hernia repairs is generally considered the standard of care when using the surgical robot unless there are extenuating circumstances. The purpose of this chapter is to identify and differentiate the products that can be used in hernioplasties. It is as complete as I could deliver but by the time of the printing of this textbook others may have become available.

I believe that the ideal material has not yet been developed. There are, however, many that have been described above that do function quite well for the surgeon and the patient. Perhaps in the future, the use of genetic engineering will produce a product that is based from the protein of the patient and will allow the patient to incorporate a "natural" and "native" product into the tissues without fear of infection or adhesions. A permanent solution to the quest of the perfect biomaterial may be the result.

Acknowledgement I want to acknowledge to the reader that all manufacturer names and products are either registered trademarks, copyrighted or exclusive to that company. These cannot be used without the permission of the respective company. Although not all of the figures have stated this, I wish to thank all of these companies for their invaluable assistance in putting the most accurate information into this chapter that I could not have obtained without their assistance.

References

1. Hesselink VJ, Luiiendijk RW, de Wilt JHW, Heide R. An evaluation of risk factors in incisional hernia recurrence. Surg Gynecol Obstet. 1993;176:228–34.
2. Luijendijk RW, Hop WCJ, van den Tol P, de Lange DC, Braaksma MM, IJzermans JN, Boelhouwer RU, de Vries BC, Salu MK, Wereldsma JC, Bruijninckx CM, Jeekel J. A comparison of suture repair with mesh repair for incisinoal hernia. N Engl J Med. 2000;34(6):393–8.
3. Kokotovic D, Bisgaard T, Helgstrand F. Long-term recurrence and complications with elective incisional hernia repair. JAMA Surg. 2016;316(15):1575–82.
4. LeBlanc KA, Booth WV. Laparoscopic repair of incisional abdominal hernias using expanded polytetrafluoroethylene: preliminary findings. Surg Laparosc Endosc. 1993;3:39–41.
5. Gonzales A, Escobar E, Romero R, Walker G, Mejias J, Gallas M, Dickens E, Johnson CJ, Rabaza J, Kudsi OY. Robotic-assisted ventral hernia repair: a multicenter evaluation of clinical outcomes. Surg Endosc. 2017;31(3):1342–9.
6. Bucknall TE, Cox PJ, Ellis H. Burst abdomen and incisional hernia: a prospective study of 1129 major laparotomies. BMJ. 1982;284:931–3.
7. Goepel R. Uber die verschliersung von bruchpforten durch einleilung gerflochtener fertiger silberdrahtnetze. Verh Deutsch Ges Pathol. 1900;29:4.
8. Kirschner M. Die praktischen Ergebnisse der freien Fascien-Tranaplantation. Arch Klin Chir. 1910;92:888–912.
9. Cumberland O. Ueber die Verschliessung von Bauchwunden und Brustpforten durch Bersenkte Siberdragrnetze. Zentralbl Chir. 1900;27:257.
10. Scales JT. Discussion on metals and synthetic materials in relation to soft tissues: tissue reactions to synthetic materials. Proc R Soc Med. 1953;46:647.
11. Kalaba S, Gerhard E, Winder JS, Pauli EM, Haluck RS, Yang J. Design strategies and applications of biomaterials and devices for hernia repair. Bioact Mater. 2016:2–17.
12. Rosen MJ, Bauer JJ, Harmaty M, Carbonell AM, Cobb WS, Matthews B, Goldblatt MI, Selzer DJ, Poulose BK, Hansson BME, Rosman C, Chao JJ, Jacobsen GR. Multicenter, prospective longitudinal study of the recurrence, surgical site infection, and quality of life after contaminated ventral hernia repair using biosynthetic absorbable mesh. Ann Surg. 2017;265:205–11.
13. LeBlanc KA. Prostheses and products for hernioplasty. In: LeBlanc KA, Kingsnorth AN, Sanders D, editors. Management of abdominal wall hernias. 5th ed. Springer; 2018. p. 109–172.
14. Cook T, LeBlanc KA. Fixation tacks add significant weight to hernia repair. SAGES Annual Meeting, Boston, MA, March 16–19; 2016.

5 Algorithm of Open/Laparoscopic/Robotic Repair

Archana Ramaswamy

Inguinal and ventral hernias are common complaints with a lifetime incidence of developing an inguinal hernia estimated at 30% for men. Umbilical and incisional hernias are also relatively common in men and women with an incidence of 10–20%.

The surgical treatment of hernias was first described with some success for inguinal hernias with the Bassini repair in 1887 [1]. Polypropylene mesh was introduced in the 1950s, and laparoscopic repair in the 1990s. Similarly, umbilical and incisional hernia repair techniques have evolved, from tissue repair to muscle release to prosthetic reinforcement [2]. Since introduction of the first robotic system in the 2000s, the procedures for abdominal wall reconstruction have been progressing to include additional minimally invasive approaches.

5.1 Inguinal Hernia

5.1.1 Indications for Repair

Patients with symptomatic inguinal hernias are routinely offered surgical repair, unless there are significant medical comorbidities where the risks potentially outweigh the benefits. It had been common practice to offer repair to all patients with an inguinal hernia, due to the concerns of development of incarceration and the risks of emergent surgery. However, as 30% of individuals present with minimally symptomatic or asymptomatic hernias, this traditional dogma was challenged and watchful waiting has been studied as an option for men with unilateral inguinal hernias.

The outcomes of the study performed in North America demonstrated a 32% crossover rate to surgery at 3.2 years and an estimated cumulative crossover rate of 68% at 10 years [3]. A UK study demonstrated similar outcomes with a crossover

A. Ramaswamy (✉)
University of Minnesota, Minneapolis VA Medical Center, Minneapolis, MN, USA
e-mail: ramaswam@umn.edu

K. A. LeBlanc (ed.), *Robotic Assisted Hernia Repair*,
https://doi.org/10.1007/978-3-030-23025-8_5

rate of 72% at 7.5 years [4]. Crossover rates seem to be higher in the older age group and the risks of emergent operation in the observation group were low. Policy change in the UK did result in slightly different outcomes compared with the randomized studies. There was a significantly higher rate of emergency operation (5.5% vs 3.6%), in addition to a higher rate of complications (18.5% vs 4.7%) and mortality (5.4% vs 0.1%) following emergency operation [5].

Recently, a study of watchful waiting from the Netherlands noted a crossover rate of 35% at 24 months [6], similar to the early outcomes from the North American and UK studies. It is important to note that the majority of the randomized population in all these studies comprise those who sought consultation for their inguinal hernia. Watchful waiting may have a higher success rate in an unselected population. A meta-analysis of the 3 studies notes lower pain scores on follow-up with surgical groups compared with the observation group [7].

Chronic pain has been recognized as being an important outcome measure and increased preoperative and postoperative acute pain scores have been shown to predict higher chronic pain scores [8]. Further studies will be required to elucidate whether watchful waiting leads to higher chronic pain prevalence. The findings of these studies highlight the need for shared decision making by improving patient health care literacy.

5.1.2 Inguinal Preoperative Imaging

The diagnosis of an inguinal hernia is most commonly made via physical exam. However, imaging of the groin is increasingly performed both prior to surgical referral, and in cases of equivocal physical exam findings. High accuracy has been noted with dynamic ultrasound with sensitivity and specificity rates over 95% [9, 10]. Ultrasonic studies can also identify other sources of inguinal pathology which are less common, such as undescended testicles, round ligament varicosities, and malignancies, to name a few [11–13].

CT scan may be a primary screening tool or may be chosen if ultrasound is nondiagnostic. CT is often performed with a Valsalva maneuver, though this does require some level of patient compliance. Another option is to proceed with a prone CT, which has been demonstrated to have higher sensitivity rates when compared with supine CT, both in the imaging of clinically detectable (100% vs 65%) and occult hernias (86% vs 34%) [14].

Preoperative imaging can be useful in assessing inguinal hernias in circumstances including groin pain without evidence of a protrusion, and where there are concerns of loss of domain. Herniography, which has demonstrated acceptable accuracy [15], is rarely used currently due to the availability, and accuracy, of the noninvasive modalities.

There is some suggestion that MRI may be the modality of choice (sensitivity: 0.91) when investigating an occult hernia in a highly selected referral population with a high proportion of women, since CT and US may both have low sensitivity (033 and 0.54 respectively) is this group [16].

5.1.3 Operative Approach

Inguinal hernias can be repaired via open or laparoscopic techniques. The open approach includes mesh and non-mesh repairs, and the laparoscopic approach includes the totally extraperitoneal (TEP) or transabdominal preperitoneal (TAPP) techniques. The use of robotics in inguinal hernia has generally been reserved for the transabdominal preperitoneal (rTAPP) technique. Mesh is routinely used in open hernia repairs, and studies suggest that it has halved the recurrence rate, in addition to decreasing neurovascular injuries, and operative times [17].

There has been an increasing interest in non-mesh hernia repairs over the last few years, with the Shouldice repair often touted as the gold standard of non-mesh hernia repair. Though low recurrence rates have been demonstrated in patients undergoing inguinal hernia repair at the Shouldice clinic [18], a Cochrane review of the Shouldice technique demonstrated a lower recurrence rate compared with other non-mesh hernia repairs, but a higher recurrence rate than with mesh hernia repairs [19]. This likely reflects the improved outcomes in a selected population undergoing a procedure in a specialized hospital (Shouldice Clinic). The Desarda non-mesh inguinal hernia repair technique is being increasingly discussed, but there is little data available regarding long term results. Short term outcomes appear to be similar to Lichtenstein in meta-analyses and systematic reviews [20, 21].

5.1.4 Laparoscopic Inguinal Hernia Repairs

Laparoscopic inguinal hernia repairs have been performed for over 20 years. Even though both TEP and TAPP procedures conclude in the placement of mesh in the preperitoneal space, access to the space varies significantly. The comparison of studies examining laparoscopic and open repair of inguinal hernias have demonstrated low recurrence rates in experienced hands.

The majority of studies demonstrate similar recurrence rates when TEP and TAPP are compared, leading the International Endohernia Society to conclude that they are both effective methods [22]. It is important to note however, that, even though recurrence rates of TAPP and open repair are similar, there is some suggestion that TEP has a higher recurrence rate compared with open repair. This has been noted in both a meta-analysis [23] and national hernia registry [24]. The higher recurrence rates of TEP likely demonstrate the significant learning curve associated with this procedure. This learning curve, in addition to the lack of familiarity with preperitoneal anatomy and endoscopic suturing, have likely contributed to the low adoption rates of TEP and TAPP. Estimates of utilization of minimally invasive techniques have remained low with recent reports of 8–48% [25, 26]. The mean rates have hovered around 20–30%.

Robotic inguinal hernia repair is most commonly laparoscopic TAPP (rTAPP) performed with the use of robotic arms. The technique is unchanged, but the improved visualization, ergonomics, and ease of suturing have made this an attractive tool to increase adoption rates of minimally invasive techniques for inguinal hernia repair. There is insufficient data at this time to identify any clear differences in outcomes between laparoscopic TAPP and rTAPP. For most of the discussion below, the comments relating to a laparoscopic approach, also apply to the robotic assisted laparoscopic approach.

As we have noted that several approaches provide relatively similar outcomes in experienced hands, the choice of procedure is dependent on surgeon expertise and must be tailored to the specific circumstances of the patient.

5.1.5 Bilateral Hernias

There seems to be little debate that bilateral inguinal hernias are better approached with laparoscopy when expertise is available [27], with the expectation of decreased post-operative pain and complications, with higher quality adjusted life years (QALY) at 1 year [28].

5.1.6 Obesity

When obesity is associated with a thick abdominal wall, this can make open, TEP and TAPP procedures more complex. Open hernia repair may require larger incisions and require a longer operative time due to the amount of tissue than needs to be divided and retracted to access the inguinal canal. TEP can also be more complex as laparoscopic instrument mobility may be limited. Difficulties with TAPP may occur as the abdominal wall may limit angulation of the instruments when closing the peritoneum. The extra degrees of freedom with robotic instruments can be helpful when approaching inguinal hernia repair in the obese patient.

5.1.7 Anticoagulated Patients

The number of patients receiving anticoagulation or antiplatelet medications seems to be constantly increasing. When the medication can be stopped perioperatively for several days, the risks of bleeding should be unchanged compared with the general population. In those who require early resumption of anticoagulation, the options should be considered in more depth. The available studies suggest that hematomas are less common in minimally invasive repairs compared with open repairs, though there is little information about clinically significant hematomas requiring intervention [27]. It is important to consider the fact that bleeding after anterior repairs is likely to be limited due to the confined space, however, preperitoneal bleeding may take longer to tamponade due to either extension into the peritoneal cavity or into the retroperitoneal space. This may lead to more clinically significant bleeding even if the chance of bleeding is decreased with minimally invasive repairs.

5.1.8 Medical Comorbidities

Open inguinal hernia repairs can be performed under general anesthesia, though the majority are likely performed under local anesthesia with or without the use of moderate or deep sedation. TAPP and TEP repairs are routinely performed under general anesthesia, though there are a few reports of both being successfully performed with regional anesthesia [29, 30]. In patients with significant comorbidities, where general anesthesia or pneumoperitoneum could lead to decompensation of chronic severe medical conditions, open hernia repair under local anesthesia should be strongly considered.

5.1.9 Women

Inguinal hernias are less frequently seen in women. The most common subtype is indirect inguinal, though femoral hernias are more frequently noted in women, and frequently not diagnosed preoperatively. At reoperation, a femoral hernia has been the noted as the "recurrence" in 30–40% when the initial direct or indirect hernia has been approached in an open fashion [31]. This leads us to question whether female gender is actually a risk factor for recurrence [32], or whether this is acting as a proxy for missed femoral hernias. There are no studies which examine the safety of watchful waiting in women, and it is not recommended.

5.1.10 Femoral Hernias

Femoral hernias may present as a protrusion on the anterior thigh, but, may also be difficult to discern on physical exam and imaging studies. Watchful waiting is not recommended as the chance of incarceration and need for bowel resection during emergent operation are higher compared with inguinal hernias. Open anterior repair is likely to miss a femoral hernia when a standard Lichtenstein repair is utilized. A femoral hernia can be repaired from a groin incision if the floor of the canal is opened and a preperitoneal repair is performed. This is not commonly performed, and many surgeons are unfamiliar with an open preperitoneal inguinal hernia repair. A minimally invasive approach is the method of choice as all hernias within the myopectineal orifice can be addressed with a standard dissection.

5.1.11 Preperitoneal Mesh/Lower Midline Surgery

Prior surgical procedures that required a lower midline incision can make inguinal hernia repair from a posterior approach more challenging. Intra-abdominal adhesions may need to be lysed prior to entering the preperitoneal space during a TAPP, and previous dissection in the preperitoneal space may have resulted in a significantly scarred space making further access complicated. Preperitoneal mesh can also render the space difficult to dissect, and therefore, the benefits of a minimally invasive operative approach may be limited due to longer operative times and risk of vascular and visceral injury. Though there are reports of using TEP to approach recurrent hernias following previous preperitoneal mesh [33], it is likely not the most expeditious approach in most surgeons' hands. Inability to create the space, adherent epigastric vessels, and large peritoneal tears are just some of the pitfalls. A recurrence following an initial laparoscopic repair can be safely approached with an open repair. If a laparoscopic repair is desired in specific situations, such as with bilateral hernias or a multiply recurrent hernia with both anterior and posterior mesh present, then a TAPP approach would be recommended to avoid the need for balloon dissection and allow a larger working space. Most robotically trained surgeons find the use of the robotic technology especially advantageous in these situations.

5.1.12 Scrotal/Nonreducible Hernia

The limited working space during a TEP can make the reduction of the scrotal hernia sac, or the reduction of visceral contents from a nonreducible hernia, much more challenging. It is often easier to approach these with either an open approach, or via the TAPP method [34].

5.1.13 Summary

Outcomes for inguinal hernia repair are strongly linked to surgeon expertise. In a healthy man with a symptomatic unilateral inguinal hernia, without any previous lower abdominal surgery, surgeons should proceed with the technique that they perform most frequently. As an increasing number of patients fall outside of the circumstances discussed above, it increases the need for the hernia surgeon to be comfortable with various methods of inguinal hernia repair. As the increasing adoption of the robotic technology proceeds, it is anticipated that there will be continued increased use of the rTAPP by more surgeons. Figures 5.1 and 5.2 summarize the points discussed above.

5.1.14 Ventral/Incisional Hernia

Ventral/Incisional hernias comprise a heterogenous group of abdominal wall defects from small umbilical hernias, to large incisional hernias and those located in atypical locations. The approach to the patient and their hernia need to tailored to both patient goals and to their comorbidities. The treatment of incisional hernias is costly, with an estimate of $3.2 billion in the US in 2006 [35]. More recently, it has been

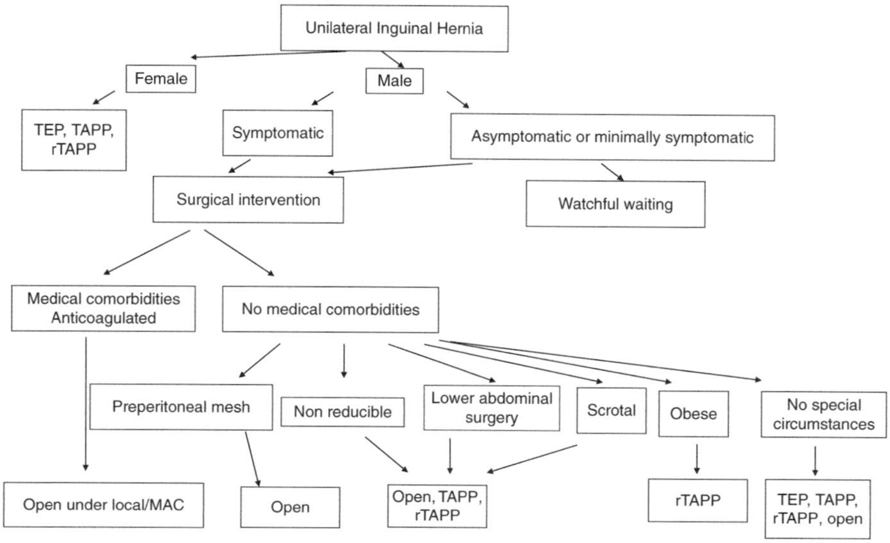

Fig. 5.1 Algorithm for the approach to unilateral inguinal hernias

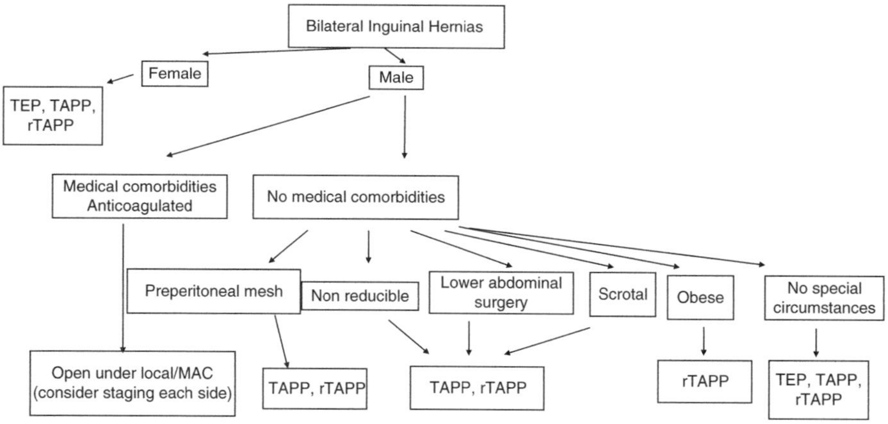

Fig. 5.2 Algorithm for the approach to bilateral inguinal hernias

estimated that over $17.5 million are being spent on hernia repair and its complications in a population of 12,000 patients undergoing elective abdominal surgery with a 3.5% incisional hernia rate [36]. Recognition of the costs and the high recurrence rates in population based studies [37] has increased interest in identification of the high risk populations and improving surgical technique in abdominal wall closure. As research continues from a prevention standpoint, the surgeon's armamentarium grows with options for repair from open to minimally invasive techniques.

5.1.15 Indication for Repair

Similar to the inguinal hernia patient population, most individuals with symptomatic ventral hernias are offered repair if they are medically fit. Watchful waiting for the asymptomatic or minimally symptomatic patient has thus far identified a need for urgent intervention of 4% of patients in longitudinal studies with follow-up of up to 5 years [38, 39]. The observation group also demonstrated a crossover rate of under 20% to surgery with similar outcomes from delayed surgery as those who underwent surgery at the outset. It is concerning, however, that when patients are placed in the observation group due to comorbidities or obesity, there seems to be a higher rate of urgent repair. In one study where 50% of the study group were placed in the observation group for the indications mentioned above, there was a 25% need for urgent repair, with a higher complication and mortality in this group [40].

It is unclear what the overall costs to the system would be when balancing the cost of surgery, emergency surgery or continued observation, with the savings associated with the avoidance of surgery. There is some concern that there might be higher healthcare utilization and days away from work in those who are being observed [41]. A randomized study is in the recruitment phase and should provide more information regarding the natural history of minimally symptomatic ventral hernias [42].

5.1.16 Preoperative Imaging

Preoperative imaging is not mandatory prior to ventral hernia repair [43], however, can be helpful in the following situations:

- Morbid obesity- the fascial defect may not be readily palpable
- Complex ventral hernias- large defects, with associated enterocutaneous fistulas or previous mesh [44]
- Concerns for loss of domain
- Atypical locations- to identify the extent of fascial defects and/or identification of muscular laxity

Radiologic imaging studies can help guide preoperative and operative planning. The component separation methods or injection of botulinum toxin into the lateral portions of the abdominal flat muscles may be considered for large defects (Chaps. 15 and 24). Additionally, the use of preoperative pneumoperitoneum may be considered for loss of domain (Chap. 14).

5.1.17 Prehabilitation

The vicious cycle of hernia repair to surgical site infection to readmission(s) and hernia recurrence needs to broken [45]. There are various risk stratification tools available to predict recurrence and postoperative complications, though only a few have been externally validated, and are likely used only in a limited fashion when making decisions with patients on a daily basis [46]. Several risk factors, however, are commonly noted in the ventral hernia population. The comorbidities most often encountered include obesity, malnutrition, uncontrolled diabetes, and smoking.

Obesity has been associated with a risk of recurrence following hernia repair of over 30%. Prehabilitation with weight loss goals within a structured program prior to hernia repair, in those with a BMI of 30–40, has been shown to have a lower rate of early complications and recurrence, but with a higher rate of a requirement for emergent hernia repair [47]. If medically supervised weight loss is unsuccessful, weight loss surgery prior to hernia repair is a viable option.

Smoking is associated with poor oxygenation at the surgical site and is associated with increased complications. Smoking cessation prior to a complex or recurrent hernia repair should likely be mandatory when clinically feasible. A four week time period is probably adequate based upon research that has demonstrated that four weeks of abstinence from smoking leads to similar wound healing as longer periods of abstinence [48].

Perioperative blood glucose control is important to decrease the risk of surgical site infection and other complications. A frequent "hard stop" for elective surgery is a hemoglobin A1c of 8 or greater. While this is important, there should also be a focus on the maintenance of euglycemia both intraoperatively and postoperatively.

Malnutrition has been noted to be present in up to 30% of patients undergoing elective gastrointestinal surgery [49]. Malnutrition can be assessed via routinely used nutritional parameters, recent weight loss, and other indices. Recently, there has been increasing interest in using sarcopenia, a depletion of lean skeletal muscle mass, to assess malnutrition. It may identify nutritional status better than acute phase reactants, and is a precursor to frailty. Sarcopenia is associated with long term morbidity and mortality at 30 days to 1–3 years [50].

Sarcopenia measurements, defined mainly within the oncology population, may not be applicable to hernia patients. A study of patients undergoing ventral hernia repair failed to note an increased complication rate in the sarcopenic patients, who comprised almost 30% of their study population [51]. Decreasing muscle mass was associated with an increasing complication rate, but more research is necessary to identify the utility of sarcopenia in this patient population. Nutritional supplementation should be instituted prior to elective hernia repair when necessary.

When making decisions with patients who have risk factors which are non-modifiable, or where symptoms do not allow the time frame to address the comorbidities, it is important to tailor procedures and set patient expectations appropriately.

5.1.18 Operative Approach

The methods of hernia repair vary mainly with the position of mesh and whether the hernia defect is closed. The Rives Stoppa repair has been considered the gold standard for hernia repair for many years. Various nomenclature has been used to describe mesh position. For the purposes of this chapter, *inlay* describes mesh sutured to the defect edges, *onlay* describes mesh overlying the anterior rectus sheath, and intraperitoneal onlay (IPOM) refers to barrier coated mesh being placed against the peritoneum with adequate overlap of mesh onto healthy fascia. Retrorectus mesh placement is self-explanatory, though the mesh placement may extend into the preperitoneal space if the repair requires more complex techniques such as transversus abdominis release to achieve fascial closure. Complete preperitoneal repairs are also performed and have become more popular with the utilization of robotic technology which has enabled the performance of transabdominal preperitoneal repairs (TAPP).

Inlay repairs have been generally been abandoned. Onlay repairs may be a good option when a hostile abdominal cavity is expected and the retrorectus space is difficult to access. Various techniques for component separation have been described, with the current interest being focused on transversus abdominis release (TAR). Open hernia repair allows the choice of all of the above techniques. The traditional laparoscopic ventral hernia repair (LVHR) did not include closure of the hernia defect (referred to as bridging the defect) and placement of intraperitoneal mesh. Closure of the hernia defect was adopted by some during LVHR, using either transfascial suture placement or intracorporeal suturing methods. The introduction of robotic technology and wristed instruments has allowed surgeons easier access to the preperitoneal and retrorectus space to be able to transition from open to minimally invasive abdominal wall reconstruction. As the focus of ventral hernia repair has gravitated toward midline closure and complex abdominal wall reconstruction, it is important to note that bridging techniques still have a role. Identification of high risk patients and selection of bridging hernia repairs for these individuals can help ensure similar post-operative complications as those noted in low risk patients [52].

5.1.19 Mesh Utilization

Mesh has become a mainstay in the repair of ventral hernias, with studies demonstrating a reduction in recurrence rates [53] even in small umbilical hernias over 1 cm in size [54]. As materials have evolved over time, surgeons have increased the use of mesh designed for intra-abdominal placement, even for open repair, due to ease of placement. Even though there is no evidence of high rates of mesh related complications in the randomized studies of suture versus mesh repair, the importance of prosthetic materials is paramount in these repairs. The follow-up in these studies has been variable, with many being limited to 12 months [55]. The long term safety of intraperitoneal mesh has been increasingly questioned with case reports of complications caused by mesh constructs [56]. Concern has also been raised that as reoperation rates for recurrence decrease, reintervention rates for mesh related complications is increasing [53]. However, the study of mesh locations for the repair of these hernias needs further evaluation to elucidate these data points.

When open repair with intraperitoneal mesh is compared with laparoscopic IPOM, it is not surprising to note that open repair is associated with longer operative times, complication rates, surgical site infections, and hospital stay [57], without any difference in recurrence rates at 5 years [58].

5.1.20 Defect Closure in LVHR

Bridging the defect in LVHR has been blamed for post-operative seroma development, mesh eventration and even for some recurrences. Closure of the defect with either transfascial externally placed sutures or with intracorporeal suturing has been described [59, 60]. A recent meta-analysis did identify lower seroma rates, in addition to lower complication rates and hospital stay, when defect closure was employed [61]. Other studies have failed to confirm an early benefit in outcomes [62] but a recent study published from the Danish Hernia database did demonstrate decreased reoperation for hernia recurrence in the cohort where defect closure was performed in addition to permanent tack fixation [63]. The available data is relatively inconclusive and has led some to close all defects, while others close only slightly larger defects, and many surgeons don't close any defects. More research is needed to allow surgeons to understand the best method to manage these options.

When defect size is considered when making a choice between operative techniques, recommendations in guidelines from several societies suggest that laparoscopic IPOM be limited to hernias which are less than 10 cm in size. This stems from findings of increased complexity of repair of these larger hernias, in addition to increased recurrence rates [64, 65]. However, the advent of robotic technology has permitted the closure of defects that could not be done by standard laparoscopic methods. Again, more research needs to be done.

5.1.21 Outcomes of Robotic Repair

Data regarding the outcomes of robotics in ventral hernia repair are emerging, with mixed results. A New York State administrative database analysis from 2010 to 2013 demonstrated higher emergency room visits, complications, readmissions, and longer length of stay following robotic repair when compared with laparoscopic repair [66]. Analysis of the Vizient database also noted higher rates of complications and postoperative infections in robotic ventral hernia repairs compared with the laparoscopic repairs [67].

Analysis of data from the nationwide inpatient sample from 2008 to 2013 did not identify any differences in patient outcomes between robotic and laparoscopic ventral hernia repair, though there was an increase in cost with the use of robotic technology [68].

Data from the Americas Hernia Society Quality Collaborative does note a reduction in the length of stay with the use of robotics for retromuscular ventral hernia repair [69]. Similarly, a single institution retrospective review also noted a decrease in hospital stay following robotic TAR compared with open TAR [70].

Robotic technology has been anticipated to increase the adoption of MIS techniques in hernia- both for inguinal hernia, with the improved visualization and ergonomics, and for ventral hernia, with the ability to performed complex abdominal wall reconstruction previously performed with open methods. The limited published data has noted that, in the time period between 2008 and 2015, growth in robotic surgery paralleled a reduction in laparoscopic surgery for 5 general surgical procedures, including inguinal and ventral hernia repair. The conclusion from this data was that laparoscopic procedures were being converted to robotic procedures rather than conversion of open procedures to robotic procedures [71]. Another consideration is that the robotic methodology was approved for hernia repair in mid-2014, making this a technology that is still in clinical development.

5.2 Conclusion

It is difficult to create an algorithm for ventral hernia repair as expertise and opinion vary significantly, even among experts. In a study of five surgeons presented with case scenarios, there was consensus on decision to operate for 56% of the scenarios, consensus on operation type in 40%, and on mesh position in 40% [72]. Even situations where an open strategy seems like the most obvious choice (significant excess skin, bowel compromise, enterocutaneous fistula, previous skin graft, excision of a large piece of mesh), there still exist options for a minimally invasive approach, or with a hybrid approach. There are several options for each patient, (see Fig. 5.3) which highlights the importance of shared decision making. Future research will determine the algorithm for each surgeon and the patient.

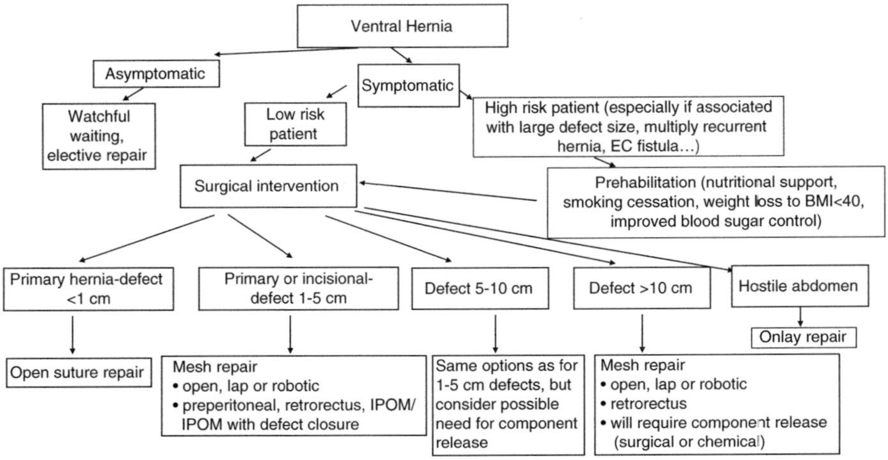

Fig. 5.3 Algorithm for the approach to ventral/incisional hernias

References

1. Bassini E. Nuovo metodo sulla cura radicale dell'ernia inguinale [New method for radical repair of inguinal hernia]. Arch Soc Ital Chir. 1887;4:80.
2. Basile F, Biondi A, Donati M. Surgical approach to abdominal wall defects: history and new trends. [Review]. Int J Surg. 2013;11(Suppl 1):S20–3.
3. Fitzgibbons RJ, Ramanan B, Arya S, et al. Long-term results of a randomized controlled trial of a nonoperative strategy (watchful waiting) for men with minimally symptomatic inguinal hernias. Ann Surg. 2013;258(3):508–15.
4. Chung L, Norrie J, O'Dwyer P. Long-term follow-up of patients with a painless inguinal hernia from a randomized clinical trial. Br J Surg. 2011;98:596–9.
5. Hwang M, Bhangu A, Webster C, Bowley D, Gannon M, Karandikar S. Unintended consequences of policy change to watchful waiting for asymptomatic inguinal hernias. Ann R Coll Surg Engl. 2014;96(5):343–7.
6. de Goede B, Wijsmuller AR, van Ramshorst GH, INCA Trialists' Collaboration, et al. Watchful waiting versus surgery of mildly symptomatic or asymptomatic inguinal hernia in men aged 50 years and older: a randomized controlled trial. Ann Surg. 2018;267(1):42–9.
7. Gonga W, Li J. Operation versus watchful waiting in asymptomatic or minimally symptomatic inguinal hernias: The meta-analysis results of randomized controlled trials. Int J Surg. 2018;52:120–5.
8. Hu QL, Chen DC. Approach to the patient with chronic groin pain. Surg Clin N Am. 2018;98(3):651–65.
9. Lee RKL, Griffith JF, Ng WHA. High accuracy of ultrasound in diagnosing the presence and type of groin hernia. J Clin Ultrasound. 2015;43:538–47.
10. Niebuhr H, König A, Pawlak M, Sailer M, Köckerling F, Reinpold W. Groin hernia diagnostics: dynamic inguinal ultrasound (DIUS). Langenbecks Arch Surg. 2017;402:1039–45.
11. Park HR, Park SB, Lee ES, Park HJ. Sonographic evaluation of inguinal lesions. Clin Imaging. 2016;40:949–55.
12. Revzin MV, Ersahin D, Israel GM, Kirsch JD, Mathur M, Bokhari J, Scoutt LM. US of the inguinal canal: comprehensive review of pathologic processes with CT and MR imaging correlation. Radiographics. 2016;36:2028–48.
13. Jacobson JA, Khoury V, Brandon CJ. Ultrasound of the groin: techniques, pathology, and pitfalls. Am J Roentgenol. 2015;205:513–23.
14. Miyaki A, Yamaguchi K, Kishibe S, Ida A, Miyauchi T, Naritaka Y. Diagnosis of inguinal hernia by prone- vs. supine-position computed tomography. Hernia. 2017;21:705–13.
15. Cohen R, Turkenburg J, Dalen AV. Herniography in 79 patients with unexplained pain in the groin: a retrospective study. Eur J Radiol. 1990;11:184–7.
16. Miller J, Cho J, Michael MJ, Saouaf R, Towfigh S. Role of imaging in the diagnosis of occult hernias. JAMA Surg. 2014;149:1077–80.
17. Lockhart K, Dunn D, Teo S, Ng JY, Dhillon M, Teo E, van Driel ML. Mesh versus non-mesh for inguinal and femoral hernia repair. Cochrane Database Syst Rev. 2018;(9):CD011517.
18. Malik A, Bell CM, Stukel TA, Urbach DR. Recurrence of inguinal hernias repaired in a large hernia surgical specialty hospital and general hospitals in Ontario, Canada. Can J Surg. 2016;59(1):19–25.
19. Amato B, Moja L, Panico S, Persico G, Rispoli C, Rocco N, Moschetti I. Shouldice technique versus other open techniques for inguinal hernia repair. Cochrane Database Syst Rev. 2012;(4):CD001543.
20. Emile SH, Elfeki H. Desarda's technique versus Lichtenstein technique for the treatment of primary inguinal hernia: a systematic review and meta-analysis of randomized controlled trials. [Review]. Hernia. 2018;22:385–95.
21. Ge H, Liang C, Xu Y, Ren S, Wu J. Desarda versus Lichtenstein technique for the treatment of primary inguinal hernia: A systematic review. [Review]. Int J Surg. 2018;50:22–7.
22. Bittner R, Montgomery MA, Arregui E, et al. Update of guidelines on laparoscopic (TAPP) and endoscopic (TEP) treatment of inguinal hernia (International Endohernia Society). Surg Endosc Other Interv Tech. 2015;29(2):289–321.

23. O'Reilly EA, Burke JP, O'Connell PR. A meta-analysis of surgical morbidity and recurrence after laparoscopic and open repair of primary unilateral inguinal hernia. Ann Surg. 2012;255:846–53.
24. Lundström KJ, Holmberg H, Montgomery A, Nordin P. Patient-reported rates of chronic pain and recurrence after groin hernia repair. BJS. 2018;105:106–12.
25. Trevisonno M, Kaneva P, Watanabe Y, Fried GM, Feldman LS, Andalib A, Vassiliou MC. Current practices of laparoscopic inguinal hernia repair: a population-based analysis. Hernia. 2015;19:725–33.
26. Vu JV, Gunaseelan V, Krapohl GL, Englesbe MJ, Campbell DA Jr, Dimick JB, Telem DA. Surgeon utilization of minimally invasive techniques for inguinal hernia repair: a population-based study. Surg Endosc. 2019;33(2):486–93.
27. The Hernia Surge Group. International guidelines for groin hernia management. Hernia. 2018;22(1):1–165.
28. Ielpo B, Nunez-Alfonsel J, Duran H, Diaz E, Fabra I, Caruso R, Malave L, Ferri V, Barzola E, Quijano Y, Vicente E. Cost-effectiveness of randomized study of laparoscopic versus open bilateral inguinal hernia repair. Ann Surg. 2018;268(5):725–30.
29. Tzovaras G, Symeonidis D, Koukoulis G, Baloyiannis I, Georgopoulou S, Pratsas C, Zacharoulis D. Long-term results after laparoscopic transabdominal preperitoneal (TAPP) inguinal hernia repair under spinal anesthesia. Hernia. 2012;16(6):641–5.
30. Baloyiannis I, Perivoliotis K, Sarakatsianou C, et al. Laparoscopic total extraperitoneal hernia repair under regional anesthesia: a systematic review of the literature. Surg Endosc. 2018;32:2184–92.
31. Burcharth J, Andresen K, Pommergaard H-C, Bisgaard T, Rosenberg J. Direct inguinal hernias and anterior surgical approach are risk factors for female inguinal hernia recurrences. Langenbeck's Arch Surg. 2014;399:71–6.
32. Burcharth J, Pommergaard H-C, Bisgaard T, Rosenberg J. Patient-related risk factors for recurrence after inguinal hernia repair: a systematic review and meta-analysis of observational studies. Surg Innov. 2015;22(3):303–17.
33. Ferzli GS, Khoury GE. Treating recurrence after a totally extraperitoneal approach. Hernia. 2006;10(4):341–6.
34. Siow SL, Mahendran HA, Hardin M, Chea CH, NikAzim NA. Laparoscopic transabdominal approach and its modified technique for incarcerated scrotal hernias. Asian J Surg. 2013;36(2):64–8.
35. Poulouse BK, Shelton J, Phillips S, et al. Epidemiology and cost of ventral hernia repair: making the case for hernia research. Hernia. 2012;16:179–83.
36. Fischer JP, Basta MN, Mirzabeigi MN, et al. A risk model and cost analysis of incisional hernia after elective, abdominal surgery based upon 12,373 cases: the case for targeted prophylactic intervention. Ann Surg. 2016;263(5):1010–7.
37. Flum DR, Horvath K, Koepsell T. Have outcomes of incisional hernia repair improved with time? A population-based analysis. Ann Surg. 2003;237(1):129–35.
38. Bellows CF, Robinson C, Fitzgibbons RJ, Webber LS, Berger DH. Watchful waiting for ventral hernias: a longitudinal study. Am Surg. 2014;80(3):245–52.
39. Kokotovic D, Sjolander H, Gogenur I, Helgstrand F. Watchful waiting as a treatment strategy for patients with a ventral hernia appears to be safe. Hernia. 2016;20(2):281–7.
40. Verhelst J, Timmermans L, van de Velde M, Jairam A, Vakalopoulos KA, Jeekel J, Lange JF. Watchful waiting in incisional hernia: is it safe? Surgery. 2015;157(2):297–303.
41. Strosberg DS, Pittman M, Mikami D. Umbilical hernias: the cost of waiting. Surg Endosc. 2017;31(2):901–6.
42. Lauscher JC, Martus P, Stroux A, Neudecker J, Behrens U, Hammerich R, Buhr HJ, Ritz JP. Development of a clinical trial to determine whether watchful waiting is an acceptable alternative to surgical repair for patients with oligosymptomatic incisional hernia: study protocol for a randomized controlled trial. Trials. 2012;13:14.
43. Bittner R, Bingener-Casey J, Dietz U, et al. Guidelines for the laparoscopic treatment of ventral and incisional abdominal wall hernias (International Endohernia Society (IEHS))—Part 1. Surg Endosc. 2013;28:2–29.

44. Halligan S, Parker SG, Plumb AA, Windsor ACJ. Imaging complex ventral hernias, their surgical repair, and their complications. Eur Radiol. 2018;28:3560–9.
45. Joslyn NA, Esmonde NO, Martindale RG, Hansen J, Khansa I, Janis JE. Evidence-based strategies for the prehabilitation of the abdominal wall reconstruction patient. Plast Reconstr Surg. 2018;142:21S–9S.
46. Bernardi K, Adrales GL, Hope WW, Keith J, Kuhlens H, Martindale RG, Melin AA, Orenstein SB, Roth JS, Shah SK, Tsuda S, Liang MK. Abdominal wall reconstruction risk stratification tools: a systematic review of the literature. Plast Reconstr Surg. 2018;142:9S–20S.
47. Liang MK, Bernardi K, Holihan JL, Cherla DV, Escamilla R, Lew DF, Berger DH, Ko TC, Kao LS. Modifying risks in ventral hernia patients with prehabilitation: a randomized controlled trial. Ann Surg. 2018;268(4):674–80.
48. Sorensen LT, Karlsmark T, Gottrup F. Abstinence from smoking reduces incisional wound infection: a randomized controlled trial. Ann Surg. 2003;238:1–5.
49. Ho JWC, Wu AHW, Lee MWK, Lau S, Lam P, Lau W, Kwok SSS, Kwan RYH, Lam C, Tam C, Lee S. Malnutrition risk predicts surgical outcomes in patients undergoing gastrointestinal operations: results of a prospective study. Clin Nutr. 2015;34(4):679–84.
50. Jones K, Gordon-Weeks A, Coleman C, Silva M. Radiologically determined sarcopenia predicts morbidity and mortality following abdominal surgery: a systematic review and meta-analysis. World J Surg. 2017;41:2266–27.
51. Siegal SR, Guimaraes AR, Lasarev MR, et al. Sarcopenia and outcomes in ventral hernia repair: a preliminary review. Hernia. 2018;22:645–52.
52. Dietz UA, Fleischhacker A, Menzel S, Klinge U, Jurowich C, Haas K, Heuschmann P, Germer CT, Wiegering A. A risk-adjusted procedure tailoring leads to uniformly low complication rates in ventral and incisional hernia repair: a propensity score analysis and internal validation of classification criteria. Hernia. 2017;21:569–82.
53. Kokotovic D, Bisgaard T, Helgstrand F. Long-term recurrence and complications associated with elective incisional hernia repair. JAMA. 2016;316(15):1575–82.
54. Kaufmann R, Halm JA, Eker HH, Klitsie PJ, Nieuwenhuizen J, Geldere DV, Simons MP, Harst EV, Riet M, Holt B, Kleinrensink GJ, Jeekel J, Lange JF. Mesh versus suture repair of umbilical hernia in adults: a randomised, double-blind, controlled, multicentre trial. Lancet. 2018;391(10123):860–9.
55. López-Cano M, Martin-Dominguez LA, Pereira JA, Armengol-Carrasco M, García-Alamino JM. Balancing mesh-related complications and benefits in primary ventral and incisional hernia surgery. A meta-analysis and trial sequential analysis. PLoS One. 2018;13(6):e0197813.
56. Muysoms FE, Bontinck J, Pletinckx P. Complications of mesh devices for intraperitoneal umbilical hernia repair: a word of caution. Hernia. 2011;15:463–8.
57. Kockerling F, Lammers B. Open intraperitoneal onlay mesh (IPOM) technique for incisional hernia repair. Front Surg. 2018;5:66.
58. Lavanchy JL, Buff SE, Kohler A, Candinas D, Beldi G. Long-term results of laparoscopic versus open intraperitoneal onlay mesh incisional hernia repair: a propensity score-matched analysis. Surg Endosc. 2019;33(1):225–33.
59. Orenstein SB, Dumeer JL, Monteagudo J, Poi MJ, Novitsky YW. Outcomes of laparoscopic ventral hernia repair with routine defect closure using "shoelacing" technique. Surg Endosc. 2011;25(5):1452–7.
60. Palanivelu C, Jani KV, Senthilnathan P, Parthasarathi R, Madhankumar MV, Malladi VK. Laparoscopic sutured closure with mesh reinforcement of incisional hernias. Hernia. 2007;11:223–8.
61. Tandon A, Pathak S, Lyons NJ, Nunes QM, Daniels IR, Smart NJ. Meta-analysis of closure of the fascial defect during laparoscopic incisional and ventral hernia repair. [Review]. Br J Surg. 2016;103(12):1598–607.
62. Papageorge CM, Funk LM, Poulose BK, Phillips S, Rosen MJ, Greenberg JA. Primary fascial closure during laparoscopic ventral hernia repair does not reduce 30-day wound complications. Surg Endosc. 2017;31(11):4551–7.

63. Baker JJ, Oberg S, Andresen K, Rosenberg J. Decreased re-operation rate for recurrence after defect closure in laparoscopic ventral hernia repair with a permanent tack fixated mesh: a nationwide cohort study. Hernia. 2018;22(4):577–84.
64. Earle D, Roth JS, Saber A, Haggerty S, Bradley JF, Fanelli R, et al. SAGES guidelines for laparoscopic ventral hernia repair. Surg Endosc. 2016;30:3163–83.
65. Bittner R, Bingener-Casey J, Dietz U, Fabian M, Ferzli GS, Fortelny RH, et al. Guidelines for laparoscopic treatment of ventral and incisional abdominal wall hernias (International Endohernia Society (IEHS))–part 1. Surg Endosc. 2014;28(2–29):3170–6.
66. Altieri M, Yang J, Xu J, Talamini M, Pryor A, Telem DA. Outcomes after robotic ventral hernia repair: a study of 21,565 patients in the state of New York. Am Surg. 2018;84(6):902–8.
67. Armijo P, Pratap A, Wang Y, Shostrom V, Oleynikov D. Robotic ventral hernia repair is not superior to laparoscopic: a national database review. Surg Endosc. 2018;32:1834–9.
68. Coakley KM, Prasad T, Lincourt AE, Augenstein V, Sing RF, Heniford BT, Colavita PD. A nationwide evaluation of robotic ventral hernia surgery. Am J Surg. 2017;214(6):1158–63.
69. Carbonell AM, Warren JA, Prabhu AS, Ballecer CD, Janczyk RJ, Herrera J, Huang LC, Phillips S, Rosen MJ, Poulose BK. Reducing length of stay using a robotic-assisted approach for retromuscular ventral hernia repair a comparative analysis from the americas hernia society quality collaborative. Ann Surg. 2108;267:210–7.
70. Bittner JG IV, Alrefai S, Vy M, Mabe M, del Prado PAR, Clingempeel NL. Comparative analysis of open and robotic transversus abdominis release for ventral hernia repair. Surg Endosc. 2018;32:727–34.
71. Armijo PR, Pagkratis S, Boilesen E, Tanner T, Oleynikov D. Growth in robotic-assisted procedures is from conversion of laparoscopic procedures and not from open surgeons' conversion: a study of trends and costs. Surg Endosc. 2018;32:2106–13.
72. Kokotovic D, Gogenur I, Helgstrand F. Substantial variation among hernia experts in the decision for treatment of patients with incisional hernia: a descriptive study on agreement. Hernia. 2017;21(2):271–8.

6 Etiology and Management of Hernia-Related Chronic Pain: Implications of Robotics

Ian T. MacQueen and David C. Chen

6.1 Background

Many techniques using open, laparoscopic, robotic, and hybrid procedures exist in the treatment of hernia with a broad variety of disease requiring many different options to address hernia type, location, patient factors, available tools, and technical expertise. The adoption of the routine use of mesh in ventral and inguinal hernia repair has improved recurrence rates. This is especially true for inguinal hernias, since tension-free, mesh-based repair has become the standard of care. High level evidence in ventral hernias supports the use of prosthetic reinforcement with significant reduction in recurrence rates [1, 2]. Postherniorrhaphy chronic pain, however, remains a prevalent complication representing a substantial burden of morbidity for patients after both ventral and inguinal hernia repair. Exact rates of postherniorrhaphy chronic pain depend on the definition used, but generally range widely in the literature from 0% to upwards of 60% [3, 4]. The Swedish Hernia Registry reports that severe or debilitating postherniorrhaphy chronic pain after inguinal hernia repair occurs at a rate of between 5% and 7% [5].

Development of postherniorrhaphy chronic pain may develop regardless of the repair technique [6–8], and as such must remain a consideration for any surgeon performing robotic-assisted ventral or inguinal hernia repair. A thorough understanding of the causes of pain, groin and abdominal wall neuroanatomy, and technical aspects of the initial operation are necessary to successfully manage this complication [8–10]. These factors determine the medical and operative interventions available to address chronic pain after hernia repair. In addition to the implications of robotic repairs on the development of chronic pain and hernia repair, the technical

I. T. MacQueen (✉) · D. C. Chen
Lichtenstein Amid Hernia Clinic, David Geffen School of Medicine at UCLA, Los Angeles, CA, USA
e-mail: dcchen@mednet.ucla.edu

K. A. LeBlanc (ed.), *Robotic Assisted Hernia Repair*,
https://doi.org/10.1007/978-3-030-23025-8_6

advantages of robotic assisted surgery including superior optics, range of motion, precision, and dexterity also play a role in the surgical treatment of this challenging problem. Effective management is crucial given the personal and societal consequences of postherniorrhaphy chronic pain on quality of life, disability, and healthcare utilization.

6.2 Pain Classification

Postherniorrhaphy pain may be divided into two broad categories: nociceptive pain and neuropathic pain. Nociceptive pain is the result of direct injury to tissue and the subsequent local inflammatory processes. Endogenous nociceptive molecules mediate the production of this pain by acting on nociceptors. Neuropathic pain, in contrast, results from nerve injury. After hernia repair, neuropathic pain symptoms may include pain with radiation (especially inguinodynia radiating to the scrotum or femoral triangle, in the case of inguinal hernia repair), hyperalgesia, hyperesthesia, hypoesthesia, paresthesia, allodynia, or hyperpathia. A positive Tinel sign may be present. Nerves may be injured by indirect or direct structural damage during the operation, or by entrapment by suture, contact with mesh (Fig. 6.1), folded mesh (Fig. 6.2), meshoma, or fixating devices. In the postherniorrhaphy patient, nociceptive and neuropathic pain exist on a spectrum with significant overlap between the categories. Somatic and visceral etiologies of pain including soft tissue and bony injury and inflammation as well as adhesions and obstruction add to the complexity of presentation, As is common in establishing the cause of any chronic pain, the diagnosis of postherniorrhaphy chronic pain is confounded by individual, social, genetic, and psychological factors.

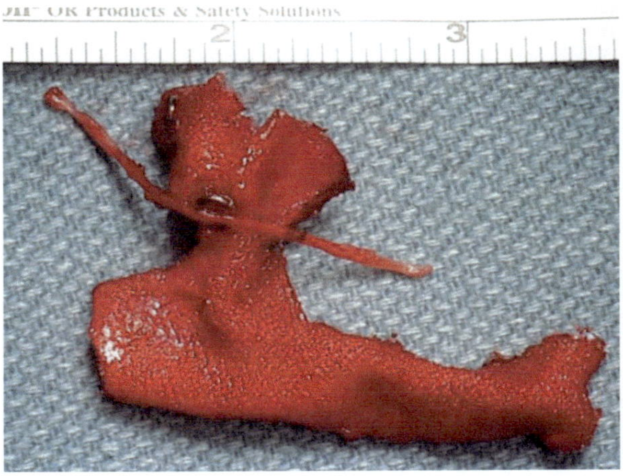

Fig. 6.1 Neuropathic pain is frequently related to nerve entrapment by suture, fixation devices, or mesh, as seen in this explanted mesh with associated injured nerve resected en bloc

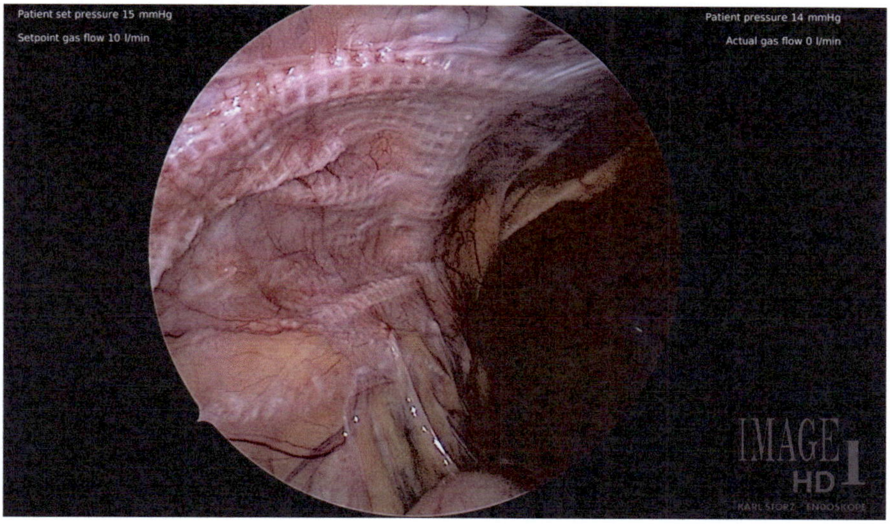

Fig. 6.2 Folded mesh (shown here), mesh migration, and meshoma may contribute to development of chronic pain.

6.3 Anatomic Considerations

Understanding the neuroanatomy of the abdominal wall and groin is crucial to preventing chronic pain, and to understanding the likely cause in the patient suffering from this complication. The anterior abdominal wall is innervated by the nerve roots from T7 at the subxiphoid position through L1 at the groin. These nerve branches travel from spinal cord to anterior midline, traveling initially along the inferior costal surface (for T7–T12), then traversing between muscle layers of the abdominal wall and giving off perforating superficial branches along the course of the nerve. Postherniorrhaphy neuropathic chronic pain in the abdominal wall above the groin is frequently caused by nerve entrapment or injury by suture, fixation devices, or by the mesh itself. While the nerves can be injured anywhere along their variable and redundant course, the proximal retroperitoneal trunks are most susceptible in flank hernia repairs while the coalescence of the perforating nerves at the semilunar line are at risk in ventral repairs. While the precision of robotic suturing may decrease the traditional risks associated with transfascial sutures and penetrating fixation with tacks or staples during intraperitoneal onlay mesh (IPOM) repair, robotic-assisted repair of ventral and flank hernias may risk nerve entrapment through other mechanisms. Robotic-assisted surgery facilitates visualization and placement of sutures with primary closure of ventral and flank defects. The use of suture through the abdominal wall especially in off-midline and flank hernias may predispose to pain related to nerve entrapment, though this is not currently well studied. During robotic-assisted ventral hernia repair, risk of nerve injury or entrapment may be minimized through careful suture placement, avoiding excessively deep suture bites, and sparing use of fixation devices, especially in the lateral areas of the abdominal wall and flank where the nerves course between the deeper muscle layers.

The neuroanatomy relevant to inguinal hernia repair extends from the retroperitoneal lumbar plexus to the terminal branches exiting through the inguinal canal. The anatomy of these nerves and nerve plexuses is complex and highly variable [11, 12]. However, meticulous identification of the relevant nerves and preventing their injury or direct contact with mesh has been demonstrated to reduce rates of post-operative chronic pain to less than 1% after open repair [7]. The three nerves most commonly contributing to chronic postherniorrhaphy inguinal pain (CPIP) are the ilioinguinal nerve, the genital branch of the genitofemoral nerve, and the iliohypogastric nerve.

The ilioinguinal nerve (IIN) originates from the L1 nerve root traversing anterior to the quadratus muscle before exiting through the transversus abdominis muscle above the level of the iliac crest. It then travels between the transversus abdominis and internal oblique muscles until it enters into the inguinal canal medial to the anterior superior iliac spine. The IIN then courses over the anterior surface of the spermatic cord, covered by the investing fascia of the internal oblique muscle. Care should be taken not to disrupt this protective fascia during open inguinal hernia repair. The iliohypogastric nerve (IHN) also originates from the L1 nerve root cephalad to the ilioinguinal nerve traversing anterior to the quadratus muscle before exiting through the transversus abdominis muscle above the level of the iliac crest. It then travels between the transversus abdominis and internal oblique muscles until it enters into the inguinal canal typically cephalad and medial to the ilioinguinal nerve. The IHN then travels between the internal and external oblique muscle layers in the medial inguinal canal exiting at the conjoined tendon. The investing fascia of the internal oblique protects the nerve from contacting an anteriorly placed mesh. Neither ilioinguinal nor iliohypogastric nerves are commonly visualized during robotic-assisted or laparoscopic inguinal hernia repair. The distal retroperitoneal course of the IIN and IHN above the iliac crest may be occasionally visualized with wide lateral dissection during an extended view total extraperitoneal (eTEP) inguinal approach or with lateral flank repairs. An understanding of their course is critical though, and care should be taken to avoid passing suture or fixation material through the anticipated course of these nerves, risking injury or entrapment of the underlying nerve.

The genitofemoral nerve typically originates from the L1 nerve root continuing its retroperitoneal course over the psoas muscle. In the preperitoneal space, the genital branch continues inferiorly and anteriorly to enter the deep inguinal ring, traversing the inguinal canal within the spermatic cord. While identification in the inguinal canal is difficult due to its diminutive size and location within the cremasteric sheath, the genital and femoral branches may be encountered with dissection lateral to the spermatic vessels. In the case of robotic-assisted or laparoscopic pre-peritoneal repair, one must additionally consider that the main trunk or femoral branch of the genitofemoral nerve, the anterior or lateral femoral cutaneous nerve, or even the femoral nerve may contribute to the development of chronic pain. During a pre-peritoneal repair, these structures typically lie within a predictable area in the surgical field, termed the "triangle of pain." The boundaries of this triangle are the iliopubic tract, the gonadal vessels, and the reflected border of peritoneum. After reflection of the peritoneum away from this area of the abdominal wall, dissection in this region should be minimized to avoid disrupting the transversalis fascia and connective tissue layer protecting these nerves from the overlying mesh. Suture and fixation material should be avoided in this area, as placement carries risk of nerve injury and resulting chronic pain. Avoidance of fixation or use of glue or self-gripping mesh in preperitoneal inguinal hernia repair is recommended to minimize the risk of developing chronic post-operative inguinal pain. Specific to robotic inguinal hernia repair is the recommendation to avoid direct suture closure of the direct and indirect hernia defect. This technique was abandoned from laparoscopic hernia surgery as it increased the risk of pain without benefit with regards to recurrence. While robotic suturing simplifies this task, it risks entrapment of the iliohypogastric nerve along the inguinal floor with direct defects. Damage to the spermatic cord, genital nerve, and ilioinguinal nerve from entrapment has also been seen from suturing. Alternative strategies such as imbrication of the transversalis fascia or suturing this to Cooper's ligament may obliterate the dead space without risking nerve entrapment.

6.4 Conservative Management of Neuropathic Pain

Most pain that develops after hernia repair is self-limited, though it may take upwards of a year to resolve. For this reason, pain is managed expectantly during this time period. Pharmacologic therapies including NSAIDs and agents for neuropathic pain, such as gabapentin and pregabalin, may be beneficial. Chronic use of narcotics should be avoided. Behavioral therapies including physical therapy, stretching, icing, and avoidance of exacerbating activities and positions should be encouraged. If pain persists for greater than 3 months, it is reasonable to consider procedural intervention. For pain that seems localized to one or more individual nerve distributions, nerve blocks using local anesthetic or steroids are a typical first step to establishing that pain is neuropathic in nature and related to injury or irritation of a particular nerve or nerves. If transient relief is gained from nerve block but symptoms remain severe, nerve ablation may be pursued for a more durable effect, or the patient may proceed to operative intervention. It is preferred that any nerve blocks and/or ablations should be performed by specialists with experience in management of neuropathic pain.

6.5 Surgical Management of Neuropathic Pain

Appropriate and effective management of postherniorrhaphy chronic pain requires a thoughtful and systematic approach. Proper identification of patients suited for operative intervention is imperative. Surgical intervention for chronic pain unresponsive to standard nonsurgical modalities should not be considered until 3 months (6 months with mesh based repairs) after the original hernia repair [3, 7]. Furthermore, surgery is not appropriate nor beneficial for all patients who fail conservative measures, and should only be sought for those patients determined to have discrete, neuroanatomic problems amenable to surgical correction. The patients most likely to benefit from operative neurectomy are those with neuropathic pain isolated to a defined distribution that was not present prior to the original operation, and that showed improvement with diagnostic and therapeutic nerve blocks. Identification of good operative candidates requires a comprehensive history characterizing symptoms, physical examination including dermatomal mapping/distribution and sensory testing, review of the prior operative report (with specific attention to the type of repair, mesh used, position of the mesh, fixation method, and nerve handling), imaging evidence of meshoma or other anatomic abnormalities, and effects of prior treatments [7, 13].

6.6 Risks of Surgery

Operative remediation of post herniorrhaphy chronic pain carries risk of complications including persistence or exacerbation of underlying pain, deafferentation hypersensitivity, abdominal wall laxity due to partial muscle denervation, and anticipated permanent numbness in the affected regions. For female patients undergoing inguinal neurectomy, the region of anticipated numbness includes the ipsilateral labia, which may contribute to sexual dysfunction. Reoperation in a field containing scar tissue carries risks of bleeding, vascular injury, disruption of the original hernia repair, hernia recurrence, vascular injury, and testicular loss. These risks should be disclosed to the patient and this discussion documented prior to the operation.

6.7 Chronic Pain After Ventral Hernia Repair

Chronic pain after ventral hernia repair is multifactorial and challenging to treat as many overlapping etiologies may exist and further intervention may not alleviate the subjective pain. Recurrence, infection, chronic inflammation, scarring and contraction, nerve entrapment, meshoma, and adhesions may all contribute to these symptoms. Neuropathic pain is typically related to nerve entrapment at site of defect closure or in the area of mesh placement. Surgical management of neuropathic pain related to ventral hernia repair has not been studied as extensively as it has in inguinal hernia repair. Unlike in inguinal hernia repair, neurectomy is not routinely performed nor recommended for chronic pain after ventral hernia repair due to the inaccessibility of the thoracic nerve roots and the unpredictable, overlapping, and redundant course of the peripheral branches. As suture and fixation devices are commonly implicated as the cause of nerve entrapment, surgical management of this pain is focused on removal of the offending suture or fixation material. While removing entrapping sutures or fixating devices may be effective, it is theorized to carry risk of persistent pain attributable to the injured nerves which are left in place [7]. Mesh-related pain caused by contraction, folding, disruption, extrusion, migration, adhesions, fistulization, hernia recurrence, and infection may lead to nociceptive pain and foreign body sensation. Use of robotic-assistance may facilitate removal of intraperitoneal or pre-peritoneal suture, fixation material, or mesh. Distribution and foci of pain should be carefully identified pre-operatively and marked in such a way that the site on the abdominal wall can be identified and confirmed intra-operatively, both internally and externally. As there is significant overlap of innervation throughout the abdominal wall sensory nerves, an attempt should be made to remove all foreign material in the area of pain in order to maximize expected relief of symptoms. In many instances, this may require completely dismantling a prior repair and performing a new repair of the hernia. This should be done again with careful attention to placement of suture and fixation material. Operative consideration for remedial surgery for ventral hernia-related pain has no specific operative algorithm and the decision to pursue intervention should be shared with the patient to establish realistic expectations. Optimally, a discrete pathology, anatomic target, and remediable problem should be present to maximize the likelihood of success. An experienced hernia specialist should consider reliable patients with severe pain that originated after surgical intervention with a reasonable mechanism of pain for operative intervention.

6.8 Chronic Pain After Inguinal Hernia Repair

For patients with neuropathic pain resulting from inguinal hernia repair that is refractory to conservative measures, neurectomy of the ilioinguinal nerve, iliohypogastric nerve, and/or genital branch of the genitofemoral nerve is a universally accepted treatment option. For patients with pain in the overlapping distribution of these three nerves in the lower groin, triple neurectomy remains the most definitive approach. This operation was pioneered in our institute in 1995, and currently remains arguably the most effective therapy available [7, 14]. Alternative but less effective options include removal of mesh and fixation material with or without revision of the prior repair, and selective neurolysis or neurectomy without triple neurectomy [7, 15–17]. The normal appearing nerves in place during single or double neurectomy often contain ultrastructural changes or microscopic neuromas, which may cause pain without overt changes to the appearance of the nerve. Furthermore, the anatomic variation and overlapping distributions of innervation of the nerves in the groin make selective neurectomy less reliable [7]. Finally, further remedial surgery following selective neurectomy increases the technical challenge increasing the risk of morbidity and decreasing the likelihood of successful intervention.

Operative triple neurectomy in conjunction with removal of meshoma, when present, is a safe, effective, and well tolerated therapy for well selected patients with refractory neuropathic inguinodynia [7]. At the Lichtenstein Amid Hernia Clinic, our experience includes over 800 patients using an open approach with a success rate of over 85%, and 100 patients using a laparoscopic retroperitoneal approach with a 90% success rate. Our current management strategy involves a tailored approach with open, laparoscopic, and hybrid techniques to address the anterior and posterior inguinal canal with tailored neurectomy, mesh removal, and subsequent hernia repair based on mechanism, anatomy, symptoms, and technical feasibility.

6.9 Technique: Neurectomy After Robotic-Assisted Preperitoneal Inguinal Hernia Repair

If no penetrating fixation was used in the original preperitoneal repair and dermatomal mapping demonstrates involvement of the genitofemoral or lateral femoral cutaneous distribution, neurectomy may be performed in the preperitoneal space or retroperitoneum via a laparoscopic approach avoiding the anterior canal and inguinal nerves. If all the ilioinguinal and iliohypogastric nerves are also involved by mechanism and dermatomal distribution, a triple neurectomy is more likely to successfully address this pain. Standard triple neurectomy after open inguinal hernia repair involves resecting segments of the ilioinguinal nerve, the iliohypogastric nerve, and the genital branch of the genitofemoral nerve. However, inguinal hernia repairs performed via a posterior approach (including robotic-assisted repairs) are most often associated with in neuropathic pain originating from the main trunk, femoral branch, and preperitoneal segment of the genital branch of the genitofemoral nerve. Neuropathic injuries of these nerves can be addressed by open extended triple neurectomy, which includes segmental resection of the main genitofemoral trunk in the retroperitoneum, or by robotic/laparoscopic preperitoneal or retroperitoneal neurectomy [18]. If all three nerves are implicated by dermatomal mapping, an open extended triple neurectomy, robotic/laparoscopic retroperitoneal triple neurectomy, or hybrid open ilioinguinal and iliohypogastric and laparoscopic preperitoneal genitofemoral neurectomy may be performed.

6.10 Open Extended Triple Neurectomy

Open Extended triple neurectomy is approached through the same incision in the case of a prior open repair, or through a standard inguinal incision in the case of a prior laparoscopic or robotic-assisted repair. The incision may be extended cephalad and lateral to facilitate exposure of the proximal portions of the ilioinguinal and iliohypogastric nerves. All nerves are resected as proximally as possible. It is our standard practice to ligate the proximal nerve stumps and place them into surrounding muscle, as intramuscular reimplantation is theorized to protect the nerve from post-operative inflammation and scarring.

The ilioinguinal nerve can be identified lateral to the deep inguinal ring and should be divided as proximally as the exposure will allow. The iliohypogastric nerve can be identified in the plane between the aponeuroses of the internal and external oblique. It should be traced proximally to the segment of the nerve that runs within the internal oblique muscle, and divided in this intramuscular segment, at a point outside the field of the original hernia repair and proximal to injury and scarring. Failure to resect the intramuscular segment may result in persistent pain due to an occult injury in this segment. Rarely, the iliohypogastric nerve runs deep to the internal oblique aponeurosis and traverses both internal and external oblique aponeuroses at a single point. If this is the case, the internal oblique aponeurosis should be split to allow division of the subaponeurotic nerve proximal to this point. Attention should be paid to any mesh or fixation material along the course of these nerves, and the nerves should be divided proximal to any such material. In respect to anterior inguinal nerve injury from a posterior preperitoneal repair, the potential sites of injury include the direct and indirect spaces from entrapment or penetrating fixation. Anterior neurectomy should be directed as proximal in the canal near the anterior superior iliac spine as possible as a posterior injury may not be as readily apparent.

The trunk of the genitofemoral nerve is exposed utilizing the same split made previously in the internal oblique muscle during resection of the iliohypogastric nerve. Extending this split exposes transversus abdominis muscle, which is similarly bluntly split along its fibers. The underlying parietal peritoneum is mobilized cephalad and medially to access the psoas muscle and main trunk of the genitofemoral nerve. Resection at this level addresses any neuropathic pain originating from the main trunk, femoral branch, or preperitoneal segment of the genital branch. Access for open extended triple neurectomy remains a challenge with preperitoneal mesh based repairs as the mesh will typically cover the entire myopectineal orifice. The genital nerve however, may still be identified as it travels between the mesh and parietal surface of the preperitoneal space.

6.11 Laparoscopic Retroperitoneal Triple Neurectomy

Laparoscopic retroperitoneal triple neurectomy involves accessing and resecting the main trunks of the ilioinguinal, iliohypogastric and genitofemoral nerves within the lumbar plexus [19]. Dividing the nerves at this site guarantees a resection proximal to the surgical field of the original hernia repair, and any associated cause of neuropathic pain. With the patient positioned in lateral decubitus position, the operating table is flexed to maximize the ipsilateral space between the costal margin and iliac crest. Initial access is achieved via a 12 mm transverse incision 4 cm above the iliac crest, in the midaxillary line. Access to the retroperitoneum is achieved by incision of the external oblique fascia and bluntly splitting the oblique muscles along their fibers. This potential space is expanded using an oval dissecting balloon placed through the incision and inflated under direct vision. After dissection, the cavity is insufflated to a pressure of 15 mm Hg. The operation typically only requires placement of one additional 5 mm port, placed 2 cm medial to the initial access port.

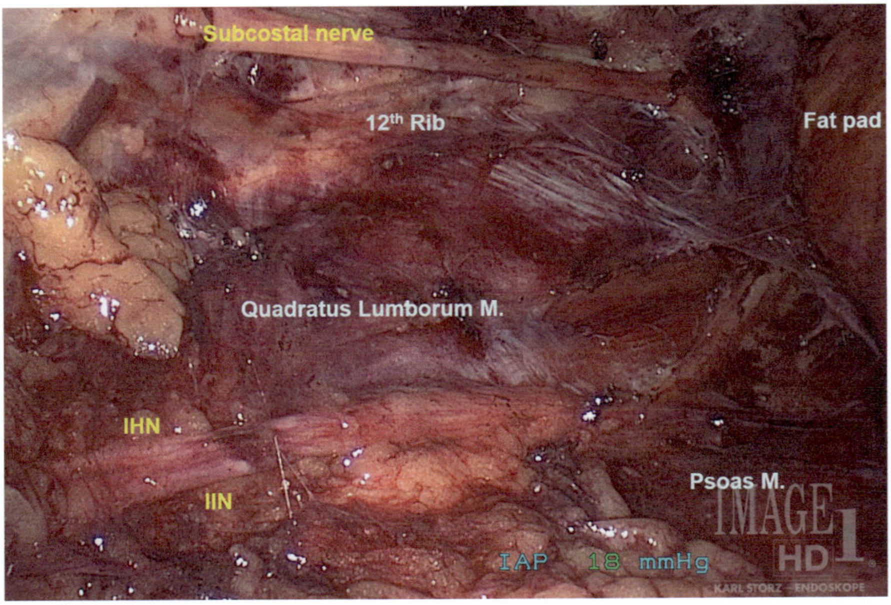

Fig. 6.3 Intraoperative identification of retroperitoneal nerve anatomy (cephalad view). Subcostal nerve at top easily identified by the 12th rib. Iliohypogastric nerve (IHN) and ilioinguinal nerve (IIN) shown here arising from a common trunk over quadratus and exiting behind psoas at L1. Retroperitoneal fat pad rotated over psoas medially

Medial dissection of the retroperitoneal fat pad provides exposure of the psoas and quadratus lumborum muscles. The iliohypogastric and ilioinguinal nerves can be identified overlying the quadratus muscle at L1 (Fig. 6.3). These nerves frequently share a common trunk.[11, 12] In order to aid identification of these nerves at L1, the T12 subcostal nerve may be identified at the T12 costal margin. Dissection is continued inferiorly to identify the genitofemoral nerve trunk running over the body of the psoas muscle (Fig. 6.4). This nerve may be a common trunk at this level, or may have already split into separate genital and femoral branches. The lateral femoral cutaneous nerve may be seen as it traverses over the iliacus muscle lateral to the psoas, below the iliac crest and may be addressed at this location if injured. The anatomy of the lumbar plexus and related structures should be clearly delineated prior to division of any nerve. The structures medial to the psoas include the ureter and iliac vessels, and should be identified and protected. Once the anatomy has been defined, the iliohypogastric and ilioinguinal nerves should be resected over the quadratus lumborum. The main trunk of the genitofemoral nerve should be resected over the psoas muscle. In rare cases of femoral nerve injury with motor deficits, removal of all offending foreign mesh, fixation material, sutures, and tacks should be performed lateral to the psoas overlying the femoral nerve ensuring that the nerve itself is preserved and the injury is not exacerbated. The primary limitation of retroperitoneal neurectomy is the wider distribution of numbness and the loss of motor innervation to the lower oblique muscles leading to bulging. While

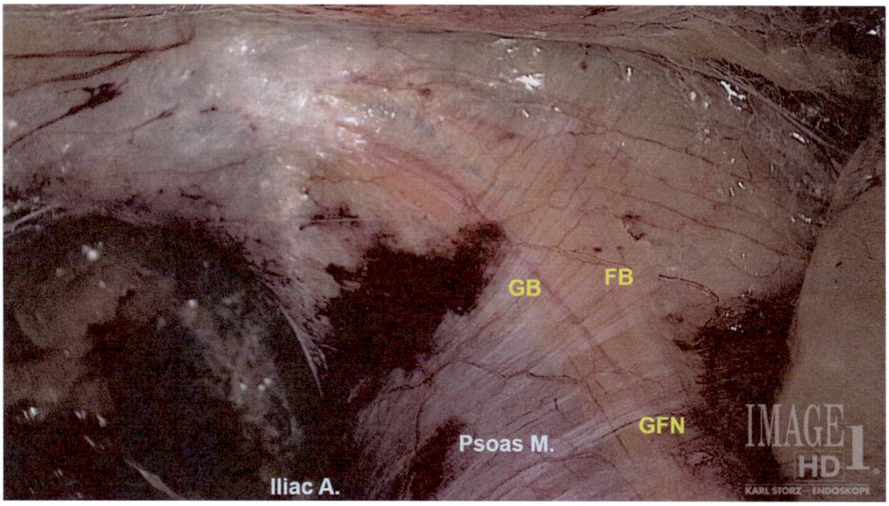

Fig. 6.4 Shown here on the patient's right side, the genitofemoral nerve (GFN) can be found in the retroperitoneum running along the psoas muscle. It splits into the genital branch (GB) and femoral branch (FB)

this has not been a significant consideration for patients in excruciating neuropathic pain, the proximal resection of the iliohypogastric and ilioinguinal nerves clearly carries more incidental morbidity and is used sparingly as needed in our experience.

For isolated genitofemoral or lateral femoral cutaneous nerve injuries, remedial surgery can be performed using a standard laparoscopic or robotic preperitoneal transabdominal (TAPP), total extraperitoneal (TEP), or extended view total extraperitoneal (eTEP) approach. These nerves may be traced cephalad and lateral to the prior repair and the likely mechanism of injury examined. Fixation material including tacks and sutures should be removed, mesh may be released or removed as indicated, and neurectomy or neurolysis may be performed depending on preoperative symptoms and intraoperative findings. This approach to the GFN and LFC nerve may be combined as a hybrid approach with an open ilioinguinal and iliohypogastric neurectomy avoiding the motor denervation and wide distribution of numbness experienced with retroperitoneal neurectomy.

6.12 Chronic Orchialgia

Orchialgia may result from open or laparoscopic inguinal hernia repair, and may be difficult to distinguish from the scrotal pain often associated with neuropathic genital inguinodynia. True orchialgia will not respond to triple neurectomy alone. Postherniorrhaphy orchialgia is thought result from injury to the paravasal and autonomic nerve fibers that accompany the cord structures. The paravasal nerves are found in the lamina propria of the vas deferens, and segmental resection of this structure has been shown to be of benefit in treating this symptom [18]. However, it

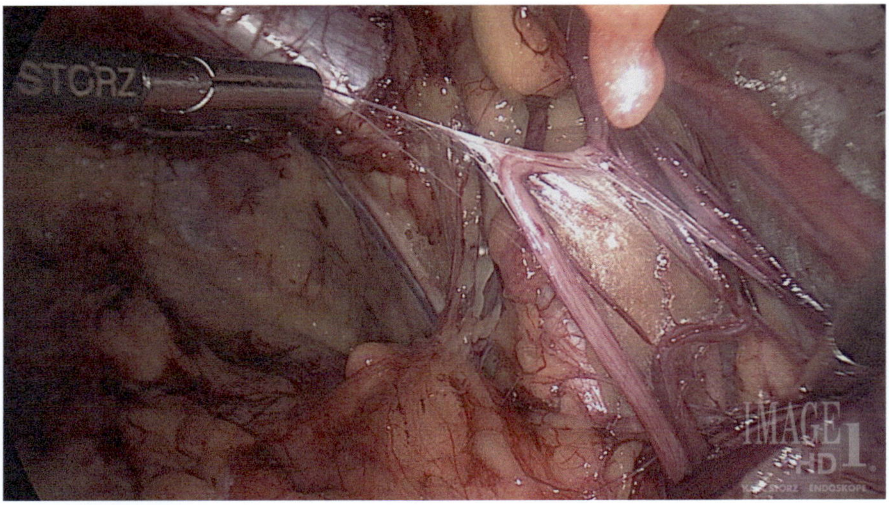

Fig. 6.5 Proximal vas deferens neurolysis

should be noted that orchialgia caused by preperitoneal mesh repair such as robotic-assisted repair is unlikely to respond to open vas neurolysis, as the affected area is commonly too proximal to be accessed via an open approach. For these patients, the autonomic nerve plexus may be accessed proximal to the mesh either laparoscopically or with robotic-assistance (Fig. 6.5).

6.13 Robotic-Assisted Surgery for Chronic Pain

There has been little study of the use of robotic-assistance for remedial surgery in cases of postherniorrhaphy chronic pain. At our institution, we have found the robot to be most useful in cases of difficult reoperative fields after posterior hernia repairs, especially in patients in whom folded mesh or meshoma seems to be the primary inciting factor causing pain. The robotic approach offers excellent visualization of the posterior groin and facilitates precise dissection of mesh that could be challenging or impossible laparoscopically (Fig. 6.6). The additional angles of traction and dissection that are possible allow the surgeon to limit the use of energy devices and associated thermal spread. Finally, use of the robot allows for suture repair of any vascular structures if necessary (Fig. 6.7). This operation may be approached with similar positioning and port placement to a robotic assisted transabdominal preperitoneal repair. The peritoneal flap is created in similar fashion and the mesh dissected from surrounding tissue. The peritoneal flap dissection may need to be widened to allow closure if any peritoneum is removed with the mesh. This approach allows for access to the genital branch of the genitofemoral nerve, and allows for paravasal neurolysis in cases of orchialgia. It does not offer easy access to the iliohypogastric

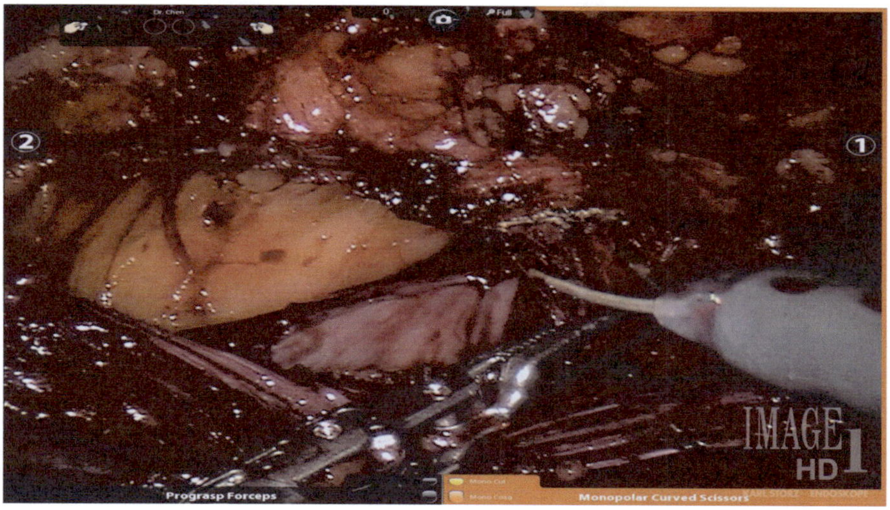

Fig. 6.6 Robotic-assisted removal of preperitoneal mesh. The robot facilitates precise dissection of the mesh from surrounding tissues

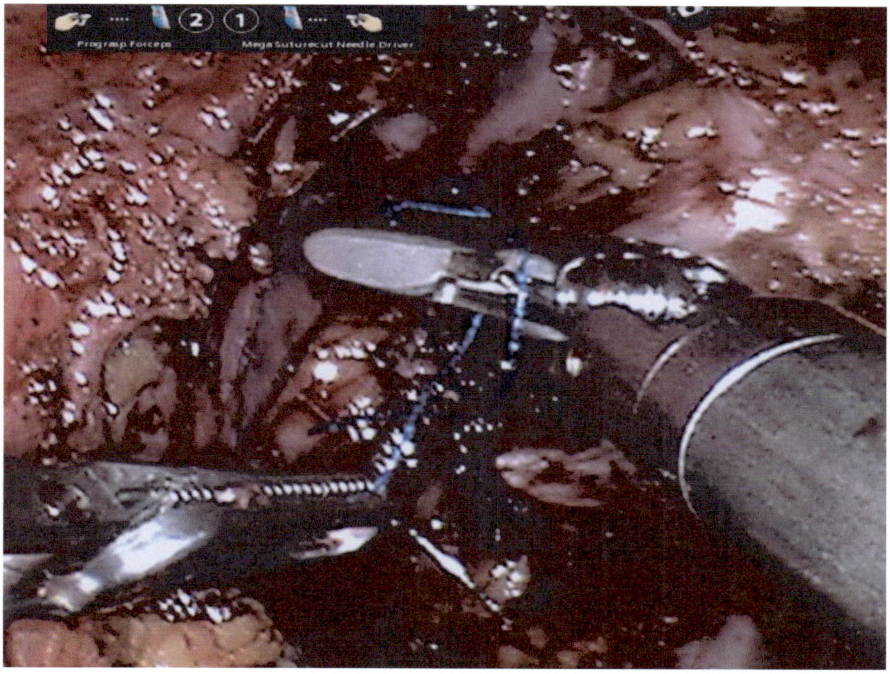

Fig. 6.7 Robotic-assisted repair of iliac vein after removal of preperitoneal split mesh

or ilioinguinal nerves, but may easily be combined as a hybrid procedure with an open inguinal neurectomy if indicated.

There is little literature regarding robotic-assisted triple neurectomy. Mahan et al. described performing this operation in 2014 [20], but no significant data exist to evaluate its the efficacy or safety. The operation is performed in the mid-lateral decubitus position via a transperitoneal approach. The posterior peritoneum is incised and medial visceral mobilization is performed to expose the retroperitoneum on the affected side. This provides exposure of the retroperitoneal structures similar to that gained during laparoscopic retroperitoneal triple neurectomy, as described above. Again, the anatomy should be carefully and completely defined prior to any resection. Clips or suture may be used to ligate the proximal and distal nerve stumps. The purported benefits of this approach, as described by Mahan et al., are technical simplicity and elegant anatomic visualization.

In our experience, any remedial operation that would be performed laparoscopically may be facilitated by robotic assistance. While we have performed posterior neurectomy, removal of plug and bilayer mesh, femoral nerve neurolysis, and subsequent hernia repair using robotic assistance, the true benefit has been in removing large, multiple, fixated, and split (encircling the cord) preperitoneal meshes that typically carry significantly more risk regarding compromise to cord and vascular structures. The robotic assisted method has allowed for precise and controlled venous and arterial repair, complete meshectomy, and preservation of entrapped cord structures. While no universal algorithm exists for management of these complex cases, robotic assistance has made these minimally invasive operations safer and more controlled in our experience, without vascular complication or cord loss.

6.14 Conclusion

There is no level 1 or 2 evidence regarding the operative management of neuropathic pain resulting from repair of ventral or inguinal hernia, by robotic-assisted or any other approach. Best practices are guided by case reports, case series, expert opinion, and expert consensus [7, 14]. At the Lichtenstein Amid Hernia Clinic, we have evaluated and treated thousands of patients with postherniorrhaphy chronic pain. Therapies have included conservative or nonoperative management, mesh removal, removal of suture and fixation material, revision of hernia repair, selective neurectomy, quadruple neurectomy and others. For pain related to ventral hernia repair, we advocate removal of meshoma, suture, and fixation material in the distribution of pain in reliable, highly symptomatic patients. For pain related to inguinal hernia repair we advocate selective neurectomy of all likely involved nerves- typically a triple neurectomy if all nerves are mechanistically and symptomatically at risk. In the case of laparoscopic or robotic-assisted repair with placement of a preperitoneal mesh, we specifically recommend open extended triple neurectomy, laparoscopic retroperitoneal triple neurectomy, or hybrid open and preperitoneal neurectomy including resection of the main trunk of the genitofemoral nerve. Patients with concurrent postherniorrhaphy orchialgia may benefit from combining paravasal neurectomy with inguinal neurectomy. We have performed over 800 open triple and open extended triple neurectomies, over 100 laparoscopic retroperitoneal triple neurectomies, and over 50 hybrid laparoscopic preperitoneal and open inguinal neurectomies making ours the largest single-institution experience. Overall success rates for open triple neurectomy are over 85% and increase to over 90% when the intramuscular segment of the iliohypogastric nerve is resected (as has been our practice since 2004) or when open extended triple neurectomy is performed. Laparoscopic triple neurectomy, performed in selected patients, has carried a similar success rate of over 90%. Our current practice does not follow a single algorithm but tailors the approach often with a hybrid minimally invasive laparoscopic or robotic and open technique to maximize the likelihood of success and minimize the morbidity of neurectomy and reoperative surgery. Acceptable outcomes are a product of careful patient selection and surgeon experience. A plan of care must reasoned for each patient based upon mechanism, symptoms, anatomy, and technical considerations. Careful attention to neuroanatomy and operative technique during initial hernia repair is the best means of preventing the development of postherniorrhaphy chronic pain and the need for remedial surgery.

References

1. Luijendijk RW, Hop WC, van den Tol MP, de Lange DC, Braaksma MM, IJzermans JN, Boelhouwer RU, de Vries BC, Salu MK, Wereldsma JC, Bruijninckx CM, Jeekel J. A comparison of suture repair with mesh repair for incisional hernia. N Engl J Med. 2000;343(6):392–8.
2. Burger JW, Luijendijk RW, Hop WC, Halm JA, Verdaasdonk EG, Jeekel J. Long-term follow-up of a randomized controlled trial of suture versus mesh repair of incisional hernia. Ann Surg. 2004;240(4):578–83.
3. Poobalan AS, Bruce J, Smith WC, King PM, Krukowski ZH, Chambers WA. A review of chronic pain after inguinal herniorrhaphy. Clin J Pain. 2003;19(1):48–54.
4. Hakeem A, Shanmugam V. Inguinodynia following Lichtenstein tension-free hernia repair: a review. World J Gastroenterol. 2011;17(14):1791–6.
5. Franneby U, Sandblom G, Nordin O, Nyren O, Gunnarsson U. Risk factors for long-term pain after hernia surgery. Ann Surg. 2006;244(2):212–9.
6. Bay-Nielsen M, Perkins FM, Kehlet H. Pain and functional impairment 1 year after inguinal herniorrhaphy: a nationwide questionnaire study. Ann Surg. 2001;233(1):1–7.
7. Alfieri S, Amid PK, Campanelli G, Izard G, Kehlet H, Wijsmuller AR, Di Miceli D, Doglietto GB. International guidelines for prevention and management of post-operative chronic pain following inguinal hernia surgery. Hernia. 2011;15(3):239–49.
8. Lichtenstein IL, Shulman AG, Amid PK, Montllor MM. Cause and prevention of postherniorrhaphy neuralgia: a proposed protocol for treatment. Am J Surg. 1988;155(6):786–90.
9. Amid PK, Hiatt JR. New understanding of the causes and surgical treatment of postherniorrhaphy inguinodynia and orchalgia. J Am Coll Surg. 2007;205(2):381–5.
10. Aavsang E, Kehlet H. Surgical management of chronic pain after inguinal hernia repair. Br J Surg. 2005;92(7):795–801.
11. Klaassen Z, Marshall E, Tubbs RS, Louis RG Jr, Wartmann CT, Loukas M. Anatomy of the ilioinguinal and iliohypogastric nerves with observations of their spinal nerve contributions. Clin Anat. 2011;24(4):454–61.

12. Rab M, Ebmer J, Dellon AL. Anatomic variability of the ilioinguinal and genitofemoral nerve: implications for the treatment of groin pain. Plast Reconstr Surg. 2001;108(6):1618–23.
13. Amid PK. Radiologic images of meshoma: a new phenomenon causing chronic pain after prosthetic repair of abdominal wall hernias. Arch Surg. 2004;139(12):1297–8.
14. Lange JF, Kaufmann R, Wijsmuller AR, Pierie JP, Ploeg RJ, Chen DC, Amid PK. An international consensus algorithm for management of chronic postoperative inguinal pain. Hernia. 2015;19(1):33–43. https://doi.org/10.1007/s10029-014-1292-y.
15. Aavsang E, Kehlet H. The effect of mesh removal and selective neurectomy on persistent postherniotomy pain. Ann Surg. 2009;249(2):327–34.
16. Zacest AC, Magill ST, Anderson VC, Burchiel KJ. Long-term outcome following ilioinguinal neurectomy for chronic pain. J Neurosurg. 2010;112(4):784–9.
17. Loos MJ, Scheltinga MR, Roumen RM. Tailored neurectomy for treatment of postherniorrhaphy inguinal neuralgia. Surgery. 2010;147(2):275–81.
18. Amid PK, Chen DC. Surgical treatment of chronic groin and testicular pain after laparoscopic and open preperitoneal inguinal hernia repair. J Am Coll Surg. 2011;213(4):531–6.
19. Chen DC, Hiatt JR, Amid PK. Operative management of refractory neuropathic inguinodynia by a laparoscopic retroperitoneal approach. JAMA Surg. 2013;148(10):962–7.
20. Mahan MA, Kader AK, Brown JM. Robot-assisted triple neurectomy for iatrogenic inguinal pain: a technical note. Acta Neurochir. 2014;156(1):171–5.

Part II

Inguinal Hernia

Operating Room Set Up for Robotic Assisted Inguinal Hernia Repair

7

Aldo Fafaj and Ajita Prabhu

Key Points

- Minimally invasive inguinal hernia repair is one of the recommended treatment modalities when expertise is available
- The transabdominal preperitoneal (TAPP) approach to inguinal hernia repair is a procedure amenable to robotic assistance
- Robotic room setup and establishing a dedicated robotic surgery team play a critical role in operating room efficiency

7.1 Introduction

Laparoscopic surgery became integrated in the field of general surgery after the development of the computer video chip, which allowed magnified images to be displayed on video monitors [1]. Since the first laparoscopic cholecystectomy in 1987, the rapid adoption of minimally invasive techniques has changed the field of general surgery dramatically [1, 2]. Traditional open procedures could be performed with small incisions which ultimately improved wound morbidity, post-operative pain and length of hospital stay. Robot assisted surgery (RAS) continues the innovations in minimal invasive techniques. Over the years RAS has evolved from movements of the endoscope to a master-slave system which allows translation of the surgeon's hand motions from a remote console to various instruments inside the patient's body [3]. The number of robot-assisted surgical procedures is increasing by 15% every year [4]. Improved outcomes from this technology have been well

A. Fafaj (✉) · A. Prabhu
Center for Abdominal Core Health, Digestive Disease and Surgery Institute, Cleveland Clinic Foundation, Cleveland, OH, USA
e-mail: fafaja@ccf.org; PRABHUA@ccf.org

K. A. LeBlanc (ed.), *Robotic Assisted Hernia Repair*,
https://doi.org/10.1007/978-3-030-23025-8_7

described in the fields of gynecology, urology and colorectal surgery [5]. Benefits include the ability for three-dimensional binocular vision, improved dexterity and ergonomics, greater range of motion and telesurgery [4, 6, 7]. Although RAS is younger in general surgery, it is quickly expanding [5].

Inguinal hernia repair is one of the most common procedures that a general surgeon performs [8]. The surgical management of inguinal hernias has paralleled the natural evolution of surgical innovations [9]. Although the Lichtenstein open mesh repairs have low rates of morbidity and mortality, the minimally invasive approach (1) is associated with less post-operative pain, numbness, hematoma formation and faster return to normal activity, (2) it has become the standard of care for many general surgeons, and (3) it is one of the recommended treatment modalities in capable hands [5, 9, 10]. Despite the aforementioned benefits, the laparoscopic technique is used in less than 28% of inguinal hernia repairs [11, 12]. One of the contributing factors to this low penetrance is the steep learning curve requiring advanced laparoscopic skills [10, 13]. The trans-abdominal pre-peritoneal (TAPP) inguinal hernia repair is a procedure amenable to robotic assistance because it overcomes the limitations in degrees of freedom and ergonomic challenges of the laparoscopic approach [5, 13].

The most utilized master-slave system is the da Vinci® Surgical System (Intuitive Surgical; Sunnyvale, CA) and over the years this system has been updated with five different models. The Xi and its predecessor Si are the two models encountered most frequently today [3]. The use of these systems is currently evolving in the field of inguinal hernia repair. One of the major hurdles to overcome is the added operative time when using the robot. The standardization of the operating room setup and the establishment of a dedicated robotic team play a critical role in the overall efficiency of the procedure. In this chapter, we will discuss the surgical personnel, operating room set up, patient and robot positioning.

7.2 The RAS Team and Operating Room

The robotic surgery team consists of the surgeon, the first assistant, the circulating nurse and the surgical technician. It is imperative for each member of the team to be thoroughly knowledgeable in robotic, laparoscopic and open surgeries [14]. There are several commercially available robotic training modules and it is recommended that all team members complete these modules prior to joining the RAS team. Because of the extra training required, it is important to have a dedicated robotic team, if possible, as this will minimize delays due to the learning curve associated with this technique.

The surgeon, as the leader of the team, should be familiar with each step of the RAS in order to troubleshoot any potential problems. The first assistant plays a critical role during the procedure and mastering not only instrument exchange but also laparoscopic skills such as retraction, suction/irrigation and clipping will improve the efficiency of the procedure [3]. The circulating nurse and the surgical technician are the other essential members of the team. They should master the set-up of all the different components, sterile draping, robot maneuvering in the operating room and docking, the various instruments available and how to perform their exchange from robotic arms. All bedside team members should be able to manually manipulate the robot arms using the clutch buttons in order to move the ports out ("burping") or in (deep seating) which will allow the surgeon to reach the target anatomy or maximize the working space. Finally, they should be able to troubleshoot collision of the arms, which can lead to instrument or drape dislodgements. Developing these skills is essential to developing an efficient RAS team as it will prevent interruptions during the surgery which will otherwise occur if the surgeon has to re-scrub.

The operating room must accommodate all of the robotic components while allowing the surgeon to have an unobstructed view of the patient, tension free cable connections and pathways for the personnel to move freely and safely around the room [3]. Some surgeons prefer to have laparoscopic instruments available in the operating room which can be used for gaining intraperitoneal access and establishing pneumo-peritoneum. These instruments can be used to lyse any adhesions before the robot is engaged and as a safety mechanism in case the RAS cannot be used as planned [2]. When compared to laparoscopic instruments the robotic ones have a more limited lifespan. The robotic arms will not function with an instrument that has surpassed the manufacturer recommended uses. It is important to have extra instrument trays available in the operating room as this will prevent delays during the operation in case this problem is encountered.

Before the case starts, a team huddle is recommended and it should include the surgeon, the anesthesiologist, the surgical assistant, the circulating nurse and the surgical technician. This is an opportunity for the team to discuss any anesthesia concerns, the operative plan, the available equipment, the position of the patient cart, and the type of mesh that will be used. While this may appear time consuming at first, it will ensure proper surgical set up and will help anticipate any potential problems. Finally, the team should discuss alternative approaches if the RAS does not go as planned, confirming that the instruments required are available in the operating room.

7.3 The Robotic Equipment

The da Vinci® Surgical System consists of three main units, the patient cart, the surgeon console and the vision cart.

a. The patient cart has the mechanical arms, usually one camera and 3–4 instrument arms, which translate the surgeon's hand movements from the surgeon console to the patient and the target anatomy. Once all the cannulas are placed, the patient cart is maneuvered into position by the operating room staff.
b. The surgeon console is the control center for the robot arms. It allows for three dimensional images delivered via two separate left and right images. In addition,

the display shows any errors encountered during the instrument exchanges, the instrument available in each arm and the energy device. Foot pedals and two arm controls allow the surgeon to remotely manipulate each arm on the patient cart. When positioning the surgeon console in the operating room, it is important to allow a direct line of sight between the surgeon and the operative field. While the three-dimensional image offers great detail of the target anatomy, the surgeon cannot visualize the position of the robot arms outside the patient's body. Ensuring a direct line of sight gives the surgeon the ability to assess the position of the arms with relation to the patient and the target anatomy.

c. The vision cart is similar to the laparoscopic monitor tower. It contains a two dimensional monitor, an insufflator and a light source. Both the vision cart and surgeon console are equipped with intercom capabilities which facilitates communication between the surgeon and the other members of the team.

7.4 Patient Position, Cannula Placement and Robot Docking

7.4.1 Patient Positioning

The patient is positioned supine on the operating room table. Both arms are tucked on the sides with foam padding, if necessary, in order to minimize pressure related injuries. The surgeon can choose the position of the patient cart, on the side (parallel dock) or between the legs, based on their level of comfort and preference. A lithotomy position will be necessary to accommodate the patient cart between the patient's legs. In our practice we find it easier and more efficient to side dock. A safety strap in applied across the lower extremities or across the chest if the patient is in lithotomy. A Foley catheter is routinely inserted in all cases. The patient is then prepped widely, and sterile drapes are applied.

7.4.2 Cannulas

Gaining access to the abdomen is done similarly to established minimally invasive techniques. These include the open cut-down (Hasson) technique and the optical trocar with or without Veress needle insufflation. Because of the number of the cannulas and their position we elect to gain entry into the abdomen via the open cut down technique. Incision is made at least 3 cm above the umbilicus and this site is used to place the 12 mm balloon cannula where the camera will be inserted. Placing the camera port in this position will allow better visualization and adequate working space especially when closing the peritoneum flap once the repair is completed. After establishing pneumo-peritoneum to a pressure of 15 mm Hg, a laparoscopic camera is inserted and the intra-abdominal contents are quickly surveyed. Under visual guidance, two additional 8 mm cannulas are inserted at the lateral edges of

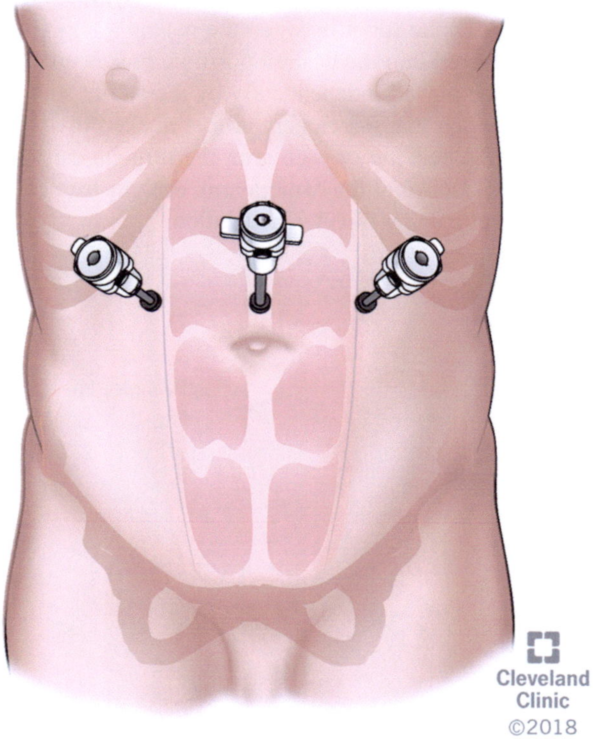

Fig. 7.1 Laparoscopic port placement for robotic inguinal hernia repair. A 12 mm balloon cannula is placed 3 cm superior to the umbilicus. Two 8 mm cannulas are placed at the lateral edges of the rectus sheath on either side and at the same level as the supraumbilical midline cannula

the rectus sheath on either side and at the same level as the supraumbilical midline cannula (Fig. 7.1). Ensuring adequate space between the 8 mm ports will maximize the range of motion of each robot arm which is important when suturing. Since we use the Si model, where the camera can be inserted through only one dedicated port, we prefer to insert the mesh and the required sutures inside the abdomen through the 12 mm port prior to docking the camera arm. This allows for minimal undocking and redocking of the robot. If desired and available, a 5 mm laparoscope can be inserted through one of the 8 mm ports to watch the mesh and sutures enter the abdomen.

7.4.3 Robot Docking

Once all the cannulas are placed the patient is positioned in slight Trendelenburg and the patient cart is moved into position. A two-person team is recommended for efficient and safe maneuvering. A non-sterile team member should push the patient cart and a second person from the team should provide audible cues in order to facilitate movements. To avoid confusion room objects should be used for direction instead of left and right cues. For inguinal hernia repairs we prefer to side dock the patient cart (Fig. 7.2). Alternatively, the lithotomy patient position can be used to dock the robot between the patient's legs (Fig. 7.3). Once the patient cart is maneuvered into the desired position, brakes are applied automatically and each arm can be moved independently by the sterile staff using the clutch buttons. It is recommended that the camera arm is docked first followed by the two additional arms. Upon docking of each arm, the surgeon can move to the surgeon's console. By taking control of the camera arm, each instrument can be safely inserted by the first assistant under direct visualization.

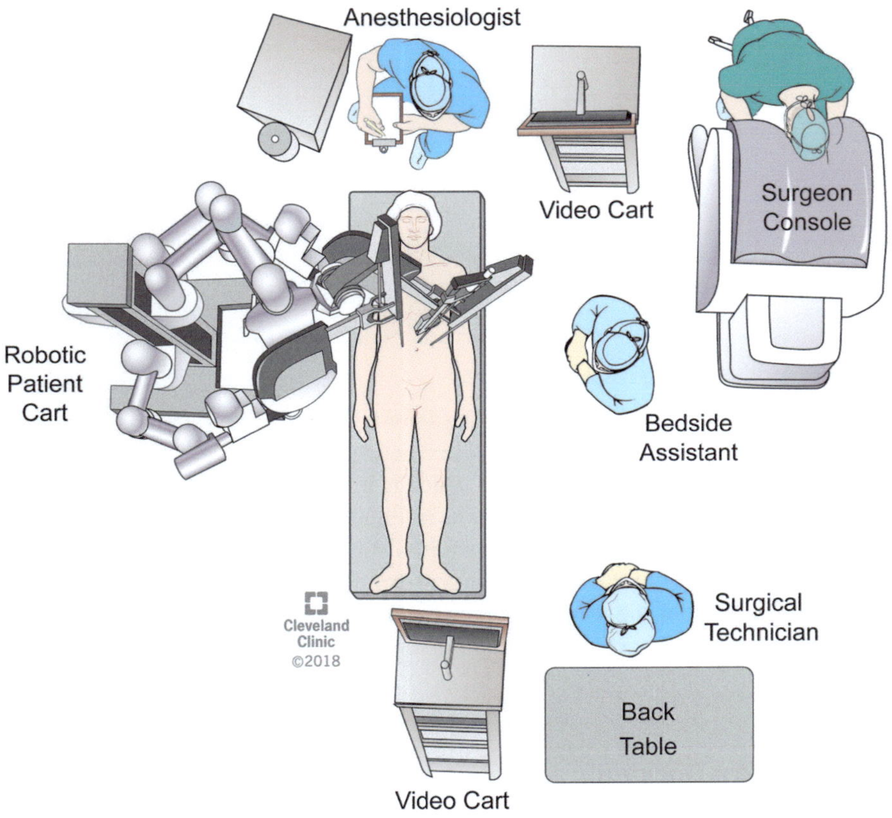

Fig. 7.2 Overhead view of the operating room set up that we use for inguinal hernia repair showing the patient cart docked on the side

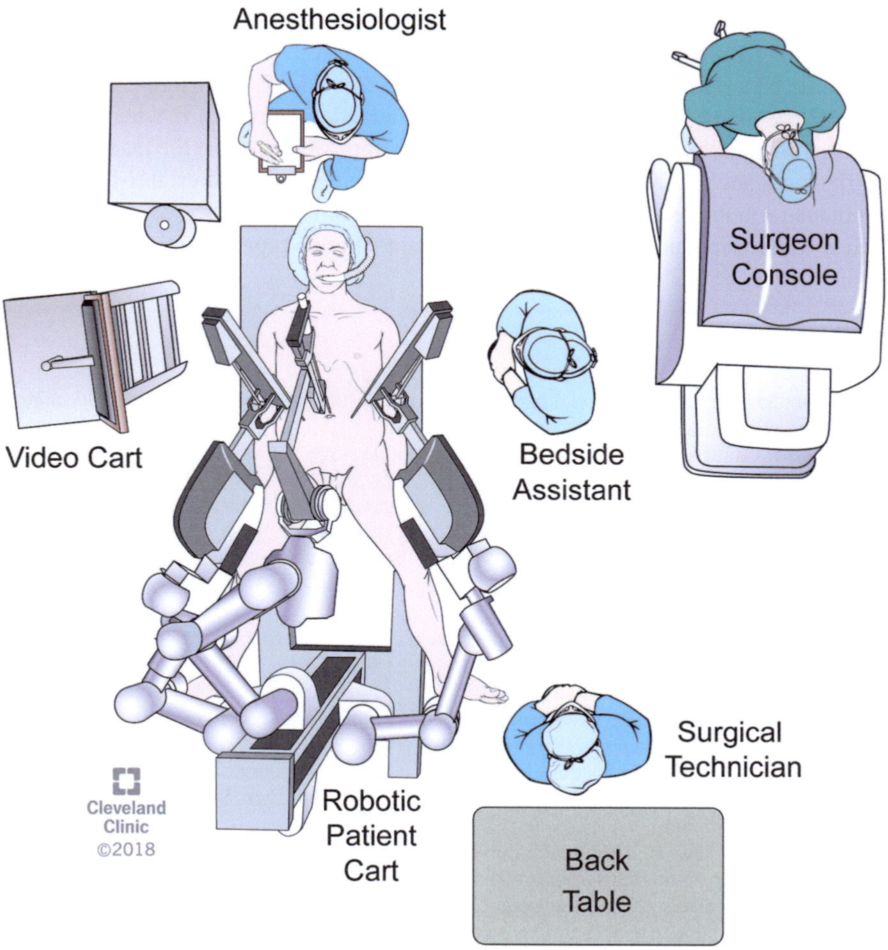

Fig. 7.3 Overhead view of operating room set up showing an alternative position for the patient cart. The patient is placed in lithotomy position and the patient cart is docked between the legs

7.5 Conclusion

Inguinal hernia repair is one of the most common procedures that the general surgeon perform. Despite the benefits that minimally invasive techniques afford, there is a slow adoption rate for inguinal hernia repairs, likely because of the advanced laparoscopic skill required. The robotic approach overcomes the limitations in degrees of freedom and ergonomic challenges of the laparoscopy while retaining the same benefits. As with any new technology, the RAS is not without challenges. One of the major hurdles to overcome is the added operative time when using the robot. The operative times have been shown to improve once past the learning curve [15]. The standardization of the operating room setup and the establishment of a dedicated robotic team play a critical role in the overall efficiency of the procedure and it will ensure success of the robotic inguinal hernia repair practice.

References

1. Spaner SJ, Warnock GL. A brief history of endoscopy, laparoscopy, and laparoscopic surgery. J Laparoendosc Adv Surg Tech A. 1997;7:369–73.
2. Kroh M, Chalikonda S, editors. Essentials of robotic surgery. Cham: Springer; 2015. https://doi.org/10.1007/978-3-319-09564-6.
3. Su L, editor. Atlas of robotic urologic surgery. Cham: Springer; 2017. https://doi.org/10.1007/978-3-319-45060-5.
4. van't Hullenaar CDP, Bos P, Broeders IAMJ. Ergonomic assessment of the first assistant during robot-assisted surgery. J Robot Surg. 2019;13(2):283–8. https://doi.org/10.1007/s11701-018-0851-0.
5. Waite KE, Herman MA, Doyle PJ. Comparison of robotic versus laparoscopic transabdominal preperitoneal (TAPP) inguinal hernia repair. J Robot Surg. 2016;10:239–44. https://doi.org/10.1007/s11701-016-0580-1.
6. Shah J, Vyas A, Vyas D. The history of robotics in surgical specialties. Am J Robot Surg. 2015;1:12–20. https://doi.org/10.1166/ajrs.2014.1006.
7. Altieri M, Yang J, Xu J, Talamini M, Pryor A, Telem D. Outcomes following robotic ventral hernia repair: A study of 21, 565 patients in the state of New York. Surg Endosc Other Interv Tech. 2016;30:S244.
8. Horne CM, Prabhu AS. Minimally invasive approaches to inguinal hernias. Surg Clin North Am. 2018;98:637–49. https://doi.org/10.1016/j.suc.2018.02.008.
9. Charles EJ, Mehaffey JH, Tache-Leon CA, Hallowell PT, Sawyer RG, Yang Z. Inguinal hernia repair: is there a benefit to using the robot? Surg Endosc. 2017;32:2131–6. https://doi.org/10.1007/s00464-017-5911-4.
10. Dickens RGE, Amico AGLD, Rabaza CRJ. Open versus robotic - assisted transabdominal preperitoneal (R - TAPP) inguinal hernia repair: a multicenter matched analysis of clinical outcomes. Hernia. 2018;22(5):827–36. https://doi.org/10.1007/s10029-018-1769-1.
11. Trevisonno M, Kaneva P, Watanabe Y, Fried GM, Feldman LS, Lebedeva E, et al. A survey of general surgeons regarding laparoscopic inguinal hernia repair: practice patterns, barriers, and educational needs. Hernia. 2015;19:719–24. https://doi.org/10.1007/s10029-014-1287-8.
12. Thiels CA, Holst KA, Ubl DS, McKenzie TJ, Zielinski MD, Farley DR, et al. Gender disparities in the utilization of laparoscopic groin hernia repair. J Surg Res. 2017;210:59–68. https://doi.org/10.1016/j.jss.2016.10.028.
13. Belyansky I, Reza Zahiri H, Sanford Z, Weltz AS, Park A. Early operative outcomes of endoscopic (eTEP access) robotic-assisted retromuscular abdominal wall hernia repair. Hernia. 2018;22(5):837–47. https://doi.org/10.1007/s10029-018-1795-z.
14. Ross H, Lee SW, Champagne BJ, Pigazzi A, Rivadeneira DE, editors. Robotic approaches to colorectal surgery. Cham: Springer; 2015. https://doi.org/10.1007/978-3-319-09120-4.
15. Muysoms F, Van Cleven S, Kyle-Leinhase I, Ballecer C, Ramaswamy A. Robotic-assisted laparoscopic groin hernia repair: observational case-control study on the operative time during the learning curve. Surg Endosc. 2018;32(12):4850–9. https://doi.org/10.1007/s00464-018-6236-7.

Routine Robotic Inguinal Hernia Repair

8

Joseph Dux, Loic Tchokouani, Erica D. Kane,
and Brian P. Jacob

8.1 Introduction

Performing inguinal hernia repairs via robotic technique has become more popular since 2013. Many debates have coincided with this growth over the value proposition of using robotic technology to perform a routine operation which already holds a standard of fast recovery and optimized outcomes. The main argument against the use of robotic technology in this setting is the concern of additional expense without the improvement of outcomes compared to its laparoscopic counterpart.

Compared to open inguinal hernia repairs, robotics can afford patients the same minimally invasive benefits as laparoscopy. Advantages of a robotic approach to a transabdominal preperitoneal (TAPP) hernia repair over laparoscopic TAPP include a steadier camera and the ability to utilize instruments that have seven degrees of freedom and enhanced ergonomics. Current literature has supported these benefits [1], though some of the publications are limited by author bias. At this time, the use of robotics remains slightly more expensive than laparoscopy in many centers [2]; though, some centers have been able to make both platforms cost neutral [3]. The robotic approach does remain more expensive than open. Long term recurrence rates and chronic pain rates are yet to be determined for robotic transabdominal preperitoneal (TAPP) hernia repair, but a randomized trial comparing robotic versus laparoscopic TAPP hernia repair is underway. The results of this study will not be available until after 2020.

J. Dux · L. Tchokouani
Department of Surgery, Icahn School of Medicine at Mount Sinai, New York, NY, USA

E. D. Kane
Department of Anesthesia, Perioperative, and Pain Medicine,
Icahn School of Medicine at Mount Sinai, New York, NY, USA

B. P. Jacob (✉)
Laparoscopic Surgical Center of New York, Icahn School of Medicine at Mount Sinai,
New York, NY, USA

K. A. LeBlanc (ed.), *Robotic Assisted Hernia Repair*,
https://doi.org/10.1007/978-3-030-23025-8_8

The technique discussed in this chapter is only for robotic TAPP. While there are benefits to performing laparoscopic or robotic total extraperitoneal (TEP) inguinal hernia, that description is beyond the scope of this chapter.

8.2 Patient Selection

Patient selection for robotic inguinal hernia repair is similar to that of laparoscopic repairs. The patient must be able to tolerate general anesthesia and abdominal insufflation. The surgery can be performed on most body mass index up to approximately 45. Once a patient is morbidly obese, it is always best to recommend weight loss prior to performing a robotic inguinal hernia repair, as obesity is directly related to an increased recurrence rate [4]. Smoking cessation of a minimum of 3–4 weeks prior to surgery is strongly advised. Ongoing smoking is not an absolute contraindication; however, it predisposes the patient to increased adverse events post-operatively.

Previous inguinal hernia surgery should be explicitly solicited from the patient, as well as their previous operative reports. In the case of a re-operation, the surgeon must become familiar with the type of previous repair, indication for repair, and type of mesh used. Patients who have undergone prior open repairs can safely be re-operated on robotically. For those patients who have undergone prior laparoscopic or robotic repairs, the surgeon should consider performing these with an open technique. This said, if the surgeon is experienced with re-do hernia repairs in the preperitoneal plane, he or she may consider approaching these robotically.

Because of the location of the preperitoneal dissection, the surgeon should also be specifically aware of any prior prostate surgery. There is a real risk of bladder injury when performing an adequate medial dissection when freeing up the pubic symphysis and Cooper's ligament. As an experienced hernia surgeon, I prefer to do these via the Lichtenstein (open) approach; nevertheless, performing the robotic TAPP in a patient with previous prostatectomy is still feasible in experienced hands. Of note, all post-prostatectomy patients should have a foley catheter placed before the surgery.

Another pre-operative concern are patients with large inguinal scrotal hernias, which are generally better repaired by an open technique with a drain in the scrotum to help minimize seroma. While not a contraindication for the robot, the risk of recurrence, hematoma, and seroma may be elevated in robotic TAPP for giant inguinal scrotal hernias. Furthermore, aggressive reduction of hernia contents can increase risk of injury.

Lower midline scars are also not a contraindication to performing robotic TAPP, but the surgeon must be aware that adhesiolysis may be required in order to safely perform the repair. Thus careful port placement is required to not cause injury.

8.3 Surgical Technique

8.3.1 Patient Set-Up and Trocar Placement

After induction of general anesthesia and endotracheal intubation, the patient is placed in the supine position with both arms tucked and padded at the patient's sides. The abdomen is prepped and draped in usual sterile fashion. Our routine is to start with a 5 mm Optiview entry using a 5 mm Optiview trocar and a zero degree 5 mm laparoscope. Once insufflated, we then insert the three 8 mm robotic trocars assuming one has access to an Xi DaVinci system, otherwise a 12 mm trocar is inserted for the camera, and two 8 mm trocars are inserted for the instruments when working on an Si system. Alternatively, access with a Veress needle maybe be established through an 8 mm supraumbilical incision if the surgeon is more comfortable with this technique.

Three 8 mm trocars are placed under direct vision: one in the supraumbilical incision, one in the right lateral abdomen, and one in the left lateral abdomen. The horizontal distance between each trocar is at least 8 cm in the same horizontal plane. Modifications to trocar placement may be made based on patient habitus; patients with less width may require less horizontal distance between trocars as the lateral trocars may be impeded by the anterior superior iliac spines. The supraumbilical port is designated as the camera port and the lateral ports as the working ports. The patient is placed in Trendelenburg position to limit obstruction of view by intraabdominal contents. A zero-degree or a 30-degree camera can be used per surgeon preference. For the majority of cases, we prefer a zero degree camera as it allows better viewing for the creation and closure of the peritoneal flap, as well as adequate dissection of the retroperitoneum. As described below, it is imperative to completely reduce the peritoneal flap to the level of the iliac vessels to decrease the risk of mesh folding.

For efficiency, the anticipated sutures and mesh may be placed intra-abdominally before docking of the robot. We elect to insert the sutures and secure them to the abdominal wall away from the dissection field but in vision prior to docking and to insert the mesh at the time of mesh placement.

8.3.2 Dissection

After docking, we inspect both groins and decide whether the procedure will be a unilateral or bilateral repair. The symptomatic side should be approached first. A curvilinear peritoneal incision is performed with monopolar curved scissors between the anterior superior iliac spine (palpated by the assistant) and the medial umbilical ligament. This will allow sufficient space for placement of an appropriately sized mesh. Using Prograsp™ Forceps and the monopolar scissors, the peritoneal flap is

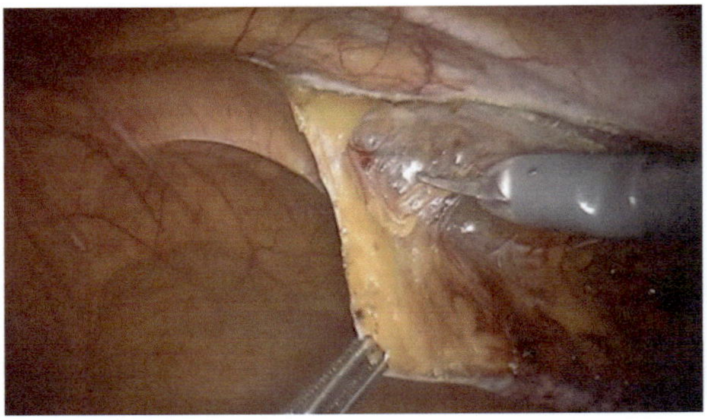

Fig. 8.1 Creation of the peritoneal flap

carefully created (Fig. 8.1). Ideally, the plane between the parietal peritoneum and the transversalis fascia is developed. This flap is usually started at the level of the ipsilateral anterior superior iliac spine laterally and carried medially to and including the ipsilateral umbilical ligament.

It is important to properly obtain the Critical View of the Myopectineal Orifice (CV of the MPO). The stepwise approach to obtain this view is as follows:

1. Identify and dissect the pubic tubercle across the midline and Cooper's ligament (CL). For large, direct hernias, extend the dissection to the contralateral CL.
2. Rule out a direct hernia. Remove any fat in the Hesselbach triangle to fully investigate.
3. Dissect at least 2 cm between CL and the bladder to facilitate flat placement of the medial and inferior edge of mesh toward the space of Retzius, thereby avoiding mesh displacement caused by bladder distention.
4. Dissect between CL and the iliac vein to identify the femoral orifice and rule out a femoral hernia.
5. Dissect the indirect sac and peritoneum sufficiently to parietalize the cord's elements (Fig. 8.2).

   This step is often not completed, especially in a small surgical field. To ensure compliance with this requirement, continue to dissect until the cord's elements lie flat. Then, visualize the psoas muscle and iliac vessels, pull the sac and peritoneum upward without triggering movement of the cord structures, and dissect between the cord structures to avoid missing a tail of the sac.
6. Identify and reduce cord lipomas (which may appear small and unimportant until reduced). They usually lie lateral to the cord's elements, they should not be confused with lymph nodes (which are generally spared). Most lipomas do not require removal, but should be placed above the mesh to help prevent mesh rolling upward.
7. Dissect peritoneum lateral to the cord structures beyond the anterior superior iliac spine (ASIS), with careful attention to make sure the edge of the peritoneal flap is dissected below the level of the iliacs, and below the inferior most edge of the mesh's inferior border (Fig. 8.3 yellow arrows).

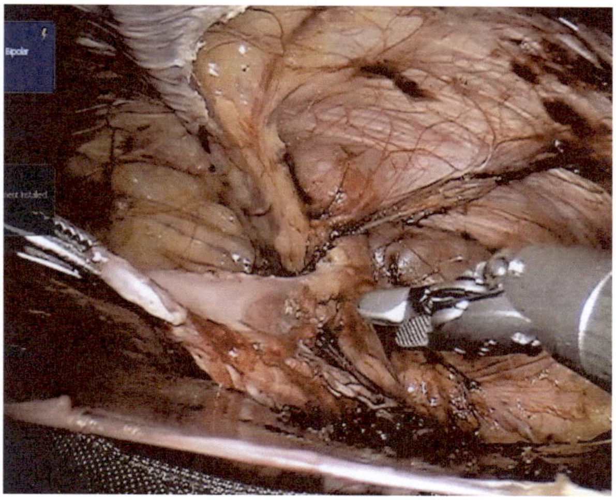

Fig. 8.2 Dissection of the indirect sac and exposure of the cord structures

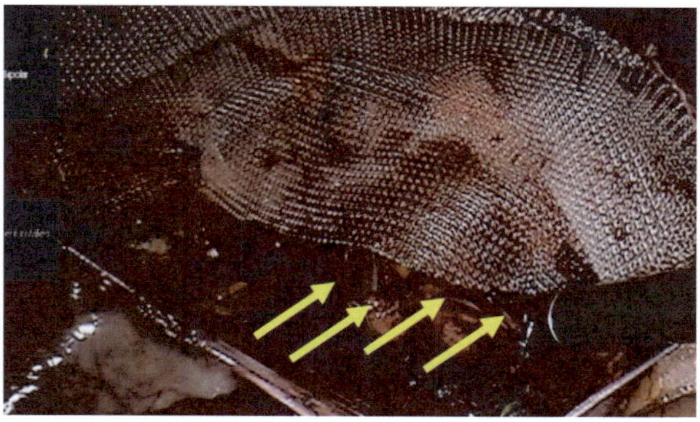

Fig. 8.3 Yellow arrows indicate the lower level of dissection of the flap

8. Provide mesh coverage and ensure that mesh and mechanical fixation are placed well above an imaginary inter-ASIS line and any defects, thereby avoiding recurrence and nerve injury, especially to the ilioinguinal nerve.

8.3.3 Mesh Placement

Once the CV of the MPO is established, the mesh can be placed (Fig. 8.4, cvmpo).

Mesh size should be at least 15 cm × 10 cm, although a larger piece of mesh is sometimes required to cover the MPO. It is our practice to use a 12 cm × 16 cm sized mesh (Fig. 8.5).

Preferably, choose mesh that adapts to the contour of the space and the cord. It should not have undue memory. Place it without creases or folds. Splitting the mesh should be avoided. Ensure that the lateroinferior corner lies deep against the wall. The mesh should adequately cover the femoral space, direct space, and

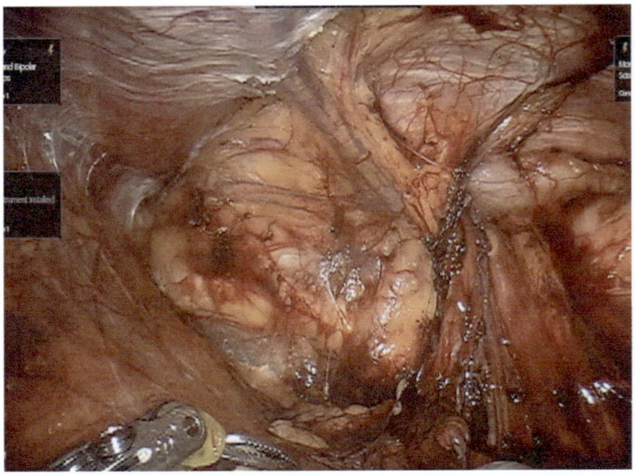

Fig. 8.4 Critical view of the myopectineal orifice (cympo)

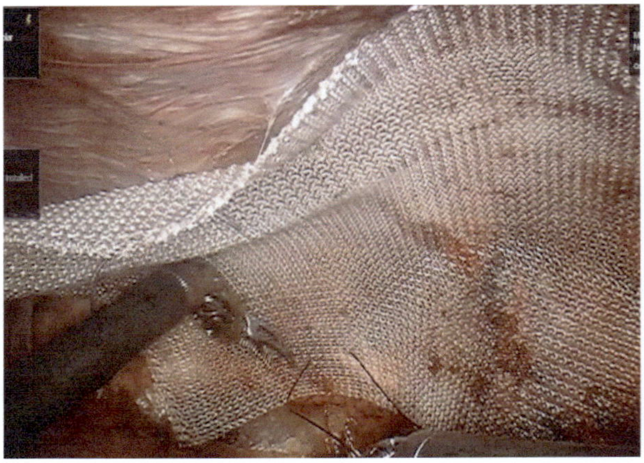

Fig. 8.5 Large mesh will be secured to Cooper's ligament

myopectineal orifice. We routinely secure the mesh to at least Cooper's or to the tubercle (Fig. 8.6 yellow arrow), with one fixation spot, and then we will occasionally add a second fixation point.

If one chooses to fix the mesh, sutures may be placed medially on the abdominal wall at Cooper's Ligament, avoiding the epigastric vessels, and laterally and above the internal ring. The latter two fixation points should be above an imaginary inter-ASIS line to avoid injury to vascular and nervous structures, as previously mentioned.

8.3.4 Peritoneal Closure

We close the peritoneal flap using a 2–0 or 3–0 slowly absorbable barbed suture, approximately 15 cm in length (eg. V-Loc™) (Fig. 8.7).

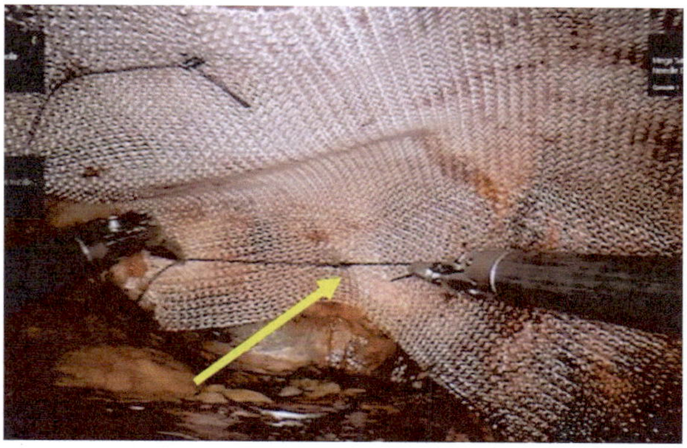

Fig. 8.6 Fixation at Cooper's ligament plus another site medial to the epigastric vessels

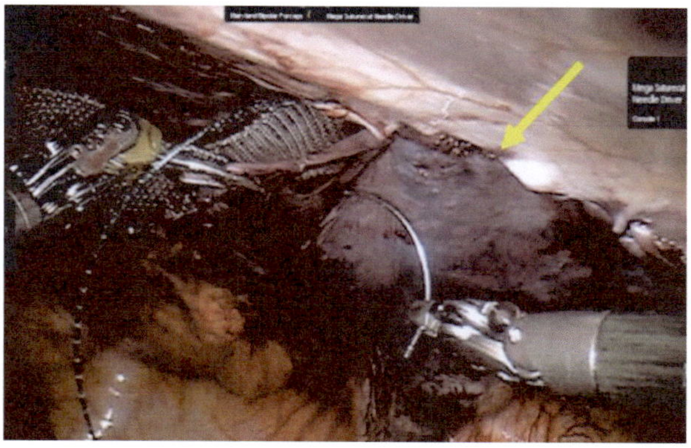

Fig. 8.7 Flap closure (yellow suture) with barbed suture

The suture is run in one direction using a Mega Suture Cut Needle. Once closed, the robot arms are undocked, the trocars are removed under direct vision, and the abdomen is desufflated.

It is important to desufflate, then reinsufflate, to confirm the mesh won't shift dramatically. This extra step takes a few seconds and is well worth it. Some surgeons aspirate the pneumo out of the preperitoneal space, which is another way to assure the mesh will not clamshell.

The fascia of the trocar sites are optionally closed with figure-of-eight sutures with 0-Vicryl, followed 4–0 Monocryl for the skin.

8.4 Recovery

The surgery is usually carried out in an ambulatory setting. The patient is monitored for a few hours in the recovery room with no ambulatory restrictions. Once patients have voided, pain is controlled, and no other issues are present, they can be discharged. Postoperative urinary retention (POUR) is reported in 1.25–8% of cases [5–7]. Minimizing POUR can be achieved by preoperative voiding, limiting administration of IV fluids, avoiding the use of tacks if possible, and minimizing opioid use. Other risk factors include male gender, age over 50, and benign prostatic hyperplasia [8]. Postoperative incisional pain is usually mild and lasts for several days. Males also may experience transient testicular pain or discomfort. Most pain can be managed with over-the-counter pain medications such as Acetaminophen or a non-steroidal anti-inflammatory. The patient may go back to their normal routine as tolerated, with no restriction on heavy lifting. The incidence for ileus after the surgery is not defined, but it is rare and usually self-limited. Routine follow up is 1–2 weeks after the surgery, with attention to wound healing and pain management. Another clinic visit is scheduled 3–6 months later, with no requirement for further routine follow-up visits.

8.5 Adverse Events

The overall complication rate is reported as 7–21%, with most of complications being grade 1–2 on the Clavien Dindo Scale. The most common complications are urinary retention (1.25–8%), seroma (0.2–2.5%), hematoma (0.7–3.8%), and surgical site infection (0.2–3%) [1, 2, 5–7, 9, 10].

8.5.1 Small Bowel Obstruction

Small bowel obstruction (SBO), as opposed to ileus mentioned before, may be a serious complication. Previously, it was attributed to migration of the intestine beneath the peritoneal flap [11]. With the adoption of sutured peritoneal flap closure the risk is minimized but still exists. Multiple reports exist of internal hernia occurring due to peritoneal flap defects formed by widely separated tacking or stapling [12, 13]. This scenario tends to cause early post-operative SBO, at an average of 8 days, compared to obstruction related to adhesive disease, which occurs around 25 days. There have been case reports of exposed peritoneal flap barbed sutures as points of obstruction as well as obstructions secondary to trocar site hernia (usually Richter's hernia)[14, 15]. Any complaint suggestive of SBO should be taken seriously and worked up with imaging as indicated. When diagnosed early, laparoscopic investigation can be performed safely with resolution of the obstruction.

8.5.2 Recurrence

Hernia recurrence can happen at any time after surgery. Early recurrence symptoms can be the result of a retained cord lipoma that was not dissected properly during the surgery [16]. Another common cause is due to "clam shelling of the mesh" from inadequate dissection of the preperitoneal space or placement of too large a piece of mesh. True recurrence can be direct or indirect and can result from mesh migration or suboptimal repair; recently reported at a rate of 0.6–4% in two recent publications [6, 7] Timing and indication for surgical repair is based on the patient symptoms, complaints, and surgeon evaluation.

8.5.3 Chronic Pain

The incidence of postoperative inguinodynia is low, but can be debilitating and cannot be ignored. A detailed history must be taken and a complete physical exam should be performed. Additionally, pain mapping is a very useful tool in investigating chronic groin pain. At times, cross sectional imaging may be necessary in elucidating the etiology of the pain. A stepwise approach to pain relief includes physical therapy, anesthetic injections, and nerve ablations. Some refractory cases, however, warrant exploration and possibly mesh removal. Surgical mesh extraction can prove to be very successful with very specific patient selection [17].

8.6 Controversies

8.6.1 Direct Hernia Defect Closure

There are a few currently debated topics in robotic hernia repair. One of these includes direct hernia defect closure. With use of the robotic platform, the surgeon is able to close the defect with excellent vision. A few studies have demonstrated a possible decrease in seroma occurrence during laparoscopic repair; however, no clear benefit exists [18] Furthermore, suturing the direct defect adds a potential risk of chronic pain, bleeding, and damage to surrounding structures [19].

8.6.2 Mesh Fixation

The choice of mesh fixation differs between surgeons. Some choose to use tackers or sutures to secure mesh and ensure adequate mesh overlap (sutures are more commonly employed in robotic repair due to technical feasibility). Others opt to use fibrin glue as their fixating agent, self-fixating mesh, or no additional means of fixation, avoiding securing agents all together. In reality, any method is feasible and appropriate depending on surgeon preference and expertise. One must also take into account the potential risks of each technique and the patients' primary complaint [20].

8.6.3 Non-Mesh Robotic TAPP Repairs

An evolving concept is non-mesh robotic TAPP repairs, which has become feasible due to the increased visualization and fine articulating capabilities of the robot. With the known complications of chronic pain, the utility of non-mesh repairs is being explored. Rates of chronic pain and recurrence after a non-mesh robotic repair has yet to be determined. As of the writing of this chapter, non-mesh robotic inguinal hernia repairs remains experimental and should best be performed as part of a long term study.

8.7 Conclusion

Robotic TAPP hernia repair is safe and feasible in the hands of an experienced surgeon. It is applicable to a variety of scenarios including previous hernia repairs (both laparoscopic and open), large scrotal hernias, previous prostatectomy, and even feasible in patients with midline scars. Despite evidence for increased operative cost, outcomes are improved compared to open techniques and may be equivalent compared to the laparoscopic TAPP technique. Trocar site hernias remain a unique risk compared to laparoscopy, given the procedure utilizes three 8 mm trocars. Surgeons early in their learning curve may have higher recurrence rates and potential complications compared to surgeons who are more experienced in this technique. As the utility of the robot platform continues to evolve, outcomes will continue to improve and options for inguinal hernia repair will expand. Further studies should be performed to investigate outcomes comparing the different hernia repair platforms.

References

1. Kudsi OY, McCarty JC, Paluvoi N, Mabardy AS. Transition from laparoscopic totally extraperitoneal inguinal hernia repair to robotic transabdominal preperitoneal inguinal hernia repair: a retrospective review of a single surgeon's experience. World J Surg. 2017; https://doi.org/10.1007/s00268-017-3998-3.
2. Waite KE, Herman MA, Doyle PJ. Comparison of robotic versus laparoscopic transabdominal preperitoneal (TAPP) inguinal hernia repair. J Robot Surg. 2016; https://doi.org/10.1007/s11701-016-0580-1.
3. Higgins RM, Frelich MJ, Bosler ME, Gould JC. Cost analysis of robotic versus laparoscopic general surgery procedures. Surg Endosc Other Interv Tech. 2017;31:185–92.
4. Rosemar A, Angerås U, Rosengren A, Nordin P, Angeras U, Rosengren A, Nordin P. Effect of body mass index on groin hernia surgery. Ann Surg. 2010;252:397–401.
5. Escobar Dominguez JE, Ramos MG, Seetharamaiah R, Donkor C, Rabaza J, Gonzalez A. Feasibility of robotic inguinal hernia repair, a single-institution experience. Surg Endosc Other Interv Tech. 2016; https://doi.org/10.1007/s00464-015-4717-5.
6. Iraniha A, Peloquin J. Long-term quality of life and outcomes following robotic assisted TAPP inguinal hernia repair. J Robot Surg. 2017; https://doi.org/10.1007/s11701-017-0727-8.
7. Kosturakis AK, Larusso KE, Carroll ND, Nicholl MB. First 100 consecutive robotic inguinal hernia repairs at a Veterans Affairs hospital. J Robot Surg. 2018; https://doi.org/10.1007/s11701-018-0812-7.
8. Patel JA, Kaufman AS, Howard RS, Rodriguez CJ, Jessie EM. Risk factors for urinary retention after laparoscopic inguinal hernia repairs. Surg Endosc Other Interv Tech. 2015;29:3140–5.

9. Muysoms F, Van Cleven S, Kyle-Leinhase I, Ballecer C, Ramaswamy A. Robotic-assisted laparoscopic groin hernia repair: observational case-control study on the operative time during the learning curve. Surg Endosc. 2018;32(12):4850–9.
10. Dickens EO, Kolachalam R, Gonzalez A, Richardson C, D'Amico L, Rabaza J, Gamagami R. Does robotic-assisted transabdominal preperitoneal (R-TAPP) hernia repair facilitate contralateral investigation and repair without compromising patient morbidity? https://doi.org/10.1007/s11701-018-0815-4.
11. Gopal SV, Warrier A. Recurrence after groin hernia repair-revisited. Int J Surg. 2013;11:374–7.
12. McKay R. Preperitoneal herniation and bowel obstruction post laparoscopic inguinal hernia repair: Case report and review of the literature. Hernia. 2008;12:535–7.
13. Agresta F, Mazzarolo G, Bedin N. Incarcerated internal hernia of the small intestine through a re-Approximated peritoneum after a trans-abdominal pre-Peritoneal procedure-Apropos of two cases: Review of the literature. Hernia. 2011;15:347–50.
14. Köhler G, Mayer F, Lechner M, Bittner R. Small bowel obstruction after TAPP repair caused by a self-anchoring barbed suture device for peritoneal closure: case report and review of the literature. Hernia. 2015;19:389–94.
15. Fitzgerald HL, Orenstein SB, Novitsky YW. Small bowel obstruction owing to displaced spiral tack after laparoscopic TAPP inguinal hernia repair. Surg Laparosc Endosc Percutan Tech. 2010; https://doi.org/10.1097/SLE.0b013e3181dfbc05.
16. Gersin KS, Heniford BT, Garcia-Ruiz A, Ponsky JL. Missed lipoma of the spermatic cord. A pitfall of transabdominal preperitoneal laparoscopic hernia repair. Surg Endosc. 1999;13:585–7.
17. Moreno-Egea A. Surgical management of postoperative chronic inguinodynia by laparoscopic transabdominal preperitoneal approach. Surg Endosc Other Interv Tech. 2016;30:5222–7.
18. Li J, Zhang W. Closure of a direct inguinal hernia defect in laparoscopic repair with barbed suture: a simple method to prevent seroma formation? Surg Endosc Other Interv Tech. 2018;32:1082–6.
19. Kane ED, Leduc M, Schlosser K, Parentela N, Wilson D, Romanelli JR. Comparison of peritoneal closure versus non-closure in laparoscopic trans-abdominal preperitoneal inguinal hernia repair with coated mesh. Surg Endosc. 2018;32:627–37.
20. Mayer F, Niebuhr H, Lechner M, Dinnewitzer A, Köhler G, Hukauf M, Fortelny RH, Bittner R, Köckerling F. When is mesh fixation in TAPP-repair of primary inguinal hernia repair necessary? The register-based analysis of 11,230 cases. Surg Endosc Other Interv Tech. 2016;30:4363–71.

Robotic Repair of Giant Inguinal Hernias

9

David S. Edelman

9.1 Introduction

Giant inguinal hernias are infrequent in developed countries, but are seen enough times that surgeons who focus their practice on the repair of hernias need to be familiar with the planning, performance, correction and treatment of this problem. In situations where access to surgical care is limited, inguinal hernias that extend into the scrotum with extension into a sac down to the mid-thigh, knee or further are more frequently encountered. The surgical management is more challenging in these situations. Having access to a broad variety of pre-operative, peri-operative and post-operative assistance cannot be overstressed. A straight forward laparoscopic repair can turn into a complicated operation that every hernia surgeon should avoid but be ready to act upon. This chapter will try to cover as many possible issues associated with the robotic repair of giant inguinal (scrotal) hernias to better prepare the surgeon and the entire team involved in the care of this problem.

9.2 History

To review the entire history of inguinal hernia repair is beyond the scope of this chapter. To not mention some of the icons associated with the progress of inguinal hernia surgery would be an oversight. In 1884, Bassini described the extraperitoneal approach of hernia repair and reconstruction of the inguinal floor. Theodor Bilroth in 1890 opined that mesh was the ideal material to close a hernia defect but his meshes failed due to infection, rejection and recurrence. In the mid 1950's, Marlex (polyolefin) and polypropylene were popularized by Francis Usher and Pierre Frauchard, separately. It was 30 years later before Stoppa and Rives

D. S. Edelman (✉)
Doctor's Hospital, Baptist Health South Florida, Miami, FL, USA
e-mail: ETSsurgeon@sweatstop.com

K. A. LeBlanc (ed.), *Robotic Assisted Hernia Repair*,
https://doi.org/10.1007/978-3-030-23025-8_9

introduced the concept of a giant prosthetic mesh reinforcement of the visceral sac using Mersilene (dacron polyester). There is an excellent review of the Stoppa groin hernia repair in the 1998 Surgical Clinics of North America by George E. Wantz that should be reviewed by any present day hernia surgeon before tackling the pre-peritoneal approach to inguinal hernias or more importantly, giant scrotal hernias. Most all of the laparoscopic methods follow the tenets set forth by these landmark papers proposing using a mesh not less than 10 × 10 cm in size but approaching a 12 × 15 cm sized mesh, if possible. The discussion goes on to point out the importance of an anatomic, suture-less and tension-free repair as to result in an effective inguinal hernia repair.

9.3 Pre-operative Preparation

The re-introduction of herniated bowel back into the abdominal cavity due to a large, scrotal hernia will alter many aspects of a patient's cardio-pulmonary and vascular systems. The diaphragm will be pushed upwards and alter lung function or decrease venous return to the heart, change portal flow to the liver or alter blood flow in and away from the kidneys. The increase in abdominal pressure can cause changes in the abdominal wall and can cause a breakdown of the skin which can lead to wound dehiscence and hernia recurrence. In addition, many patients with scrotal hernias are older and have associated cardiovascular or respiratory diseases. Placing them under a general anesthesia will affect their peri-operative and post-operative course. Patients may need to be maintained on a ventilator after surgery. Informing the patient of these possibilities can help them participate in their pre- and postoperative care. Lastly, the risk of colon cancer is rising in many parts of the world and patients over 45 or who have a family history of colon cancer cannot be overlooked or avoided in the preoperative work up; in other words a colonoscopy, barium enema or CT enterography may be needed before surgery.

The surgeon who is treating this type of hernia will need to coordinate numerous pre-operative evaluations. A concise, complete history and physical exam with clear documentation of these findings is the first step. There is a need to include medications, allergies, family and social history to fully understand all of the patient's problems. Baseline blood work must be done which should include a complete blood count (CBC with platelets), comprehensive metabolic panel (CMP-25: electrolytes, liver function, renal function and protein), coagulation profile (PT, PTT) as well as a chest X-ray and an electrocardiogram (EKG). Routine cardiology and pulmonary consultation are frequently necessary. If an abnormality with the patient's renal function is noted on the chemistry panel, one should consider a pre-operative nephrology consultation to allow the kidney specialist an opportunity to become familiar with this patient before surgery and make any necessary changes in the diet and fluid balance. The knowledge that forcing the intestine back into the abdominal cavity can decrease blood flow from the lower extremities and pelvis should alert the surgeon to the risk of deep vein thrombosis. Placement of an IVC filter should be considered in such situations. Some of the percutaneous filters can be removed in the post-operative period and this can be discussed with the medical consultants prior to hernia repair. Gastrointestinal (GI) consultation may be needed for assistance in the determination and completion of needed colonic endoscopic screening and gastro-esophageal endoscopy. A barium small bowel evaluation or CT scan with contrast may be necessary if there is any question about the contents within the hernia sac (bowel and/or urinary bladder) and how the surgery may alter or deal with them.

Lastly, urology and plastic surgery evaluation is commonly necessary to assist with the operation. A massive scrotum may also cause the penis to be retracted and make it difficult to find it or access the urinary bladder during an operative procedure. It is not uncommon to need a cystoscopy in order to place a urinary catheter at the start of surgery. An evaluation by the urologist prior to the day of surgery may alleviate this disconcerting situation. Additionally, the urologist will have insight into the proper reconstruction of the scrotum at the conclusion of the operation. Most importantly, the spermatic cord and testicle may be involved in the hernia sac to a point of being seriously injured during this type of hernia repair. The availability of the urologist at the time of the scrotal hernia repair could be beneficial during and after surgery if there is a question of testiclicular viability, as well.

Depending on the size of the scrotum, a scrotoplasty may be necessary. Surgeon comfort with this along with an urologist may suffice, but if there is any question of the need or extent of this problem when the scrotum is massive, the assistance of a plastic surgeon is welcomed.

The ability to reduce the hernia into the abdominal cavity prior to surgery cannot be overemphasized. *Type 1* giant, scrotal hernias which may reach down to the mid-thigh and are reducible, usually can be approached without many alterations in pre-operative planning or surgical care. If the hernia reaches below the mid-thigh to the knee, a *Type 2* giant hernia, or below the knee, a *Type 3* giant hernia, reduction of the hernia contents becomes unlikely and increased intra-abdominal pressure and loss of abdominal domain are issues that must be considered. Type 2 and Type 3 hernias are most likely better approached with open hernioplasty and scrotal reduction procedures. However, once the open procedure is completed, a robotic, laparoscopic re-inforcement of the posterior inguinal floor may be a consideration is selected instances.

9.4 Operative Techniques

Progressive pneumoperitoneum is a technique that, when combined with Botulinum Toxin A (Botox), can increase the abdominal wall musculature length and act as a chemical component separation. It should be started 5–6 weeks prior to surgery. Using ultrasonic or CT scan guidance, an Interventional Radiologist should inject 100–300 units of Botox on each side of the abdominal wall. Stated in another way, 50 units of Botox can be injected into each of the Internal Oblique, External Oblique and Transverse abdominis muscles in the anterior axillary line on both the right and left abdominal wall. This procedure is tolerated very well under conscious sedation.

One of the main disadvantages to the use of Botox is deep muscle injury and muscle weakness. Caution should be exercised in patients with chronic respiratory dysfunction as there have been instances of prolonged postoperative ventilation and the need for abdominal musculature recruitment for ventilation. Inactivation of the lateral abdominal muscles may make coughing, sneezing and deep breathing difficult. The use of an incentive spirometer device can assist the patient during this time and is helpful to increase breathing capacity and decrease postoperative compression atelectasis.

The effects of abdominal wall elongation from Botox will start about 2 weeks after instillation which is when Progressive Pneumoperitoneum (if needed) should be initiated. A percutaneous or laparoscopic assisted peritoneal dialysis catheter (or Hickman Catheter) can be placed at the same time as the Botox injection allowing 2 weeks for healing. For the initial pneumoperitoneum, it is done once or twice a day for the first week and weekly thereafter for a total of 4 weeks. Patients may need to be hospitalized or monitored as an outpatient to assess toleration of the progressive pneumoperitoneum. Usually within a week, the patient's abdominal wall will expand to accommodate the one liter of ambient air that is injected. Alternatively, some centers will introduce the air every 2–3 days in a clinic situation after the initial introduction is completed. During the course of progressive pneumoperitoneum, the hernia contents may be able to be reduced. If this occurs, the repair of the inguinal hernia may proceed without he need for open surgery and/or a scrotoplasty. Bowel prep and colonoscopy can be considered a day or two prior to operative repair of the inguinal hernia.

Complications from progressive pneumoperitoneum are not common but do occur. Adhesions from previous surgery may be a reason for failure to establishment of the pneumoperitoneum. Epigastric pain and the sensation of gastric fullness is not uncommon at the time the establishment of the pneumoperitoneum. Organ rupture, bowel injury, hematoma formation, air emboli and subcutaneous emphysema are a few of the uncommon complications that can occur from this procedure.

Performance of a robotic inguinal hernia should be the same as described in an earlier chapter of this book. There may need to be modifications to the techniques which will include steep Trendelenburg position, placement of the cannulas higher and above the umbilicus than one would use for a more straight forward robotic inguinal hernia and the use of a 4th, accessory cannula for use of a grasper or fan retractor to hold back the intestinal contents or to introduce mesh. This fourth port, usually an 8 mm cannula, may be as large as a 12 mm cannula and the surgeon should select an appropriate cannula. Usually, the 12 mm cannula site may need to be closed at the completion of the operation. I do not routinely close the 8 mm cannula sites except when it is located at the umbilicus or within an abdominal wall hernia.

The patient should be intubated under general endotracheal anesthesia and supine on the operating room table. The arms are usually tucked but may have to be on arm boards if the patient is too large. With sequential compression devices (SCD's) on the calves, the bed should be put into as steep a Trendelenburg position that can be tolerated. An initial effort at hernia reduction may be attempted at this time. The cautery return pad is placed per hospital protocol with the cautery settings selected as low as possible to prevent inadvertent arcing of the current to the intestines or other abdominal organs. The prepping and draping should be done very widely to include the scrotum. A urinary drainage catheter should be considered as many of these procedures are longer than 90 min. As mentioned earlier, if the penis is retracted, an urologist may be needed to place the catheter using cystoscopic guidance.

Selection of the cannula sites should be far enough away from the anticipated arcuate ligament and may be 6–8 cm above the umbilicus. Accessory cannulas on either side of the midline camera port are placed about 8–10 cm laterally. If a fourth port is deemed necessary, it can be placed in the right lower abdomen above and away from the anterior superior iliac spine. Either a 0 ° or 30° laparoscope will be selected depending on the comfort of the surgeon but I generally use a 0° laparoscope. Once the site is selected for the camera, I recommend on open approach into the abdominal cavity but the operative surgeon can use a Veress needle technique or an optical trocar. I will set the insufflator to a pressure under 15 mm Hg and use the lowest possible setting due to the head-down position and the ability of anesthesia to adequately ventilate the patient. A large grasper is used in the left hand, but it is not uncommon for me to use a regular, robotic needle holder instead. The right hand instrument should have cautery ability and although I use the cautery hook (set at 20 watts coagulating current), it is not unusual for many surgeons to use cautery scissors or bipolar graspers instead.

All of the intestine must be reduced from the hernia sac before going any additional dissection occurs. If the bowel is adherent to the inside the hernia sac, it will be extremely difficult to reduce it thereby increasing the risk of an injury to the bowel. The assistant may need to push on the scrotum at this point while the surgeon gently retracts and pulls on the mesentery of the bowel to allow the intestines to be reduced into the abdominal cavity. It is advisable to set a timer and not labor at this point for more than 10–15 min. If the bowel cannot be reduced, consideration should be made to temporarily stop laparoscopy and open the inguinal region with a transverse, inguinal or lower midline incision. In this instance, it may be easier to open, reduce the hernia, do a simple Bassini closure of the inguinal floor prior to placing a large piece of mesh behind the hernia repair.

Once the intestine and urinary bladder are reduced, the peritoneum can be opened lateral to the umbilical ligament at the arcuate ligament. The peritoneal dissection is carried further laterally to the anterior axillary line (about 8–10 cm). The epigastric vessels need to be identified at this point and the dissection carried down inferiorly, along these vessels to their takeoff from the femoral vessels. Medial to the epigastric vessel origin, the pubic bone is identified and dissection is carried out below and past the midline on the side of the hernia. Lateral to the epigastric vessels, any indirect hernia sac or cord lipoma are meticulously removed from the spermatic cord or round ligament with the understanding that the femoral artery and vein are directly below. Once the iliopubic tract is identified, the hernia sac can be followed down along the spermatic cord or round ligament and dissected free. I do not transect the round ligament, but some surgeons do. It is wise to assess the viability of the testicle at this time since large scrotal hernias stretch the spermatic cord structures. The release of the tension on the spermatic cord can precipitate thrombosis of the spermatic vasculature. Intra-operative ultrasound, if available, can be used if there is question of vascular integrity.

If you have been successful up to this point, repair of the hernia can proceed. Most times, the hernia defect is quite large and the additional placement of a suture to reconstruct and imbricate the transversalis fascia to act as a "back-stop" is recommended. There are many ways to re-create a tension-free inguinal floor using robotic needle holders in both hands (one may be a suture-cutter). For a direct hernia, I will use a 0 braided polyester suture and either do a purse string stitch tying it to itself or a running suture by making a simple knot medially, then running the suture lateral to the epigastric vessels and back to where I started and finally tying an intra-corporeal knot. Alternatively, a "Barbed" suture (V-loc or Stratafix) of 2–0 or 0 size, either absorbable or non-absorbable can be run by suturing the sac to itself or the posterior pubic bone. For an indirect hernia, I start laterally with interrupted figure 8 sutures of 0 braided polyester suture but this could be used as a running suture. If this is chosen the surgeon should look cautiously for the nerves at the internal ring and leave adequate spacing for the spermatic cord at the internal ring and not place undo tension on the closure.

Finally, I will introduce a ruler and measure the operative site to use the largest piece of soft polypropylene mesh that I can safely place. From Stoppa's and Wantz's work, a 12 × 15 cm or larger piece of mesh is ideal. Selection of mesh is the surgeon's preference and there are many types available that work well. Once the mesh is rolled up into a "cigarette" shape, it can pass through an 8 mm cannula or the accessory 12 mm cannula without much difficulty. Using two needle holders or a grasper and a needle holder, the mesh is opened completely and placed behind the hernia repair below the pubic bone, lateral to the midline and as far lateral as possible to the edge of the arcuate ligament onto the cord structures and iliofemoral vessels. I prefer to spray the mesh with fibrin sealant, but many surgeons will place a suture or two to prevent the mesh from moving or have the surgical assistant place a few tacks. Some surgeons will use self-adhering mesh for this part of the procedure.

I will close the peritoneum with a running 3–0 absorbable, barbed suture. If a 12 mm cannula was used, a port closure device or a simple suture closure should be made. I will close the midline "umbilical" port site, as well. Skin closure is a surgeon's preference, but I have used an absorbable subcuticular skin closure followed by tissue skin adhesive for many years.

9.5 Post-operative Issues and Recommendations

Intensive care unit (ICU), a step-down "progressive care unit" (PCU) or routine floor care should be discussed with the anesthesiologist or a pulmonologist before the patient leaves the Post Anesthesia Care Unit (PACU). I will leave the Foley catheter in overnight, start prophylactic anticoagulation (if an IVC filter was not used) and monitor the patient carefully for the first night or two.

Complications that need to be monitored for include:

- Elevation of the hemidiaphragm with decreased pulmonary function, rapid heart and respiratory rate;
  - post-operative portable *Chest X-ray* and *Arterial Blood Gas* in the PACU
- Increased abdominal pressure leading to lower venous return and lower cardiac output;
- Abdominal compartment syndrome and mesenteric ischemia;
  - intra-abdominal hypertension is defined as a pressure over 12 mm Hg in adults. However, if the pressure continues to rise over 20 mm Hg and organs begin to fail, the syndrome has now progressed to the end stage of the highly fatal process termed abdominal compartment syndrome- measure *lactic acid*
- Low urine output due to third spacing of fluids from a large operative area of dissection or Hematoma from a large dissection area;
  - post-operative *serum chemistries* and a complete blood counts-*CBC*
- Small and large bowel adhesions which may have been injured by adhesiolysis that may cause an ileus or a post-operative intestinal obstruction;
  - *serial plain abdominal X-ray- KUB*
- Deep vein thrombosis, pulmonary emboli or pelvic venous stasis due to return of the intestine into the abdominal cavity;
  - *venous sonogram* of the pelvis and lower extremity
- Urinary bladder injury or an atonic bladder when the bladder is reduced out of the hernia defect;
- Orchitis, testicular atrophy or ischemia from the manipulation or the effects of shortening the spermatic cord;
  - *testicular sonogram*
- Edema of the scrotum, wound ischemia or mesh infection.

9.6 Summary

Large scrotal hernias can be approached using robotic and laparoscopic techniques. Preparation is paramount to a successful repair, no matter what technique or approach is selected. It is not considered a complication to add an open inguinal or midline abdominal incision to the repair of these complex hernias as there are times when the surgeon cannot determine that the open approach is safer until the time of surgery. A careful and well thought out pre-operative approach can optimize the operative repair. Using appropriate consultations is encouraged. Post-operative issues develop, not infrequently, and it may be wise to consider placement of the patient for a day or two in the Intensive Care Unit to monitor for minor problems before they become serious issues.

Acknowledgments A special thanks to Charlotte Klienman and Simone Baldeon, at the Baptist Health Library for their assistance with this chapter.

References

1. Patas A, Tsiaousis P, Papaziogas B, et al. Repair of a inguinoscrotal hernia. Hernia. 2010;14:305–7.
2. Wantz GE. Giant prosthetic reinforcement of the visceral sac, The Stoppa groin hernia Repair. Surg Clin N Am. 1998;78(6):1075–87.
3. Coetzee E, Price C, Boutall A. Simple repair of a giant inguinoscrotal hernia. Int J Surg Case Rep. 2011;2:32–5.
4. Trakarnsagna A, Chinswangwatanakul V, Methasate A, et al. Giant inguinal hernia: report of a case and reviews of surgical techniques. Int J Surg Case Rep. 2014;5:868–72.
5. Karthikeyan VS, Sistla SC, Ram D, Ali SM, Rajkumar N. Giant inguinoscrotal hernia- report of a rare case with literature review. Int Surg. 2014;99:560–4.
6. Vagholkar K, Vagholkar S. Surgical management of giant inguinoscrotal hernias. Int Surg J. 2015;2(4):693–5.
7. Sturniolo G, Tonante A, Gagliano E, et al. Surgical treatment of the giant inguinal hernia. Hernia. 1999;3:27–30.
8. Tahir M, Ahmed FU, Seenu V. Giant inguinoscrotal hernia: case report and management principles. Int J Surg. 2008;6:495–7.
9. Weissler JM, Lanni MA, Tecce MG, et al. Chemical component separation: a systemic review and meta-analysis of botulinum toxin for management of ventral hernia. J Plast Surg Hand Surg. 2017;51(5):366–74.
10. Soltanizadeh S, Helgstrand F, Jorgensen LN. Botulinum toxin A as an adjunct to abdominal wall reconstruction for incisional hernia. Plast Reconstr Surg Glob Open. 2017;5(6):e1358.
11. Moreno IG. Chronic eventrations and large hernias: preoperative treatments by progressive pneumoperitoneum. Surgery. 1947;22:945–53.
12. Koontz AR, Graves JW. Preoperative pneumoperitoneum as an aid in the handling of gigantic hernias. Ann Surg. 1954;140:759–62.
13. Edelman DS. Robotic inguinal hernia repair. Am Surg. 2017;83(12):1418–21.
14. Kolachalam R, Dickens E, D'Amico L, Richardson C, et al. Early outcomes of robotic-assisted inguinal hernia repair in obese patients: a multi-institutional retrospective study. Surg Endosc. 2018;32(1):229–35.

Pelvic Hernias

10

Ricardo Zugaib Abdalla and Thiago Nogueira Costa

10.1 Introduction

Pelvic hernia is diagnosed as a protrusion of anatomical contents through the pelvic floor. The pelvic floor is a complex anatomical environment, composed of several overlapping myopectineal tissues, joints and bones at the base of the cavity to assist in supporting the organs of the abdomen. All this complex reference is important to remember when we are working on the reconstruction of pelvic anatomy [1]. The pelvic defects realize some hernia types, such as, the sciatic, obturator, para-vesical and perineal hernias. The first three are rare entities, mostly primary hernias [2, 3]. Primary defects are congenital, because of anatomical predisposing factors. The urogenital perineal floor has a different structure from posterior pelvic floor. Although these types of diseases are different, they have similarities in their treatment, but without standardization, because of their rare presentations. Perineal or secondary hernias are usually incisional hernias following proctectomy or abdominal perineal excision (APE) [4, 5]. They account for 1–7% of the incisional hernias, with a rare incidence [6]. APE is the surgical treatment for patients with distal rectal cancer in whom an anterior resection (AR) of the rectum with anastomosis cannot be performed, leaving them with a terminal colostomy and a blind-end pelvic floor. Even though it is a radical procedure, it has a high incidence of local recurrence, due to the extended invasion those types of cancer possess [7]. Therefore, other techniques were created to try to get optimal oncologic results. This was how the extralevator abdominal perineal excision (ELAPE) was created, with a larger margin of resection in the attempt to have better oncologic outcomes. However, with the increased resection, the incidence of perineal hernia became higher, leading to the discussion of prevention

R. Z. Abdalla (✉) · T. N. Costa
Department of Digestive Surgery, Hospital das Clinicas of University of Sao Paulo Medical School, Sao Paulo, Brazil
e-mail: ricardo.abdalla@hc.fm.usp.br

K. A. LeBlanc (ed.), *Robotic Assisted Hernia Repair*,
https://doi.org/10.1007/978-3-030-23025-8_10

and possible treatments of this disease [8, 9]. Both can be treated either from the abdominal cavity or from the outside, but this chapter focuses on incisional and intra cavitary approach.

The main risk factors of the development of a perineal hernia (other than the type of surgery performed) include: female gender (five times more common than men), neoadjuvant chemoradiation (very common in these types of disease), poor nutrition, use of tobacco, wound infection and the failure to close the perineal defect [10]. Other factors, such as, obesity and age have lower impact on hernia formation [11]. There are no classifications regarding perineal or sciatic hernias, since they are rare; and their main treatment is not well standardized.

Symptoms range from bowel obstruction, obstipation, skin erosion, and slight bulging in these regions. The patients can exhibit urinary problems, perineal pain or other types of skin lesions [12]. Intractable pain must be considered as a diagnosis of recurrent tumor. In the case of perineal hernias, most plastic surgeons can construct rotational tissue flaps or primary closure, to treat them locally. Surgery from the inside could be considered the best approach because of minimally invasive procedure principles, with less infection, decreased recovery time, and visualization of the defect origin. This leads to better disease understanding, because there is no subcutaneous or myoaponeurotic tissue interposition. Therefore, the repair can respect a physiologic recovery, with the help of the use of mesh [13–15]. Even though there are a variety of procedures, the recurrence rate can still be as high as 16% [16].

Benefits of the minimally invasive surgery are proven for abdominal wall defects, however, the laparoscopic approach has only a few cases reported for this problem due to the difficulties of the deep dissection, distant adhesions, straight forward non-articulating instruments, 2D view, difficult mesh placement and fixation. The robotic dissection is at its dawn, but working with irradiated tissue is, probably, easier to do when compared with rigid, non-articulating laparoscopic instruments. Robotic arm torque helps to reach more areas with less fatigue, as well as, the relative frictionless movement can facilitate difficult dissections [17, 18]. The ideal mesh and ideal pelvic fixation of the mesh are obstacles to face with every patient, meaning that each one must be treated with individually [19–21]. The decision varies per patient, due to their unique pathologies, with the goal of the recovery of the whole diaphragmatic pelvis [14, 22]. With the advent of the robotic technologies, the articulated forceps and 3D view optics, many problems can be better solved [23]. Thus, in this chapter we present a concept-based technique of robotic treatment of the pelvic defects.

10.2 Technique

Before commencement of the procedure, the patient must be evaluated and prepared. It must be emphasized that these are mostly oncologic patients after chemotherapy and/or radiotherapy. First, a good history of symptoms and comorbidities must be acquired from the patient. Performance status is very important, because of the post-operative risks for complications (seroma, hematoma, post-operative

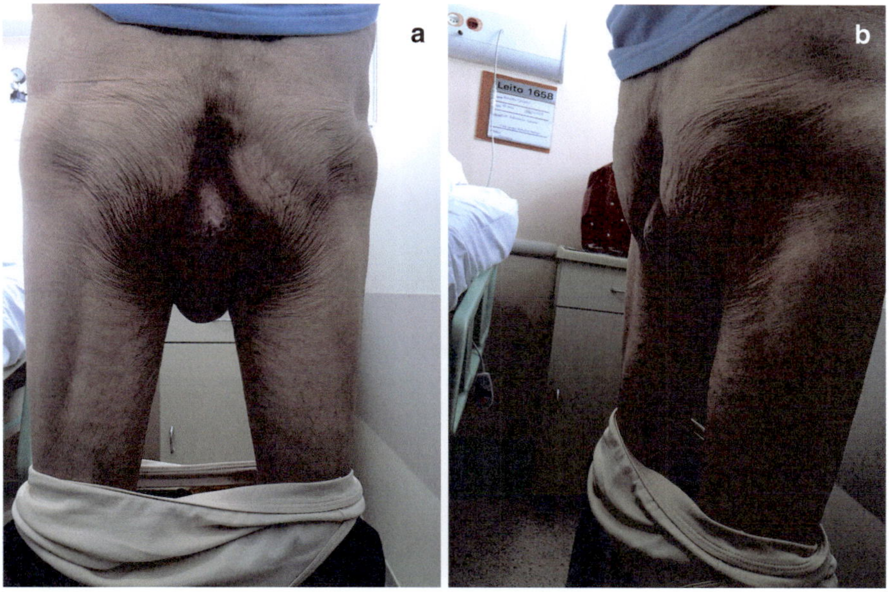

Fig. 10.1 (**a**, **b**) Physical exam

infection, etc.). Physical examination in performed with the patient in different positions. (Fig. 10.1a, b). In order to confirm the diagnosis, a Computed Tomography (CT) of the abdomen and pelvis should be done (Fig. 10.2a, b).

When the diagnosis is made the patient must be prepared for surgery. Additional hernia possibilities must be considered and investigated, such as parastomal hernia or midline incisional hernia. The importance of the identification of these other defects is to provide the team with a complete understanding of all pathologies that need to be treated. Therefore, during the intra-abdominal view, the best repair can be made for each case and potentially the need for more than one procedure at a later time to repair all the hernias that are found. The robot with its longer instruments and with more freedom of movements than traditional laparoscopic instrumentation can be located on the contralateral side of the ostomy and further away from the pelvis. This allows more possibility to determine which repair should be done at the time of operation.

10.3 Patient Preparation and Positioning

The patient is hospitalized on the same day of the surgery. In most cases, there is no need for bowel preparation. Once in the operating room (OR) appropriate preparation is noted in Table 10.1. General anesthesia is applied with endotracheal intubation. Next, the patient receives prophylactic antibiotics and the urinary catheter as well as the placement of peripheral lines.

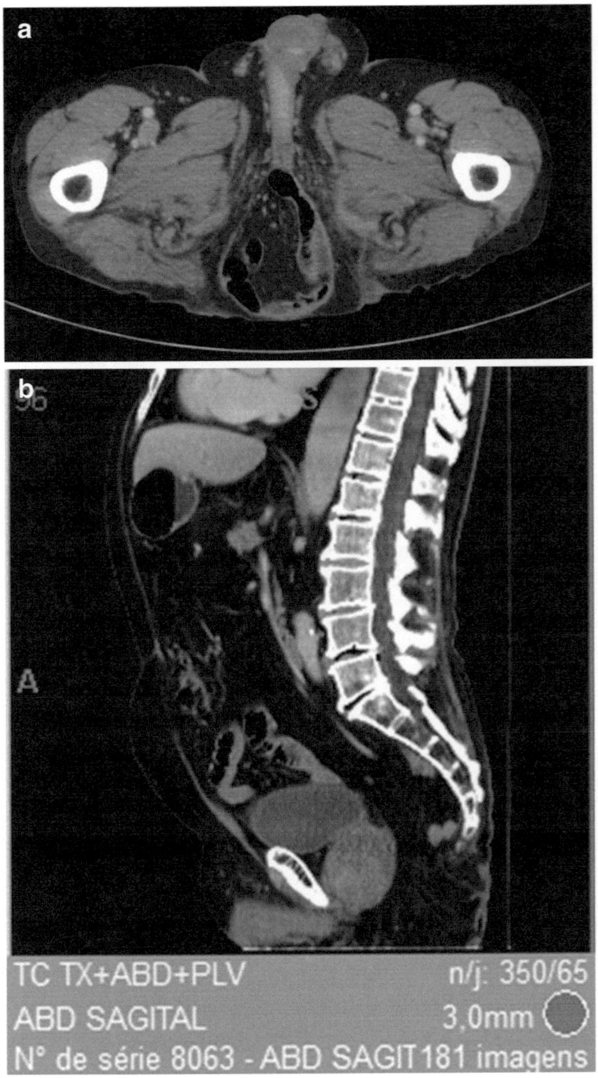

Fig. 10.2 (**a**, **b**) Computed tomography showing perineal hernia. (Axial and Sagittal)

The patient is placed on the surgical table with both arms tucked and legs close together, slightly spread or in lithotomy position, depending upon the necessity to reach the perineal protrusion from the outside, especially in larger hernias. Sometimes the legs can be spread to dock the robotic cart between them.

The patient is always secured to the table with fixation straps and well protected with chest and a head/eye protectors. A warming device placed on the chest to maintain body temperature (Fig. 10.3).

Table 10.1 Patient's preparation

Patient's preparation
Antibiotics
Urinary catheter
Peripheral lines
Fixation strap
Chest protector
Head/eye protector
Endotracheal cannula
Anesthesia cannulas
Energy Cables
Colostomy closure (sterile drape) Surgical drapes
Sterile film
Heater device

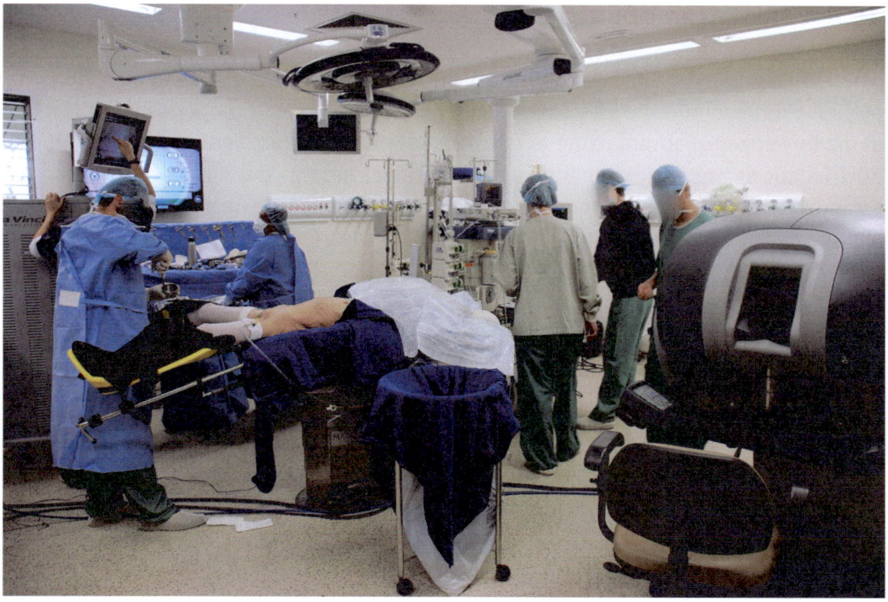

Fig. 10.3 Patient position

The surgical skin preparation is done using chlorhexidine. The surgical drapes are wide placed exposing all the abdominal area, extending laterally to expose both flanks. The colostomy, if present, is closed using a separate sterile surgical drape (Fig. 10.4a, b). After these steps, the anesthesia cannulas, energy cables and other parts of the OR are secured for surgery.

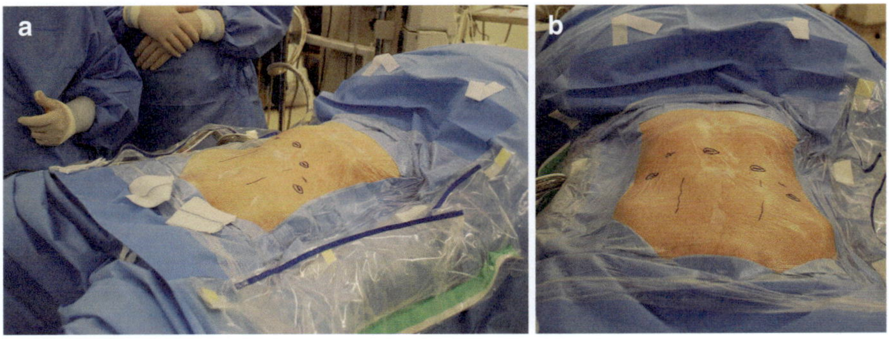

Fig. 10.4 (**a**, **b**) Drapes and marks

10.4 Initiation of Surgery

The surgery is ready to begin after all the preparations described above are completed. Entrance into the abdominal cavity to create the pneumoperitoneum is made at the left upper quadrant using a Veress needle with the pressure of 12 mm Hg. The port locations are selected choosing the perineal area as the target. When a colostomy is present, all the cannulas are placed to the right side or the fourth cannula is changed to contralateral side. The first cannula inserted is the optical one, 12 mm, positioned at 2 cm above umbilical scar and 2 cm to the patient's right; respecting a 20 cm distance from the target and aligned with the Si or Xi robotic cart.

When the camera is inserted, an initial evaluation of the abdominal cavity is done, looking at its entirety, from liver to pelvis, searching for adhesions, the primary hernia and other possible defects, such as: inguinal hernias, midline, parastomal or lateral incisional/ventral hernias [24]. The newest robotic generation makes it easier to investigate the cavity and/or work viewing all of the abdomen, because of the lighter camera.

The other 8 mm cannulas are placed in a slight curve, following the rule of 8–10 cm distance from each other to avoid collision during the procedure. The newer (Xi) generation is placed in a straight line at the same level of the camera with 6–8 cm distance from each other. This will facilitate manipulation and dissection closer to the instruments, when other abdominal wall hernias are noted. Arm 1 is placed in the right patient flank, arm 2 at the mid clavicular line on the patient's left side and arm 3 in the left iliac fossa or contralaterally when needed to be placed away from a colostomy. A fifth cannula for the assistant can be placed in the upper right quadrant (Fig. 10.4b). Caution must be taken to avoid injury to the colostomy when it exists.

In other cases, such as sciatic hernias, the optical cannula can be placed 4–5 cm above the umbilicus. In this setup the arm 1 can be placed at the right upper quadrant, arm 2 in the left upper quadrant and arm 3 in the left flank. The assistant port can be between the arms 2 and 3 at left side of the patient. In these types of hernias there is no concern of the colostomy, and most of the patients have not had previous surgeries. The working space is more cephalad than for the perineal incisional hernias. Because the perineal hernias require more posterior pelvic adhesiolysis which is more distal in the abdomen cavity, the robotic instruments will go deeper into the pelvis during the procedure.

10.5 Docking

When the cannulas are in place and position checked, it is time to dock the robot. Using the pelvic defect as the target, the robot can dock in many positions, but mainly from the "leg" approach. It is important that the patient extremities (head and feet) are at the table limits as this will give more room to the robotic patient cart approach. The arm joints should not collide with the patient's body or operative table if we respect the operative table borders corresponding to the patient limits.

Figures 10.5a–d show the possible dockings that can be done in the pelvic hernia repair (the new robot generation is easier to dock, because the boom comes from above the patient). It is beneficial to repeat the same docking position, as many times as possible.

The robot patient cart can come from the left side, with the legs close together, pointing a little lateral: this type of docking is used to treat left sciatic hernias and

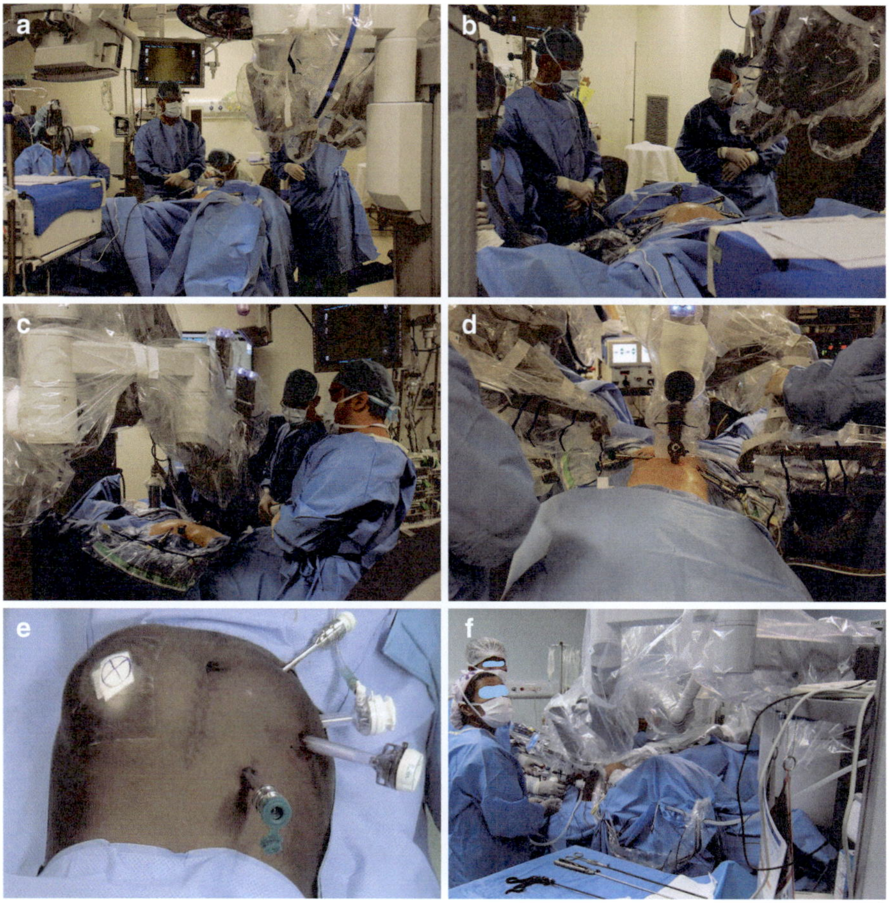

Fig. 10.5 (a–f) Docking

perineal hernias in order to protect the colostomy and treating possible paracolostomy defects, often present in patients that have undergone APE or ELAPE (Fig. 10.5e).

In the case of a right sciatic hernia the patient cart can come from the right with the legs close together. The third option is the docking between the legs, like it is used in prostatectomies (Fig. 10.5f). In event that an emergency situation develops, the assistant must be ready to undock the robot and take whatever action is necessary to solve the problem.

10.6 Surgical Technique

The surgical technique can be divided into sections for better understanding of the procedure. Hence, it will be separated in: dissection/adhesiolysis, consideration of defect closure when possible, mesh placement and fixation.

10.7 Dissection/Adhesiolysis

One of the most important parts about the dissection is the identification of the structures to be separated. Since one of the major complications of the perineal hernia repair is bowel injury, the adhesiolysis becomes even more important. The perineal defects are often accompanied by strong adhesions, mainly in the pelvic area, but the entire abdominal cavity can present them. The robotic instruments with wrist movements along with the 3D view can facilitate the management of these adhesions, diminishing lesion incidence and making the process faster. The CO_2 plays an important role penetrating between tissues, making a "gas dissection", sometimes revealing a safe plan to work.

The instruments used are: (Figs. 10.5 and 10.6)

- Monopolar scissors
- Maryland bipolar
- Cadiére with or without energy
- Double fenestrated
- Needle driver

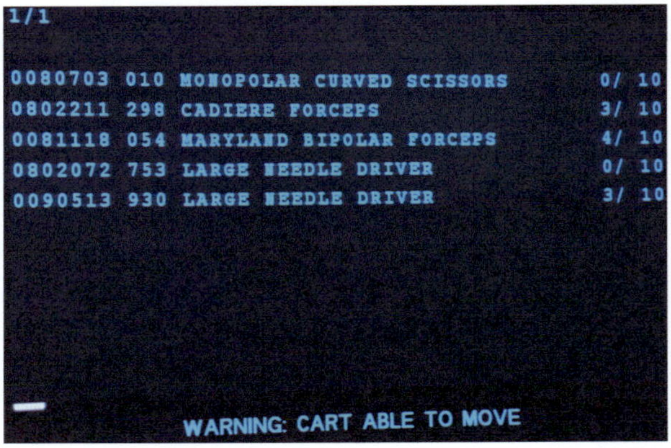

Fig. 10.6 Instruments

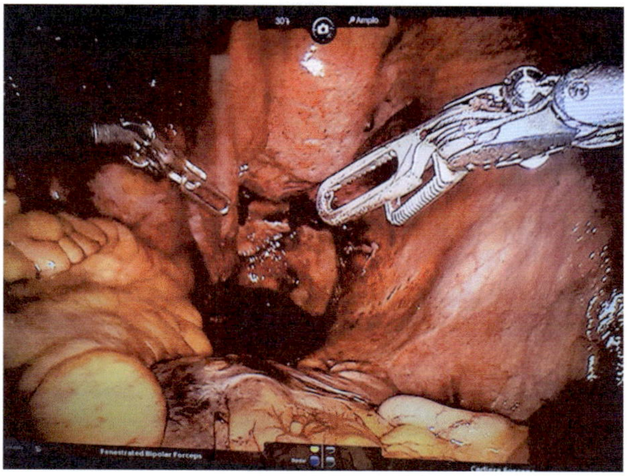

Fig. 10.7 Perineal defect (internal view)

The whole dissection is made using cautery, blunt dissection or cold scissors, depending on the location and type of adhesion. In the perineal area is sometimes difficult to have the right angle to work on, but with the robotic technology, the instruments' wrists can overcome this problem and the surgeon can dissect deeper into the pelvis and obturator space. The assistant can push the defect from the outside, with a lower intraabdominal pressure to reach deeper adhesions. Another important part about the perineal hernias, is that these patients can have concomitant hernias, such as paracolostomy or inguinal, so caution must be taken not to induce injuries.

After dissecting and lysis of all the adhesions, the defect can be seen, like any other laparoscopic incisional hernioplasty. (Fig. 10.7) At this time, it is important to have a good description of the hernia, with accurate measurement and correct vision of the edges, in order to choose the correct type of repair, reconstruction and fixation.

10.8 Defect Closure

There is a big discussion regarding whether to close the defect or not, in different types of hernia (ventral, inguinal). In recent years, the majority of the papers tend to favor the hernia closure, mainly in ventral hernias, for the mesh to lay flat and against the abdominal wall. In the perineal and obturator defects, this could be challenging, since there are few tissues to approximate and close.

Sometimes, in small defects, using the robotic instruments, such as the needle driver, the surgeon can approximate the edges of the defect with suture and trying to provide as little tension as possible. However, in most of the cases reported in the literature, regarding pelvic hernias, there is no closure of the defect. In our experience, the defect is only closed when we can provide no tension with surrounded tissues.

10.9 Mesh Placement and Fixation

After dissecting and exposing the defect it is time to understand the situation and plan its repair. There are surgical groups that repair these types of hernia from the perineum using surgical flaps without any meshes [2, 25–28]. But when this repair is approached from the abdominal cavity it is recommended to use a mesh, since in the majority of the times, the defect cannot be closed [6, 29–31].

The preferred type of mesh is coated mesh or double layer (i.e. tissue separating), because there is no tissue or peritoneum to cover the mesh and they will be exposed to the bowel. The mesh must have 3–5 cm wide overlap than the original defect, in all directions, with or without closing it. The most overlap that is obtainable is preferred.

Fixation can be done by hernia stapler (tackers) or by suture. Tackers are under a higher risk of bleeding, because of the pelvic vessels. Suture can be done under direct vision with delicate movements, choosing the border to pass the stitches. A big mesh can be fixed around the pelvis with a running suture over muscles posteriorly and laterally. When the mesh goes anterior, it can stay behind the bladder, over the urogenital ligament (when it is possible to dissect and visualize) or even can go over the bladder and fixate at Cooper's ligaments, on both sides. There are few studies comparing the type of fixation in other types of concomitant hernias, such as inguinal and ventral [32]. At this time, the recommendation is to consider each case individually. In the perineal hernia repair, the authors prefer to use tackers when the pelvic wall is seen, with good results. The tackers are applied at the peripheral part of the defect and 5 cm wider in a double crown technique, with direct vision (Fig. 10.8a, b).

10.10 Complications

All the types of surgery have their potential complications. In hernia surgery, those complications can impact the treatment, the return to normal activities and the rate of recurrence [33, 34].

One of the most common complications in laparoscopic and robotic hernia repair is the seroma. This is caused by a fluid collection localized mainly between the repair (mesh or closure) and the skin/hernia sac. In the perineal area this is very common due to the space and size of the hernia sac. In an effort to decrease the risk of this development, a good practice could be plication of the hernia sac in an effort to eliminate the dead space within the sac itself. It is essentially placing sutures in subcutaneous tissue, what is not always possible. However, most of the seromas are treated without any intervention [35–37].

Other major complication is bowel injury. This type of problem can lead to reoperations and even death. In the pelvic area it is important to do the adhesiolysis carefully so as to avoid any bowel lesions.

Clinical complications such as pulmonary infections and embolism must be remembered and care must focus on prevention with the use of prophylaxis an anti-coagulant of choice.

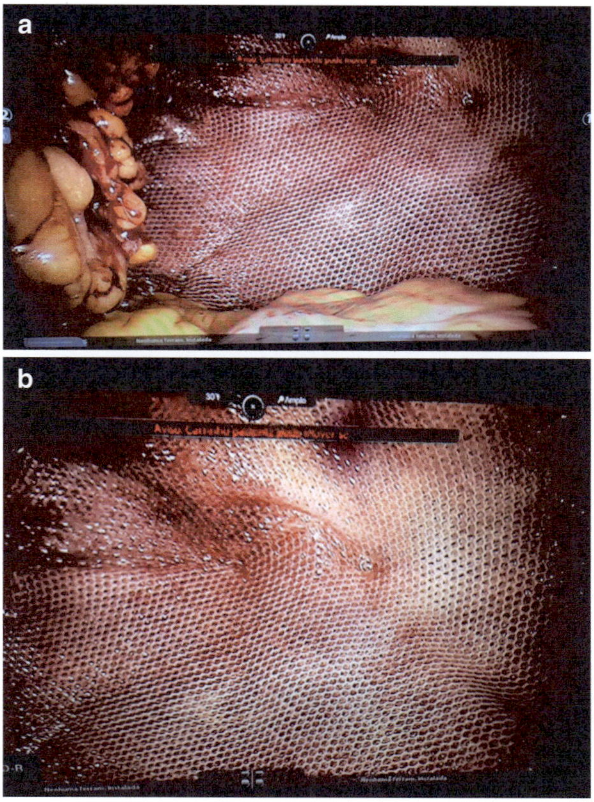

Fig. 10.8 Final view of the repair, with the mesh placed. (**a**) Internal view with colostomy. (**b**) Close internal view

Other complications such as infection, bleeding and adynamic ileus can be difficult to appreciate in some cases. The main complications can be seen in Table 10.2. Seroma, infection and patient clinical decompensation must be considered in these patients as most are at higher risk of these adverse events because they have had previous oncologic treatment(s).

Table 10.2 Surgical complications

Surgical complications
Seroma
Infection
Mesh migration
Bleeding
Adynamic ileus
Bowel injury
Care with colostomy
Clinical complications—Pulmonary and urinary

10.11 Results and Perspectives

There is little evidence until now regarding the minimally invasive treatment of pelvic hernias, including the robotic assisted repair. Although there are a short number of cases reported it appears that recurrence rates are lower, with good clinical results regarding time of hospital stay, pain and other complications [37]. Even the costs look better or lower when compared to pure laparoscopic procedures in more difficult cases as robotic surgery can decrease the length of stay and use of pain medication. It has also be noted that there are shorter operative times, less dissection and scars regarding robotic technology as this appears to facilitate the hernia repair technique.

However, it continues to be costly per procedure. Nonetheless, with major clinical trials comparing the robotic approach to pelvic hernias with the traditional surgeries (open repair and/or laparoscopic) this data will be confirmed or refuted. However, it currently appears that the total costs can be lower as the outcomes and benefits are confirmed.

10.12 Summary

Perineal/pelvic hernias have a rare incidence, achieving from 1% to 3% of the surgeries done in the pelvic floor [6, 7]. With the development of larger techniques to try to treat the distal rectal cancer, such as ELAPE, the incidence of that type of hernia is increasing.

There are different types of surgical procedures to repair the perineal hernia, but they are not standardized and can be done either from the perineum or from the abdominal cavity [33, 38]. With the advent of the minimally invasive surgery (MIS) the hernia repair could be taken to another level, with the understanding of anatomy and good technique to dissect the adhesions. Limitations such as 2D view and lack of articulated movements have lead the laparoscopic repair to be limited to only a few case reports.

Thus, by using the robotic technology those problems can be overcome and better results achieved in the treatment of perineal hernias. Caution and care must be taken to prepare the patient and the equipment to be used in these procedures.

10.13 Concluding Remarks

- Pelvic hernias are a rare presentation and high recurrence rate after repair.
- Patient preparation before and during the surgery is important in the surgical setup.
- Robotic arms, cannulas position and 3D view can improve the technique and the surgical outcomes.
- Caution must be taken to avoid early and late surgical complications.

Glossary

Abdominoperineal Excision (APE) Surgical procedure to treat distal rectal and anal carcinoma, in which an anastomosis cannot be done.

Extralevator APE (ELAPE) Surgical procedure proposed by Holms. et al., to improve local tumor control and with the aim to reduce local recurrence.

References

1. DeSilva JM, Rosenberg KR. Anatomy, development, and function of the human pelvis. Anat Rec (Hoboken). 2017;300(4):628–32.
2. Salum MR, Prado-Kobata MH, Saad SS, Matos D. Primary perineal posterior hernia: an abdominoperineal approach for mesh repair of the pelvic floor. Clinics (Sao Paulo). 2005;60(1):71–4.
3. Sorelli PG, Clark SK, Jenkins JT. Laparoscopic repair of primary perineal hernias: the approach of choice in the 21st century. Color Dis. 2012;14(2):e72–3.
4. Van Damme JP, Timmermans T. Primary closure of the perineal wound after abdominoperineal amputation for adenocarcinoma. Acta Chir Belg. 1980;79(5):327–32.
5. Rodriguez-Wong U. Primary posterior perineal hernia. Case report and review of the literature. Cir Cir. 2014;82(1):93–7.
6. Beck DE, Fazio VW, Jagelman DG, Lavery IC, McGonagle BA. Postoperative perineal hernia. Dis Colon Rectum. 1987;30(1):21–4.
7. Aboian E, Winter DC, Metcalf DR, Wolff BG. Perineal hernia after proctectomy: prevalence, risks, and management. Dis Colon Rectum. 2006;49(10):1564–8.
8. Patel RK, Sayers AE, Gunn J. Management of a complex recurrent perineal hernia. J Surg Case Rep. 2013;2013(8). https://doi.org/10.1093/jscr/rjt056.
9. Sayers AE, Patel RK, Hunter IA. Perineal hernia formation following extralevator abdominoperineal excision. Color Dis. 2015;17(4):351–5.
10. Mjoli M, Sloothaak DA, Buskens CJ, Bemelman WA, Tanis PJ. Perineal hernia repair after abdominoperineal resection: a pooled analysis. Color Dis. 2012;14(7):e400–6.
11. Skipworth RJ, Smith GH, Anderson DN. Secondary perineal hernia following open abdominoperineal excision of the rectum: report of a case and review of the literature. Hernia. 2007;11(6):541–5.
12. Ogilvie JW, Ricciardi R. Complications of perineal surgery. Clin Colon Rectal Surg. 2009;22(1):51–9.
13. Abbas Y, Garner J. Laparoscopic and perineal approaches to perineal hernia repair. Tech Coloproctol. 2014;18(4):361–4.
14. Allen SK, Schwab K, Day A, Singh-Ranger D, Rockall TA. Laparoscopic repair of postoperative perineal hernia using a two-mesh technique. Color Dis. 2015;17(3):O70–3.
15. Alvarez Garzon HJ, Maubon T, Jauffret C, Vieille P, Fatton B, de Tayrac R. Synthetic mesh repair of an anterior perineal hernia following robotic radical urethrocystectomy. Int Braz J Urol. 2017;43(5):982–6.
16. Holm T, Ljung A, Haggmark T, Jurell G, Lagergren J. Extended abdominoperineal resection with gluteus maximus flap reconstruction of the pelvic floor for rectal cancer. Br J Surg. 2007;94(2):232–8.
17. Baek SJ, Kim SH. Robotics in general surgery: an evidence-based review. Asian J Endosc Surg. 2014;7(2):117–23.
18. Diana M, Marescaux J. Robotic surgery. Br J Surg. 2015;102(2):e15–28.
19. d'Acampora AJ, Joli FS, Tramonte R. Expanded polytetrafluoroethylene and polypropylene in the repairing of abdominal wall defects in Wistar rats. Comparative study. Acta Cir Bras. 2006;21(6):409–15.

20. Berger D, Bientzle M. Polyvinylidene fluoride: a suitable mesh material for laparoscopic incisional and parastomal hernia repair! A prospective, observational study with 344 patients. Hernia. 2009;13(2):167–72.
21. Imagawa Y, Tomita K, Kitahara K, Yano K, Hosokawa K. Repair of symptomatic perineal hernia with a titanium mesh. Hernia. 2014;18(4):587–90.
22. Dietz UA, Spor L, Germer CT. Management of mesh-related infections. Chirurg. 2011;82(3):208–17.
23. Fisher RA, Dasgupta P, Mottrie A, Volpe A, Khan MS, Challacombe B, et al. An over-view of robot assisted surgery curricula and the status of their validation. Int J Surg. 2015;13:115–23.
24. Schoonderwoerd L, Swank DJ. The role of optical access trocars in laparoscopic surgery. Surg Technol Int. 2005;14:61–7.
25. Rasmussen HM, Frederiksen HJ. Perineal hernia after rectal extirpation. Ugeskr Laeger. 1993;155(36):2817–8.
26. de Campos FG, Habr-Gama A, Araujo SE, Sousa AH Jr, Nahas CR, Lupinacci RM, et al. Incidence and management of perineal hernia after laparoscopic proctectomy. Surg Laparosc Endosc Percutan Tech. 2005;15(6):366–70.
27. Remzi FH, Oncel M, Wu JS. Meshless repair of perineal hernia after abdominoperineal resection: case report. Tech Coloproctol. 2005;9(2):142–4.
28. Morcos BB, Al-Masri M, Baker B. Perineal hernia, another incisional hernia? Indian J Surg. 2009;71(3):112–6.
29. Dulucq JL, Wintringer P, Mahajna A. Laparoscopic repair of postoperative perineal hernia. Surg Endosc. 2006;20(3):414–8.
30. Ruiz DE, Khaikin M, Vivas D, Newman M, Wexner SD. Multimedia article. Recurrent postoperative perineal hernia: transperineal redo mesh repair. Dis Colon Rectum. 2007;50(7):1080–1.
31. Stamatiou D, Skandalakis JE, Skandalakis LJ, Mirilas P. Perineal hernia: surgical anatomy, embryology, and technique of repair. Am Surg. 2010;76(5):474–9.
32. Rayhanabad J, Sassani P, Abbas MA. Laparoscopic repair of perineal hernia. JSLS. 2009;13(2):237–41.
33. Chelala E, Declercq S. Laparoscopic repair of post-abdominoperineal resection hernia: biological mesh and augmentation technique. Hernia. 2015;19(5):853–6.
34. Sarr MG, Stewart JR, Cameron JC. Combined abdominoperineal approach to repair of postoperative perineal hernia. Dis Colon Rectum. 1982;25(6):597–9.
35. Franklin ME Jr, Abrego D, Parra E. Laparoscopic repair of postoperative perineal hernia. Hernia. 2002;6(1):42–4.
36. Kramer BA, Whelan CM, Powell TM, Schwartz BF. Robot-assisted laparoscopic sacrocolpopexy as management for pelvic organ prolapse. J Endourol. 2009;23(4):655–8.
37. So JB, Palmer MT, Shellito PC. Postoperative perineal hernia. Dis Colon Rectum. 1997;40(8):954–7.
38. Lee TG, Lee SJ. Mesh-based transperineal repair of a perineal hernia after a laparoscopic abdominoperineal resection. Ann Coloproctol. 2014;30(4):197–200.

Adverse Events of Robotic Transabdominal Preperitoneal Inguinal Hernia Repair

11

Matthew Sharbaugh, Liam Knott, and T. Paul Singh

11.1 Introduction

The robotic transabdominal preperitoneal (rTAPP) inguinal hernia repair is a durable long-term solution for inguinal hernias with less postoperative pain, quicker return to work and an extremely low recurrence rate [1]. The addition of the robotic platform has proven to be both safe and cost effective in the repair of indirect, direct, femoral, and obturator hernias [1–3]. Laparoscopic transabdominal preperitoneal (lTAPP) hernia repair can be cumbersome with straight laparoscopic instruments. The wristed articulation and three dimensional magnification of the robotic system allows for easier dissection of the preperitoneal plane, improved visualization of the cord structures and hernia sac, and more efficient closure of the peritoneal flap. The robotic platform does help significantly in the completion of the procedure however, intraoperative problems and complications still occur. The intraoperative complications for rTAPP are inherently the same as they are for the laparoscopic version of the procedure but their repair varies vastly with the aid of wristed instrumentation. Primarily, the intraoperative injury of vascular structures, urogenital structures, and injuries to the bowel are of utmost concern. The majority of these complications have previously been researched and discussed extensively in the laparoscopic literature [4]. In this chapter, we will discuss the specifics to management of these injuries on the robotic console.

Inguinal hernia anatomy can be challenging for the novice surgeon or trainee and mastery of this region is critical before undertaking this complex operation. Consideration of the possible injuries and complications that can occur during rTAPP, it is best to break down the anatomy to specific regions and consider the complications within those defined anatomic zones.

M. Sharbaugh (✉) · L. Knott · T. Paul Singh
Department of Robotic and Minimally Invasive Surgery, Albany Medical Center, Albany, NY, USA

K. A. LeBlanc (ed.), *Robotic Assisted Hernia Repair*,
https://doi.org/10.1007/978-3-030-23025-8_11

11.2 Triangle of Doom

The triangle of doom is appropriately named as this area contains some of the largest vascular structures of the human body, which when injured can lead to torrential and catastrophic bleeding. The aptly named triangle lies between the vas deferens medially, the spermatic vessels laterally, and the peritoneal reflection inferiorly with the deep inguinal ring at the apex. This triangle lies below the iliopubic tract, and any dissection in this area must be carefully considered as the inadvertent complications can be life threatening. Large scrotal hernias, recurrent hernias, and previous pelvic surgery can skew the anatomy and lead to inadvertent forays into this dangerous region. As the inferior epigastric artery and veins branch directly off of the external iliac vessels, keeping them in view and awareness of their location can help orient the surgeon and reduce the risk of injury to the iliac artery and vein. While injury is rare to these major vascular structures during robotic TAPP, when dissection is carried below the iliopubic tract, the risk of iliac injury is increased significantly. If brisk bleeding is encountered, there are a number of measures that can be taken to help control and correct the issue. A sponge should be inserted into the abdomen and used to apply firm pressure to the area of bleeding. If this pressure is able to control the bleeding, time is available to prepare for the next set of maneuvers. The intra-abdominal pressure from the insufflation can be increased, as this will decrease venous return as well as cardiac output and will help in slowing the bleed if venous. The anesthesia team and the personnel in the room should be notified of the issue at hand and should rapidly prepare for a conversion to open surgery. The blood bank should be notified so that blood products will be made available. Depending on the experience and comfort level of the operator, assistance from other available general or vascular surgeons should be sought at this time. If the surgeon is experienced in advanced laparoscopic and robotic suturing techniques, attempts at primary repair of the injury can be made. If only two operating arms of the robot are employed, placing a fourth port to bring in the fourth arm of the robot or adding an assistant port can be of great assistance for retraction and visualization. Primary repair of the injury may be feasible at this point. Similar to open surgery, proximal and distal control of the vessel should be obtained. A small laceration can be fixed primarily with Prolene suture (Ethicon, Inc., Sommerville, NJ). The wristed instrumentation of the robotic platform allows these sutures to be placed precisely on the vessel to avoid narrowing these critical structures. This repair is feasible for the most skilled robotic surgeons and has been described in the literature during pelvic surgery [5]. Larger injuries or inadvertent thermal injury to the iliac vessels should be debrided back to healthy tissue and an anastomosis performed. The use of prosthetic conduit may be needed to bridge larger gaps and avoid a repair with tension. If immediate control and repair is not possible, the decision to convert to an open procedure should be made quickly, as life threatening bleeding and the risks of a CO_2 air embolism are very real.

In addition to the iliac artery and vein, the inguinal region is a highly vascularized area with a number of substantial vessels that can cause significant bleeding and obscure the operative field. The main landmark in the dissection of the preperitoneal plane is the inferior epigastric vessels emanating directly from the external iliac vessels. As mentioned previously the inferior epigastric vessels should be visualized through the peritoneum before the plane is initially dissected and used as a landmark throughout the dissection. As the median umbilical ligament is grasped and retracted medially to incise the peritoneum, the inferior epigastric vessels are visible lateral to this fold. As the peritoneal flap is raised, care must be taken to avoid injury to the inferior epigastric artery and vein. Situations such as recurrent hernias and previous pelvic surgeries can complicate the dissection and make injury to these vessels more likely. In the event of an injury to the inferior epigastric vessels, simple ligation is the preferred management strategy. When this occurs we typically use the Robotic Weck clip applier (Intuitive Surgical: Sunnyvale, California) and hem-o-lock clips (Teleflex Incorporated: Wayne, PA). Suction irrigation from one of the port sites and a sponge inserted into the abdomen can aid with visualization and exposure. If clips are unavailable, simple suture ligation is straightforward with the wristed articulation and is a viable option for control of the inferior epigastric vessels.

Other structures that may lead to major bleeding events during the rTAPP include the corona mortis and the spermatic vessels. The corona mortis, or crown of death, is present in about one third of patients and is a collateral connection of arteries and veins between the inferior epigastric and obturator vessels running obliquely over the lateral portion of Cooper's ligament [6]. The arcade got its name due to the difficult nature of control bleeding from an anterior open approach as the vessel retracts deep into the operative field. There is significant variation in this vascular anatomy. The corona mortis can be venous, arterial, and may actually be an aberrant obturator artery. Knowledge of the anatomy and of the possible variants is essential. During the exposure of Cooper's ligament, there is a risk of injury to the corona mortis. The robotic approach allows improved visualization and the presence and course of this vessel is more apparent. If injury to this vessel is identified, bipolar energy, hemostatic clips, or suture ligation should be employed without delay to attain homeostasis and prevent retraction and devastating hemorrhage.

The spermatic cord is a significant structure in which rare but potentially significant postoperative hemorrhage or hematoma can occur from either the testicular artery or the pampiniform plexus. Increased traction to these vessels during the dissection of the spermatic cord and reduction of the peritoneal hernia sac can lead to troublesome bleeding which is more likely to occur with a large scrotal component of the hernia. If the testicular artery is torn or cut, it should be clipped or ligated for hemostasis. The testicle will most likely survive with collateral flow from the cremasteric artery and the artery to the vas deferens. The pampiniform plexus is a very delicate arcade of small veins and rough handling of the fatty tissue of the spermatic cord will invariably cause bleeding. This bleeding will stain the field and make further dissection significantly more difficult. For these tears, cautious use of bipolar energy is usually sufficient for hemostasis. Testicular pain and swelling that continues to increase in the postoperative period should prompt an urgent scrotal duplex ultrasound to check for flow in the testicular artery and pampiniform plexus to identify potential resultant causes of ischemic orchitis.

The vas deferens traverses the triangle of doom from medial to lateral rising out of the pelvis and entering the deep inguinal ring. Injury to this structure is rare and can be avoided with minimal gentle traction applied in this region. We use the Fenestrated Bipolar instrument (Intuitive Surgical: Sunnyvale, California) as opposed to the Prograsp (Intuitive Surgical: Sunnyvale, California) for its decreased crushing force. At our institution we strive to teach trainees the proper handling of tissues during rTAPP. Extensive scarring, previous pelvic injury and reoperative surgery can lead to tethering and misidentification of the vas deferens putting it at risk for injury [7]. If an injury is identified intraoperatively the vas deferens can be safely ligated in patients without desired future fertility. For those patients who desire future fertility a two-layered vasovasostomy is feasible on the robotic platform and has been described in various case reports [8, 9]. This complex reanastomosis should only be performed by the most experienced and technically gifted robotic surgeons with experience handling urogenital injuries. If such a surgeon is not present, urologic consultation is recommended.

11.3 Triangle of Pain

The triangle of pain is located lateral to the triangle of doom and is bordered by iliopubic tract, the testicular vessels and the peritoneal fold. It obtained its name as many critical nerves run through this zone. Injury to these nerves present across a spectrum, from minimal discomfort to debilitating neuropathic pain and muscle atrophy. The avoidance of dissection and injury to the nerves in the triangle of pain is imperative during the rTAPP inguinal hernia repair. Injury to the lateral femoral cutaneous nerve remains a rare complication during this operation. This nerve originates from L2 and L3 and upon exiting the spinal cord traverses along the lateral edge of the psoas muscle. It then passes inferiorly to the inguinal ligament and innervates the skin to the lateral portion of the thigh. Injury to this nerve can be quite debilitating as it causes sharp shooting pain down the lateral side of the thigh, hampering ambulation.

The genitofemoral nerve arises from the L1 and L2 nerve roots. It pierces the psoas muscle and splits into the genital branch medially and the femoral branch laterally. The genital branch enters the deep inguinal ring and travels within the spermatic cord in men and alongside the round ligament in women. This nerve innervates the skin of the scrotum and provides motor signaling to the cremasteric muscle. In women, the nerve provides sensory innervation of the mons pubis and labia majora. The femoral branch of the genitofemoral nerve travels laterally under the inguinal ligament and through the femoral canal, lateral to the femoral vessels. This nerve provides sensory innervation to the anterior medial thigh. Injury to either branch of the genitofemoral nerve may lead to painful neuralgia and troubling sensory loss.

Sensory cutaneous nerve injury is rarely diagnosed intraoperatively and is more likely to be identified in the postoperative setting. If the injury is noticed during the hernia repair, it is appropriate to ligate the nerve to avoid postoperative neuralgia. A good physical exam postoperatively, along with ultrasound guided local anesthetic injection, can pinpoint nerve injury. Computed topography or magnetic resonance imaging can help by elucidating recurrence as the cause of increased postoperative pain. The first step in treating cutaneous nerve injuries is to manage these patients with anti-inflammatory medications, gabapentin, acupuncture, tricyclic antidepressants, nerve blocks done under ultrasound guidance and referral to a chronic pain management team [10]. If less invasive options are unsuccessful and the pain is present for greater than 12 months, robotic assisted triple neurectomy should be performed [11]. During triple neurectomy, the improved visualization and wristed instrumentation of the robotic platform allows easy identification of the cutaneous nerves, precise ligation and avoidance of the ureter and vascular structures. The robotic platform also allows for proximal crush injuries to be applied to the nerves which decreases painful neuroma formation [11].

Femoral nerve injury during rTAPP carries a different morbidity than the cutaneous nerves listed above. The femoral nerve arises from the second through fourth lumbar nerve roots of the spinal cord and provides the majority of motor and sensory function to the anterior compartment of the lower extremity. It traverses this area lateral to the femoral vessels in the femoral canal and is responsible for flexion of the hip joint and extension of the knee. The nerve can be injured by dissection below the iliopubic tract or by placement of sutures or tacks in this location [12]. Injury to the femoral nerve is an extremely rare occurrence with the robotic TAPP surgery but can lead to devastating loss of ambulatory function, muscle atrophy and chronic paresthesia. The diagnosis can be made by physical exam and electrophysiology [13]. Treatment usually requires reexploration to evacuate any hematoma or removal of offending agent whether it be a tack, mesh, or suture [13]. The improved optics of the robotic system greatly improves the visualization and identification of an offending agent after femoral nerve injury.

11.4 Other

The most widely described injuries occur in the triangles listed above. However, an often documented cause of bleeding during laparoscopic TAPP hernia repairs has been produced by the placement of mesh anchoring tacks. It is our practice to use a self-adhesive mesh thereby eliminating the use of any tacks in this area (Covidien: ProGrip polyester mesh). Tacks have been shown to decrease operative times in laparoscopic TAPP at the expense of increased cost [14]. The wristed instrumentation of the robotic platform and the self-adhering mesh eliminates this step, time, and cost. For those surgeons that prefer a mesh that requires fixation, anchoring sutures are more easily placed with robotic articulation. The control and depth of suture placement is superior than the use of a tacker, which requires manual pressure on the abdominal wall and can easily slip during deployment causing inadvertent injury [15]. When performing a robotic inguinal hernia repair, we would advise against any tacking device and rely solely on suture fixation, if at all necessary.

The bladder is often encountered during robotic inguinal hernia repairs. Our practice is to not place foley catheters pre-operatively, but all patients are instructed to void prior to entering the operating room. In small inguinal hernias, encountering the bladder is less likely. The rTAPP allows direct visualization and avoids the blind balloon dissection seen during TEP repair. There are case reports of this balloon dissection leading to bladder injury [16, 17]. The rTAPP does not eliminate this risk however. If the initial peritoneal incision is made lateral to the median umbilical fold, and dissection of the peritoneal flap is not carried medially to the umbilical fold, the bladder can usually be safely avoided. However, in large inguinal defects, especially direct defects, the presence of the bladder within the hernia is common. The bladder should be identified and returned to the appropriate medial location during reduction of the hernia sac. If there is an injury to the bladder during this reduction, the bladder should be repaired primarily. This repair can be done in one or two layers [16, 17]. Bladder injury in this location is considered an "extraperitoneal" injury. Suturing of the bladder defect is significantly easier robotically, and conversion to an open procedure is rarely necessary. A foley catheter should be placed at the conclusion of the case and remain for seven to ten days. The completion of the hernia repair with prosthetic mesh has been shown to be safe after a small bladder injury [16].

There are a number of steps during any minimally invasive inguinal hernia repair that are prone to bowel injury. The majority of these injuries occur during the first trocar insertion [4]. At our institution we perform an open cutdown off the midline under direct visualization to minimize injuries seen by the optical trocar or Veress needle techniques. The usual care for safe entry into the abdomen is essential to avoiding a bowel injury. If a bowel injury is encountered and the injury is full thickness with the spillage of enteric contents, we recommend repairing the bowel injury and aborting the case, as continuing at this point may lead to an unnecessarily high risk of mesh infection. The wristed instrumentation of the robotic platform allows for this repair to be performed with ease and precision.

Another step in the rTAPP where a bowel injury may be encountered is during the reduction of a large incarcerated scrotal hernia. Typically, after insufflation and the placement of the patient in the Trendelenburg position, we will gently reduce the bowel contents of the hernia. However, we will only reduce the contents of the hernia that will come without much force, as the reduction of the contents will be facilitated by the reduction of the hernia sac itself. Bowel injuries can occur during this step of reduction of the hernia contents. These injuries are often times traction injuries causing serosal tears. If this does occur the limbert suture repair and continuation of the case is appropriate. We avoid use of the Prograsp and instead prefer the Fenestrated Bipolar instrument (Intuitive Surgical: Sunnyvale, California) or other atraumatic graspers. This avoids undue trauma to the bowel and helps to prevent injuries. For full thickness tears, the decision has to be made based on level of contamination whether or not to proceed with placement of a prosthetic mesh.

During laparoscopic TAPP repairs, especially for extremely large scrotal hernias, complete reduction of the hernia sac can be extremely difficult and at times impossible. In these situations, transection of the sac and leaving the hernia sac in situ in the scrotum is a viable option but may lead to increased seroma formation. However, during robotic repairs, sac transection is less often necessary. The wristed articulation allows for easier manipulation of the sac within the defect. Grasping and retraction of the sac can be facilitated by the insertion of a fourth port and third working arm. This allows the operator to maintain continuous traction on the sac as the dissection of the distal sac continues. We have rarely needed to transect the sac during robotic repairs. It is our practice to reduce as much of the sac as possible to prevent postoperative seroma formation. If a portion of the sac is left in place, it is important to remember to close the defect in the sac to prevent mesh interaction with the abdominal contents once the peritoneal flap is closed. The percentage of seromas after rTAPP is very low [2] and most resolve spontaneously. For seromas that persist, compression, percutaneous aspiration, drain placement, or sclerosing agents may be utilized.

There are a number of other complications such as urinary retention, mesh infection and small bowel obstruction that are seen after robotic inguinal hernia repair. Robotic TAPP remains a mainstay in the armamentarium to minimize these complications. Urinary retention occurs 2% of the time after rTAPP [1]. Open inguinal hernia repair can have up to a 15% rate of urinary retention [18]. Better visualization and atraumatic manipulation of the tissues in the preperitoneal plane may account for this difference. The majority of infectious agents found in mesh infections are skin pathogens and the rTAPP minimizes exposure of the mesh to such organisms. The mesh should never touch the patients skin and the corresponding rate of mesh infection is minimal. Many large series have been published without a mesh infection [2, 19]. Hematoma is a rare complication rTAPP occurring in 3.9% of patients [2] and can be seen up to 6% in open surgery [20]. Hematomas are mostly self-limiting and only rarely require scrotal evacuation. The delicate grasping mechanisms of the robotic platform and the ease of controlling hemorrhage described above help to minimize this complication.

It is our practice to be meticulous during the closure of the peritoneum after rTAPP. This is because there are reported instances of small bowel obstruction (SBO) through peritoneal defects, termed peritoneal pocket hernia (PPH) [21]. The wristed articulation of the robotic system allows such defects to be closed with ease and should not be overlooked. In larger series, SBO occurred 0.6% of the time after rTAPP [1] and in addition to PPH has been reported to be caused by exposed barbed suture or by misplaced tacks [22].

11.5 Conclusion

The intraoperative complications of the robotic transabdominal preperitoneal inguinal hernia repair mirror those encountered during the laparoscopic version of the repair. The knowledge of the surrounding anatomy and meticulous surgical dissection is required to avoid the many pitfalls. If an intraoperative complication is encountered, conversion to an open procedure should always be considered, however the improved visualization and articulation of the robotic system provides a minimally invasive approach to combat these challenging complications.

References

1. Iraniha A, Peloquin J. Long-term quality of life and outcomes following robotic assisted TAPP inguinal hernia repair. J Robot Surg. 2018;12(2):261–9.
2. Dominguez JEE, Ramos MG, Seetharamaiah R, Donkor C, Rabaza J, Gonzalez A. Feasibility of robotic inguinal hernia repair, a single-institution experience. Surg Endosc. 2016;30(9):4042–8.
3. Waite KE, Herman MA, Doyle PJ. Comparison of robotic versus laparoscopic transabdominal preperitoneal (TAPP) inguinal hernia repair. J Robot Surg. 2016;10(3):239–44.
4. Lomanto D, Katara AN. Managing intra-operative complications during totally extraperitoneal repair of inguinal hernia. J Minim Access Surg. 2006;2(3):165.
5. Menderes G, Clark M, Tower A, Azodi M. External iliac vein injury and repair during robotic-assisted pelvic lymphadenectomy. J Minim Invasive Gynecol. 2015;22(5):718.
6. Ates M, Kinaci E, Kose E, Soyer V, Sarici B, Cuglan S, Korkmaz F, Dirican A. Corona mortis: in vivo anatomical knowledge and the risk of injury in totally extraperitoneal inguinal hernia repair. Hernia. 2016;20(5):659–65.
7. Flechner L, Smith J, Treseler P, Maa J. Vasal injury during inguinal herniorrhaphy: a case report and review of the literature. Perm J. 2014;18(4):85.
8. Barazani Y, Kaouk J, Sabanegh ES Jr. Robotic intra-abdominal vasectomy reversal: a new approach to a difficult problem. Can Urol Assoc J. 2014;8(5–6):E439.
9. Trost L, Parekattil S, Wang J, Hellstrom WJG. Intracorporeal robot-assisted microsurgical vasovasostomy for the treatment of bilateral vasal obstruction occurring following bilateral inguinal hernia repairs with mesh placement. J Urol. 2014;191(4):1120–5.
10. Ferzli GS, Edwards ED, Khoury GE. Chronic pain after inguinal herniorrhaphy. J Am Coll Surg. 2007;205(2):333–41.
11. Mahan MA, Kader AK, Brown JM. Robot-assisted triple neurectomy for iatrogenic inguinal pain: a technical note. Acta Neurochir. 2014;156(1):171–5.
12. Keating JP, Morgan A. Femoral nerve palsy following laparoscopic inguinal herniorrhaphy. J Laparoendosc Surg. 1993;3(6):557–9.
13. Garcia-Urena MA, Vega V, Rubio G, Velasco MA. The femoral nerve in the repair of inguinal hernia: well worth remembering. Hernia. 2005;9(4):384–7.
14. Agresta F, Marzetti A, Andrea Verza L, Prando D, Azabdaftari A, Rubinato L, Vacca U, Roveran A, Porfidia R, Maria Vigna SA. Laparoscopic TAPP inguinal hernia repair: mesh fixation with absorbable tacks, initial experience. J Minim Invasive Surg Sci. 2016;5(2):e35609.
15. Moreno-Egea A, Paredes PG, Perello JM, Campillo-Soto A, Baena EG, Muñoz JRO, Aguayo-Albasini JL. Vascular injury by tacks during totally extraperitoneal endoscopic inguinal hernioplasty. Surg Laparosc Endosc Percutan Tech. 2010;20(3):e129–31.
16. Chow P-M, Su Y-R, Chen Y-S. A rare complication from total extraperitoneal (TEP) laparoscopic inguinal hernia repair: bladder rupture associated with a balloon dissector. Hernia. 2013;17(6):797–9.
17. Dalessandri KM, Bhoyrul S, Mulvihill SJ. Laparoscopic hernia repair and bladder injury. JSLS. 2001;5(2):175.
18. Hudak KE, Frelich MJ, Rettenmaier CR, Xiang Q, Wallace JR, Kastenmeier AS, Gould JC, Goldblatt MI. Surgery duration predicts urinary retention after inguinal herniorrhaphy: a single institution review. Surg Endosc. 2015;29(11):3246–50.
19. Edelman DS. Robotic Inguinal Hernia Repair. Am Surg. 2017;83(12):1418–21.

20. Zeb MH, Pandian TK, El Khatib MM, Naik ND, Chandra A, Morris DS, Smoot RL, Farley DR. Risk factors for postoperative hematoma after inguinal hernia repair: an update. J Surg Res. 2016;205(1):33–7.
21. Narayanan S, Davidov T. Peritoneal pocket hernia: a distinct cause of early postoperative small bowel obstruction and strangulation: a report of two cases following robotic herniorrhaphy. J Minim Access Surg. 2018;14(2):154.
22. Peach G, Tan LC. Small bowel obstruction and perforation due to a displaced spiral tacker: a rare complication of laparoscopic inguinal hernia repair. Hernia. 2008;12(3):303–5.

Re-operation After Robotic Inguinal Hernia Repair

12

Jordan A. Bilezikian, Robert G. Johnson, and William W. Hope

12.1 Introduction

Robotic surgical techniques are increasingly used for hernia repair, and robotic minimally invasive inguinal hernia repair is an area of significant growth. This requires that surgeons know the most appropriate techniques for reoperations. Unfortunately, there are no published long term outcome studies. However, recurrence rates are assumed similar to be to the laparoscopic inguinal hernia repair recurrence rates of 1–3% in large series [1–3]. Despite a low recurrence rate for robotic inguinal hernia repairs, the number of repairs annually requires that surgeons successfully evaluate and treat patients that need reoperation after a robotic inguinal hernia repair.

12.2 Rationale for Robotic Inguinal Hernia Repair

Robotic surgical techniques were initially used in gynecologic and urologic surgery. The advantages of robotic surgery compared with traditional laparoscopic surgery include better visualization with a high definition magnification lens and 3-dimensional viewing, better dexterity with 360 degrees of instrument rotation with seven planes of translated wrist motion, and better ergonomics due to a more comfortable posture for the operating surgeon [4]. Robotic hernia repairs were first described in conjunction with robotic prostatectomy [5]. One of the few reports investigating transabdominal preperitoneal (TAPP) robotic inguinal hernia repair without prostatectomy was published by Escobar Dominguez et al. and was a case series of 78 patients at a single institution [6]. The study concluded that robotic

J. A. Bilezikian (✉) · R. G. Johnson · W. W. Hope
New Hanover Regional Medical Center, Wilmington, NC, USA
e-mail: Jordan.Bilezikian@nhrmc.org; Bobby.Johnson@nhrmc.org; William.Hope@nhrmc.org

K. A. LeBlanc (ed.), *Robotic Assisted Hernia Repair*,
https://doi.org/10.1007/978-3-030-23025-8_12

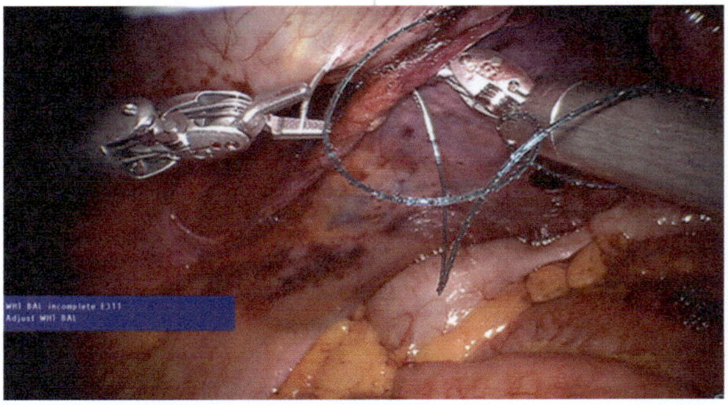

Fig. 12.1 Robotic suture closure of peritoneum during robotic inguinal transabdominal preperitoneal (TAPP) hernia repair

TAPP inguinal hernia repair was a safe approach with several advantages compared with the laparoscopic approach [6].

Robotic inguinal hernia repair is based on the principles of the laparoscopic TAPP and is well described elsewhere in this book (Chaps. 8 and 9). Proposed benefits for robotic inguinal hernia repair include easier suturing compared with the laparoscopic approach and potential for avoiding the use of penetrating tacker fixation and the ease of closing/suturing the peritoneum compared with laparoscopic suturing or tacker fixation. Barbed suture has gained popularity with surgeons as the suture of choice for the peritoneal closure; however, more research is needed to compare this with traditional methods (Fig. 12.1). Another potential advantage is that it can facilitate the use of a minimally invasive approach for operations that are too technically difficult for a laparoscopic approach.

12.3 Indications for Reoperative Inguinal Hernia Repair

The most common reason for reoperation after inguinal hernia repair is recurrence (Fig. 12.2). Despite many improvements in the repair technique, recurrences still occur, and there is no current evidence to support watchful waiting in patients with recurrence, so reoperation is usually recommended [3].

Reoperation is indicated for other reasons such as infection, bowel obstruction, and chronic pain. Discussion of these indications is outside the scope of this chapter. However, chronic groin pain, which occurs less often after minimally invasive repairs than after open repairs, is a complex chronic problem [3]. Although chronic groin pain is still not entirely understood, there are several treatment algorithms to guide surgeons with managing this complex problem (see Chap. 6) [3, 7].

12.4 Reasons for Failure of Robotic Inguinal Hernia Repair

Robotic inguinal hernia repairs and laparoscopic inguinal hernia repairs fail for similar reasons. Intrinsic/demographic risk factors for recurrence include anatomy, female gender, and abnormal collagen metabolism [3]. Obesity is an

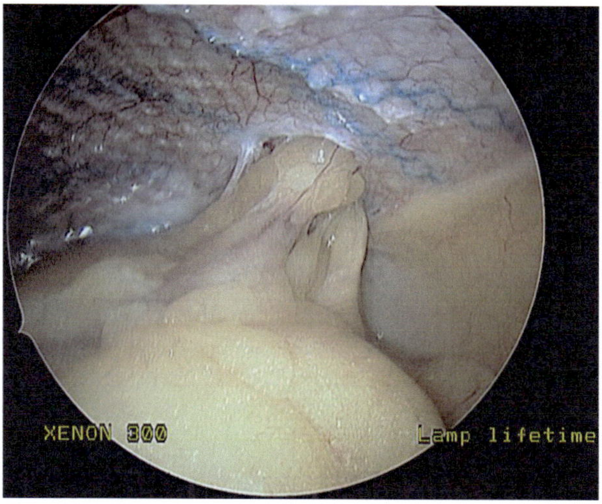

Fig. 12.2 Recurrent inguinal hernia following a robotic repair. A medial defect is present just underneath the previously placed mesh. This was likely due to inadequate fixation or poor placement of the initial mesh

acquired risk factor for recurrence [3]. Perioperative risk factors for recurrence include poor surgical technique, low surgical volume, and/or surgical inexperience. [3]. Poor surgical technique leading to recurrence often includes medial recurrence at the angle between the rectus sheath and the inguinal ligament, which is often a consequence of inadequate mesh fixation, inadequate mesh size, or inadequate hernia defect coverage due to poor location the mesh over the defect [8].

12.5 Strategies for Reoperative Surgery

Because there is no literature to support the use of watchful waiting in recurrent inguinal hernias, most patients without contraindications should be offered surgery [3].

When planning reoperative inguinal hernia repair surgery, apply the same principles as any reoperative surgery. Obtain and review the operative report from the original surgery. Specifically, note the surgical technique, type of mesh, type of fixation, and closure of peritoneum employed (for example, if a TAPP was used). These are important pieces of information to acknowledge when planning a laparoscopic or robotic reoperation.

Some patients needing reoperative hernia surgery following failed robotic repair have already undergone an open repair with mesh, which may have been the reason robotic repair was recommended. These operations can be challenging and have high complication rates. Due to many clinical variables that complicate decision making, these patients should be treated individually with no clear recommendation for one specific technique or method. Surgeons treating these patients should be well versed in many inguinal hernia repair methods/techniques. Recent guidelines recommend referral of these patients to an expert hernia surgeon [3].

12.6 Treatment Options for Recurrent Inguinal Hernia Following Robotic Repair

12.6.1 Open Repair

An open repair is the easiest and most often used method for reoperation after a failed robotic inguinal hernia repair. However, this is often debated. Recent international guidelines for hernia management recommend that a laparoscopic/minimally invasive repair be used after a failed open repair, and an open repair should be used after a failed laparoscopic/minimally invasive repair [3]. By extending the understand that a robotic inguinal hernia repair is a minimally invasive repair, many surgeons agree with the option of an open repair after a failed robotic repair.

The justification for this is avoidance of scar tissue at the time of reoperation, which some published case series have reported to increase complications [3]. Because robotic inguinal hernia repair requires taking down the peritoneum and placing mesh in the preperitoneal space, reoperation in this area can be difficult due to scar tissue. This plane filled with scar tissue is avoided by approaching the inguinal hernia recurrence anteriorly.

The most common anterior approach for hernia repair after failed robotic/minimally invasive hernia repair is the Lichtenstein hernia repair (Fig. 12.3). This approach avoids entering the preperitoneal space, which can be scarred from previous surgery [3]. However, if surgeons choose an open repair, they should use the anterior approach of their choice.

12.6.2 Laparoscopic Repair

Laparoscopic repair is not generally recommended due to the potentially higher rate of complications and difficulties associated with reoperative laparoscopic hernia surgery after failed laparoscopic/minimally invasive repairs. Although it is not

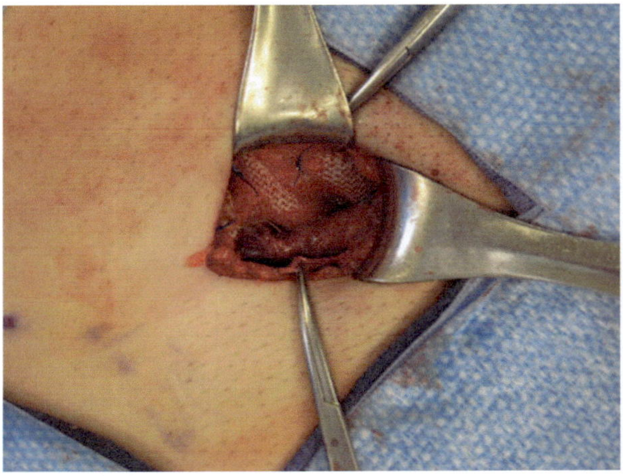

Fig. 12.3 Open anterior Lichtenstein repair of recurrent inguinal hernia following a robotic inguinal hernia repair. Surgeons should use the open anterior technique of their choice following a failed minimally invasive repair

recommended, it is still an option chosen by some surgeons. There can be several drawbacks to this option including the difficulty with scar tissue and dissection planes especially around important areas such as the iliac vein, iliac artery, spermatic cord vessels, and vas deferens. One commonly encountered problem associated with reoperative minimally invasive hernia repair in the TAPP approach is management of the peritoneum. The peritoneum can be densely adherent to the previous mesh, which can cause large holes in the peritoneum and can be very difficult to close laparoscopically. In cases when one is unable to completely cover the newly placed mesh with peritoneum, coated mesh products should be used.

12.6.3 Robotic Repair

Although an open repair is the most common and most commonly recommended operation following a failed laparoscopic/minimally invasive inguinal hernia repair, surgeons experienced with robotic surgery have approached these robotically (Fig. 12.4). Several reasons are used to justify a robotic reoperation including better visibility and dexterity as well as the improved ability to close large holes in the peritoneum with suturing. However, there are no published studies to support these claims. Additionally, it is not uncommon to have a patient present that has undergone failed open and laparoscopic hernia repairs.

A robotic reoperative hernia repair can be very complex and have many possible complications including injury to the spermatic cord, vas deferens, and an increased risk of bleeding [9, 10].

One potential benefit of the robotic reoperative approach is the ability to clearly identify the mechanism of failure of the previous robotic repair. Although some information can be gleaned from an open repair, in our experience, placing a laparoscope for diagnostic laparoscopy often provides a clear picture of the mechanism of recurrence. Better visualization for the surgeon, which has been well described, is another potential benefit of using robotic technology for reoperation [4]. This is important to evaluate vascular structures and nerves, which can be distorted due to the scar tissue and mesh.

A major difficulty with reoperative laparoscopic inguinal hernia repair for recurrence is management of the peritoneum during TAPP repairs. Due to scar tissue and

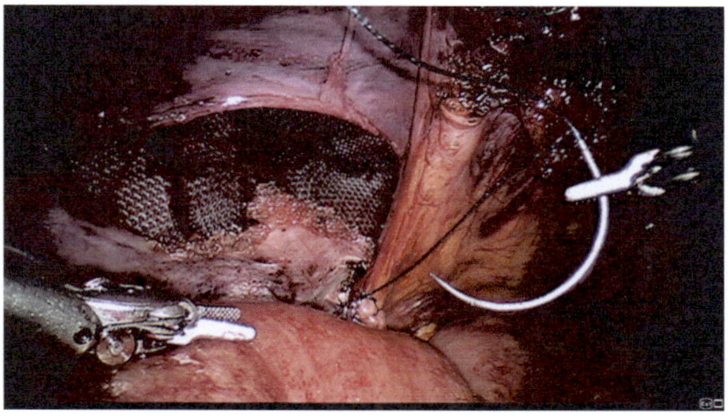

Fig. 12.4 Robotic reoperative inguinal hernia repair following previous robotic inguinal hernia repair. The previous mesh/peritoneum was dissected and a new mesh placed to cover the recurrent defect. The old mesh is seen incorporated into the robotic peritoneal closure

mesh, maintenance of a good preperitoneal plane is difficult, and holes or tears in the peritoneum can occur. While there are methods to help close these using the laparoscopic technique (suturing, Endoloops, tacks), these maneuvers can be challenging and time consuming. The improved ability to suture using robotic technology and easier recreation/repair of the peritoneum are important factors when deciding which technique to use when a difficult operation is expected.

12.7 Special Considerations

Although robotic inguinal hernia repair is based on the laparoscopic TAPP repair, there are subtle differences that can impact reoperative surgery. However, very little is known about this topic due to the paucity of literature.

One interesting issue related to robotic inguinal hernia repair is peritoneal closure using a barbed suture (i.e., V-lock, Medtronic, Minneapolis, MN). This is a fairly new technique and was popularized by the robotic technique. As with all new techniques, new challenges and complications have been reported including peritoneal disruption [11, 12]. During initial experiences with robotic inguinal hernia repair, some surgeons did not use the barbed suture as intended and did not "back-track" or tie the suture. This was thought to cause some of the peritoneal breakdowns. These breakdowns in the peritoneum can cause small bowel obstructions when bowel herniates in the preperitoneal space and is called a preperitoneal hernia [12].

Another reported complication associated with barbed suture use is the bowel or omentum adhering to the barbs of the suture when a large amount of extra suture is left in the peritoneal cavity [13] (Fig. 12.5). To date, there has been no reported erosion of barbed suture into the intestine; however, one should be aware of potential complications associated with this new technique of closing the peritoneum.

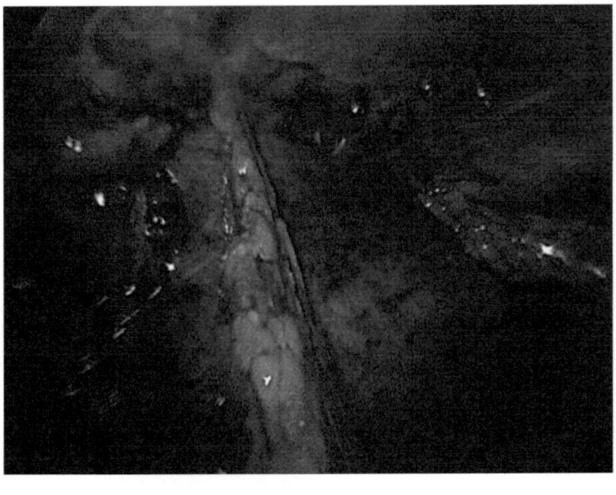

Fig. 12.5 Omentum adherent in two places to barbed sutures previously placed during a robotic inguinal hernia repair

12.8 Conclusions

Failed robotic inguinal hernia repairs are usually caused by technical issues. In general, the repairs should be done using an anterior (Lichtenstein) approach. In certain patients, a minimally invasive approach can be considered. In these patients, robotic reoperation is recommended due to better visibility and improved ability to suture the peritoneum.

References

1. Wauschkuhn CA, Schwarz J, Boekeler U, Bittner R. Laparoscopic inguinal hernia repair: gold standard in bilateral hernia repair? Results of more than 2800 patients in comparison to literature. Surg Endosc. 2010;24:3026–30. https://doi.org/10.1007/s00464-010-1079-x.
2. Bittner R, Schwarz J. Inguinal hernia repair: current surgical techniques. Langenbeck's Arch Surg. 2012;397:271–82. https://doi.org/10.1007/s00423-011-0875-7.
3. HerniaSurge G. International guidelines for groin hernia management. Hernia. 2018;22:1–165. https://doi.org/10.1007/s10029-017-1668-x.
4. Lanfranco AR, Castellanos AE, Desai JP, Meyers WC. Robotic surgery: a current perspective. Ann Surg. 2004;239:14–21. https://doi.org/10.1097/01.sla.0000103020.19595.7d.
5. Finley DS, Rodriguez E Jr, Ahlering TE. Combined inguinal hernia repair with prosthetic mesh during transperitoneal robot assisted laparoscopic radical prostatectomy: a 4-year experience. J Urol. 2007;178:1296–9; discussion 9–300. https://doi.org/10.1016/j.juro.2007.05.154.
6. Escobar Dominguez JE, Ramos MG, Seetharamaiah R, Donkor C, Rabaza J, Gonzalez A. Feasibility of robotic inguinal hernia repair, a single-institution experience. Surg Endosc. 2016;30:4042–8. https://doi.org/10.1007/s00464-015-4717-5.
7. Hu QL, Chen DC. Approach to the patient with chronic groin pain. Surg Clin North Am. 2018;98:651–65. https://doi.org/10.1016/j.suc.2018.02.002.
8. Gopal SV, Warrier A. Recurrence after groin hernia repair-revisited. Int J Surg. 2013;11:374–7. https://doi.org/10.1016/j.ijsu.2013.03.012.
9. Kockerling F, Bittner R, Kuthe A, Stechemesser B, Lorenz R, Koch A, et al. Laparo-endoscopic versus open recurrent inguinal hernia repair: should we follow the guidelines? Surg Endosc. 2017;31:3168–85. https://doi.org/10.1007/s00464-016-5342-7.
10. Haapaniemi S, Gunnarsson U, Nordin P, Nilsson E. Reoperation after recurrent groin hernia repair. Ann Surg. 2001;234:122–6.
11. Cueto J, Vazquez JA, Solis MA, Valdez G, Valencia S, Weber A. Bowel obstruction in the postoperative period of laparoscopic inguinal hernia repair (TAPP): review of the literature. JSLS. 1998;2:277–80.
12. McKay R. Preperitoneal herniation and bowel obstruction post laparoscopic inguinal hernia repair: case report and review of the literature. Hernia. 2008;12:535–7. https://doi.org/10.1007/s10029-008-0341-9.
13. Tagliaferri EM, Wong Tavara SL, Abad de Jesus JL, Bergmann H, Hammans S, Seidlmayer CM. Small bowel obstruction SBO after TAPP repair caused by a self-anchoring barbed suture device for peritoneal closure: case report. J Surg Case Rep. 2018;2018:rjy165. https://doi.org/10.1093/jscr/rjy165.

Part III

Ventral and Incisional Hernia

Botulinum Toxin Aided Hernia Repair

13

Talar Tejirian and Louise Yeung

13.1 Introduction

Botulinum neurotoxin, one of the most potent biologic toxins, has been found to have a broad degree of versatility in clinical applications. Initial ideas for therapeutic use emerged as early as 1817, when the toxin was first extracted from infected sausage and found to cause paralysis of skeletal muscle. The causative agent, *clostridium botulinum*, was finally elucidated in 1895. It was given its name due to its association with sausage (*botulus*, sausage in Latin) [1]. Now, over a hundred years later, botulinum toxin has a vast array of clinical uses in the fields of neurology, ophthalmology, gastroenterology, urology, orthopedics, dermatology, pain management, plastic surgery and increasingly, general and hernia surgery.

13.2 Background and Pharmacology

Botulinum toxin products consist of a botulinum neurotoxin component and various non-toxic complexing proteins. The pharmacological structure of botulinum is made up of an interconnected heavy and light amino chain acid with a disulfide bridge [2].

By binding with high affinity to the glycoprotein structures of the cholinergic nerve terminals, botulinum temporarily interrupts the transmission through the synapse and inhibits the release of acetylcholine from the presynaptic terminal. Botulinum toxin also has the ability to block the cholinergic autonomic innervation of various glands and smooth muscles. Studies have also shown the effect of botulinum toxin on pain transmitters. Effects of botulinum blockade have been described for substance P, glutamate, calcitonin gene related peptide and noradrenaline [2].

T. Tejirian (✉) · L. Yeung
Department of Surgery, Kaiser Permanente Los Angeles Medical Center,
Los Angeles, CA, USA

K. A. LeBlanc (ed.), *Robotic Assisted Hernia Repair*,
https://doi.org/10.1007/978-3-030-23025-8_13

While the toxin first starts taking action within two to three days, effects build up gradually and maximal response occurs at around 2 weeks. The overall effect will start declining at around 2.5 months, with fair consistency. Despite repeat or prolonged usage, no habituation effects are usually seen, although muscles consistently exposed to BTA may atrophy.

Because botulinum toxin consists of foreign proteins, antigens may be formed against them. These antibodies may induce therapy failure by blocking the effects of the toxin. Only antibodies against the botulinum toxin itself (rather than those against the complexing proteins) will block the biologic activity and so are referred to as neutralizing antibodies. Risk factors for antibody-induced therapy failure include use of single dose regimens and injection interval, but do not include cumulative dose, treatment time and patient age. While previously it was thought that there may be higher rates of immunogenicity, current studies show a frequency of immunogenicity of only 1–5% [3]; thus studies are emerging that support more frequent (<12 weeks) or higher doses without as much fear of inducing nonresponsiveness [4, 5].

Botulinum toxin has a fairly good safety profile, as the toxin binds with high affinity to the cholinergic nerve terminal and thus is quite well contained. However, local effects and unintended diffusion into adjacent sites may cause weakness in and around the target area [6]. It is possible for small amounts of BTA to be distributed throughout the body via systemic circulation. This is usually only clinically apparent when extremely large amounts of botulinum toxin are used, and is detected as increased jitter in muscles distant from the injection site [2]. Other systemic adverse effects are rare, but include allergic reactions, generalized weakness and influenza-like symptoms. BTA can worsen symptoms for patients with existing pareses such as myasthenia gravis, Lambert-Eaton syndrome, amyotrophic lateral sclerosis or other myopathies or motor neuropathies [7]. Therefore caution should be used and risks clarified if BTA will be used in these cases.

While there are seven serotypes of botulinum toxin, only types A and B are approved for medical targeting. Four commercial botulinum toxin preparations are approved and available in the United States and European countries. Onabotulinumtoxin A (trade name Botox, Allergan Inc., Irvine, California), abobotulinumtoxin A (trade name Dysport, Ipsen Ltd., Slough, UK), incobotulinumtoxin A (trade name Xeomin, Merz Pharmaceuticals, Frankfurt, Germany) and rimabotulinumtoxin B (trade name Myobloc® or NeuroBloc®, US World Meds, Louisville, Kentucky) have varying shelf-lives between 24–36 months. Botox, Dysport and Xeomin act by cleaving synaptosomal-associated protein 25 on the A serotype, whereas Myobloc® or NeuroBloc® cleaves the vesicle-associated membrane protein on the B serotype. Additional preparations available elsewhere internationally include Prosigne (Lanzhou Biological Products, China, Lanzhou, Gansu, China), Meditoxin or Neuronox (Medy-Tox, Seoul, Korea), and Botulax (letibotulinumtoxin A; Hugel Inc., Chuncheon, Korea).

13.3 Existing Clinical Applications

The clinical uses of botulinum toxin are numerous and span across multiple fields of medicine. Table 13.1 lists some of the more common applications from various specialties.

Many of the uses listed in Table 13.1 above may be classified as "Level B—probably effective" or "Level C—possibly effective" despite widespread use and expert

Table 13.1 Common clinical indications for botulinum toxin—adapted from Dressler D. Clinical applications of botulinum toxin. Curr Opin Microbiol. 2012;15 (3):325–336

Specialty field	Condition
Ophthalmology	Strabismus
	Ptosis
	Entropion
Neurology	Dystonias – Blepharospasm, oromandibular dystonia, lingual dystonia, tardive dystonia, bruxism, cervical dystonia, occupational dystonias, Hallervorden-Spatz syndrome
	Spasticity – Focal (arm, leg) – Non-focal (hemispasticity, paraspasticity, tetraspasticity)
	Hemifacial spasm
	Tics
	Migraine
	Cerebral palsy
	Hyperhidrosis
	Hypersalivation – Parkinsonian syndromes
	Tremors
	Pain – Muscular (dystonia, spasticity, piriformis syndrome, thoracic outlet syndrome, epicondylitis syndrome, possibly chronic pain syndromes)
	Raynaud phenomenon
Urology	Detrusor sphincter dyssynergia
	Idiopathic detrusor hyperactivity
	Neurogenic detrusor overactivity
	Urinary retention
	Bladder pain syndrome
	Pelvic floor spasms
	Benign prostate hyperplasia
Otorhinolarynology	Laryngeal/pharyngeal dystonia
	Gustatory sweating
	Crocodile's tears
	Chronic rhinitis
Pediatrics	Infantile cerebral palsy

(continued)

Table 13.1 (continued)

Specialty field	Condition
Gastroenterology	Achalasia
	Cricopharyngeal achalasia
	Esophageal spasms
	Gastroparesis
	Sphincter of Oddi spasms
Plastic surgery	Muscular wrinkles, glabellar lines
General surgery	Anal fissure
	Hernia surgery

acceptance as standard of care. Additionally many indications are still considered off-label but have been seen to have effectiveness and positive outcomes. Not all of the available BTA formulations have been studied and evaluated with randomized controlled clinical trials in all applications, therefore published guidelines such as those from the American Academy of Neurology [8] demonstrate a lower level of support than some expert opinion.

13.4 Applications in Hernia Surgery

Hernia surgery is a rapidly developing sub-field within the specialties of general and plastic surgery. With the popularity of laparoscopic and now increasingly robust interest in robotic technologies, as well as advances made in biomedical technology and mesh development, evolving techniques are allowing surgeons to tackle more challenging and more complex hernias than ever before, while still striving for improving long-term outcomes.

Large ventral hernias, whether primary or incisional in origin, pose a difficult challenge for repair. Up to 20% of patients undergoing laparotomy may develop an incisional hernia [9], with rates as high as 35% for those patients needing emergency procedures [10]. Additionally, factors such as obesity, diabetes, wound infection, immunosuppression, malignancy, smoking and previous laparotomy will increase the risk of hernia development [11]. Simply performing a bridging repair, or closing an abdominal defect under too much tension, has a high rate of failure. Each previous failed hernia repair places a patient at increasingly higher risk of recurrence as the quality of the tissue declines from repeated dissection, mesh explantation and fascial debridement and retraction [12]. The recurrence rate of incisional hernia has been reported as 24% after first repair, increasing to 35% after second and 39% after third attempted repair [13]. Hernia repair can be further complicated if the patient has “loss of domain”. While there is no explicit definition or precise measurement method for this, a generally accepted definition is when 50% of the abdominal viscera reside outside the abdominal cavity [14]. The upper size limit of hernias that can be repaired takes many factors into consideration apart from absolute size, including the location of the hernia, orientation and number of defects, amount and compressibility of intra-abdominal contents and the quality and compliance of the abdominal wall. If closure of the abdominal fascia is successfully accomplished, additional risks remain. These include abdominal compartment syndrome if intra-abdominal pressures are too high after closure, or flap necrosis and donor site morbidity in the case of myofascial cutaneous flap closure [15].

To ease hernia repair and potentially lower some of these morbidities, there has been interest in increasing abdominal wall compliance or expanding the existing abdominal wall. Lengthening the abdominal wall musculature may allow for primary fascial closure and thus, lower the chance of mesh eventration whilst achieving a more functional abdominal wall. This is currently described in the literature by using one of three methods – progressive preoperative pneumoperitoneum (PPP) [16, 17], tissue expanders [16, 18] and botulinum toxin A (BTA) [19, 20]. The remainder of this chapter will focus on the role of botulinum toxin A in hernia repair.

13.5 Technique of Injection

13.5.1 Anatomy

The abdominal wall musculature is divided into the medial and lateral components. Medially, the rectus abdominis muscle is surrounded by the anterior and posterior fascia. At the lateral edge of the rectus abdominis muscle, the fascial layers fuse to form the linea semilunaris, then split to surround the muscles of the lateral compartment. Three muscle layers comprise the lateral abdominal wall, which is the focus of the area of the BTA injection. Anterior to posterior the muscular layers are as follows: external oblique, internal oblique, transversus abdominis.

13.5.2 Our Technique

One month before planned incisional hernia repair, BTA injection is performed under sterile technique using ultrasound guidance in the interventional radiology suite. The entire abdomen and bilateral flanks are prepped and draped after midazolam and fentanyl are administered. The planned tract is anesthetized with 1% lidocaine. BTA solution is prepared by diluting 100–150 units of Botox® into 100 units of preservative-free sterile saline. Three locations are chosen along the lateral abdominal wall utilizing ultrasound guidance to identify all three muscle layers. Using a 21 gauze, 7 cm long needle attached to the BTA/saline solution, the three layers of the abdominal wall are traversed at an angle while visualized under ultrasound. Care is taken not to violate the peritoneum. Injection is started in the transversus muscle, visualizing the solution bathing the muscle fibers. The injection is continuous as the needle is slowly pulled back into the internal oblique and then external oblique muscles, with uninterrupted ultrasound visualization of the injection. This is repeated for the two other locations on the unilateral side. The identical procedure is performed on the contralateral lateral abdominal wall, totaling six injections sites and 200–300 units of BTA. Three hundred units are chosen unless the patient is small and frail with very thin muscle layers.

13.6 Data and Outcomes

The first trial experimenting with the use of botulinum toxin for the abdominal wall was performed in 2006. In this study, BTA was injected into the abdominal wall of rats to evaluate if muscle paralysis can decrease intraabdominal pressure and increase intraabdominal volume. Despite only a 3-day study period, the authors found there were significant differences in the pressure and volume in the control and BTA groups [21]. In 2009, Ibarra-Hurtado et al. published the landmark paper describing BTA injection before abdominal wall reconstruction for hernia repair. Twelve patients had bilateral BTA injection under electromyographic guidance. The first two patients underwent weekly transverse hernia measurements and the authors noted reduction in the size of the hernia up to 4 weeks after injection. The next ten patients underwent a CT scan 4 weeks after BTA injection and noted a mean decrease of over 5 cm for the transverse hernia defect. There were no complications related to the BTA injection [19]. Since this publication, the literature for the use of BTA on the abdominal wall is increasing, however the research is heterogeneous.

13.6.1 Studies Involving Ventral/Incisional Hernia Repair and BTA

After the landmark study mentioned above, additional studies showed the abdominal wall changes that occur after BTA injection. Pre and post BTA injection CT scans have shown an increase in the length of the abdominal wall. Ibarra-Hurtado showed a mean increase in muscle length of about 2.5 cm per side. Sequential studies by Ibrahim as the senior author showed an increase of 4 cm per side [12, 22–24] except for one of the publications that demonstrated a mean unstretched length gain of 2.8 cm per side [25]. Ibarra-Hurtado also showed a reduction of the lateral abdominal muscle thickness by 1 cm [26]. This translates into an increase in the intraabdominal volume and more compliance. Both Ibarra-Hurtado studies reported they were able to close the abdominal wall defect either by open simple closure or Rives-Stoppa in many cases, however some patients did require abdominal wall component separation. Four studies published in 2016 and 2017, all with the same senior author, include 16, 27, 32, and 56 patients. Each subsequent study seems to be an update of the previous one, expanding on the results. While some of the specific details are missing individually in each of the papers, the most recent study with 56 patients allows for a more detailed breakdown of the several arms of treatment. It included patients who received 200 units of BTA versus 300 units of BTA and also looked at another group who underwent BTA administration and PPP. CT scan measurements were done for all participants before and after BTA to check the amount of muscle lengthening and the size of the defect. In all the studies with Ibrahim as the senior author, the patients underwent laparoscopic or a hybrid laparoscopic-open-laparoscopic repair of the hernia with intraperitoneal onlay mesh. If they were not able to close the defect primarily, then an endoscopic components release was performed [12, 22–25, 27]. In an additional study, Elstner and Jacombs et al. reported up to a 58% decrease in the hernia defect size on CT scan [12].

A meta-analysis analyzing the data of several studies showed a mean hernia width reduction of 5.79 cm and a mean lateral abdominal wall muscular lengthening of 3.33 cm after BTA injection [28].

13.6.2 Studies Involving a Combination of BTA and PPP

Studies have been published where BTA injection was coupled with PPP when repairing larger hernias. The data in these papers is difficult to interpret as it is unclear how much each of the two adjuncts individually contributed to reestablishing enough domain to repair the complex hernias [12, 29, 30].

13.6.3 Timing of Injection

As BTA does not work immediately, the timing of the injection in relation to the hernia repair needs to be considered. It takes 2 weeks to get the maximal clinical effectiveness of BTA, however Ibarra-Hurtado et al. found that the changes in the abdominal wall could take place up to 4 weeks. Therefore their recommendation was to perform the operation 1 month after BTA injection, which was their practice in both studies [19, 26]. The studies authored by Ibrahim reported injection 1–4 weeks prior to the planned repair [12, 22–24]. In contrast, Zendejas et al. published results of 22 patients who underwent BTA injection, where 13 patients had the injection the same day as the operation [31]. Only nine patients underwent preoperative injection 1–19 days beforehand. As it is unlikely that the benefits of the BTA injection where present during the operation for most of these patients, the authors could not comment on hernia defect or abdominal wall musculature changes. Their focus was on evaluating postoperative pain and finding decreases in pain on hospital day #2 and #5 compared to controls.

13.6.4 Other Uses

BTA has also been evaluated in patients with an acute open abdomen. Zielinski et al. performed BTA injection in 18 patients with an open abdomen resulting from acute surgical diseases. After patients underwent initial laparotomy, a negative pressure dressing or Wittman patch was placed and resuscitation completed for at least 12–24 hours. BTA injection was performed after resuscitation was complete. The lateral abdominal muscle complex on either side was injected with 150 units of Botox® divided into three locations for a total of 300 units of Botox. The authors reported half the patients underwent BTA injection within 24 h of the first laparotomy and overall they achieved an 83% fascial closure rate with 1–8 subsequent serial abdominal explorations [32]. A follow-up study by Zielinski et al. published in 2016 randomized 46 patients to placebo versus BTA injection after damage control laparotomy. Although there were no complications attributed to BTA or the injection, the authors reported no benefit from the BTA injection with regards to primary fascial closure, length of stay or pain modulation after decompressive laparotomy [33]. These two papers by the same institution with differing results leads to some confusion when evaluating the use of BTA for patients with an acute open abdomen.

In addition to aiding the closure of the abdominal wall, BTA injection has other potential benefits as well. One benefit may result from the fact that BTA paralysis lasts 3–6 months, working not only preoperatively but extending benefits postoperatively as well. Normally, the lateral abdominal wall muscle complex, when active, leads to forces of lateral retraction which is opposed by the linea alba [34]. When the linea alba is reapproximated with the hernia repair, it needs time to remodel and scar together. With the lateral paralysis in place, it allows the linea alba to heal for several months without the constant lateral forces. This can theoretically decrease hernia recurrence or separation of the reapproximated linea alba. A study utilizing an established rat model for incisional hernias randomized rats to sham surgery (control group) versus BTA treated plus laparotomy versus laparotomy alone. Results demonstrated reduced number and size of incisional hernias after laparotomy for BTA treated rats. Additionally, the BTA treated rats had weaker abdominal wall muscles [35]. The results support the theory that abdominal wall paralysis decreases incisional hernias due to the decrease in lateral abdominal wall muscle contraction.

A second potential benefit is in the ability of BTA to modulate pain. BTA is known to inhibit substance P and calcitonin gene related peptide. These molecules are factors involved in inflammation and pain sensation. BTA has already been shown to help in other myofascial and muscular pain syndromes, therefore it is very possible that the BTA injection can decrease postoperative pain and potentially lower opioid requirements [36–39]. A case report of a patient who received 300 units of Botox® after laparoscopic ventral hernia repair reported a significant and durable decrease in pain [40]. Another case report describes injection of BTA at the time of abdominal wall reconstruction in a patient with a history of liver transplant. The authors reported the patient did not require any opioid analgesics postoperatively [41]. Additionally, BTA injection has been described for abdominal cutaneous nerve entrapment syndrome, however the effects of BTA in this syndrome were not evaluated in this article [42].

13.6.5 Reported Techniques of Injection and Formulations

The original description of the injection by Ibarra-Hurtado et al. involved using electromyography to identify 5 points of maximum activity on each side of the lateral abdominal muscle complexes. Each side was injected with 250 units of Dysport® with 50 units at each site. Total amount of bilateral Dysport® was 500 units diluted in 5 ml of saline for a concentration of 100 units/ml. The second study by Ibarra-Hurtado et al. describes the same technique but with ultrasound guidance injection at 5 points placing the injection between the external and internal oblique muscles. Other authors all describe a similar technique of injecting 150 units of Botox® diluted in saline to a concentration of 2 units/ml into each lateral abdominal wall muscular complex at 3 points, totaling 300 units injected bilaterally at 6 points in total. At each point, ultrasound guidance is used to insure injection into all three muscle layers [12, 22–24, 31, 33, 40]. Ibrahim does report some use of an equivalent dose of Dysport® instead of Botox®. There is one paper with CT comparisons of patients who received 200 units versus 300 units of Botox®. Average gain in the lateral muscle length was 3.6 cm in the 200 unit group and 4.4 cm in the 300 unit group, as established by CT scan measurement. This was noted to be a statistically significant difference [24]. There are no reports on the use of Xeomin® for the abdominal wall.

13.6.6 Specific Safety Considerations in Abdominal Hernia Use

None of the published papers have described any complications from the use of BTA injections. There are potential risks that should be disclosed to all patients. As with any procedure there are always risks of infection, bleeding and pain. There is also a low but possible risk of violation of peritoneum and damage to structures such as intestine. Overall BTA has a very good safety profile but it should be noted that injection of the abdominal wall for hernia repair is an off-label use. Theoretically, there is a risk of BTA spreading from the injection site leading to symptoms of botulism such as asthenia, generalized muscle weakness, diplopia, ptosis, dysphagia, dysphonia, dysarthria, urinary incontinence and difficulty breathing. The highly unlikely but possible risk of death from any side effect does exist. There are several contraindications for the use of BTA. Patients who have hypersensitivity reactions such as anaphylaxis or urticaria may not be eligible to receive BTA. Caution is necessary for patients with pre-existing neuromuscular disorders as they are at increased risk of clinically significant effects similar to botulism. A careful history to rule out peripheral motor neuropathic diseases, amyotrophic lateral sclerosis or neuromuscular junction disorders such as myasthenia gravis or Lambert-Eaton syndrome is important. BTA should not be used in women that are pregnant or breastfeeding. Botox®, Xeomin®, and Dysport® contain albumin which is a derivative of human blood so there are very unlikely but theoretical risks of transmission of illnesses. Additionally, there is the potential of developing antibodies against Botox® and Dysport® which may reduce the efficacy of future use. While Xeomin® has a much lower reported rate of antibody formation, it has been observed [43]. Antibody formation increases when higher doses are given at shorter intervals. For Botox® specifically, the label recommends that adult patients receive no more than 400 units in a 3 month period. Administering BTA and aminoglycosides such as gentamicin can potentiate the toxin effects. Dysport® has unique contraindications as well. Dysport® may contain trace amounts of cow's milk protein, so caution should be used with those who are allergic. The units of Dysport® and Xeomin® are unique to their preparation and therefore are not interchangeable with other BTA medications such as Botox®. Additionally, Dysport® warnings include potential immune reaction with intradermal use only.

13.7 Conclusion

BTA holds a promising role in complex hernia repair. Although data is limited, all evidence points to a good safety profile and there are both subjective and objective benefits to its use. Future directions for investigation would need to elucidate optimum dosage, timing of administration and further clarification on patient selection in order to achieve the most beneficial circumstances.

References

1. Jankovic J. Botulinum toxin: state of the art. Mov Disord. 2017;32(8):1131–8.
2. Dressler D. Clinical applications of botulinum toxin. Curr Opin Microbiol. 2012;15(3):325–36.
3. Dressler D, Bigalke H. Immunological aspects of botulinum toxin therapy. Expert Rev Neurother. 2017;17(5):487–94.
4. Sethi KD, Rodriguez R, Olayinka B. Satisfaction with botulinum toxin treatment: a cross-sectional survey of patients with cervical dystonia. J Med Econ. 2012;15(3):419–23.
5. Evidente VG, Truong D, Jankovic J, Comella CL, Grafe S, Hanschmann A. IncobotulinumtoxinA (Xeomin®) injected for blepharospasm or cervical dystonia according to patient needs is well tolerated. J Neurol Sci. 2014;346(1–2):116–20.
6. Ramirez-Castaneda J, Jankovic J, Comella C, Dashtipour K, Fernandez HH, Mari Z. Diffusion, spread, and migration of botulinum toxin. Mov Disord. 2013;28(13):1775–83.
7. Erbguth F, Claus D, Engelhardt A, Dressler D. Systemic effect of local botulinum toxin injections unmasks subclinical Lambert-Eaton myasthenic syndrome. J Neurol Neurosurg Psychiatry. 1993;56(11):1235–6.
8. Simpson DM, Hallett M, Ashman EJ, et al. Practice guideline update summary: botulinum neurotoxin for the treatment of blepharospasm, cervical dystonia, adult spasticity, and headache: report of the guideline development Subcommittee of the American Academy of neurology. Neurology. 2016;86(19):1818–26.
9. Diener MK, Voss S, Jensen K, Büchler MW, Seiler CM. Elective midline laparotomy closure: the INLINE systematic review and meta-analysis. Ann Surg. 2010;251(5):843–56.
10. Deerenberg EB, Timmermans L, Hogerzeil DP, et al. A systematic review of the surgical treatment of large incisional hernia. Hernia. 2015;19(1):89–101.
11. Fink C, Baumann P, Wente MN, et al. Incisional hernia rate 3 years after midline laparotomy. Br J Surg. 2014;101(2):51–4.
12. Elstner KE, Jacombs AS, Read JW, et al. Laparoscopic repair of complex ventral hernia facilitated by pre-operative chemical component relaxation using botulinum toxin a. Hernia. 2016;20(2):209–19.
13. Flum DR, Horvath K, Koepsell T. Have outcomes of incisional hernia repair improved with time? A population-based analysis. Ann Surg. 2003;237(1):129–35.
14. Novitsky YW. Hernia surgery: current principles. Cham: Springer; 2016.

15. Novitsky YW, Elliott HL, Orenstein SB, Rosen MJ. Transversus abdominis muscle release: a novel approach to posterior component separation during complex abdominal wall reconstruction. Am J Surg. 2012;204(5):709–16.
16. Caldironi MW, Romano M, Bozza F, et al. Progressive pneumoperitoneum in the management of giant incisional hernias: a study of 41 patients. Br J Surg. 1990;77(3):306–7.
17. Dumont F, Fuks D, Verhaeghe P, et al. Progressive pneumoperitoneum increases the length of abdominal muscles. Hernia. 2009;13(2):183–7.
18. Admire AA, Dolich MO, Sisley AC, Samimi KJ. Massive ventral hernias: role of tissue expansion in abdominal wall restoration following abdominal compartment syndrome. Am Surg. 2002;68(5):491–6.
19. Ibarra-Hurtado TR, Nuño-Guzmán CM, Echeagaray-Herrera JE, Robles-Vélez E, de Jesús González-Jaime J. Use of botulinum toxin type a before abdominal wall hernia reconstruction. World J Surg. 2009;33(12):2553–6.
20. Jankovic J. Botulinum toxin : therapeutic clinical practice and science. Philadelphia, PA: Saunders/Elsevier; 2009.
21. Cakmak M, Caglayan F, Somuncu S, et al. Effect of paralysis of the abdominal wall muscles by botulinum a toxin to intraabdominal pressure: an experimental study. J Pediatr Surg. 2006;41(4):821–5.
22. Elstner KE, Read JW, Rodriguez-Acevedo O, et al. Preoperative chemical component relaxation using botulinum toxin a: enabling laparoscopic repair of complex ventral hernia. Surg Endosc. 2017;31(2):761–8.
23. Elstner KE, Read JW, Rodriguez-Acevedo O, Ho-Shon K, Magnussen J, Ibrahim N. Preoperative progressive pneumoperitoneum complementing chemical component relaxation in complex ventral hernia repair. Surg Endosc. 2017;31(4):1914–22.
24. Rodriguez-Acevedo O, Elstner KE, Jacombs ASW, et al. Preoperative botulinum toxin a enabling defect closure and laparoscopic repair of complex ventral hernia. Surg Endosc. 2018;32(2):831–9.
25. Farooque F, Jacombs AS, Roussos E, et al. Preoperative abdominal muscle elongation with botulinum toxin a for complex incisional ventral hernia repair. ANZ J Surg. 2016;86(1–2):79–83.
26. Ibarra-Hurtado TR, Nuño-Guzmán CM, Miranda-Díaz AG, Troyo-Sanromán R, Navarro-Ibarra R, Bravo-Cuéllar L. Effect of botulinum toxin type a in lateral abdominal wall muscles thickness and length of patients with midline incisional hernia secondary to open abdomen management. Hernia. 2014;18(5):647–52.
27. Elstner KE, Read JW, Jacombs ASW, et al. Single port component separation: endoscopic external oblique release for complex ventral hernia repair. Surg Endosc. 2018;32(5):2474–9.
28. Weissler JM, Lanni MA, Tecce MG, Carney MJ, Shubinets V, Fischer JP. Chemical component separation: a systematic review and meta-analysis of botulinum toxin for management of ventral hernia. J Plast Surg Hand Surg. 2017;51(5):366–74.
29. Bueno-Lledó J, Torregrosa A, Ballester N, et al. Preoperative progressive pneumoperitoneum and botulinum toxin type a in patients with large incisional hernia. Hernia. 2017;21(2):233–43.
30. Bueno-Lledó J, Torregrosa Gallud A, Jiménez Rosellón R, et al. Preoperative preparation of "loss of domain" hernia. Progressive pneumoperitoneum and botulinum toxin type a. Cir Esp. 2017;95(5):245–53.
31. Zendejas B, Khasawneh MA, Srvantstyan B, Jenkins DH, Schiller HJ, Zielinski MD. Outcomes of chemical component paralysis using botulinum toxin for incisional hernia repairs. World J Surg. 2013;37(12):2830–7.
32. Zielinski MD, Goussous N, Schiller HJ, Jenkins D. Chemical components separation with botulinum toxin a: a novel technique to improve primary fascial closure rates of the open abdomen. Hernia. 2013;17(1):101–7.
33. Zielinski MD, Kuntz M, Zhang X, et al. Botulinum toxin A-induced paralysis of the lateral abdominal wall after damage-control laparotomy: a multi-institutional, prospective, randomized, placebo-controlled pilot study. J Trauma Acute Care Surg. 2016;80(2):237–42.

34. Brown SH, McGill SM. Transmission of muscularly generated force and stiffness between layers of the rat abdominal wall. Spine (Phila Pa 1976). 2009;34(2):E70–5.
35. Lien SC, Hu Y, Wollstein A, et al. Contraction of abdominal wall muscles influences size and occurrence of incisional hernia. Surgery. 2015;158(1):278–88.
36. Durham PL, Cady R. Regulation of calcitonin gene-related peptide secretion from trigeminal nerve cells by botulinum toxin type a: implications for migraine therapy. Headache. 2004;44(1):35–42; discussion 42–33
37. Göbel H, Heinze A, Reichel G, Hefter H, Benecke R, Dysport myofascial pain study group. Efficacy and safety of a single botulinum type a toxin complex treatment (Dysport) for the relief of upper back myofascial pain syndrome: results from a randomized double-blind placebo-controlled multicentre study. Pain. 2006;125(1–2):82–8.
38. Childers MK, Wilson DJ, Gnatz SM, Conway RR, Sherman AK. Botulinum toxin type a use in piriformis muscle syndrome: a pilot study. Am J Phys Med Rehabil. 2002;81(10):751–9.
39. Perez D, Wildi S, Demartines N, Bramkamp M, Koehler C, Clavien PA. Prospective evaluation of vacuum-assisted closure in abdominal compartment syndrome and severe abdominal sepsis. J Am Coll Surg. 2007;205(4):586–92.
40. Smoot D, Zielinski M, Jenkins D, Schiller H. Botox a injection for pain after laparoscopic ventral hernia: a case report. Pain Med. 2011;12(7):1121–3.
41. Oliveira LT, Essu FF, de Mesquita GHA, et al. Component separation of abdominal wall with intraoperative botulinum a presents satisfactory outcomes in large incisional hernias: a case report. Int J Surg Case Rep. 2017;41:99–104.
42. Weum S, de Weerd L. Perforator-guided drug injection in the treatment of abdominal wall pain. Pain Med. 2016;17(7):1229–32.
43. Dressler D, Adib Saberi F, Bigalke H. IncobotulinumtoxinA (Xeomin(®)) can produce antibody-induced therapy failure in a patient pretreated with abobotulinumtoxinA (Dysport(®)). J Neural Transm (Vienna). 2014;121(7):769–71.

Pneumoperitoneum Aided Hernia Repair

14

Yohann Renard, Cheryne Hammoutene, and Jean-Pierre Palot

14.1 Introduction

Most incisional hernias are classified according to the size of the hernia defect, in particular to their width [1–3] and not by the difficulties in reduction of the herniated content. However, some of them, 5% in our experience [4], cannot be restored into the abdominal cavity. These giant incisional hernias with loss of domain (IHLD) imply that a proportion of the abdominal content, 20% according to Kingsnorth [5], fills permanently the extraperitoneal hernia sac [6, 7], thereby leading to a "second abdominal cavity" [8] (Fig. 14.1).

Recently, a group of expert surgeons has proposed loss of intra-abdominal domain as a common criterion to define a complex ventral hernia [9]. In case of IHLD, the massive visceral protrusion presents a major therapeutic challenge due to the difficulty to restore the volume of the herniated content into the abdomen and complete closure of the abdominal wall myofascial layers [10, 11]. Further, IHLD development is associated with lateral wall shortening and oblique muscle atrophy with decreased extensibility and compliance [12]. The replacement of the viscera within an unyielding and stiff abdominal wall may compromise the perfusion of the intestines, elevate the diaphragm [13] and may lead to subsequent intra-abdominal hypertension [14]. This situation may induce acute pulmonary complications and even a postoperative abdominal compartment syndrome [15–17].

Y. Renard (✉) · C. Hammoutene · J.-P. Palot
Department of General, Digestive and Endocrine Surgery, Robert-Debre University Hospital, University of Reims Champagne-Ardenne, Reims, France

K. A. LeBlanc (ed.), *Robotic Assisted Hernia Repair*,
https://doi.org/10.1007/978-3-030-23025-8_14

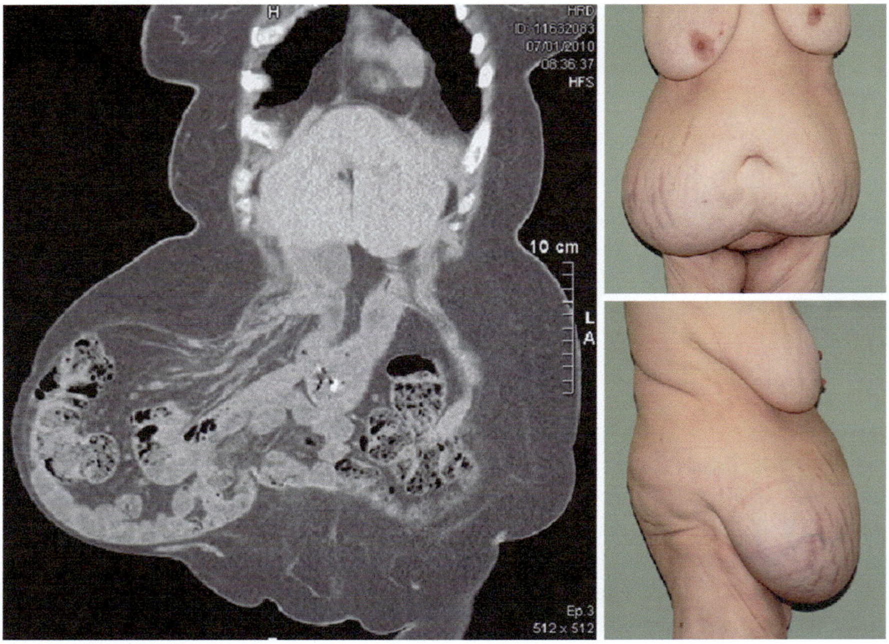

Fig. 14.1 Example of giant incisional hernias with loss of domain (IHLD), leading to a real "second abdominal cavity"

14.1.1 Preoperation Treatment Options

Several techniques have been described to increase the abdominal cavity volume [18], including tissue expanders, botulinum toxin, component separation techniques (CST) and progressive preoperative pneumoperitoneum (PPP).

The different component separation techniques (CST) are extensively reported and well described for the surgical treatment of IHLD [19–28] and are rapidly becoming the technique of choice in complex ventral hernia repair, even sometimes considered as a standard for the repair of all midline incisional hernias [25, 29–31]. The first technique described was anterior CST, reported by Ramirez et al. [32, 33]. In this technique, the external oblique muscle aponeurosis is sectioned near the semilunar line, allowing advancement of the composite flap of the ipsilateral rectus muscle medially to the midline. More recently, Novitsky et al. [19] described the transversus abdominis release (TAR). This technique consists in an extension of the Rives-Stoppa technique where the transversus abdominis muscle insertion is sectioned near the semilunar line, allowing the creation of a plane laterally between the transversus abdominis muscle and the transversalis fascia. The TAR, also called "perforator preserving CST" [29], is a safe alternative to the posterior component separation described by Carbonell et al. [20] where the lateral plane is created between the internal oblique and the transversus abdominis muscle, thus affecting the abdominal perforator nerves and vessels.

Anterior CST seems more able than the TAR to achieve the objective of closure of the midline since it allows an advancement of the rectus muscle medially up to 10 cm in length on both sides [32]. It has also been shown to increase the abdominal cavity volume by an average of 7% [13]. Of note, however, comparable outcomes of TAR and anterior CST have been reported in meta-analysis [30].

Nevertheless, anterior CST requires the lateral dissection of the subcutaneous space, leading to an increased risk devascularized skin flaps and impairment of the wound healing process with the subsequent risk of skin necrosis [24]. Further, both the anterior CST and TAR significantly alter the normal anatomy of the abdominal wall since these methods intentionally disrupt the integrity of the musculofascial components of the abdominal wall [13]. These factors may explain why CST is associated with a rate of wound complications as great as 26–42% and a recurrence rate up to 30% in large series [11, 19, 20, 34].

14.2 Progressive Preoperative Pneumoperitoneum (PPP)

First described in 1947 by Moreno [35], PPP represents an interesting alternative for surgical repair of IHLD without permanent alteration of the musculo-aponeurotic integrity of the abdominal wall [4]. It involves the progressive insufflation of the abdominal cavity. Prior to the surgical repair of IHLD. This is undertaken with the purpose of the complete reduction of the hernia content without division of any muscle or its associated aponeuroses, thus achieving a reduction of the post-operative complication rate [4, 18, 36, 37].

Contrary to CST, PPP involves a long preoperative preparation of the patients before IHLD repair, also called “Goni Moreno protocol”. Indeed, we think that the preparation of these patients, including careful pulmonary, cardiac and anesthesiologic evaluations, as well as appropriate skin preparation, is essential and should be, in fact, as crucial as the operation itself [4, 27, 36].

This technique has been used for a long time by specialized teams [38–45] but is still not extensively performed in the majority of hospitals. Nevertheless, specialized teams have reported good results with acceptable risk rate [4, 11, 36, 44, 46, 47]. Even if their series included limited number of patients [4, 11, 48], they have recently published objective data. However, no recommendation has been published until now about the indication of PPP, neither the precise protocol nor the method of repair.

14.2.1 Prior Evaluation of the Loss of Domain

The indication of PPP is usually based on clinical examination, ie, any incisional hernia that could not be reduced on physical exam [4, 44]. Nevertheless, it is sometimes difficult to clinically estimate the exact size of the incisional hernia, due to bowel adhesion or obesity [4]. Preoperative CT measurements of hernia defect sizes and abdominal wall thickness is mandatory for all complex incisional hernia [49].

In addition, in case of IHLD, preoperative CT-scan, with valsalva maneuver whenever possible, allows objective measures of the volume of the incisional hernia. Tanaka et al. [47] were the first team to report an objective method to calculate the exteriorized volume of the abdominal content on CT-scan. The hernia sac volume (*VIH*) and the abdominal cavity volume (VAC) were approximated by using their diameter within the three planes of space and using the mathematical formula of an ellipse ($4/3 \times \pi \times r1 \times r2 \times r3$), considering the shape of the two abdominal compartments as elliptic (Fig. 14.2). Using the Archimedes theory in the rat model, the efficiency of this method has been validated [50]. The exact VIH and VAC are now routinely calculated directly on CT-scan using volumetric software, as it is performed for hepatic volumetry (Fig. 14.3). The volume of the peritoneal cavity is calculated as the sum of VAC + VIH. The ratio of the volume of the hernia content was calculated according to the ratio VIH/(VAC + VIH), representing 45% on the specific example in Fig. 14.3.

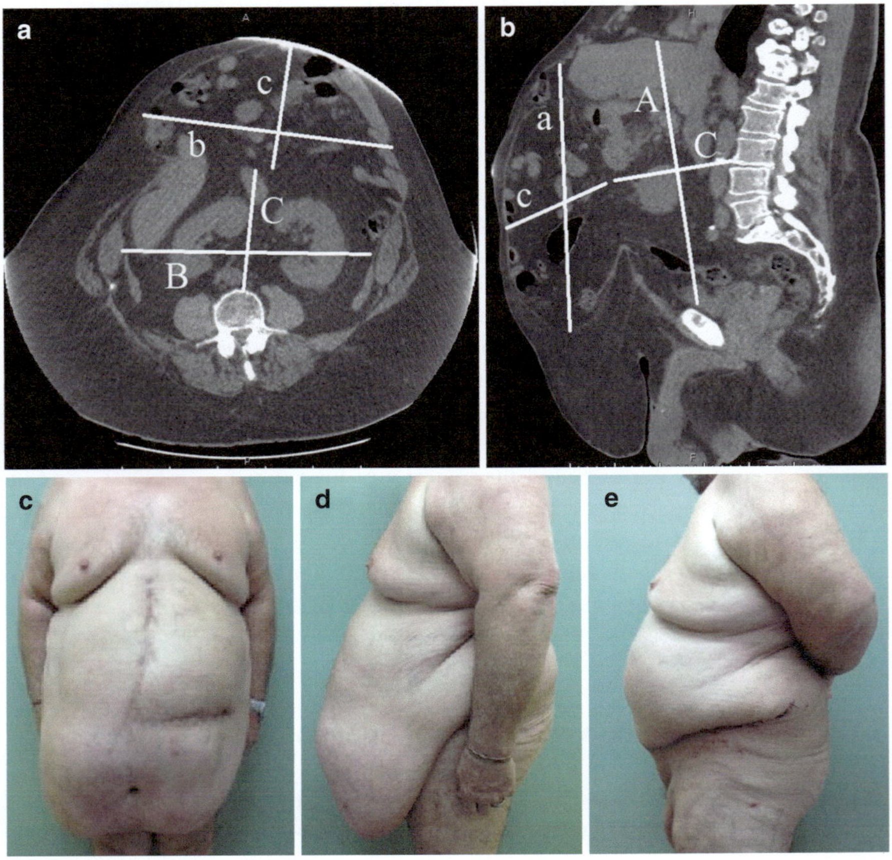

Fig. 14.2 Method to calculate VIH and VAC according to Tanaka on CT-scan (**a**, **b**) from a patient with median IHLD (**c**, **d**). VIH = $4/3 \times \pi \times a \times b \times c$. VAC = $4/3 \times \pi \times A \times B \times C$. (**e**) Result after PPP and surgery

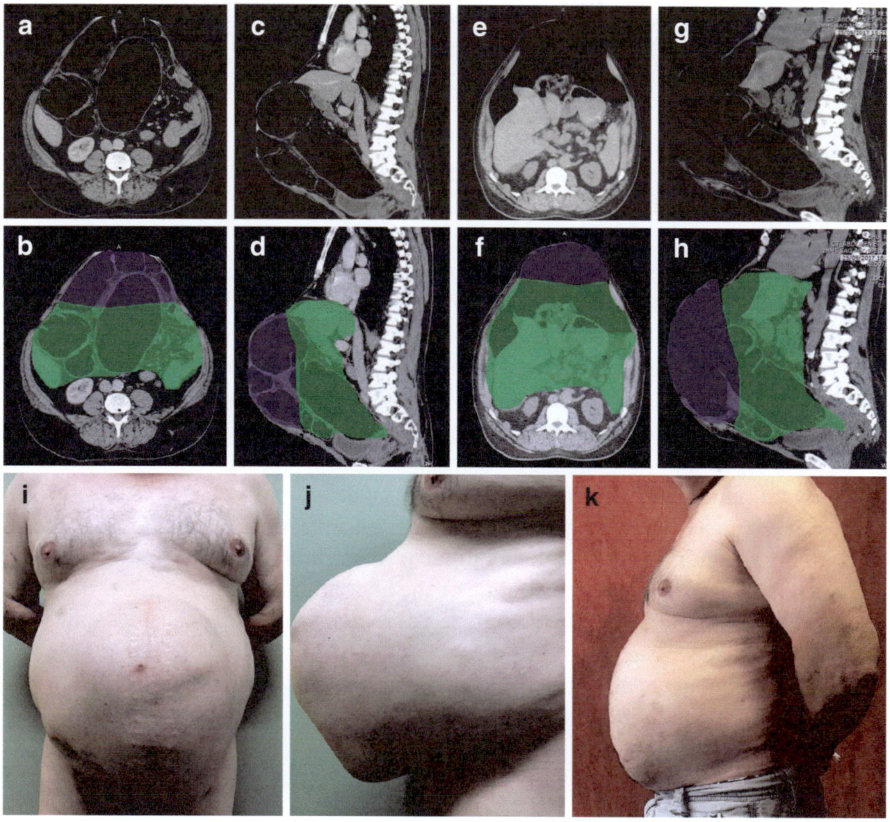

Fig. 14.3 CT volumetric measurements before PPP (**a**, **b**: Axial CT slide; **c**, **d**: Sagittal CT slice) in a patient presenting with a median giant IHLD (**i**, **j**). The VIH was measured at 3820 mL. The VAC was measured at 4653 mL. The ratio of the exteriorized visceral volume was calculated at 45% in this patient before surgery. CT volumetric measurements after progressive preoperative pneumoperitoneum and before surgery (**e**, **f**: Axial CT slide; **g**, **h**: Sagittal CT slice). The VAC was measured at 6951 mL which represented a mean VAC increase of 49%. (**k**) Results 6 months after surgery

14.2.2 Is There a Percentage of Herniated Volume from Which a PPP Is Indicated?

This exact determination is not clearly defined. Tanaka et al. [47] suggested that PPP should be performed when the ratio was at least 25%. Kingsnorth et al. [5] considered that a respiratory prehabilitation (smoking cessation, respiratory adaptation with intensive respiratory physiotherapy) should be performed in patients with a ratio of 15–20%. However, abdominal volumetry was not performed in the latter study. We consider that a IHLD with an exteriorized ratio of 20% should be prepared using PPP since recent prospective studies have shown that an exteriorized volume <20% of the entire peritoneal volume was predictive of a relative tension-free fascia closure and was associated with less postoperative pulmonary complications [9, 48, 51].

14.2.3 Objectives of the PPP

PPP has many potential and/or theoretical advantages [4, 18, 36, 37], including:

- The progressive distension of the lateral abdominal wall muscle will enlarge the abdominal cavity and allow the complete reduction of the herniated content and subsequent ability to close the defect completely.
- The PPP will cause progressive abdominal hypertension thereby resulting in diaphragmatic rehabilitation before surgery to improve ventilatory function. In other words, this can act as a pre-operative respiratory tolerance test. Some authors argue that PPP should be contraindicated in patients suffering from cardiac and pulmonary insufficiency without evidence-based data [38, 52–55]. In our experience, this pre-operative test will allow a surgical repair for patients with high comorbidities, without cardiac or respiratory failure [4].
- The resultant increase in the volume of the abdominal cavity can allow the complete reduction of the herniated organs without alteration of the abdominal wall (i.e. no CST necessary).
- The consequent pneumatic dissection of visceral adhesions facilitates the required dissection during the operation.

14.2.4 PPP Protocol

PPP can be either performed by repetitive percutaneous punctures with a Palmer needle under local anesthesia or with a percutaneous catheter implanted into the peritoneal cavity [4, 36, 43, 52, 56–58]. The use of a permanent catheter facilitates the entire process until the surgical intervention, but leads to the increased risk of infection of the catheter that may delay the operation for several months if this occurs. Repeated punctures lead to less infection rate but increase the risk of perforation of any of the contents of the abdominal cavity. Mougin published a complication rate of 20% during the PPP procedure [59]. The majority of these were minor events, without difference between the use of a catheter or repetitive puncture. More recently, catheter placement under ultrasound or CT-scan guidance has been described, which may provide better control over localization but requires good, available and motivated radiologists [60].

Each PPP procedure consists in the injection of ambient air into the peritoneal cavity through a microporous antibacterial filter after skin disinfection (Fig. 14.4a–d). A 3-way valve attached to a 60 ml syringe is a very effective and accurate method to infiltrate the air into the abdominal cavity. The procedure should be repeated every 1–3 days for 15–30 days. The volume of air injection during each procedure (500–2000 ml) and the duration of the entire procedure will depend upon the volume of the

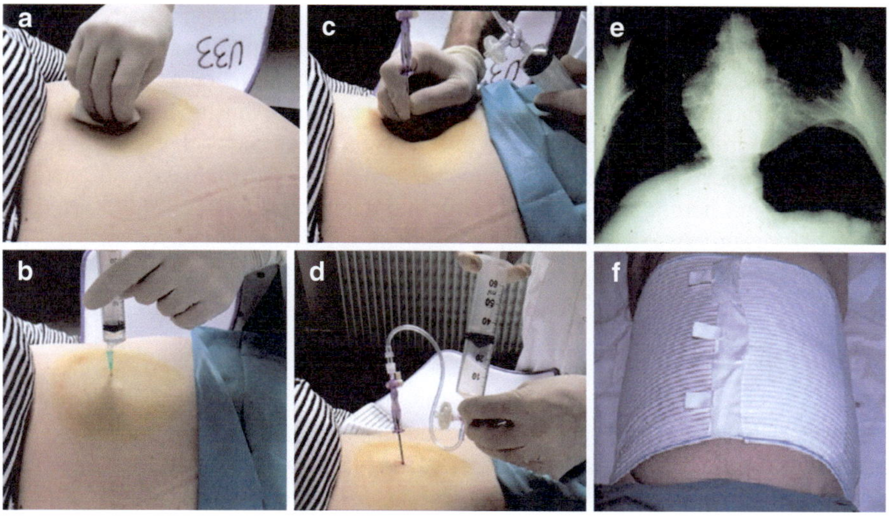

Fig. 14.4 PPP procedure using iterative puncture with a palmer needle. (**a**) Skin disinfection. (**b**) Local anesthesia. (**c**) Insertion of the palmer needle. (**d**) Insufflations of the cavity with ambient air. (**e**) Plain abdominal X-Ray showing the pneumoperitoneum under the diaphragm. (**f**) From the first session and until the day of the operation, all patients are equipped with an abdominal belt

VIH [47] and patient tolerance to each instillation. This will be manifested by either scapular or abdominal pain and/or dyspnea which can limit the amount of air and/or result in the need for administration of an analgesic agent [4].

After the initial procedure, a plain abdominal x-ray should be performed to check the presence of a pneumoperitoneum indicated by free air under both hemidiaphragms. (Fig. 14.4e). During the PPP and until the day of the operation, all patients should be equipped with an abdominal belt for active respiratory therapy in attempt to tolerate the progressive abdominal hypertension and to increase the respiratory capacity (Fig. 14.4f). In case of any dermatologic or septic skin condition, every attempt was made using detergent and antiseptic topical agents to eradicate and prevent further infectious complications. This can oftimes be avoided the use of skin lubricants or creams on the abdominal skin.

The protocol should include prophylactic subcutaneous anticoagulation starting at the time of the first PPP; the prophylactic dose may need to be increased in cases of obesity [4]. The administration of a broad spectrum antibiotic therapy should be evaluated on a case-by-case basis [36]. The first two or three procedures can be performed during conventional hospitalization to evaluate the initial tolerance to PPP [42, 61] but the subsequent ones can be performed in a outpatient surgery setting [4].

To the best of our knowledge, there is no consensus published regarding the quantity of air to insufflate, nor the length of time for this preparation. Some argue that the PPP should be stopped when excessive abdominal tension is observed [35, 41, 58]. Tanaka et al. insufflated the volume equivalent to the VIH calculated on pre-operative CT-scan [47] whereas Bueno-Lledo et al. insufflated three times this volume in consideration that, at least, some of the injected air is partially resorbed [36]. The preparation time varies greatly among the series published, ranging from 4 to 64 days, allowing the final insufflation total volume to range from 1400 to 38,000 cc (Table 14.1). Future studies are needed to clarify this precise aspect of the method. Regardless, once the selected time or volume has been achieved it is generally recommended that a new CT-scan is performed so that calculations of the new volumetry and hernia size after the procedure can be calculated. This should be done before surgery to verify the significant and sufficient increase of the VAC [4, 36, 41, 44, 46, 47].

14.2.5 Efficacy of PPP

As noted above, the pre-operative CT-scan allows calculation of objective data regarding the efficacy of the PPP [4, 36, 44, 46]. Dumont et al. [46] have reported an increase of the length of the right and left anterolateral muscles by an average of 83 mm on each side. Most importantly, the efficacy of PPP might be assessed by the increase of the VAC, by comparing pre- and post-PPP CT-scan volumetries, which might also be predictive of the success of the hernia repair. Sabbagh et al. [44, 48] and our team [4] reported an increase of the VAC by 22% and 53% respectively. These objective data may explain that PPP can lead to the spontaneous reduction of the herniated viscera, as shown on the post-PPP CT-scan (Figs. 14.3e and 14.5). For comparative purposes, the increase of VAC has also been reported after anterior CST in two series of 19 and 10 patients: the mean increase of VAC was 6% and 10%, respectively, which appears modest compared to PPP results.

Individual and pooled data of the three main studies that reported the volumetric results and efficacy of PPP in patients with giant IHLD are reported in Table 14.2 [4, 44, 47].

14.3 Surgical Repair: Minimally Invasive

To the best of our knowledge, no recommendation can be performed to date about the surgical technique. For an incisional hernia repair, the retromuscular sublay procedure (Rives-Stoppa), has been demonstrated by several authors to have a lower recurrence rate (3–7%) and is considered by many to be the gold standard technique [68]. For this reason, we advise this technique for the repair of an IHLD whenever possible [4].

To date, large series reporting minimally invasive approach of IHLD repair has not been published yet. It has been recently shown that transabdominal preperitoneal repair (TAPP), intraperitoneal onlay mesh (IPOM) or posterior CST can be easily accomplished using robotic surgery [69]. Nevertheless, application of laparoscopic or robotic ventral hernia repair is often limited by hernia morphology [70]. We argue that a minimally invasive repair of IHLD does not allow the complete closure of the defect to be guaranteed. If this cannot be accomplished there will be

Table 14.1 Series reporting the use of PPP for the repair of IHLD of hernias with loss of domain (Since 1985, including five patients or more)

Author	IHLD/VH/IH	Insufflation time (days)	Insufflated volume (cc)	Surgical success (reduction) (n,%)	Recurrence rate (n,%)	Morbidity (n,%)	Mortality (n,%)	Follow-up (months)
Raynor et al. [62]	8 VH	7	NA	100	3(37.5)	NA	NA	12
Astudillo et al. [63]	12 IHLD	7	NA	100	1(8.3)	NA	NA	12
Caldironi et al. [56]	41 VH	5.5	23,200	100	2(4.8)	NA	NA	25.3
Luder et al. [64]	11 IHLD	14–21	12,000	NA	0	NA	NA	12
Coelho et al. [65]	36 VH	6–15	7700	83.3	2(5.5)	NA	NA	10
Toniato et al. [66]	77 IHLD	11	23,200	90.1	2(2.6)	NA	NA	38.3
Mayagoitia et al. [58]	8 IHLD, 1 VH, 1 IH	9.3	7000–20,000	87.5	NA	2(25)	NA	12
Beitler et al. [67]	25 IH	7–18	4000–9000	100	2(8)	NA	NA	24
Mcadory et al. [40]	8 IHLD, 1 IH	22.4	NA	100	1(11.1)	NA	NA	17.6
Minossi et al. [45]	4 IHLD, 1 VH, 1 IH	11.6	15,000	100	0	1(25)	1(25)	4–36
Tanaka et al. [47]	23 IHLD	10	4000	100	1(4.3)	6(26)	2(8.7)	24
Sabbagh et al. [44]	19 IHLD	15.5	14,700	100	NA	7(36.8)	NA	NA
López Sanclemente et al. [61]	8 IHLD	15	666–18,000	100	1(12.5)	6(75)	NA	12
Oprea et al. [42]	14 IHLD, 3 IH	21.6	13,590	NA	NA	NA	NA	NA
Cavalli et al. [55]	5 IH			100	0			18–96
Renard et al. [4]	45 IHLD	15.7	6138	93	3(8)	15(41)	1(2)	18.6

IHLD incisional hernia with loss of domain, *VH* ventral hernia, *IH* inguinal hernia

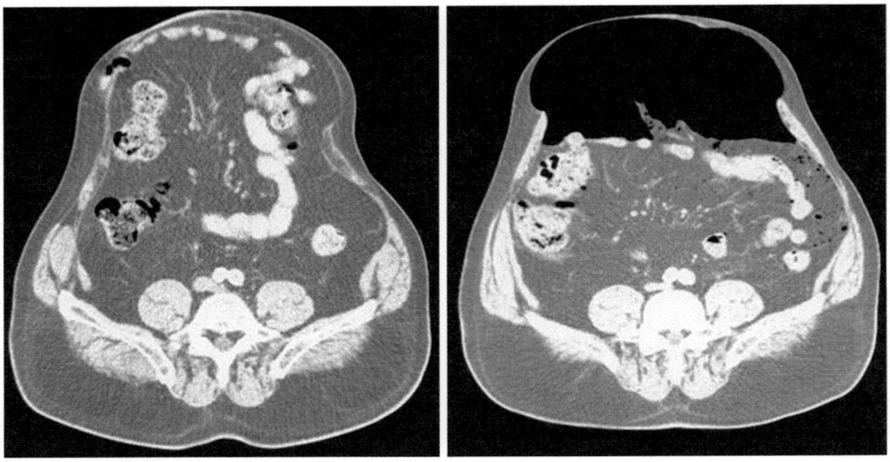

Fig. 14.5 CT-scan before (left) and after (right) PPP showing the spontaneous reintegration of herniated organs

Table 14.2 Individual and pooled data of the 3 main studies that reported the volumetric results of PPP and the efficacy and tolerance of subsequent reintegration surgery in patients with giant IHLD

	Sabbagh et al. [44]	Tanaka et al. [47]	Renard et al. [4]	Pooled results
Setting of the study	Prospective	Retrospective	Prospective	
Number of patients	19	23	45	87
VIH before PPP (cc)	1420	4500	4012	3575
VAC before PPP (cc)	9083	9410	6309	7735
VIH/(VAC + VIH) ratio before PPP (%)	14	36	38	32
VAC after PPP (cc)	11,104	NA	9603	10,112
Mean increase in the VAC (%)	22	NA	53	42.4
Success of surgical reintegration, n (%)	19 (100)	23 (100)	42/45 (93)	84/87 (97)
Non-absorbable meshes, n (%)	18 (95)	23 (100)	37 (82)	78 (93)
Specific surgical complications; n (%)	7 (37)	6 (26)	15 (41)	28 (36)
Rate of recurrence with non absorbable meshes; n (%)	NA	1 (4)	3 (8)	
Follow-up		2 years	18 months	
Global mortality, n (%)	2 (11)	2 (9)	1 (2)	5 (6)

NA not available, *VIH* volume of the incisional hernia, *VAC* volume of the abdominal cavity, *PPP* progressive preoperative pneumoperitoneum

a risk of the use of a bridging repair which may lead to higher post-operative complication and recurrence rate [71]. Even though minimally invasive hernia repair continues to gain in popularity rapidly, general surgeons have yet to develop the ideal, standardized method that adequately decreases common postoperative complications, such as wound failure, hernia recurrence and pain. The advent of robotics has made some complex repairs more feasible, but only time and well-designed clinical studies will tell if this will be a durable modality for ventral and incisional hernia with loss of domain repair [72].

14.4 Results of Surgery

Table 14.1 reports the series published about the use of PPP, on patients with IHLD and ventral hernias with loss of domain. Briefly, regarding long-term efficacy, hernia repair preceded by PPP seems to yield a low rate of hernia recurrence. Tanaka et al. reported only one recurrence (4%) after two years of follow-up [47]. Our team noticed three recurrences (8%) after a mean follow-up of only 18 months with the use of a nonabsorbable mesh [4]. The crucial point highlighted in Table 14.1 is represented by the excellent rate of surgical success, i.e. the complete closure of the defect in almost all cases after PPP. Nevertheless, recurrence, morbidity and mortality rates are still scarcely reported in the available literature concerning the treatment of IHLD, in particular after preparation with PPP.

14.5 Conclusion

CT scan with volumetry allows objective measurement of the exteriorized volume thereby aiding in the diminution of the risk of post-operative respiratory complications and appreciation of the efficacy of the preparation. The PPP, also called "Goni Moreno protocol", is a useful alternative technique to CST inducing a significant extension of the anterolateral abdominal muscles and increasing the abdominal cavity volume allowing an "ideal" treatment of IHLD.

PPP is relatively well tolerated by patients treated for an IHLD, and hernia repair preceded by PPP seems to yield good outcomes with low rate of hernia recurrence and serves to minimize the risk of postoperative abdominal compartment syndrome. PPP serves in the capacity of both a therapeutic endeavor and a pre-operative test for tolerance of the surgical repair. The main advantage of PPP compared with CST is the possibility to close large defects without transection of any abdominal wall muscle. If one is surgically unable to effect a closure of the midline, CST can be always be performed in addition to the PPP. To our knowledge, no study to date has compared PPP with CST. Overall, the studies reporting separately on PPP and on CST are not directly comparable, and whether PPP should be a relevant alternative or an adjunct to component separation needs to be discussed. PPP can be performed for all IHLD whatever the abdominal location, whereas CST is primarily designed for median IHLD and can be performed in emergency. The use of PPP preoperatively for robotic assisted hernia repair needs further elucidation but with the expansion of robotic component separation, future study needs to be performed.

References

1. Chevrel JP, Rath AM. Classification of incisional hernias of the abdominal wall. Hernia. 2000;4(1):7–11. https://doi.org/10.1007/BF01230581.
2. Muysoms FE, Miserez M, Berrevoet F, et al. Classification of primary and incisional abdominal wall hernias. Hernia. 2009;13(4):407–14. https://doi.org/10.1007/s10029-009-0518-x.
3. Luijendijk RW, Hop WC, van den Tol MP, et al. A comparison of suture repair with mesh repair for incisional hernia. N Engl J Med. 2000;343(6):392–8. https://doi.org/10.1056/NEJM200008103430603.
4. Renard Y, Lardière-Deguelte S, de Mestier L, et al. Management of large incisional hernias with loss of domain: a prospective series of patients prepared by progressive preoperative pneumoperitoneum. Surgery. 2016;160(2):426–35. https://doi.org/10.1016/j.surg.2016.03.033.
5. Kingsnorth AN, Sivarajasingham N, Wong S, Butler M. Open mesh repair of incisional hernias with significant loss of domain. Ann R Coll Surg Engl. 2004;86(5):363–6. https://doi.org/10.1308/147870804236.
6. Bauer JJ, Harris MT, Gorfine SR, Kreel I. Rives-Stoppa procedure for repair of large incisional hernias: experience with 57 patients. Hernia. 2002;6(3):120–3. https://doi.org/10.1007/s10029-002-0071-3.
7. Stoppa R, Ralaimiaramanana F, Henry X, Verhaeghe P. Evolution of large ventral incisional hernia repair. The French contribution to a difficult problem. Hernia. 1999;3(1):1–3. https://doi.org/10.1007/BF01576729.
8. Kingsnorth A. The management of incisional hernia. Ann R Coll Surg Engl. 2006;88(3):252–60. https://doi.org/10.1308/003588406X106324.
9. Slater NJ, Montgomery A, Berrevoet F, et al. Criteria for definition of a complex abdominal wall hernia. Hernia. 2014;18(1):7–17. https://doi.org/10.1007/s10029-013-1168-6.
10. Lipman J, Medalie D, Rosen MJ. Staged repair of massive incisional hernias with loss of abdominal domain: a novel approach. Am J Surg. 2008;195(1):84–8. https://doi.org/10.1016/j.amjsurg.2007.02.017.
11. Eriksson A, Rosenberg J, Bisgaard T. Surgical treatment for giant incisional hernia: a qualitative systematic review. Hernia. 2014;18(1):31–8. https://doi.org/10.1007/s10029-013-1066-y.
12. DuBay DA, Choi W, Urbanchek MG, et al. Incisional herniation induces decreased abdominal wall compliance via oblique muscle atrophy and fibrosis. Ann Surg. 2007;245(1):140–6. https://doi.org/10.1097/01.sla.0000251267.11012.85.
13. Agnew SP, Small W, Wang E, Smith LJ, Hadad I, Dumanian GA. Prospective measurements of intra-abdominal volume and pulmonary function after repair of massive ventral hernias with the components separation technique. Ann Surg. 2010;251(5):981–8. https://doi.org/10.1097/SLA.0b013e3181d7707b.
14. Trivellini G, Zanella G, Danelli PG, Pratolongo D, Ferri O. Surgical treatment of large eventrations. Study of a technic adapted to disorders of respiratory compliance. Chirurgie. 1984;110(2):116–22.
15. Oliver-Allen HS, Hunter C, Lee GK. Abdominal compartment syndrome as a rare complication following component separation repair: case report and review of the literature. Hernia. 2015;19(2):293–9. https://doi.org/10.1007/s10029-015-1362-9.
16. Mavrodin CI, Pariza G, Ion D, Antoniac VI. Abdominal compartment syndrome -- a major complication of large incisional hernia surgery. Chirurgia (Bucur). 2013;108(3):414–7.
17. De Santis L, Frigo F, Bruttocao A, Terranova O. Pathophysiology of giant incisional hernias with loss of abdominal wall substance. Acta Biomed. 2003;74(Suppl 2):34–7.
18. Alam NN, Narang SK, Pathak S, Daniels IR, Smart NJ. Methods of abdominal wall expansion for repair of incisional herniae: a systematic review. Hernia. 2016;20(2):191–9. https://doi.org/10.1007/s10029-016-1463-0.
19. Novitsky YW, Elliott HL, Orenstein SB, Rosen MJ. Transversus abdominis muscle release: a novel approach to posterior component separation during complex abdominal wall reconstruction. Am J Surg. 2012;204(5):709–16. https://doi.org/10.1016/j.amjsurg.2012.02.008.

20. Carbonell AM, Cobb WS, Chen SM. Posterior components separation during retromuscular hernia repair. Hernia. 2008;12(4):359–62. https://doi.org/10.1007/s10029-008-0356-2.
21. Appleton ND, Anderson KD, Hancock K, Scott MH, Walsh CJ. Initial UK experience with transversus abdominis muscle release for posterior components separation in abdominal wall reconstruction of large or complex ventral hernias: a combined approach by general and plastic surgeons. Ann R Coll Surg Engl. 2017;99(4):265–70. https://doi.org/10.1308/rcsann.2016.0241.
22. Fayezizadeh M, Majumder A, Belyansky I, Novitsky YW. Outcomes of retromuscular porcine biologic mesh repairs using transversus abdominis release reconstruction. J Am Coll Surg. 2016;223(3):461–8. https://doi.org/10.1016/j.jamcollsurg.2016.06.008.
23. Jones CM, Winder JS, Potochny JD, Pauli EM. Posterior component separation with transversus abdominis release: technique, utility, and outcomes in complex abdominal wall reconstruction. Plast Reconstr Surg. 2016;137(2):636–46. https://doi.org/10.1097/01.prs.0000475778.45783.e2.
24. Loh CYY, Nizamoglu M, Shanmugakrishnan RR, et al. Comparing transversus abdominus release and anterior component separation techniques in reconstructing midline hernias: a cadaveric study. J Plast Reconstr Aesthet Surg. 2018; https://doi.org/10.1016/j.bjps.2018.06.005.
25. Novitsky YW, Fayezizadeh M, Majumder A, Neupane R, Elliott HL, Orenstein SB. Outcomes of posterior component separation with transversus abdominis muscle release and synthetic mesh sublay reinforcement. Ann Surg. 2016;264(2):226–32. https://doi.org/10.1097/SLA.0000000000001673.
26. Pauli EM, Rosen MJ. Open ventral hernia repair with component separation. Surg Clin North Am. 2013;93(5):1111–33. https://doi.org/10.1016/j.suc.2013.06.010.
27. Torregrosa-Gallud A, Sancho Muriel J, Bueno-Lledó J, et al. Modified components separation technique: experience treating large, complex ventral hernias at a University Hospital. Hernia. 2017;21(4):601–8. https://doi.org/10.1007/s10029-017-1619-6.
28. Winder JS, Behar BJ, Juza RM, Potochny J, Pauli EM. Transversus abdominis release for abdominal wall reconstruction: early experience with a novel technique. J Am Coll Surg. 2016;223(2):271–8. https://doi.org/10.1016/j.jamcollsurg.2016.04.012.
29. Punjani R, Shaikh I, Soni V. Component separation technique: an effective way of treating large ventral hernia. Indian J Surg. 2015;77(Suppl 3):1476–9. https://doi.org/10.1007/s12262-015-1265-0.
30. Hodgkinson JD, Leo CA, Maeda Y, et al. A meta-analysis comparing open anterior component separation with posterior component separation and transversus abdominis release in the repair of midline ventral hernias. Hernia. 2018;22(4):617–26. https://doi.org/10.1007/s10029-018-1757-5.
31. Cornette B, De Bacquer D, Berrevoet F. Component separation technique for giant incisional hernia: A systematic review. Am J Surg. 2018;215(4):719–26. https://doi.org/10.1016/j.amjsurg.2017.07.032.
32. Ramirez OM, Ruas E, Dellon AL. "Components separation" method for closure of abdominal-wall defects: an anatomic and clinical study. Plast Reconstr Surg. 1990;86(3):519–26.
33. Ramirez OM. Inception and evolution of the components separation technique: personal recollections. Clin Plast Surg. 2006;33(2):241–6. https://doi.org/10.1016/j.cps.2005.12.011.
34. Ennis LS, Young JS, Gampper TJ, Drake DB. The "open-book" variation of component separation for repair of massive midline abdominal wall hernia. Am Surg. 2003;69(9):733–42; discussion 742–743.
35. Moreno IG. Chronic eventrations and large hernias; preoperative treatment by progressive pneumoperitomeum; original procedure. Surgery. 1947;22(6):945–53.
36. Bueno-Lledó J, Torregrosa Gallud A, Jiménez Rosellón R, et al. Preoperative preparation of "loss of domain" hernia. Progressive pneumoperitoneum and botulinum toxin type A. Cir Esp. 2017;95(5):245–53. https://doi.org/10.1016/j.ciresp.2017.04.006.
37. Geffen HJAAV, Simmermacher RKJ. Incisional hernia repair: abdominoplasty, tissue expansion, and methods of augmentation. World J Surg. 2005;29(8):1080–5. https://doi.org/10.1007/s00268-005-7972-0.

38. Koontz AR, Graves JW. Preoperative pneumoperitoneum as an aid in the handling of gigantic hernias. Ann Surg. 1954;140(5):759–62.
39. La Meir M, Vierendeels T, Poortmans M. Pneumoperitoneum in repair of giant hernias and eventrations. Acta Chir Belg. 2002;102(4):263–5.
40. Mcadory RS, Cobb WS, Carbonell AM. Progressive preoperative pneumoperitoneum for hernias with loss of domain. Am Surg. 2009;75(6):504–8; discussion 508–509.
41. Quraishi AHM, Borkar MM, Mastud MM, Jannawar GG. Pre-operative progressive pneumoperitoneum for repair of a large incisional hernia. Updat Surg. 2013;65(2):165–8. https://doi.org/10.1007/s13304-012-0134-7.
42. Oprea V, Matei O, Gheorghescu D, et al. Progressive preoperative pneumoperitoneum (PPP) as an adjunct for surgery of hernias with loss of domain. Chirurgia (Bucur). 2014;109(5):664–9.
43. Raynor RW, Del Guercio LR. The place for pneumoperitoneum in the repair of massive hernia. World J Surg. 1989;13(5):581–5.
44. Sabbagh C, Dumont F, Fuks D, Yzet T, Verhaeghe P, Regimbeau J-M. Progressive preoperative pneumoperitoneum preparation (the Goni Moreno protocol) prior to large incisional hernia surgery: volumetric, respiratory and clinical impacts. A prospective study. Hernia. 2012;16(1):33–40. https://doi.org/10.1007/s10029-011-0849-2.
45. Minossi JG, Oliveira WK, Llanos JC, Ielo SM, Hasimoto CN, Pereira RS. Preoperative progressive pneumoperitoneum in voluminous abdominal wall hernias. Arq Gastroenterol. 2009;46(2):121–6.
46. Dumont F, Fuks D, Verhaeghe P, et al. Progressive pneumoperitoneum increases the length of abdominal muscles. Hernia. 2009;13(2):183–7. https://doi.org/10.1007/s10029-008-0436-3.
47. Tanaka EY, Yoo JH, Rodrigues AJ, Utiyama EM, Birolini D, Rasslan S. A computerized tomography scan method for calculating the hernia sac and abdominal cavity volume in complex large incisional hernia with loss of domain. Hernia. 2010;14(1):63–9. https://doi.org/10.1007/s10029-009-0560-8.
48. Sabbagh C, Dumont F, Robert B, Badaoui R, Verhaeghe P, Regimbeau J-M. Peritoneal volume is predictive of tension-free fascia closure of large incisional hernias with loss of domain: a prospective study. Hernia. 2011;15(5):559–65. https://doi.org/10.1007/s10029-011-0832-y.
49. Blair LJ, Ross SW, Huntington CR, et al. Computed tomographic measurements predict component separation in ventral hernia repair. J Surg Res. 2015; https://doi.org/10.1016/j.jss.2015.06.033.
50. de Araújo LMG, Serigiolle LC, Gomes HMP, Rodrigues DAB, Lopes CM, Leme PLS. Volume calculation of rats' organs and its application in the validation of the volume relation between the abdominal cavity and the hernial sac in incisional hernias with "loss of abdominal domain". Arq Bras Cir Dig. 2014;27(3):177–81.
51. Petro CC, Raigani S, Fayezizadeh M, et al. Permissive intra-abdominal hypertension following complex abdominal wall reconstruction. Plast Reconstr Surg. 2015; https://doi.org/10.1097/PRS.0000000000001621.
52. Willis S, Conze J, Müller S, Klosterhalfen B, Schumpelick V. Progressive pneumoperitoneum in treatment of inguinal and scar hernias. Results of animal experiments and clinical applications. Langenbecks Arch Chir. 1996;381(3):132–7.
53. El Saadi AS, Al Wadan AH, Hamerna S. Approach to a giant inguinoscrotal hernia. Hernia. 2005;9(3):277–9. https://doi.org/10.1007/s10029-004-0291-9.
54. Valliattu AJ, Kingsnorth AN. Single-stage repair of giant inguinoscrotal hernias using the abdominal wall component separation technique. Hernia. 2008;12(3):329–30. https://doi.org/10.1007/s10029-008-0346-4.
55. Cavalli M, Biondi A, Bruni PG, Campanelli G. Giant inguinal hernia: the challenging hug technique. Hernia. 2015;19(5):775–83. https://doi.org/10.1007/s10029-014-1324-7.
56. Caldironi MW, Romano M, Bozza F, et al. Progressive pneumoperitoneum in the management of giant incisional hernias: a study of 41 patients. Br J Surg. 1990;77(3):306–7.
57. Näslund E, Backman L, Melcher A. A novel use for the Port-a-Cath: pneumoperitoneum in the repair of giant hernia. Eur J Surg. 1996;162(4):335–6.

58. Mayagoitia JC, Suárez D, Arenas JC, Díaz de León V. Preoperative progressive pneumoperitoneum in patients with abdominal-wall hernias. Hernia. 2006;10(3):213–7. https://doi.org/10.1007/s10029-005-0040-8.
59. Mougin N. Is progressive preoperative pneumoperitoneum (PPP) really safe? Assessment of its specific morbi-mortality in a retrospective study over 152 patients. Hum Health Pathol. 2015;35.
60. Alyami M, Passot G, Voiglio E, et al. Feasibility of catheter placement under ultrasound guidance for progressive preoperative pneumoperitoneum for large incisional hernia with loss of domain. World J Surg. 2015;39(12):2878–84. https://doi.org/10.1007/s00268-015-3206-2.
61. López Sanclemente MC, Robres J, López Cano M, et al. Progressive preoperative pneumoperitoneum in patients with giant hernias of the abdominal wall. Cir Esp. 2013;91(7):444–9. https://doi.org/10.1016/j.ciresp.2012.08.004.
62. Raynor RW, Del Guercio LR. Update on the use of preoperative pneumoperitoneum prior to the repair of large hernias of the abdominal wall. Surg Gynecol Obstet. 1985;161(4):367–71.
63. Astudillo R, Merrell R, Sanchez J, Olmedo S. Ventral herniorrhaphy aided by pneumoperitoneum. Arch Surg. 1986;121(8):935–6.
64. Luder PJ, Haller BG, Gertsch P, Blumgart LH, Lerut JP. Pneumoperitoneum and Mersilene mesh in the treatment of giant abdominal wall hernias. Helv Chir Acta. 1990;56(6):927–30.
65. Coelho JC, Brenner AS, Freitas AT, Campos AC, Wiederkehr JC. Progressive preoperative pneumoperitoneum in the repair of large abdominal hernias. Eur J Surg. 1993;159(6–7):339–41.
66. Toniato A, Pagetta C, Bernante P, Piotto A, Pelizzo MR. Incisional hernia treatment with progressive pneumoperitoneum and retromuscular prosthetic hernioplasty. Langenbecks Arch Surg. 2002;387(5–6):246–8. https://doi.org/10.1007/s00423-002-0316-8.
67. Beitler JC, Gomes SM, Coelho ACJ, Manso JEF. Complex inguinal hernia repairs. Hernia. 2009;13(1):61–6. https://doi.org/10.1007/s10029-008-0432-7.
68. Poghosyan T, Veyrie N, Corigliano N, Helmy N, Servajean S, Bouillot J-L. Retromuscular mesh repair of midline incisional hernia with polyester standard mesh: monocentric experience of 261 consecutive patients with a 5-year follow-up. World J Surg. 2012;36(4):782–90. https://doi.org/10.1007/s00268-012-1443-1.
69. Tian W, Fei Y. [Application of Da Vinci robotic surgery to hernia repair]. Zhonghua Wei Chang Wai Ke Za Zhi Chin. J Gastrointest Surg. 2018;21(7):740–3.
70. Warren JA, Love M. Incisional hernia repair: minimally invasive approaches. Surg Clin North Am. 2018;98(3):537–59. https://doi.org/10.1016/j.suc.2018.01.008.
71. Suwa K, Okamoto T, Yanaga K. Closure versus non-closure of fascial defects in laparoscopic ventral and incisional hernia repairs: a review of the literature. Surg Today. 2016;46(7):764–73. https://doi.org/10.1007/s00595-015-1219-y.
72. Vorst AL, Kaoutzanis C, Carbonell AM, Franz MG. Evolution and advances in laparoscopic ventral and incisional hernia repair. World J Gastrointest Surg. 2015;7(11):293–305. https://doi.org/10.4240/wjgs.v7.i11.293.

Operating Room Setup and Intraoperative Considerations for Robotic Ventral Hernia Repair

15

Jefferson Tyler Watson and Karl A. LeBlanc

15.1 Introduction

There are multiple benefits to the robotic surgical system when compared to conventional laparoscopy. Surgical visualization is enhanced by the system's three-dimensional capabilities. The surgeon drives the camera from his or her console, thus obviating the need for an experienced laparoscopic camera driver. Furthermore, the instrumentation has fully articulating wrists, thus diminishing the constraints of traditional laparoscopic instruments. These cumulative benefits result in a more efficient, ergonomic and flexible process, allowing the surgeon to approach larger and more complex hernias in a minimally invasive fashion. There is also evidence that the robotic platform may decrease certain complications associated with traditional laparoscopic ventral hernia repair [2, 3]. The laparoscopic approach as described by Karl LeBlanc involves placement of intraperitoneal mesh without closure of the hernia defect; this has remained the most commonly performed minimally invasive approach to incisional ventral hernia repair for over two decades [4, 5]. Studies have shown that recurrence, pseudo-recurrence, or bulging occurs in 17% of these patients. Closure of the fascia laparoscopically has been described in the literature, but requires significant technical expertise. The articulating arms of the robot allow for a more technically feasible facial closure, thereby decreasing this risk to approximately 0–5%. Primary fascial closure is also associated with a decrease in seroma formation from 27% to 11% [6–9].

J. T. Watson (✉)
Division of Advanced Gastrointestinal Surgery, Duke University, Durham, NC, USA

Division of Trauma Surgery, Duke University, Durham, NC, USA
e-mail: Jefferson.watson@duke.edu

K. A. LeBlanc
Our Lady of the Lake Physician Group, Baton Rouge, LA, USA

Louisiana State University Health Sciences Center, New Orleans, LA, USA

K. A. LeBlanc (ed.), *Robotic Assisted Hernia Repair*,
https://doi.org/10.1007/978-3-030-23025-8_15

However, to optimize these benefits, methodical and wise selection of patients, preoperative preparation, instrument selection, room coordination and device positioning must be employed. The preferred techniques of the authors for these steps are described in the following sections. The statements and recommendations of this chapter reflect the available technology of the Intuitive Surgical robotic systems (Intuitive Surgical, Inc., Sunnyvale, CA). Future technologies may modify some of these considerations in this chapter but none are available at the time of this writing.

15.2 Patient Selection

Successful outcomes of robotic ventral hernia repair depend upon the appropriate selection of candidates. When making this clinical decision, one must consider the size of the hernia and the comorbidities of the patient. One must also address modifiable risk factors, including tobacco use and obesity. Attenuating these risks, if possible, is a key component to improving post-operative outcomes, both in terms of wound healing and prevention of hernia recurrence. It is preferable that the patient has not smoked for at least one month, a criterion that can be confirmed using a nicotine test. Weight loss should also be achieved prior to undergoing elective hernia repair, particularly if a patient has a BMI over 50. If prior operations have left significant abdominal scarring or skin defects, the patient may not be the ideal robotic surgical candidate.

Prior operative reports of any previous abdominal surgery, particularly hernia operations, should be reviewed to gauge the size and location of previous defects, as well as the type of mesh and method of fixation(s) utilized. The authors often find clinical utility in a preoperative CT scan on patients as well, to evaluate size and location of hernia, which can aid in port placement, particularly in obese patients or those who have suffered recurrent hernias.

15.3 Preoperative OR Setup and Selection of Instruments

Having an established operative room set-up with designated staff who are familiar with the robotic surgical system and the specific technique employed to perform robotic hernia repairs can be extremely helpful in ensuring efficiency and quality of care. The robotic surgical system is ideally placed in a larger operating room to facilitate ease of patient cart positioning. With a little forethought, the patient cart can be situated in the most convenient position possible to allow for the most direct path to the patient when it is time to dock. This planning decreases excessive or complicated movements required by the circulator nurse. For example, the author routinely approaches his ventral hernias with his ports placed in the right anterior axillary line (Fig. 15.1).

In that case, the patient cart should be situated immediately to the patient's left. Also, before the patient enters the room, it is imperative that all extra trocars, sutures

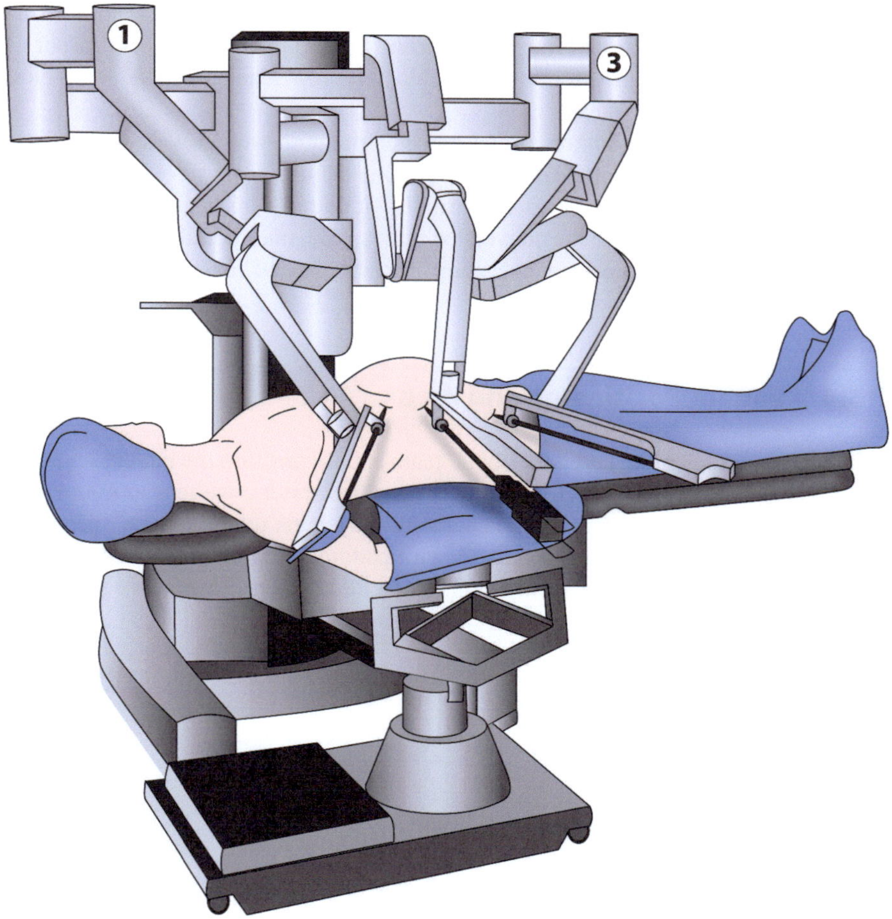

Fig. 15.1 Typical trocar and robot positions

and appropriate mesh sizes are available to avoid intraoperative delays. The CO_2 tanks should be routinely assessed preoperatively to have adequate supply. One must have both robotic and laparoscopic monitors and/or monitors that have the capacity for both modalities. Optimally, they should be easily viewable by the surgeon, surgical technician, circulator and surgical assistant, if present.

These cases require open, laparoscopic, and robotic surgical instrumentation; however, it is important to minimize the numbers of trays and instruments to only those that will be pertinent to the case. This restriction decreases count time, turnover time and table clutter. As an example, key instruments for the robotic ventral hernia repair include:

- Laparoscopic Instruments: Zero degree camera, optical view trocar for entry, laparoscopic graspers, scissors for adhesiolysis, locking single action laparoscopic grasper for mesh passage, laparoscopic suture passer (Carter-Thomason or other) and needle holders for passage of sutures

- Robotic Instruments: Robotic 30 degree camera, fenestrated bipolar, scissors, mega, mega suture cut or large needle drivers, and possibly a Cartier grasper
- Sutures: #1 double-armed, non-absorbable polypropylene barbed suture to close fascia and the secure mesh
- Mesh Selection: The authors prefer a coated medium-weight wide-pore permanent mesh for intraperitoneal placement. One should always double check that the mesh is the correct size prior to bringing it onto the operative field
- Open Options: Although the conversion rate is <5%, one should have all standard open equipment available if necessary in case of need for conversion to open operation.

15.4 Patient Positioning and Prep

Once the patient is intubated, the robotic team should position the patient appropriately to ensure the most effective use of the robotic system, while also minimizing the potential risk of injury. The patient should be supine under general anesthesia. Preferably, both arms should be tucked, with padding around hands and elbows to protect the ulnar nerve, wrists and fingers as pictured in Fig. 15.2.

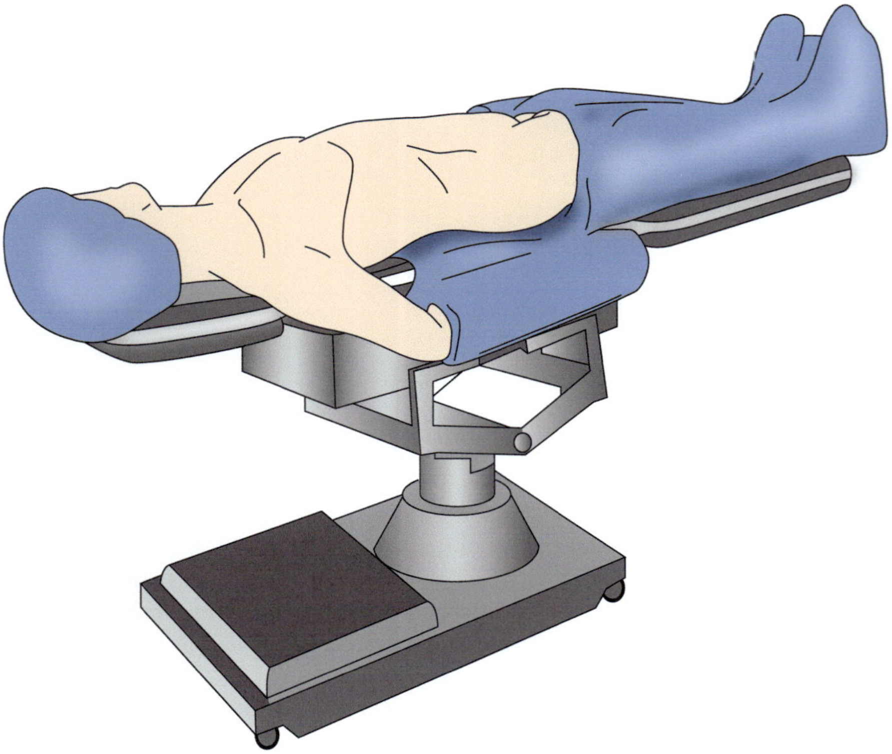

Fig. 15.2 Typical patient position

If tucking both arms is not possible secondary to body habitus, then it is advisable to tuck the arm on the side where one plans to place the robotic ports. Pubic and abdominal hair should be clipped, and the patient should be prepped using chlorhexidine from the pubis to nipples, and as far laterally as possible. A nasogastric tube and use of urinary drainage catheter is recommended. The patient should be paralyzed by anesthesia during the entire procedure.

15.5 Port Placement

Well-designed port placement is a critical step to performing an efficient robotic ventral hernia repair. If planning to place ports in the right anterior axillary line, the author gains access in the right upper quadrant (unless prior operations make this location prohibitively risky), immediately adjacent to the costal margin, using an optical view trocar and a zero degree laparoscopic camera. Once the abdomen is insufflated, you will have a better understanding of the best locations for insertion of the robotic ports. For most procedures, the fourth arm will not be needed and can be stowed prior to docking the robot. This author would also encourage using a 12 mm balloon bariatric length trocar for the camera port if using the SI. It is important to be at least two centimeters superior and medial to the ASIS with the inferior port. Although, almost all midline hernias may be approached from the vertically oriented trocars in the anterior axillary line, the small lower midline hernia or epigastric hernia may be optimally approached with the robotic trocars situated laterally across the upper abdomen or lower abdomen respectively. Alternatively, the robotic trocars can be placed on the left side of the patient if adhesions prevent the location on the right (Fig. 15.3).

15.6 Intraoperative Considerations

The patient cart, as previously discussed, should be placed in the most optimal room location to allow straight-line access to its planned bedside position. In the majority of cases, the cart should be placed at a ninety-degree angle to the patient. Arm adjustment should be considered to ensure equal spacing and minimize inter-arm collision. "Burping" the arms after attachment to the ports gives more room and alleviates the pressure applied to the patient. It is important to leave access to the assistant port for the surgical assistant for passage of mesh and sutures. If required by the room configuration, the laparoscopic camera towers and room lights can be removed prior to robot docking.

The circulating nurse and surgical technician should master the assembly and docking of both the laparoscopic and robotic components needed for the operation. This assures an efficient transition from laparoscopic to robotic equipment after gaining access to the abdomen. Although the surgeon's ability to drive the camera from the console obviates the need for an experienced laparoscopic camera driver, the presence of a well-trained and technically excellent robotic scrub assistant is crucial. The scrub

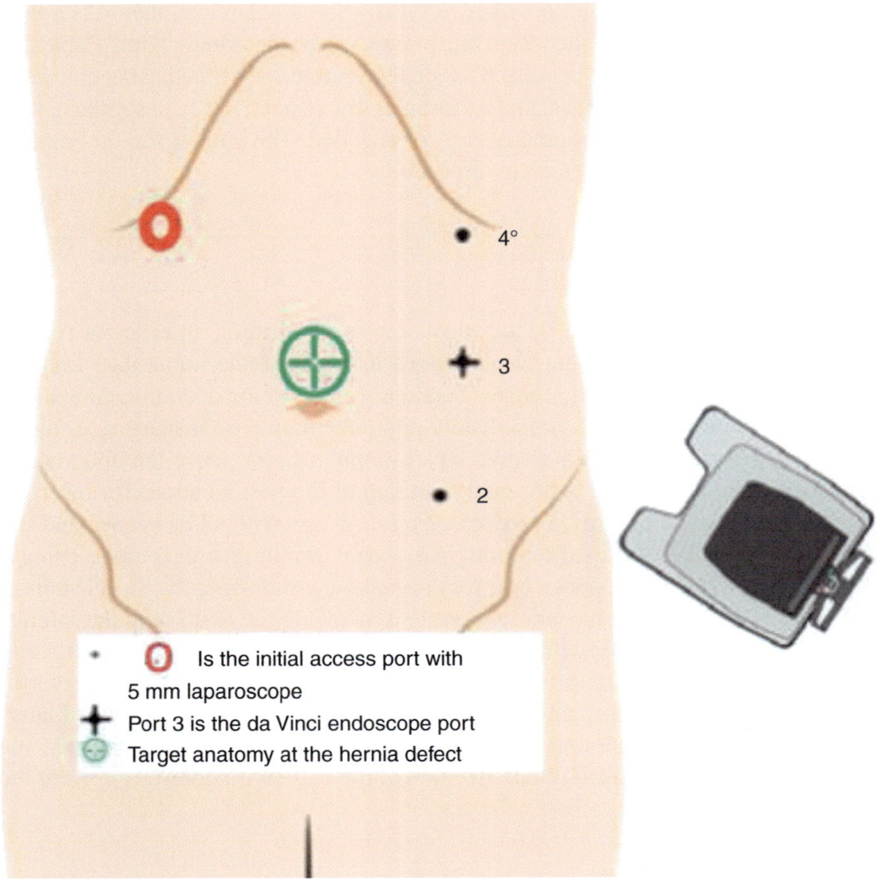

Fig. 15.3 Alternate trocar positions if unable to access the right side of the abdominal cavity

assistant should be able to manipulate the arms of the robot intra-operatively to assist in minimization of arm collision and/or enhancement of optical visualization. The assistant should also be skilled in introduction of sutures and mesh and the retrieval of needles from the ports using laparoscopic instruments. An assistant that is able to accomplish these tasks will diminish the need for the robotic surgeon to scrub throughout the case.

15.7 Conclusion

The robotic approach is an efficient and safe technique to ventral hernia repair. It allows for an easier primary facial closure, potentially decreasing the risk of recurrence, pseudo-recurrence and seroma formation as compared to a traditional laparoscopic approach in which the fascial defect is not closed. It is a more ergonomically sound platform for the surgeon and allows for increased autonomy regarding visualization and camera manipulation. Articulation of the arms may also allow for more precise lysis of adhesions or hernia reduction. Despite these benefits, the operative room setup and turnover can be a frustrating aspect of this repair modality. The authors hope that the content of this chapter may assist others in developing streamlined processes for operative preparation that could improve intraoperative and postoperative outcomes.

References

1. Deldi G, Ipaktchi R, Wagner M, et al. Laparoscopic ventral hernia repair is safe and cost effective. Surg Endosc. 2006;20:92–5.
2. Gonzalez A, Escobar E, Romero R, Walker G, Mejias J, Gallas M, Dickens E, Johnson CJ, Rabaza J, Kudsi OY. Robotic-assisted ventral hernia repair: a multicenter evaluation of clinical outcomes. Surg Endosc. 2017;31(3):1342–9.
3. Gonzalez AM, Romero RJ, Seetharamaiah R, Gallas M, Lamoureux J, Rabaza JR. Laparoscopic ventral hernia repair with primary closure versus no primary closure of the defect: potential benefits of the robotic technology. Int J Med Robot. 2015;11(2):120–55.
4. LeBlanc KA. Incisional hernia repair: laparoscopic techniques. World J Surg. 2005;29(8):1073–9.
5. LeBlanc KA. Robotic ventral hernia repair. In: Kingsnorth A, LeBlanc KA, Sanders DL, editors. Management of abdominal hernias: Springer; 2018.
6. Liang MK, Subramanian A, Awad SS. Laparoscopic transcutaneous closure of central defects in laparoscopic incisional hernia repair. Surg Laparosc Endosc Percutan Tech. 2012;22(2):e66–70.
7. Liang MK, Holihan JL, Itani K, Alawadi ZM, Gonzalez JR, Askenasy EP, Ballecer C, Chong HS, Goldblatt MI, Greenberg JA, Harvin JA, Keith JN, Martindale RG, Orenstein S, Richmond B, Roth JS, Szotek P, Towfigh S, Tsuda S, Vaziri K, Berger DH. Ventral hernia management: expert consensus guided by systematic review. Ann Surg. 2017;265(1):80–9.
8. Nguyen DH, et al. Primary fascial closure with laparoscopic ventral hernia repair: Systemic Review. World J Surg. 2014;38:3097–104.
9. Orenstein SB, Dumeer JL, Monteagudo J, Poi MJ, Novitsky YW. Outcomes of laparoscopic ventral hernia repair with routine defect closure using "shoelace" technique. Surg Endosc. 2011;25(5):1452–7.

Diastasis Recti: Robotic Extended-View Totally Extraperitoneal (eTEP) Access Hernia Repair Technique

16

Igor Belyansky, Richard Lu, and Alex Addo

16.1 Robotic Extended-View Totally Extraperitoneal Access Rives-Stoppa Technique (r-eTEP)

The eTEP technique was popularized by Dr. Jorge Daes in 2012 as an enhanced approach to conventional TEP procedures. This approach was expanded to ventral and incisional hernia repairs by Belyansky and colleagues in 2017.

Table 16.1 lists preferences in equipment when performing robotic eTEP access for Rives-Stoppa repairs.

16.2 Operative Technique

16.2.1 Patient Positioning and Operating Room Setup

Patients are positioned supine with both arms tucked at the sides in order to facilitate docking on either side. The patient is extended to approximately 30° to maximize the distance between the anterior superior iliac spine and subcostal margin, thus preventing robotic arm collision (Fig. 16.1).

Before incision, we recommend marking the relevant anatomy to identify the xiphoid process, bilateral subcostal margins, symphysis pubis, linea alba, and linea semilunaris (Fig. 16.2).

I. Belyansky (✉)
Abdominal Wall Reconstruction Program, General Surgery, Anne Arundel Medical Center, Annapolis, MD, USA

Department of Surgery, Anne Arundel Medical Center, Annapolis, MD, USA
e-mail: ibelyansky@aahs.org

R. Lu · A. Addo
Department of General Surgery, Anne Arundel Medical Center, Annapolis, MD, USA
e-mail: rlu@aahs.org; aaddo@aahs.org

K. A. LeBlanc (ed.), *Robotic Assisted Hernia Repair*,
https://doi.org/10.1007/978-3-030-23025-8_16

Table 16.1 Recommended equipment for robotic eTEP access

Laparoscopic equipment	• 5-mm 30-degree scope • Monopolar hook dissector • Laparoscopic needle driver • Two blunt graspers • 5-mm Kii Fios First Entry® (Applied Medical, Rancho Santa Margarita, CA) port (also used for robotic approach)
Robotic equipment	• 10-mm 30-degree and 0-degree scopes • Two 8-mm robotic ports (three for the da Vinci Xi system) • 12-mm bariatric port for robotic camera • *ProGrasp*™ grasper (Intuitive Surgical, Sunnyvale, CA) • Monopolar scissors • Mega Suture Cut™ needle driver (Intuitive Surgical) • Monopolar cord • Bipolar cord (optional if bipolar fenestrated grasper is used)

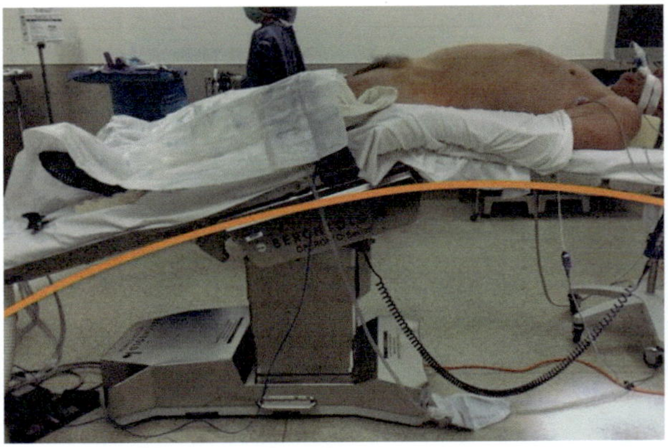

Fig. 16.1 The patient is placed in 30° extension to expand the retrorectus space and to prevent robotic arm collision

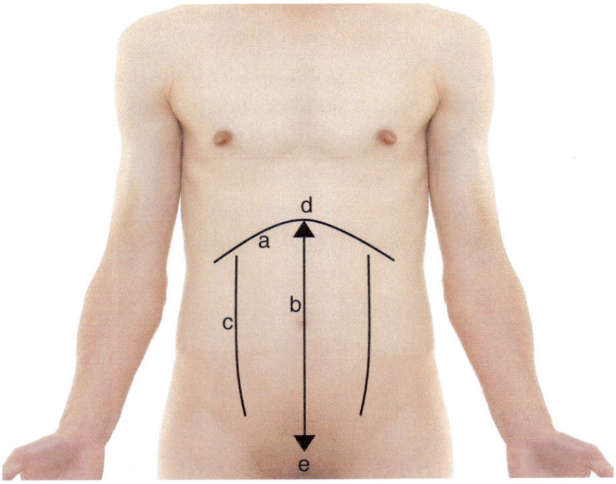

Fig. 16.2 Relevant Landmarks. (**a**) Subcostal margins, (**b**) Linea alba, (**c**) Linea semilunaris, (**d**) Xiphoid, (**e**) Pubis

16.2.2 Access

Initial entry and port placement is done with standard laparoscopy. A 5-mm skin incision is made in the area overlying the anterior rectus sheath. The position of this incision is dependent upon robot docking which will be discussed later in this chapter. An optical trocar is used to penetrate the anterior rectus sheath (Fig. 16.3a). Once the muscle fibers of the rectus abdominis are visualized, the surgeon's hand is dropped such that the direction of port advancement is almost parallel to the abdominal wall. This prevents inadvertent entry into the peritoneal cavity, which may greatly complicate the remainder of the procedure. The posterior rectus sheath is encountered and the retrorectus space is developed using blunt dissection of the areolar tissue with the laparoscope (Fig. 16.3b). Care is taken to not avulse the crossing branches of the inferior epigastric vessels, which should be carefully dissected off of the posterior rectus sheath.

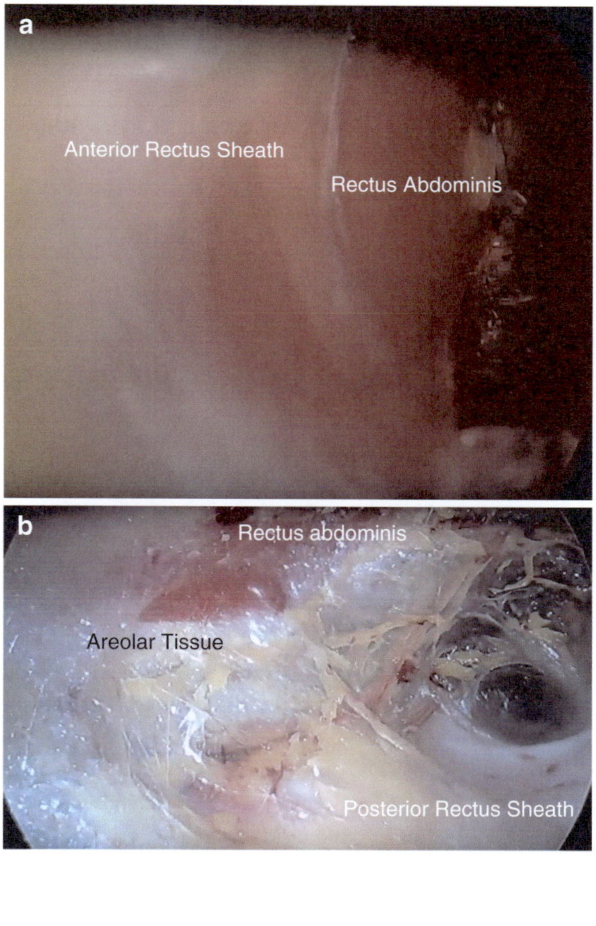

Fig. 16.3 (**a**) Entry of anterior rectus sheath with direct visualization. (**b**) Initial blunt dissection of retromuscular space

Table 16.2 Port placement and relative contraindications

Defect location	Docking position	Relative contraindications to port placement
Upper midline	Bottom docking below umbilicus/side docking	History of Caesarean section, pelvic surgery, or prostatectomy, or morbidly obese habitus with large pannus
Lower midline	Upper docking above umbilicus/side docking	History of upper midline surgeries, or Kocher or chevron subcostal incisions
Paraumbilical	Lower/upper/side docking positions	Narrow retrorectus space (specific to side docking)

16.2.3 Port Placement

Dynamic port placement, based on the area of interest, is perhaps the most important concept to understand for the performance of a successful eTEP dissection. Consideration of relevant anatomy, location of the defect, and past surgical history is critical in determining port placement. Physical examination and CT imaging are used to elucidate anatomy preoperatively. Table 16.2 lists the most common port placement based on defect location and relative contraindications.

16.2.4 Relevant Anatomy and the Principles of *Crossover*

Understanding of the preperitoneal space in relation to the retrorectus space is paramount. The peritoneal layer is the most posterior layer of the abdominal wall. Medially, prominent adipose contributions are given by the falciform ligament and the umbilical ligament.

16.2.5 Upper Midline Defects (Lower Dock Setup)

When dealing with upper midline defects, we prefer to perform the crossover to the contralateral retrorectus space below the level of the umbilicus. Relative contraindications to docking the robot inferior to the umbilicus for upper midline defects include history of caesarean section, pelvic surgery, prostatectomy, or morbidly obese habitus with large pannus (Table 16.2). Figure 16.4 demonstrates the port position for upper midline defects. Four trocars are usually placed. For a right-handed surgeon, we recommend that the first incision be made in the right upper quadrant (RUQ) in the region overlying the right rectus muscle. An optical entry technique is used to enter the right retrorectus space, as outlined in Fig. 16.3. Figure 16.5a–d demonstrate the typical sequence of port placement.

The first port (RUQ) is used as an assistant port later in the procedure. Attention should be given to locate the right inferior epigastric vessels, which travel parallel and medial to the linea semilunaris (Fig. 16.5a). Next, under direct vision, a right lower quadrant (RLQ) port is placed just lateral to the inferior epigastric vessels and approximately 3–4 cm below the level of the umbilicus (Fig. 16.5b). The RLQ port

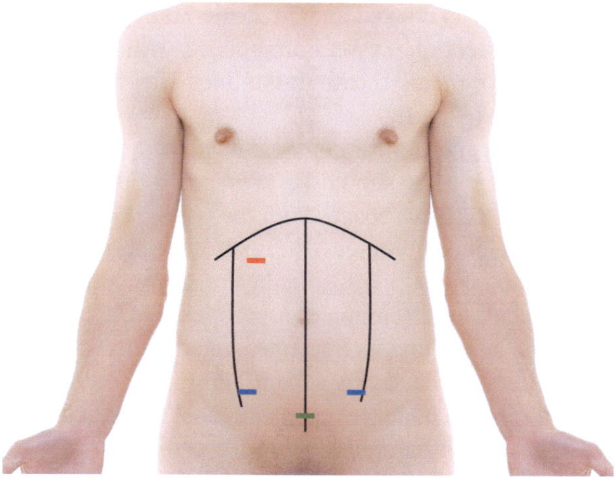

Fig. 16.4 Port placement for lower docking. Red: assistant port, Blue: robotic working ports, Green: camera port

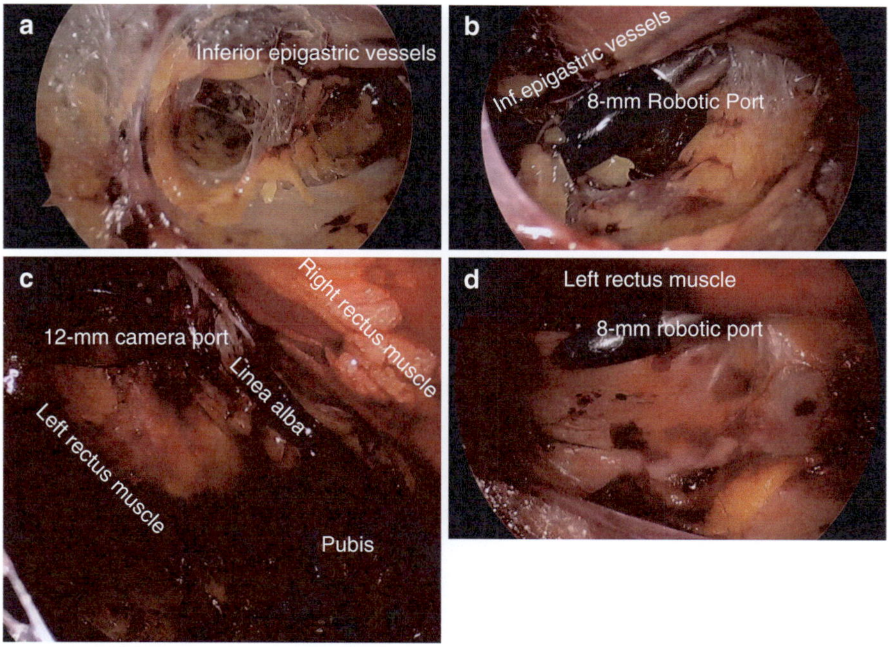

Fig. 16.5 (**a**) A RUQ port is placed for initial dissection of the right retrorectus space. (**b**) Insertion of a RLQ robotic port lateral to the inferior epigastric vessels. (**c**) Insertion of a lower midline 12-mm camera port. (**d**) Insertion of a LLQ robotic port

is further used to develop the space of Retzius with a blunt grasper. A 12-mm camera port (used with the Si) is then placed under direct vision in the lower midline, followed by placement of the left lower quadrant (LLQ) port entering the space just lateral to the left inferior epigastric vessels (Fig. 16.5c, d).

The robot is docked and a robotic 30-degree scope in the *up* position is used to start the dissection. Dissection proceeds with division of the medial contributions of the posterior rectus sheath to the linea alba bilaterally from the caudal to cephalad direction (Fig. 16.6).

Medially, peritoneal contributions by the falciform and umbilical ligaments to the posterior layer should be preserved. Continuation of this dissection joins the bilateral retrorectus spaces with the preperitoneal space medially.

As dissection continues, the neck of the hernia sac will be encountered (Fig. 16.7). In a true incisional hernia, the layers surrounding the neck of the sac may be fused and difficult to differentiate. A preoperative CT scan is an invaluable aid for identifying the hernia and its contents. An attempt may be made in some cases to reduce the entirety of the sac by separating it from its distal attachments; however, this is commonly not done in our practice. We frequently consider sharply opening the peritoneal layer just proximal to the neck of the sac to reduce the visceral contents under direct visualization and perform adhesiolysis as needed. Any defects in the posterior layer can be fixed primarily with a 2-0 absorbable suture. Once the hernia contents are reduced, retromuscular dissection continues to the level of the xiphoid process (Fig. 16.8).

The linea alba is then reconstructed using 0 V-Loc™ (Medtronic, Minneapolis, MN) suture, medializing the healthy edges of rectus abdominis muscle to oppose each other. The hernia defect is closed as part of the linea alba reconstruction (Fig. 16.9). Decreasing insufflation pressure from 15 mm Hg to 10 mm Hg or less assists in cinching of the suture line. The suture is cut after taking at least three bites with the V-Loc™ suture over the previous suture line. A ruler is then used to measure the entire retromuscular space and a medium-weight macroporous mesh is trimmed to size. This mesh is then advanced into the retromuscular space and

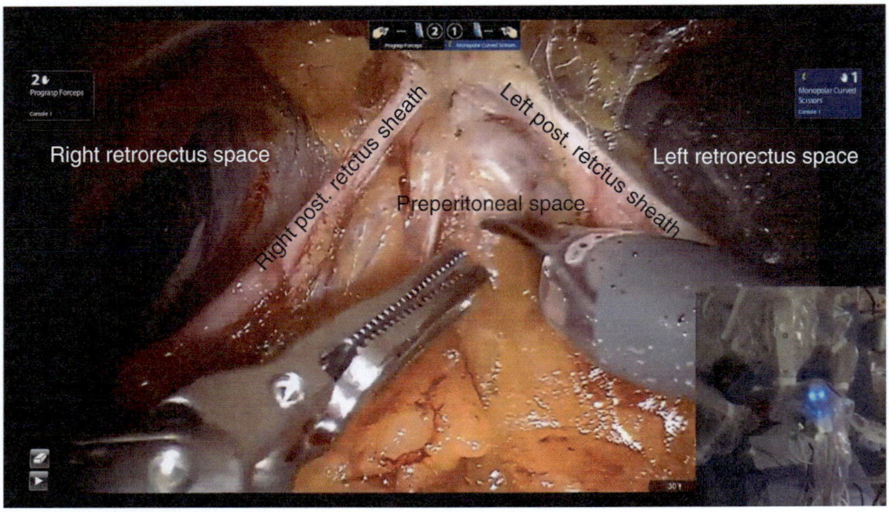

Fig. 16.6 Division of bilateral posterior rectus sheaths

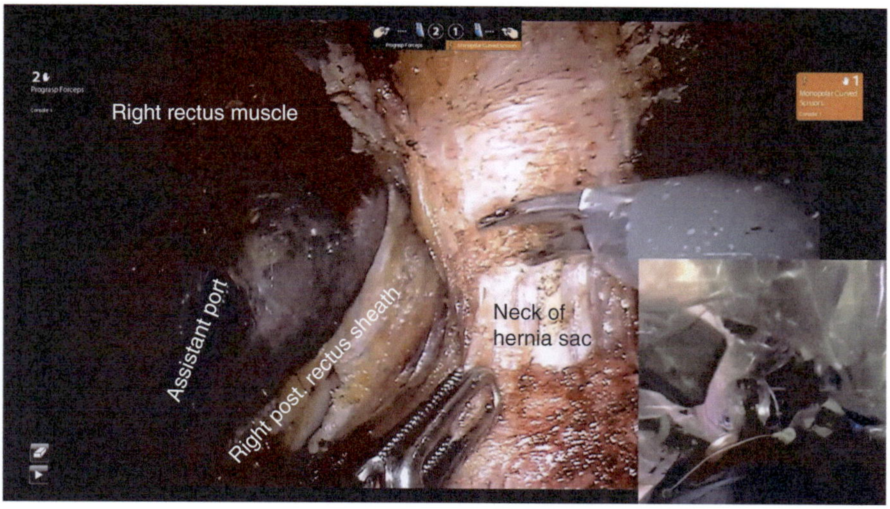

Fig. 16.7 Division of hernia sac

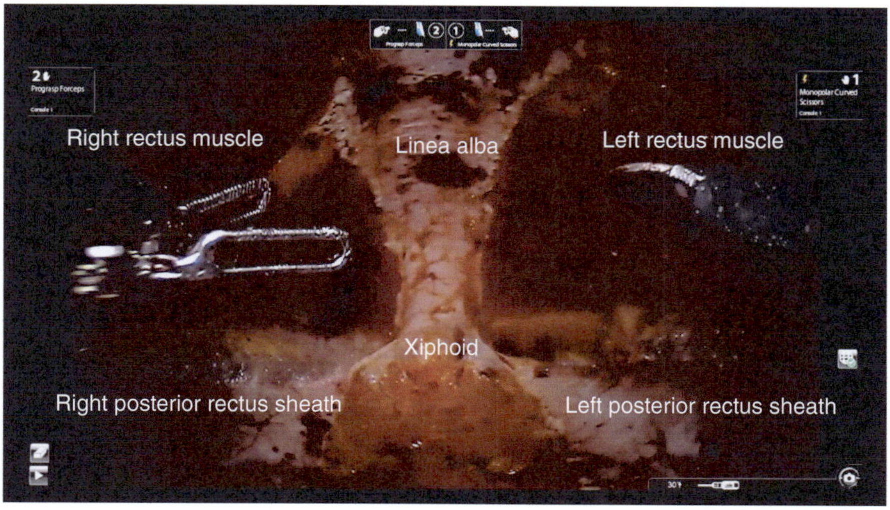

Fig. 16.8 Cephalad development of retrorectus space

positioned such that it seats flat on the posterior layer. In our practice, we do not use any penetrating fixation. Insufflation is then released and ports are removed.

16.2.6 Lower Midline Defects (Upper Dock Setup)

Figure 16.10 demonstrates the typical port approach for lower midline defects. Relative contraindications to docking the robot superior to the umbilicus for lower

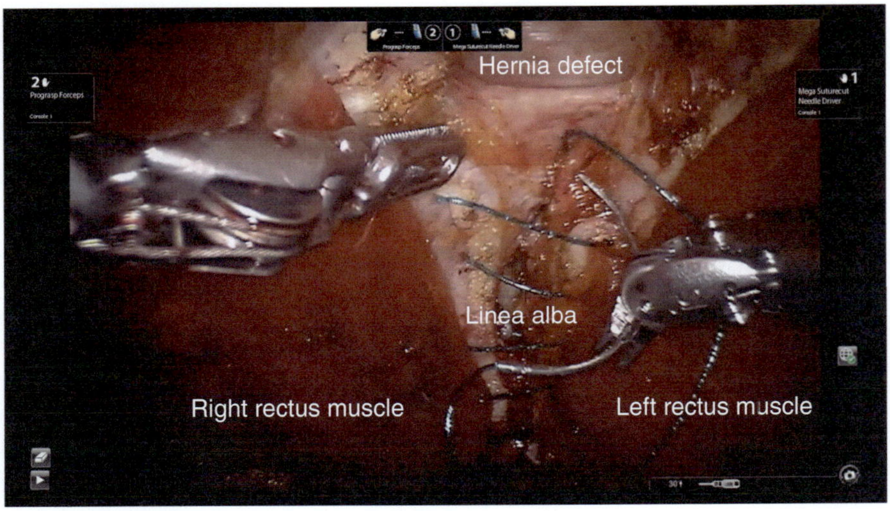

Fig. 16.9 Closure of linea alba and hernia defect

Fig. 16.10 Port placement for upper docking. Red: assistant port, Blue: robotic working ports, Green: camera port

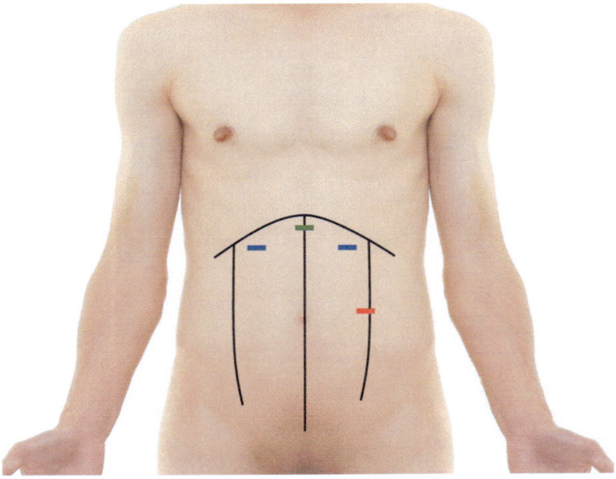

midline defects include history of upper midline surgeries, or past Kocher or chevron subcostal incisions (Table 16.2). Using the technique demonstrated in Fig. 16.3, the first port is positioned in the uppermost aspect of the left upper quadrant (LUQ), just inferior and to the left of the subxiphoid region. The port enters the left retrorectus space which is developed further with a 5-mm angled laparoscope. An 8-mm robotic port and an assistant port are placed under direct vision into the developed retrorectus space. The initial port is exchanged for a 12-mm bariatric port, to be used as the robotic (Si) camera port. The 5-mm laparoscope is placed through the assistant port, thus visualizing the medial aspect of the left posterior rectus sheath in the upper midline. The left posterior rectus sheath is incised with hook cautery near

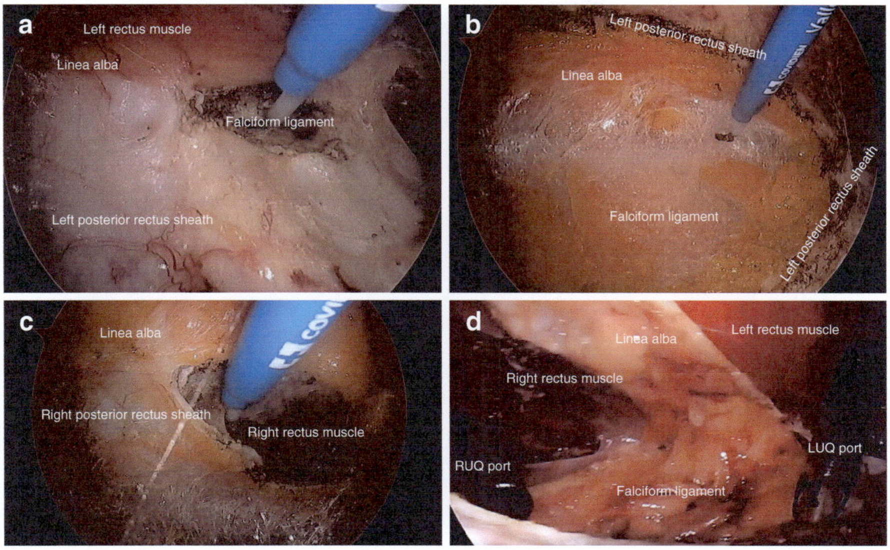

Fig. 16.11 (**a**) Incision of ipsilateral posterior rectus sheath. (**b**) Plane of dissection between linea alba and falciform ligament. (**c**) Crossover to contralateral retrorectus space. (**d**) Insertion of robotic port in contralateral retrorectus space

its medial attachment until adipose tissue from the falciform ligament is encountered. This adipose tissue is swept down bluntly with care not to cause injury to the overlying linea alba. The contralateral rectus sheath is encountered and incised. The contralateral retrorectus space is then bluntly developed until enough space is present to place a RUQ robotic port (Fig. 16.11a–d).

Once all the ports are in position, the robot is docked. Retrorectus dissection is carried out in the caudal direction, completing bilateral release of the posterior rectus sheaths. The hernia sac is encountered and sharp dissection is employed to mobilize it downwards. Alternatively, the sac can be sharply entered and adhesiolysis performed as needed. The steps and landmarks of dissection, as well as posterior layer closure and linea alba reconstruction, are identical to what has been described in the earlier section on upper midline defects.

16.2.7 Side Dock Setup

Direct retrorectus docking from a lateral approach is also possible in elective cases. Port placement is demonstrated in Fig. 16.12. The consistent reproducibility of this approach depends on the width of the retrorectus space and the patient's surgical history. The retrorectus space should be at least 7 cm wide on preoperative imaging to comfortably proceed with this approach. Table 16.2 lists some relative contraindications to this approach.

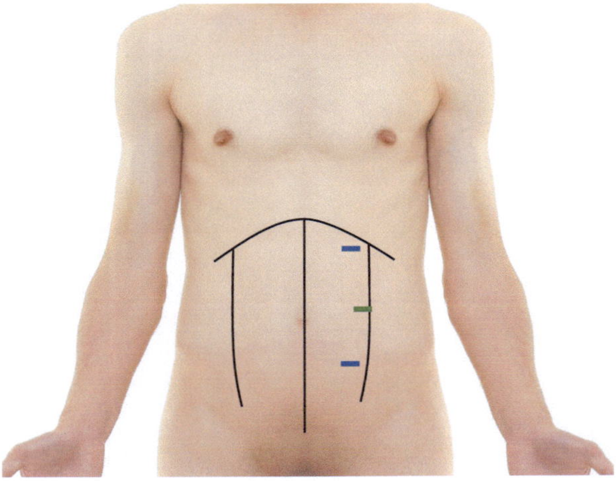

Fig. 16.12 Port placement for side docking. Blue: robotic working ports, Green: camera port

As demonstrated in Fig. 16.3, the LUQ port is placed and initial development of the retrorectus space with the laparoscope is done in a similar fashion as described above. Blunt dissection of the retrorectus space with the camera is performed, followed by placement of a 12-mm robotic camera port and an 8-mm robotic LLQ port under direct vision into the developed left retrorectus space. The LUQ port is exchanged for a robotic 8-mm port. The robot is docked, and surgical dissection begins. With this setup, the crossover is achieved robotically, not laparoscopically, as described in the previous methods.

16.2.8 Conclusion

This novel technique has begun to receive increasing traction and excitement at hernia meetings. With this in mind, longer follow up and elucidation of potential unique complications associated with this technique is of utmost importance moving forward. The eTEP approach addresses many concerns acknowledged in laparoscopic IPOM, allowing extraperitoneal mesh placement, elimination of penetrating fixation, and consistent defect closure with diastasis repair.

Robotic IPOM-Plus Repair

17

Eduardo Parra-Davila, Carlos Hartmann,
and Juan Maldonado

17.1 Introduction

Ventral hernia repair is one of the most common surgical procedures world wide; however, the complexity is increasing and the repair remains a constant challenge [1–3].

Karl LeBlanc introduced the laparoscopic approach for ventral hernia repair in 1993.

Laparoscopic recurrence rates are similar to open ventral hernia repair. The laparoscopic approach leads to improvements in recovery time, decrease in hospital length of stay and complication rates. The initial technique described detailed placement of mesh after reducing the contents of the hernia, but did not include closure of the abdominal wall defect [1–3].

Defect closure via laparoscopy requires a high degree of specialized dexterity and incurs a significantly longer procedure time, which can deter the method. The bridging technique for hernia repair can cause functional problems with patients, due to no musculo-aponeurotic coverage, resulting in adynamic areas of the abdominal wall. The bulging of the mesh into the hernia sac and development of a seroma at the created "dead" space are the most common complications with the bridging technique [1, 2, 4, 5].

With the advent of robotic surgery, larger and more complex hernia repairs are being approached in a minimally invasive fashion, with the benefits of fascial

E. Parra-Davila (✉)
Minimally Invasive and Colorectal Surgery, Florida Hospital Celebration Health, Kissimmee, FL, USA
e-mail: eduardo.parradavila.md@flhosp.org

C. Hartmann
Celebration Center for Surgery, Florida Hospital Celebration Health, Kissimmee, FL, USA

J. Maldonado
Florida Hospital Celebration Health, Kissimmee, FL, USA

K. A. LeBlanc (ed.), *Robotic Assisted Hernia Repair*,
https://doi.org/10.1007/978-3-030-23025-8_17

closure, retrorectus placement of mesh, posterior and anterior component separation techniques and intraperitoneal suturing of the mesh. These are facilitated by the minimally invasive robot platform, accomplishing the major goal of any ventral or incisional hernia repair that is to restore the integrity of the abdominal wall anatomy and medialization of the rectus muscles.

17.2 Definition

IPOM-Plus repair, is described in the guidelines for laparoscopic treatment of ventral and incisional abdominal wall hernias of the International Endohernia Society. It is a superior repair in that it closes the fascial defect with two options: running suture intraabdominally or interrupted transfascial suture transabdominally [1]. The IPOM-Plus technique reduces recurrence rates as compared with classical IPOM, mimicking open repair [1, 4].

The robotic approach allows the operator to offer traditional open repair techniques through minimally access incisions, smoother and easier intracorporeal suturing of the fascia allowing primary repair. This can result in improved physiologic abdominal wall movements and greater overlap of the mesh surrounding the defect edges. Robot-assisted laparoscopic ventral hernia repair also offers enhanced suturing options because of the afforded excellent visualization for repair of difficult hernias with bony margins, such as lumbar, suprapubic and subcostal hernias [6–8].

The IPOM-Plus technique can reduce the hernia defect by closing it completely, resulting in the elimination of postoperative bulging, reduction in the rate of seromas and improvement in the postoperative discomfort of the patient [1, 2].

Limitations of this technique are clear. Large defects are not feasibly closed without tension. Occasionally a combination with the endoscopic component separation technique or a transversus abdominal release may be required to lower the tension and enable the closure. Defects >20 cm in length should not be approached routinely by robotic techniques except in few selected cases [2, 9]. Other challenges include trocar placement, instrument collisions, difficulty with angulations, and removal of soft tissue when indicated.

17.3 Surgical Technique

17.3.1 Preoperative Care

A complete medical history along with radiologic imaging offers the opportunity for surgeons to construct a risk/benefit ratio and to coordinate an operative plan. Known risk factors for incisional hernia include male sex, advanced age, obesity, tobacco use, chronic obstructive pulmonary disease, immunosuppression, diabetes mellitus, and history of an emergent operation [6, 7, 10]. A computerized tomography scan of the abdomen and pelvis should be done for the preoperative planning and remains the most appropriate preoperative radiologic test. This exam can delineate the location of the hernia, size, contents and often (but not always) identify the location of any previously placed mesh(es).

17.3.2 Patient Positioning

For the procedure, the patient is given general anesthesia with endotracheal intubation. Intravenous prophylactic antibiotics are given. The preferred position is the patient placed supine with the arms tucked laterally on the side, unless trocar access to the lateral abdomen is obscured by this position. The patient must be always be fully secured to the operating table to prevent any incident with any changes in the table position.

17.3.3 Trocar Placement

Achievement of safe intra-abdominal access remains the first step in minimally invasive surgery. This can be challenging in patients with multiple abdominal surgeries. The sites of previous operative intervention will certainly influence the strategy to gain initial access. A popular method of access to the peritoneal cavity is the use of a Veress needle placed in the left upper quadrant subcostal region at the midclavicular line or an area where no previous surgeries are noted in order to avoid adhesions. After adequate pneumoperitoneum is established, a 5-mm optical viewing port is placed in the lateral position on the opposite side of the hernia. It is critical to place the ports as far from the defect as possible to allow for increased range of motion, operative effectiveness and avoidance of the mesh covering the ports and camera when deployed. This is not avoidable in all cases.

Depending on the size of the abdomen and location of the hernia, three or four robotic arms are used, and additional placement of an assistant port is common. The most lateral position of the camera and two instrument arms will allow for full range of motion to facilitate dissection and suture closure of the hernia defect. A 8 or 12 mm trocar for the camera is placed as far lateral to the ipsilateral edge of the defect as feasible. This usually obviates the need to place trocars on the contralateral abdomen when securing the mesh to the ipsilateral abdominal wall. An 8 mm trocar is placed in the lower lateral abdomen and the initial 5 mm optical trocar is then replaced with an 8 mm trocar or by the camera trocar. The type and location of the trocars will be influenced by the type of robot used.

The accessory port is used to aid with mesh introduction, traction, suction, suture cutting, and suture removal. Using the accessory trocar for the larger mesh introduction under direct visualization is safer and more efficient than introducing the mesh and sutures through the 12 mm camera port. This accessory port is less useful for the repair of smaller ventral hernias and the location must also be determined in relationship to the daVinci arms. The trocar site position can be located opposite the defect between one instrument arm and the camera arm trocar or can be placed through the

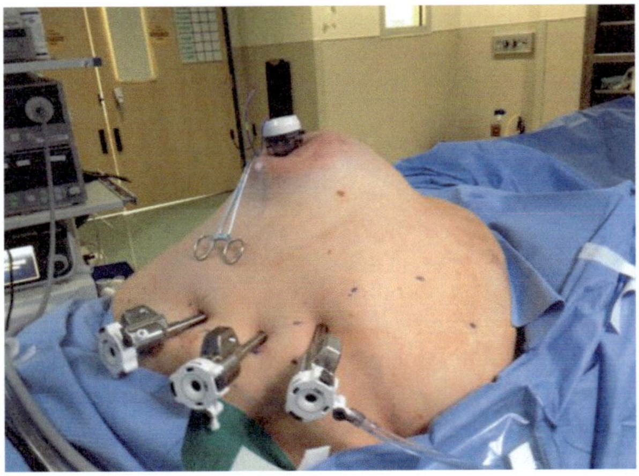

Fig. 17.1 Trocars placement and trocar placement in hernia defect

defect and be covered at the end with the mesh. If needed for double docking may be necessary for a large hernia and can be placed at the subxiphoid or suprapubic area and in that way can be utilized for both sides. it is crucial to place the accessory port as far from the defect as possible to allow for increased range and motion and effectiveness; occasionally this can be placed in the hernia itself (Fig. 17.1).

17.3.4 Docking

Patient position manipulation must be performed prior to docking of the robot. The robotic cart is driven directly towards the abdomen and over the trocar sites. The robotic docking is done from the side of the hernia to align the center column of the robot with the target and the camera.

17.3.5 Instrumentation

For right-handed surgeons, a dV Prograsp (or fenestrated bipolar) is placed on arm #2, 12 mm 30' up camera in the camera port, and the dV monopolar scissors is placed in arm #1. The dV needle holder is used to primarily close the hernia defect as well as fixating the mesh to the abdominal wall.

17.3.6 Adhesiolysis

Adhesiolysis of the abdominal wall to isolate the hernia defect must be performed meticulously so as to avoid iatrogenic injury to the abdominal viscera. For laparoscopic surgery lysis of adhesions is the most challenging, but the Da Vinci Surgical System platform facilitates adhesiolysis through its 3-D visualization, extended range-of-motion, tremor-less precision, and superior ergonomics (Fig. 17.2).

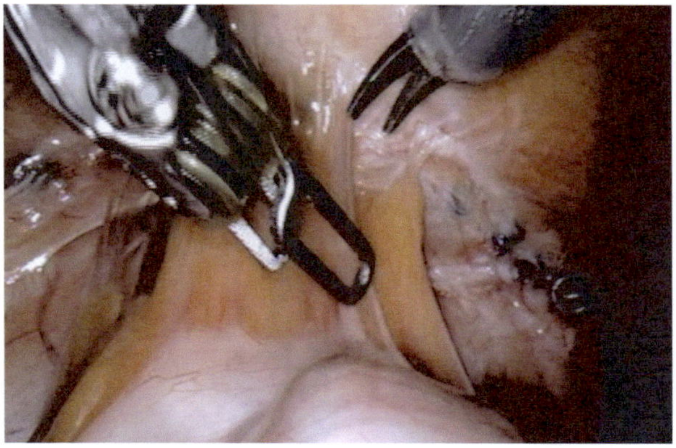

Fig. 17.2 Adhesiolysis of abdominal wall

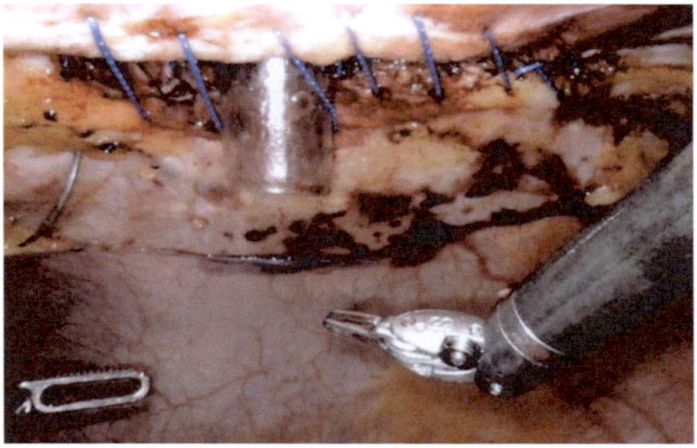

Fig. 17.3 Closure of the defect with 10 mm trocar to deploy the mesh

Complete adhesiolysis is mandatory to insure complete evaluation of the abdominal wall. If necessary, the falciform ligament is taken down to allow the placement of mesh against the abdominal wall. In the setting of dense adhesions the robotic harmonic scalpel or daVinci vessel sealer may facilitate hemostasis.

The entire repair is performed under direct visualization, with precise placement and confirmation of depth into the posterior fascia for all sutures placed. The ability to primarily close defects without component separation is based on the principles of Ramirez regarding width and location of the hernia defect (Fig. 17.3).

Of course, this is based on open technique and not working against the forces of pneumoperitoneum. As a general rule, a defect that is <10 cm wide is amenable to primary closure but this is also dependent on body habitus, age of the patient and abdominal wall compliance. Desufflation of the abdominal cavity to 6–8 mm Hg pneumoperitoneum may be necessary for less resistance during the closure. The fascial sutures should encompass 0.5–1-cm bites of fascia. Successful primary closure of the defect is facilitated by the use of the barbed V-loc suture (Medtronic, Minneapolis, MN) or other barbed sutures (Fig. 17.4). The ability to minimize tissue trauma to the abdominal wall with the robotic platform also allows the surgeon to take precise bites of tissue to anchor the mesh during the repair.

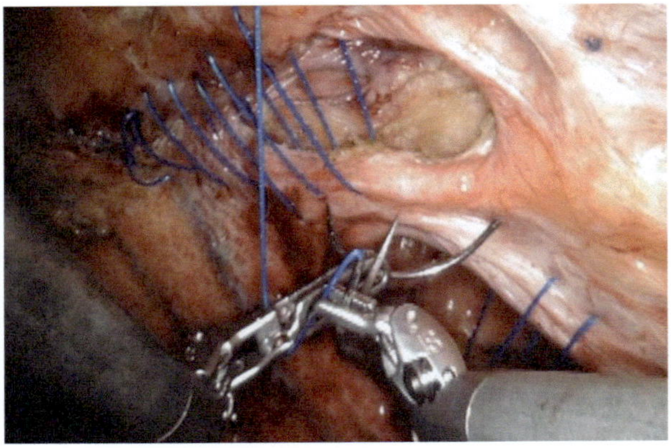

Fig. 17.4 Closure multiple defects

The suture is introduced into the intraabdominal cavity through the 8 mm dV trocar or the accessory port. Bending the needle slightly will facilitate both introduction and subsequent removal of the suture if an 8 mm trocar is used. This will not be necessary if a 12 mm trocar is used for the accessory port.

17.3.7 Selection of Mesh

An ideal mesh has sufficient strength, is chemically stable, is easily sterilized, resists infections, is non-carcinogenic, limits inflammatory foreign body reactions, and incorporates well into the abdominal wall [11]. While manufacturers are trying to produce such a product, the ideal mesh doesn't exist, but there have been a lot of improvements since the original polypropylene mesh was created in 1959. Since then several other materials have been produced such as other non-absorbable meshes, absorbable products and tissue-based biologic implants.

Permanent meshes, such as polypropylene and polyester, were used when laparoscopic hernia repair first started. However uncoated meshes were soon abandoned due to the large number of visceral adhesion related complications, such as fistula, bowel obstruction, and complications during re-operative adhesiolysis [12]. Composite meshes were developed for laparoscopic intraperitoneal onlay placement; they combine the strength of permanent mesh with an "anti-adhesion" barrier and are the ones that are most often used in robotic ventral hernia repair, most especially for the IPOM technique. Mesh technology continues to develop ahead of validating research as has been the practice for many years. As always, there are new meshes that are being developed for potential use in minimally invasive ventral hernia repair.

17.3.8 Mesh Fixation with Running Suture

The mesh is unrolled and oriented. The size of the mesh should uphold the principle of maintaining at least 5 cm overlap in all directions [10]. With the mesh positioned on the abdominal wall by using a scroll technique or the self expanding device (Echo PS, Davol, Warwick, RI), a full length non-absorbable monofilament suture (00 or 0 Prolene, Ethicon, Inc., Somerville, NJ) is introduced into the intra-abdominal cavity through the trocar of the needle holder or the accessory port depending on the size of the prosthetic. Because the mesh is placed during full insufflation, it is likely that as the abdomen is desufflated the mesh will loosen a bit. A tacking device and/or transfascial suture maybe used to secure the mesh to the anterior abdominal wall. Another commonly used option is the use of suture to fixate the midportion of the mesh to the anterior abdominal wall, which obviates the use of the other fixation methods that could potentially increase the incidence of chronic postoperative pain.

In a running fashion, the suture is then placed around the circumference of the mesh. It may be necessary to use one or two sutures for larger prosthetics (Figs. 17.5 and 17.6).

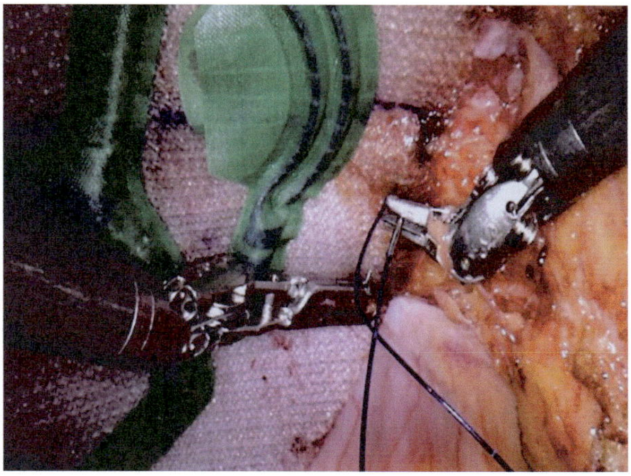

Fig. 17.5 Placement of a running suture for mesh fixation

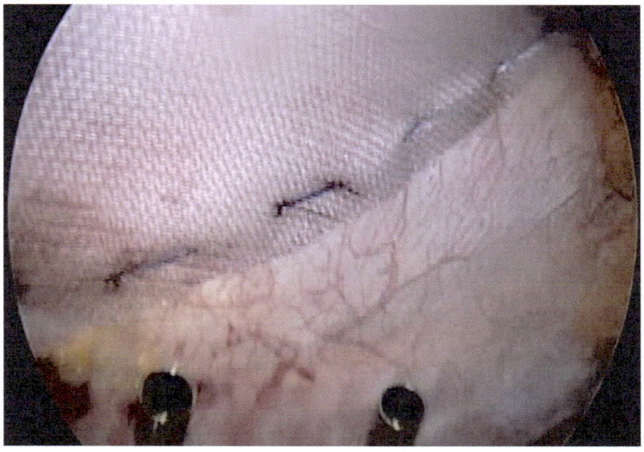

Fig. 17.6 Final appearance of the running suture fixation of the mesh

17.3.9 Closure of the Port Defects

Upon completion of mesh fixation, the robot is undocked. Only the larger 10–12 mm trocar fascial sites are closed with a suture passer under direct laparoscopic vision if not already covered by the mesh.

17.4 Postoperative Care

After surgery immediate unrestricted mobilization is encouraged as well as DVT prophylaxis. Diet is started as soon as the patient gets to the ward and advanced as tolerated depending upon the extent of adhesiolysis or concomitant procedures performed.

17.5 Conclusions

Robotic ventral hernia repair allows the operator to offer traditional open repair techniques through minimally invasive incisions.

The robotic approach visualizes the entire abdominal wall, thus detecting any impalpable hernia defect that also may be repaired at the same time. Successful primary closure of the defect is facilitated and accomplished in majority of the hernia repairs differentiating from the smaller rate done by laparoscopy alone.

Reconstruction of the linea alba in robotic assisted ventral or incisional hernia repair improves the functionality of the abdominal wall.

When necessary, the component separation option facilitates the closure and should be used for larger defects. This is further discussed in Chap. 22.

References

1. Bittner R, Bingener-Casey J, Dietz U. Guidelines for laparoscopic treatment of ventral and incisional abdominal wall hernias (International Endohernia Society [IEHS])—part 1. Surg Endosc. 2014;28:2–29.
2. Orenstein SB, Dumeer JL, Monteagudo J. Outcomes of laparoscopic ventral hernia repair with routine defect closure using “shoelacing” technique. Surg Endosc. 2010;25(5):1452–7.
3. Heniford BT, Park A, Ramshaw BJ, et al. Laparoscopic ventral and incisional hernia repair in 407 patients. J Am Coll Surg. 2000;190:645–50.
4. Bittner R, Bingener-Casey J, Dietz U. Guidelines for laparoscopic treatment of ventral and incisional abdominal wall hernias (International Endohernia Society [IEHS])—part III. Surg Endosc. 2014;28:380–404.
5. Earle D, Seymour N, Fellinger E, et al. Laparoscopic versus open incisional hernia repair: a single-institution analysis of hospital resource utilization for 884 consecutive cases. Surg Endosc. 2006;20:71–5.
6. Schluender S, Conrad J, Divino CM. Robot-assisted laparoscopic repair of ventral hernia with intracorporeal suturing. An experimental study. Surg Endosc. 2003;17:1391–5.

7. Ballantyne GH, Hourmont K, Wasielewski A. Telerobotic laparoscopic repair of incisional ventral hernias using intraperitoneal prosthetic mesh. JSLS. 2003;7:7–14.
8. Tayar C, Karoui M, Cherqui D, et al. Robot-assisted laparoscopic mesh repair of incisional hernias with exclusive intracorporeal suturing: a pilot study. Surg Endosc. 2007;21:1786–9.
9. Vasilescu D, Paun S. Surgical treatment of parietal defects with "da Vinci" surgical robot. J Med Life. 2012;5(2):232–8.
10. LeBlanc KA. Mesh overlap is a key determinant of hernia recurrence following laparoscopic ventral and incisional hernia repair. Hernia. 2016;20(1):85–9.
11. Shankaran V, Weber DJ, Reed RL, Luchette FA. A review of available prosthetics for ventral hernia repair. Ann Surg. 2011;253:6–26. https://doi.org/10.1097/SLA.0b013e3181f9b6e6.
12. Jenkins ED, Yom V, Melman L, Brunt LM, Eagon JC, Frisella MM, Matthews BD. Prospective evaluation of adhesion characteristics to intraperitoneal mesh and adhesiolysis-related complications during laparoscopic re-exploration after prior ventral hernia repair. Surg Endosc. 2010;24:3002–7.

Transabdominal Preperitoneal (rTAPP) Repair

18

Fahri Gokcal and Yusef Kudsi

18.1 Introduction

Abdominal wall hernia repair is probably the most common surgical procedure performed by general surgeons during daily surgical practice worldwide with an estimated rate of 348,000 people in the USA undergoing this surgical treatment in 2006 [1]. Ventral hernia is one of the most commonly seen types of abdominal wall hernias. Ventral hernias can be divided into two categories: primary ventral hernias (epigastric, umbilical, Spigelian etc.) and secondary ventral hernias (trocar site, incisional etc.) [2].

As the last decades have seen important advances in application of modern technology to surgical procedures, surgical tools and prosthetic materials for ventral hernia repair has expanded over time. With the help of developing technology, minimally invasive techniques have gained popularity with the advantages of preventing some of the complications of the wide dissection related to open surgery. Robotic hernia repair is an emerging technique based on the well-established principles of both laparoscopic and open ventral hernia repair. The main advantages of this platform are the availability of three-dimensional vision and easier instrument manipulation as compared to the standard laparoscopy.

Due to the fact that the use of prosthetic materials has a lower rate of recurrence as compared to suture repair, mesh placement should be considered for ventral hernia repair. There are several mesh placement methods that can be used in such patients. As intraperitoneal mesh placement, even a coated mesh, has potential complications such as fistula, adhesions complicating future surgeries, preperitoneal mesh reinforcement should be considered for ventral hernia repair.

F. Gokcal (✉)
Department of General Surgery, Van Regional Training and Research Hospital, Van, Turkey

Y. Kudsi
Tufts University School of Medicine, Boston, MA, USA

K. A. LeBlanc (ed.), *Robotic Assisted Hernia Repair*,
https://doi.org/10.1007/978-3-030-23025-8_18

In this chapter, we will provide the technical aspects of the robotic transabdominal preperitoneal (rTAPP) mesh repair in ventral and incisional hernias (VIH), with a special emphasis on preoperative evaluation, intraoperative considerations and issues, and postoperative care.

18.2 Surgical Anatomy

As understanding of the layers of the abdominal wall is critical in order to perform robotic surgery properly, surgical anatomy should be discussed.

The anterior abdominal wall can be thought of as having two parts: The anterolateral part includes the external oblique, internal oblique, and transversus abdominis muscles. These muscles are also referred to as the three flat muscles of the anterior abdominal wall. The other part is the middle portion, which is composed of the rectus abdominis and pyramidal muscles.

The aponeuroses of the above mentioned three flat muscles lie on each side of the rectus muscles. They split, pass anteriorly and posteriorly around the rectus muscle, to form a stout sheath enclosing in it. This sheath attaches medially to the linea alba in the midline, which is formed by decussation of all aponeuroses. In the lower two-thirds of the infra-umbilical anterior abdominal wall, the aponeuroses of the internal oblique and transversus abdominis muscles pass anterior to the rectus muscle, which is bounded posteriorly by the transversalis fascia only. The linea semicircularis of Douglas is the dividing line, which marks the level at which the rectus sheath loses its posterior wall. The peritoneum is the innermost layer of the abdominal wall. It is loosely connected with the transversalis fascia in most areas. Fat and other connective tissue lie within a space between the transversalis fascia and the peritoneum [3].

18.3 Mesh Selection and Placement

Different mesh positions can be performed in primary mesh reinforcement. Despite the inconsistent nomenclature of mesh positioning in the literature, it has recently been defined as following; in the onlay position, the mesh is laid on top of the external oblique fascia over the defect. In the inlay repair, mesh is the same size as the hernia defect and the edges are sutured to the hernia neck and acts as a bridge. The sublay technique implies the positioning of the mesh posterior to the rectus muscles and anterior to the posterior rectus sheath. In the underlay technique, mesh is placed anterior to the peritoneum and posterior to the rectus sheath. This is also called the preperitoneal repair. In intraperitoneal onlay mesh (IPOM), as the name implies, mesh is inserted into the abdominal compartment and laid on the anterior abdominal wall deep to the peritoneum [4]. As the anatomical terms are less open to misinterpretation, most hernia surgeons prefer to use the anatomical terms retro-muscular or retro-rectus, preperitoneal and intraperitoneal) as opposed to the colloquial terms (sublay, underlay and IPOM) in the three deepest abdominal wall planes [5]. Figure 18.1 represents the preperitoneal mesh placement.

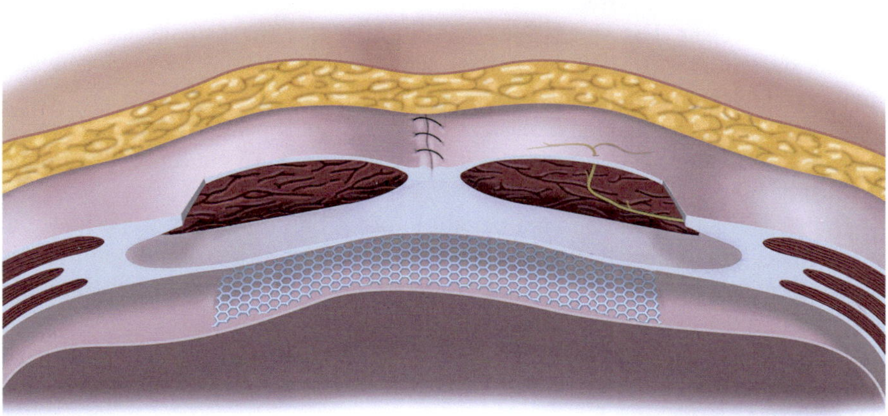

Fig. 18.1 Preperitoneal mesh placement (Reprinted with permission from Atlas of Robotic Surgery, Kudsi et al. Cine-Med, 2018. Copyright of the book and illustrations are retained by Cine-Med)

Mesh selection and mesh positioning are other points of ongoing discussion. In general, the primary function of a surgical mesh material is to provide biomechanical strength to the weakened fascial tissues. There are a wide variety of mesh options available to use in ventral hernia repair. We prefer to categorize them as synthetic non-composite, composite and biological meshes.

Composite meshes (absorbable or non-absorbable) are also known as barrier coated meshes, and have been designed for intraperitoneal placement during ventral hernia repair (IPOM) in order to reduce the risks of postsurgical complications related to adhesion formation in situations where the mesh is in contact with the abdominal viscera [6]. Although they generally have antiadhesive properties, composite mesh related adhesions have also been reported at various densities in patients requiring subsequent abdominal surgery after a prior mesh-based ventral hernia repair. This could be related to mesh eversion at the periphery of the biomaterial thereby exposing the bare polypropylene of the mesh [7].

Since the peritoneal layer is located between the viscera and the mesh in the preperitoneal ventral hernia repair technique (described below), the potential complications due to adhesion are potentially reduced to a minimum. Therefore, there is no necessity of using a coated mesh as in IPOM technique [8]. In addition, these are more expensive meshes rather than a lower cost option of bare polypropylene mesh in the preperitoneal space [9].

18.4 Patient Selection

Appropriate patient selection is essential for rTAPP VIH repair. Besides the medical status of the patient (discussed below), there are several factors which may directly affect the surgical technique such as the size and the location of the hernia defect, and prior history of VIH repair.

It is important to consider the size of the hernia defect when contemplating a rTAPP VIH repair. For single-dock rTAPP approach, the patients should have smaller defects, typically <5 cm as there is less tension on the defect closure and myofascial release is not usually required.

rTAPP approach is limited to the size of the peritoneal pocket thus in the experience of the authors the upper size limits have been 20 × 15 cm especially around midline defects.

Body mass index (BMI) is not helpful in predicting the ability to perform the preperitoneal dissection. Body habitus is very important for the ability to offer this approach as it could be very limiting if there is no space to place ports at proper distance in order to raise the flaps.

18.5 Preoperative Evaluation

Before considering rTAPP VIH repair, a thorough history and physical examination is required. Modifiable risk factors such as smoking, obesity, malnutrition, diabetes mellitus are all deleterious to wound healing and should be addressed and corrected before the elective operation, if possible [10]. Evaluation for potential reversal of provocative factors which can cause high intraabdominal pressure (e.g. the prostate hypertrophy, chronic cough, severe constipation, rectal cancer, and ascites) is also important.

Preoperative routine imaging is generally not required in the normal workup of a hernia. Because of its superior anatomic detail, cross-sectional abdominal imaging with computed tomography (CT) may be performed in patients with small to moderate incisional hernia and an atypical hernia. The CT scan is essential in defining the hernia in many obese patients, since physical exam is generally not adequate for assessment of the presence of a hernia, quantity of abdominal structures in the hernia sac, size of the hernia neck, or the width of the hernia sac. Furthermore, imaging data may also allow the surgeon to determine the docking position of robot.

Once the decision has been made to proceed and robotically repair, patient education is also an important issue to provide realistic expectations. All complications should be discussed, with a special emphasis on the risk of hematoma and seroma formation, postoperative pain, potential unexpected enterotomy, management options, and possibility of conversion to laparoscopy or open. After discussing the advantages and disadvantages of planned operation, appropriate informed consent should be obtained.

18.6 Equipment

The robotic platform equipment includes surgical cart, vision cart and surgeon console. The da Vinci® Surgical System (Intuitive Surgical Inc., Sunnyvale, CA), was approved by the Food and Drug Administration (FDA) in 2000, is by far the most widespread robotic surgical system commercially available. There are four different generations of the da Vinci® Surgical System since the first model was launched in 2001, so the following descriptions will all relate to the currently approved models (S, Si, X and Xi). In order to use the robotic da Vinci® Surgical System, EndoWrist® (Intuitive Surgical Inc., Sunnyvale, CA) instruments were designed to mimic the wrist of the surgeon's hand. These are supplied with a wide selection of different specialized tips. Of these, the authors usually prefer to use the bipolar Maryland and monopolar scissors for adhesiolysis and developing of peritoneal pocket, and large needle driver for mesh fixation and peritoneal flap closure in rTAPP VIH repair.

18.7 Surgical Technique

18.7.1 Preparation, Positioning and Access

Standard operative protocols are utilized including antibiotic prophylaxis, hair clipping, and placement of sequential compression devices. A Foley catheter is not usually required, however the surgeon may decide according to the location of hernia (especially suprapubic) and the anticipated duration of the operation. For draping, authors prefer an iodophor-impregnated sterile drape as a part of standard skin preparation, although some surgeons do not believe that this is necessary.

The patient is positioned supine on the operating table under general anesthesia. Depending on patient- and hernia-related factors, as well as the preferences of surgeon and anesthesiologist, the patient's arms is placed on the board set at 90° abduction. In order to increase the distance between the anterior superior iliac spine and the costal margin, slight flexing of the bed may be beneficial for the patients who have a short torso or limited space to adequately insertion of trocars (Fig. 18.2). Slight tilting of the operating table toward the cart of the robot may contribute to better visualization of the abdominal wall by the camera and increase the range of the robotic arms' motion without obstacle.

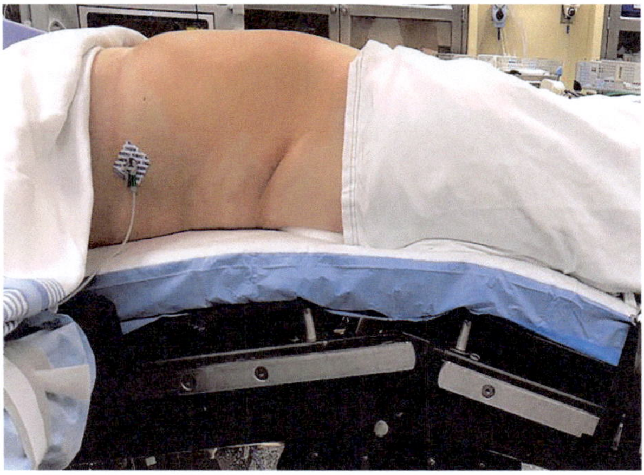

Fig. 18.2 Slightly flexion of the bed

With respect to individual surgeon preference, gaining access to the abdomen and initiation the pneumoperitoneum may be obtained by either closed (a Veress needle and/or an optical view trocar) or an open (Hasson) techniques.

Since inadvertent viscera injury is most likely to occur during initial access, the patient's surgical history and anatomy as well as the localization and size of hernia should be taken into account in the decision of the location of initial abdominal access. The authors prefer direct trocar insertion for initial access into an appropriate site after establishment of pneumoperitoneum through a Veress needle inserted at Palmer's point.

18.7.2 Trocar Placement, Adhesiolysis, Preperitoneal Dissection

One of the most important parts of the robotic operations is proper trocar placement. Three trocars, two of which are for instruments and one of which is for a camera, are usually used. The extent of the defect, anticipation of the edge of the planned flap and/or mesh and maintenance of free movement of the robotic arms should be considered when determining the position of trocars. The suggested trocar layout should positioned one on either side of the camera trocar, such that the 'Double Triangle' rule can be ensured. They should also be placed at a distance of at least 8 cm from one another in order to minimize the mechanical interference of the robotic arms with each other. The camera trocar is also recommended to be placed away from the surgical target to achieve the maximal surgical view, ideally 8–10 cm away from the proximal edge of the mesh or flap. The first trocar should be placed in the left upper quadrant along the anterior axillary line and the remaining two other trocars are placed roughly 6–8 cm apart preferably taking a "C" shape knowing the limitation of the most inferior trocar (Fig. 18.3). The authors prefer, if

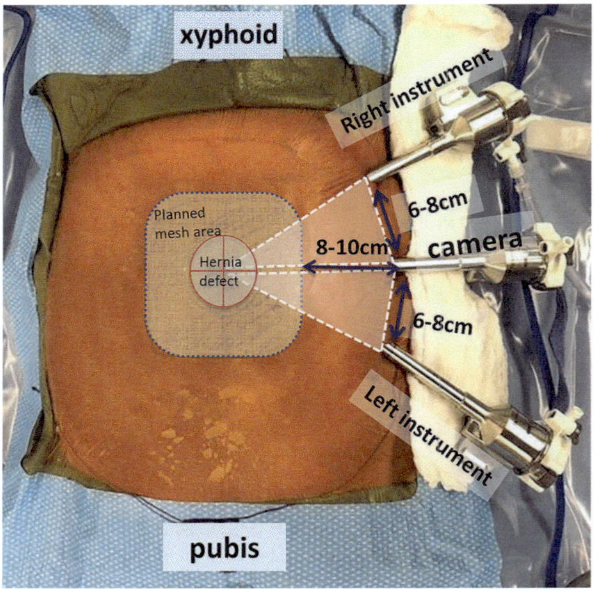

Fig. 18.3 Trocar positioning and 'Double Triangle'

possible, not to place the inferior trocar below the level of the umbilicus due to limitation related to the body habitus. In the repair of peri-umbilical hernias, we prefer another port placement to allow an oblique view; the first trocar is placed mid-clavicular line closer to the midline and the second trocar is subcostal at the level of anterior clavicular line 6–8 cm away with the remaining trocar 6–8 cm inferior and lateral (Fig. 18.4).

For a centrally located hernia defect, any port placed below the level of the umbilicus near the anterior superior iliac spine (ASIS) often results in arm collision and extensive trouble shooting. Consequently, the authors prefer to avoid that location for trocar placement for these hernias (Fig. 18.5a, b). For suprapubic, subxiphoid, or more lateral defects, the port positions vary accordingly, but similar principles are followed (Fig. 18.6).

Review of the patient's records can provide insight about into the possibility of any severe adhesions that might have been developed after peritonitis, previous surgery etc. These adhesions might occur between anterior abdominal wall peritoneum and bowel or omentum, and they should be completely dissected to expose the planned hernia defect as well as to provide an adequate area for the peritoneal flap. It is also necessary to be sure that there is not an occult hernia defect requiring repair. Careful sharp dissection with sparing use of monopolar energy and gentle traction of the bowel are essential to avoid inadvertent bowel injury during adhesiolysis. In the event of severe adhesions within the hernia sac, external gently

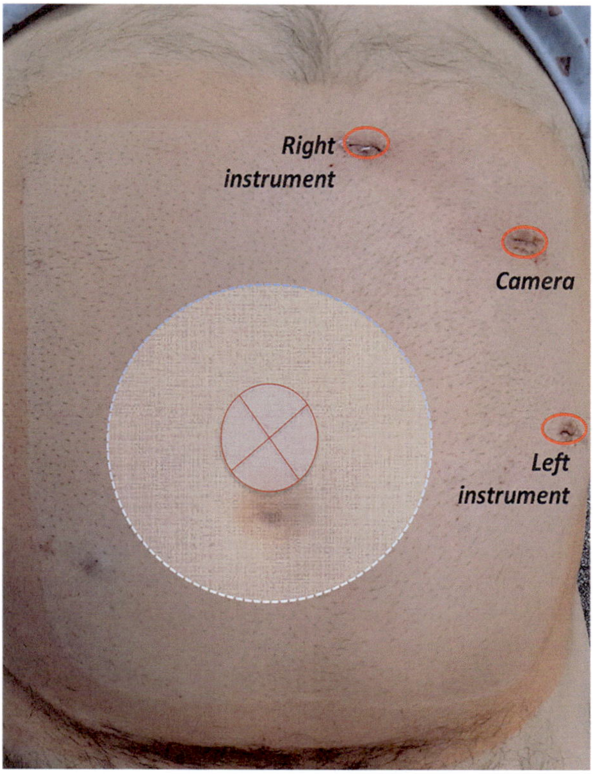

Fig. 18.4 Trocar positioning with oblique approach for centrally located hernias

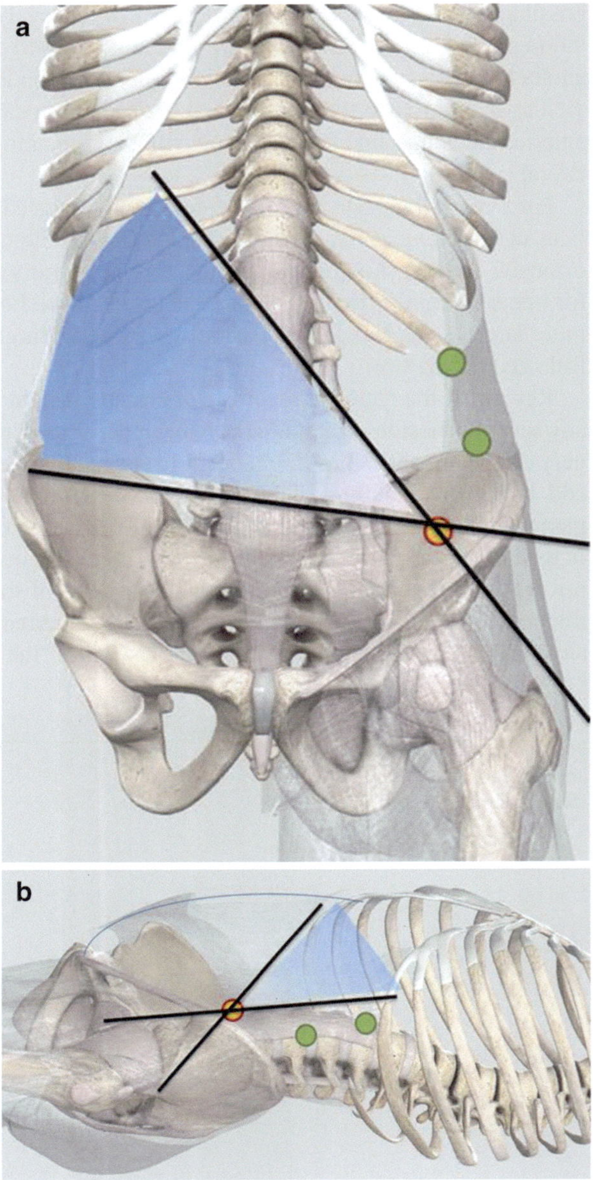

Fig. 18.5 (**a**, **b**) Limitation of instrument movement and the collision of the robotic arm when trocar is placed close to ASIS

compression of the hernia sac by the bedside assistant might aid the vision of surgeon. In general, the bipolar Maryland instrument is preferred if there is a need to control bleeding near the bowel. Subsequent to the adhesiolysis and identification of all defects, the peritoneal flap will be created.

With the use of monopolar scissors and a bipolar Maryland, the peritoneum is grasped and cut at least 5 cm from the defect on the side ipsilateral to the trocars to

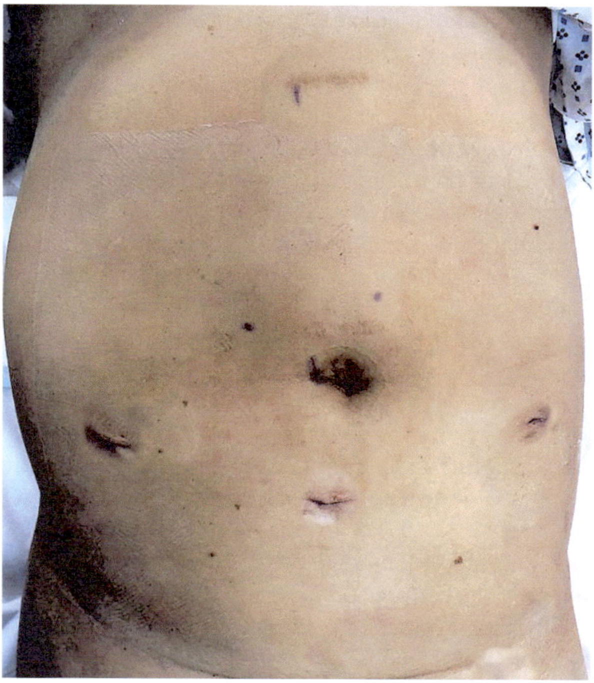

Fig. 18.6 Trocar incisions for subxiphoid hernia

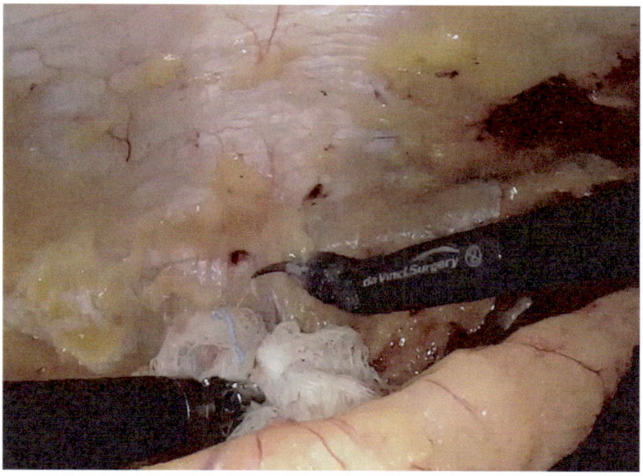

Fig. 18.7 Preperitoneal dissection and use of a sponge on the peritoneal flap

enter the preperitoneal space. Throughout the preparation of the peritoneal flap, the peritoneum traction should be gentle to avoid tearing. For this purpose, dissection of the peritoneal flap with an intra-abdominal sponge helps both to control minor bleeding and minimizes the risk of peritoneal injury (Fig. 18.7). During the dissection of the peritoneum of the hernia sac, separation of tissues without creation of peritoneal defects may not be always possible. If disruption of peritoneal integrity, occurs, this should be repaired with absorbable sutures. Peritoneal defects can result in the creation of an intraparietal hernia, which can result in acute incarceration or strangulation of omentum or intestine. Preperitoneal dissection should extend at least 5 cm in all directions around the defect to provide adequate areas for proper mesh positioning. It should be kept in mind that the wide dissection of the preperitoneal space allows a large, mobile peritoneal flap for covering the mesh. In some cases, it may not be possible to prepare the appropriate peritoneal flap due to the fact that the peritoneum is very thin. In this situation, as an alternative technique, retromuscular mesh placement should be considered after closure of the hernia defect. It should be noted that it can be problematic during robotic TAPP that this dissection can be especially difficult if one cannot remove any prior integrated mesh. Such material can become part of the posterior layer as it is often fused and difficult to separate.

18.7.3 Hernia Defect Closure, Mesh Placement, Peritoneal Flap Closure

The purpose of the hernia defect closure is to make the abdominal wall anatomy closer to the native and improve abdominal wall functions. Furthermore, closure of the defect allows more fascial contact area for the mesh and leads to equalizing the pressure and tension along the mesh and the abdominal wall. The choice of suture material may vary, but in our practice, primary closure of the hernia defect is accomplished by running a long-lasting absorbable barbed suture (Stratafix 0 on CT-1 needle, Ethicon, Somerville, NJ). Before closing the hernia defect, pneumoperitoneum is reduced to 6–8 mmHg, anesthesiologist is asked for maximal relaxation of the patient's muscle tissues. The fascial defect size is then directly measured by an intraperitoneally placed ruler. The authors follow the same guideline used for laparotomy closure which is the small bite technique. This is accomplished by taking "bites" of fascia approximately 5–8 mm from the fascial edge and placing these stitches 5 mm apart in a shoelace fashion [11] (Fig. 18.8).

The robotic platform offers the ergonomic movements and dexterity of wristed instrumentation that provides a strong technical ability to close the defect, which is typically a challenge for the laparoscopic surgeons. It has been reported that the closure of the fascial defect is accomplished in 69.3% of cases, even though many robotic surgeons are at their initial experience [12, 13].

Following hernia defect closure, the next phase is mesh placement. The length and width of the hernia defect are taken into account when determining the size of the mesh to be implanted. The size of the mesh should provide the principle of maintaining at least 5 cm overlap in all directions.

The rolled or folded non-coated mesh is introduced into intraabdominal cavity through one of the trocars. The robotic instruments are used to unroll or unfold the mesh in the preperitoneal space without any wrinkles or folds. The aim of mesh fixation is to provide adequate tissue integration. In the TAPP ventral hernia repair approach fixation of the mesh is necessary in order to prevent mesh migration. For this purpose many different techniques have been described such as tacker fixation,

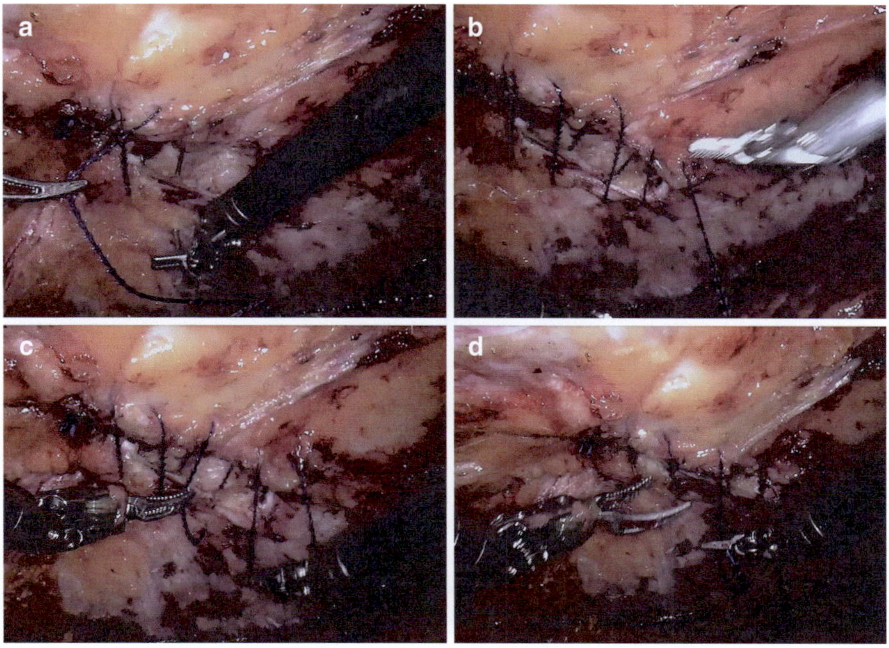

Fig. 18.8 Hernia defect closure with the use of the small stitch technique in shoelace fashion

Fig. 18.9 Mesh suture fixation

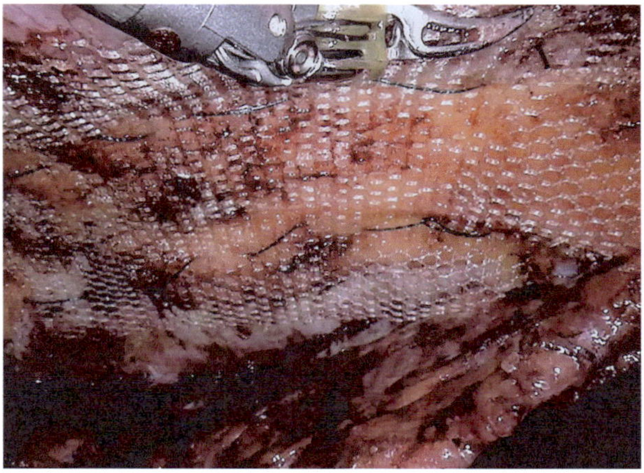

trans-fascial suturing, aerosolized fibrin sealant etc. The use of the circumferential fascial suture technique with using barbed absorbable sutures may be the preferred to secure the mesh to the posterior fascia (Fig. 18.9).

After adequate mesh fixation and control of any bleeding control are achieved, the next step is the closure of the peritoneal flap. Rapidly absorbable barbed suture (2–0 V-lock; Medtronic, New Haven, CT) may be used for this purpose. A running

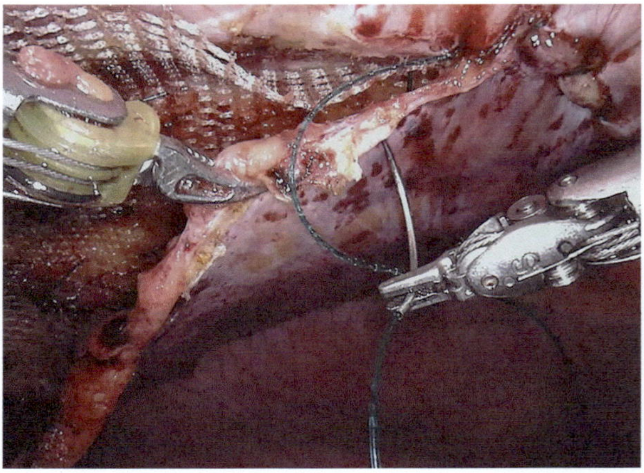

Fig. 18.10 Peritoneal defect closure

short stitch fashion reduces the chance for intraparietal hernia (Fig. 18.10). During this closure and at the end of the procedure, one must assure that the entire mesh is covered with the peritoneal flap to protect the intra-abdominal structures from any exposed mesh. The abdominal cavity is also evaluated for signs of bleeding or other adverse events. The trocars are removed and the pneumoperitoneum is released. We chose to close to suture close any trocar sites that are 10 mm or larger to decrease the risk of potential incisional hernia development in the future. A long acting local anesthetic agent is injected to the trocar sites for management of postoperative pain.

18.8 Postoperative Care

The majority of patients who undergo rTAPP VIH repair are discharged home on the same day after routine early postoperative care. Patients who require a hospital stay are usually those with have preexisting comorbidities that need to be monitored after general anesthesia.

In our experience, postoperative pain in the majority of patients is well controlled with oral nonsteroidal anti-inflammatory agents (NSAIDS). A minority of patients requires narcotics that average 20 tablets for these patients. Patients are encouraged to resume normal activity after operation. It is advised to avoid lifting heavy objects and doing exhausting activities for 4–6 weeks.

18.9 Complications

18.9.1 Bleeding-Hematoma

Trocar bleeding usually stops with tamponade from the trocar itself. During adhesiolysis, bleeding may occur from the cut omentum or adhesive bands and it can be controlled carefully with the use of a thermal energy device such as monopolar scissors or bipolar Maryland. During mesh fixation, identification of the epigastric vessels to prevent injury is very important. Therefore these use of any deep sutures near then should be avoided. If the vessel is injured, the bleeding is often controlled by ligation of it with simply with the use of a “figure of eight” trans-fascial suture. The hematoma, which is noticed during the postoperative period, usually self-limiting and generally requires no intervention unless infective complications occur [14].

18.9.2 Seroma

The seroma is caused by a fluid collection localized generally between the mesh and the hernia sac. It usually appears at postoperative week one or two and usually does not require any intervention. Mostly, it reabsorbs and the cavity obliterates within 4–6 weeks. For the patients who have symptomatic seroma formation and/or persist for more than 3 months, drainage or repeated aspirations of the seroma can be performed under sterile conditions. In case of complex sero-hematoma, an excision might be necessary after 4–5 months. As a preventative strategy, some surgeons prefer to place an abdominal binder for the compression of the hernia sac area, starting immediately postoperatively and continuing for at least 2 weeks [14]. As mentioned earlier, closure of the hernia defect before mesh placement effectively obliterates the anterior dead space, which may significantly reduce or eliminate the risk of seroma formation.

18.9.3 Intestinal Injury

Intestinal injuries might occur during trocar insertion or adhesiolysis. Despite the rate of enterotomy reported in the literature was 1.78%, probably the true rate is higher. The overall mortality of uncomplicated ventral hernia patients is 0.05%. The mortality increases to 2.8% if an enterotomy complication occurs. An unrecognized enterotomy is associated with higher mortality rate compared to a recognized enterotomy, 7.7% and 1.7% respectively [15]. Therefore, the surgeon should perform an intra-abdominal inspection in order to identify any bowel injury that may have heretofore been unrecognized, once following adhesiolysis and once again upon completion of entire procedure. In the event of the recognition of intestinal injury intraoperatively, a tailored approach should be used based upon the operative findings and degree of contamination. Continuation of rTAPP VIH repair may be performed in the event of a bowel injury repaired immediately with minimal spillage. If severe enteric contamination occurs and after bowel injury is repaired robotically, a delayed hernia repair may be performed according to an observation period of 3–7 days on intravenous antibiotic therapy if no evidence of infection is observed [16]. During postoperative period, if any local or systemic infection sign occurs, the surgeon should vigilant to recognize delayed enterotomy, which may include intraoperative intestinal injuries that were unnoticed or thermal injuries that were not full thickness at the time of the procedure. These patients should be returned to the operating room for intestinal repair, resection, and/or GI tract diversion. Strong consideration should be given to mesh removal at the time of re-operation [17].

18.9.4 Chronic Pain

In laparoscopic surgery, acute and chronic postoperative pain is often associated with the use of tack and trans-fascial suture fixation of the mesh. One of the major advantages of rTAPP VIH repair is that it eliminates the need for full-thickness trans-facial suture fixation. However, the fact remains that, during mesh fixation, the surgeon should avoid the use of deeply placed stitches at the lateral border of rectus sheath where the intercostal nerves are most vulnerable for nerve entrapment.

18.9.5 Recurrence

It has been well known that the recurrence of the repaired hernia may occur due to inadequate mesh fixation, inadequate mesh overlap, or mesh failure. Recurrence rates after ventral hernia repair are similar for laparoscopic and open methods, and range from 1% to 17% [18]. Information regarding the recurrence rate of hernias following robotic repair is limited as few centers have reported the results of the technical feasibility of robotic ventral hernia repair in their cohort. For our initial cohort of 46 cases completed entirely with the rTAPP VIH repair, all the patients (100%) reached their 1-year follow-up and, when contacted, reported no hernia recurrence [8].

18.10 Limitations

Limitations of the robotic technology include access to the robot, a steep learning curve, the use of a specialized surgical team, and increased cost of robotic platform and instrumentations. Other considerations are the need for the ability to trouble shoot any issues whether they be technical or computer generated with the robot itself.

With regard to the limitation of rTAPP VIH repair technique, large ventral hernias requiring the use of a flap that reaches over 15–20 cm become technically challenging. In this situation the authors prefer the use of a retro-muscular repair.

18.11 Conclusion

The transabdominal preperitoneal (TAPP) repair has long been utilized for inguinal hernia repair and is now being applied to VIH repair. The preperitoneal placement of the mesh not only prevents the direct contact of the prosthesis with intraabdominal structures, but also eliminates the requirement for placing more costly coated intraperitoneal mesh, and potentially minimizes the risk of complications with their use. Future multicenter prospective trials could further elucidate the potential benefits and the long-term outcomes of all types of robotic hernia repair surgery.

References

1. Poulose BK, et al. Epidemiology and cost of ventral hernia repair: making the case for hernia research. Hernia. 2012;16(2):179–83.
2. Malangoni MA, Rosen MJ. Hernias. In: Townsend CM, et al., editors. Sabiston textbook of surgery: the biological basis of modern surgical practice. Philadelphia: Elsevier Saunders; 2017. p. 1092–119.
3. Flament JB, Avisse C, Delattre JF. Anatomy of the abdominal wall. In: Bendavid R, et al., editors. Abdominal wall hernias: principles and management. New York: Springer; 2001. p. 39–63.
4. Parker SG, et al. Nomenclature in abdominal wall hernias: is it time for consensus? World J Surg. 2017;41(10):2488–91.
5. Parker SG, et al. Comment on: international hernia collaboration consensus on nomenclature of abdominal wall hernia repair: reply. World J Surg. 2018;42(1):305.
6. Sanders DL, Kingsnorth AN. Prosthetic mesh materials used in hernia surgery. Expert Rev Med Devices. 2012;9(2):159–79.
7. Jenkins ED, et al. Prospective evaluation of adhesion characteristics to intraperitoneal mesh and adhesiolysis-related complications during laparoscopic re-exploration after prior ventral hernia repair. Surg Endosc. 2010;24(12):3002–7.
8. Orthopoulos G, Kudsi OY. Feasibility of robotic-assisted transabdominal preperitoneal ventral hernia repair. J Laparoendosc Adv Surg Tech A. 2018;28(4):434–8.
9. Prasad P, et al. Laparoscopic transabdominal preperitoneal repair of ventral hernia: a step towards physiological repair. Indian J Surg. 2011;73(6):403–8.
10. Liang MK, et al. Ventral hernia management: expert consensus guided by systematic review. Ann Surg. 2017;265(1):80–9.
11. Muysoms FE, et al. European hernia society guidelines on the closure of abdominal wall incisions. Hernia. 2015;19(1):1–24.
12. Gonzalez A, et al. Robotic-assisted ventral hernia repair: a multicenter evaluation of clinical outcomes. Surg Endosc. 2017;31(3):1342–9.
13. Gonzalez AM, et al. Laparoscopic ventral hernia repair with primary closure versus no primary closure of the defect: potential benefits of the robotic technology. Int J Med Robot. 2015;11(2):120–5.
14. Alexander AM, Scott DJ. Laparoscopic ventral hernia repair. Surg Clin North Am. 2013;93(5):1091–110.
15. LeBlanc KA, Elieson MJ, Corder JM 3rd. Enterotomy and mortality rates of laparoscopic incisional and ventral hernia repair: a review of the literature. JSLS. 2007;11(4):408–14.
16. Bittner R, et al. Guidelines for laparoscopic treatment of ventral and incisional abdominal wall hernias (International Endohernia Society [IEHS])-part 2. Surg Endosc. 2014;28(2):353–79.
17. Earle D, et al. SAGES guidelines for laparoscopic ventral hernia repair. Surg Endosc. 2016;30(8):3163–83.
18. Warren JA, Love M. Incisional hernia repair: minimally invasive approaches. Surg Clin North Am. 2018;98(3):537–59.

Stapled Closure for Mid-Line Hernia Repair

19

Thiago Nogueira Costa and Ricardo Zugaib Abdalla

19.1 Introduction

Innovative surgical procedures envolve in the operative room because current procedural limitations expose technical demands that have an opportunity of improvements. In the operating room, surgeons combine their skill, knowledge, technical acumen and the advent of new technologies to improve safety and provide better results to their patients. The opportunity to solve problems makes all surgeons a natural innovator. However, there is an enormous lag from the innovation to actual procedure implementation. Recent innovations such as the benefits of minimally invasive video surgery with good anatomical reconstruction without the need to deconstruct the components of the wall structures present opportunities.

The use of synthetic prostheses associated with video surgery has revolutionized a previously undefined treatment that was dependent, almost exclusively, on the experience and expertise of each hernia surgeon [1]. Professor LeBlanc brought intracavity mesh hernioplasty to video surgery in 1993 [2]. The laparoscopic treatment of abdominal wall weakness, with ventral and incisional hernias, has been greatly used nowadays, but without a standard procedure [3].

Details of technique can be simulated in the laboratory, where anatomical references can be compared with "wet models". This results of such studies are heavily dependent upon multiple predisposing and precipitating factors, with subjective, objective and variable characteristics [4]. Our project was developed from the use of robotic technology for repair of anterior abdominal wall defects. We studied this technique in a cadaver lab with the robot initially and subsequently simulated the procedure in a porcine lab [5].

T. N. Costa · R. Z. Abdalla (✉)
Department of Digestive Surgery,
Hospital das Clinicas of University of Sao Paulo Medical School, Sao Paulo, Brazil
e-mail: ricardo.abdalla@hc.fm.usp.br

K. A. LeBlanc (ed.), *Robotic Assisted Hernia Repair*,
https://doi.org/10.1007/978-3-030-23025-8_19

The operative approach to repair the abdominal wall is based on the retromuscular, pre-peritoneal reinforcement Rives-Stoppa Principles [6]. The procedure was designed to reconstruct the mid-line from the peritoneal cavity, approximating the rectus abdominal muscles at the same time that reconstructs the posterior sheath suture line with a retro muscular space. Within this created space a mesh will be inserted, using video surgery and linear stapling to avoid greater tissue detachments and more difficult suturing efforts by the surgeon.

19.2 Background

Incisional ventral hernia has increased as midline laparotomies have become more prevalent. Laparoscopy, minimal invasive surgery (MIS), can avoid such complications, but it is estimated that up to 50% of open surgical patients develop incisional hernias, with different presentations [7–10]. Multiple concomitant procedures can develop ventral defects and incisional hernias with more than one areas of defects such oncologic patients with a multitude of procedures involved in the treatments of their disease. Bariatric surgery has been shown a high rate of ventral hernias and wound occurrences especially when performed non-laparoscopically [11]. It is clear that the most effective method of prevention of such hernias is an effective method to close the midline incision [12]. Laparoscopic repair of incisional hernias has grown significantly in the last 20 years but technical challenges are still under consideration. It has become that the combination of laparoscopy, use of a large mesh, fascial closure with suture and preoperative patient optimization are mandatory for these challenging presentations [13]. However there is no standardization of these methods and techniques that are consistently used to repair these hernia defects [14].

It is has been affirmed that defect closure with sublay mesh positioning has consistently shown good results when performed with the technical demands of the Rives-Stoppa repair [15–17]. The challenge has always been that it is technically difficult to close the fascial defects laparoscopically compared to open surgery [18]. Thus, in the era of robotic technology this procedure is a lot easier to perform than before introduction of this platform [19, 20]. We have developed this technique to supplement the need of the robot, especially in situations where access is difficult.

19.3 History

This methodology grew from our desire to develop new procedures using the robotic technology in the cadaver lab. Many instruments and devices were tested to help the procedure. During this process it appeared that the use of the endo-stapler was considered a viable option to close the defect of the anterior abdominal wall in a manner similar to the method used in other organs such as the bowel or vascular structures.

With that in mind we brought the stapler to the animal lab in order to see its characteristics and possibilities regarding the closure of abdominal wall defects. Figure 19.1a shows the abdominal wall open after laparoscopic stapling. Figure 19.1b is another view of the same open abdominal wall after stapling. Figure 19.1c shows the device being used in pigs for laparoscopic methods. After these studies we identified that the best method was to place the stapler in a sublay position, inserting each jaw of the stapler behind the left and right rectus abdominis muscles (Fig. 19.2) [9].

Once the best location was identified we evaluated the various types of cartridge in the dry lab followed by use in living tissue in the porcine model. This allowed an evaluation of the correct type of staple load for use at the aponeurosis. A pilot study was undertaken in pigs to evaluate the safety and feasibility of the procedure. Once we were assured of the safety and efficacy the first case in a patient was undertaken [21]. The first case series was attempted were in post bariatric surgery patients because of their propensity to develop supraumbilical midline hernias. The proved to be the first indication for the new technique [22].

The technique was shown to the scientific community and other colleagues tried various methods for use which resulted in an evolution of the surgical procedure,

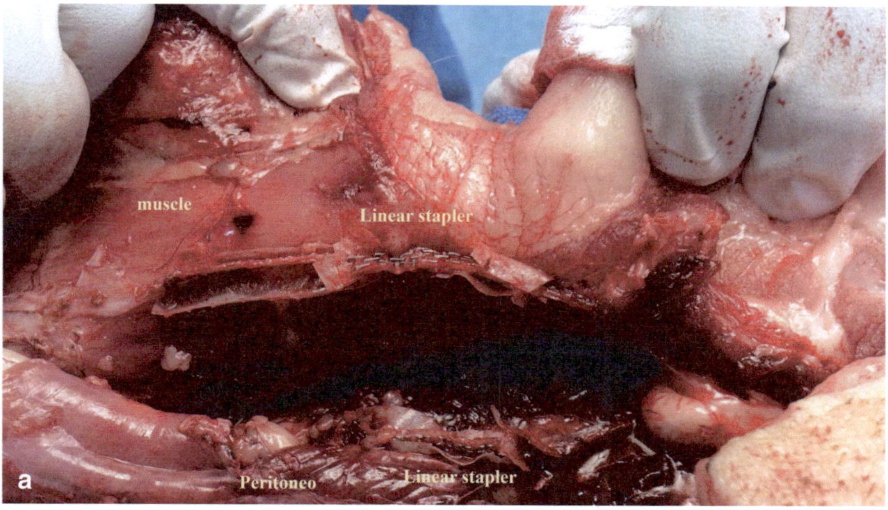

Fig. 19.1 Animal lab. (**a**) open (**b**) laparoscopic (**c**) pig lab

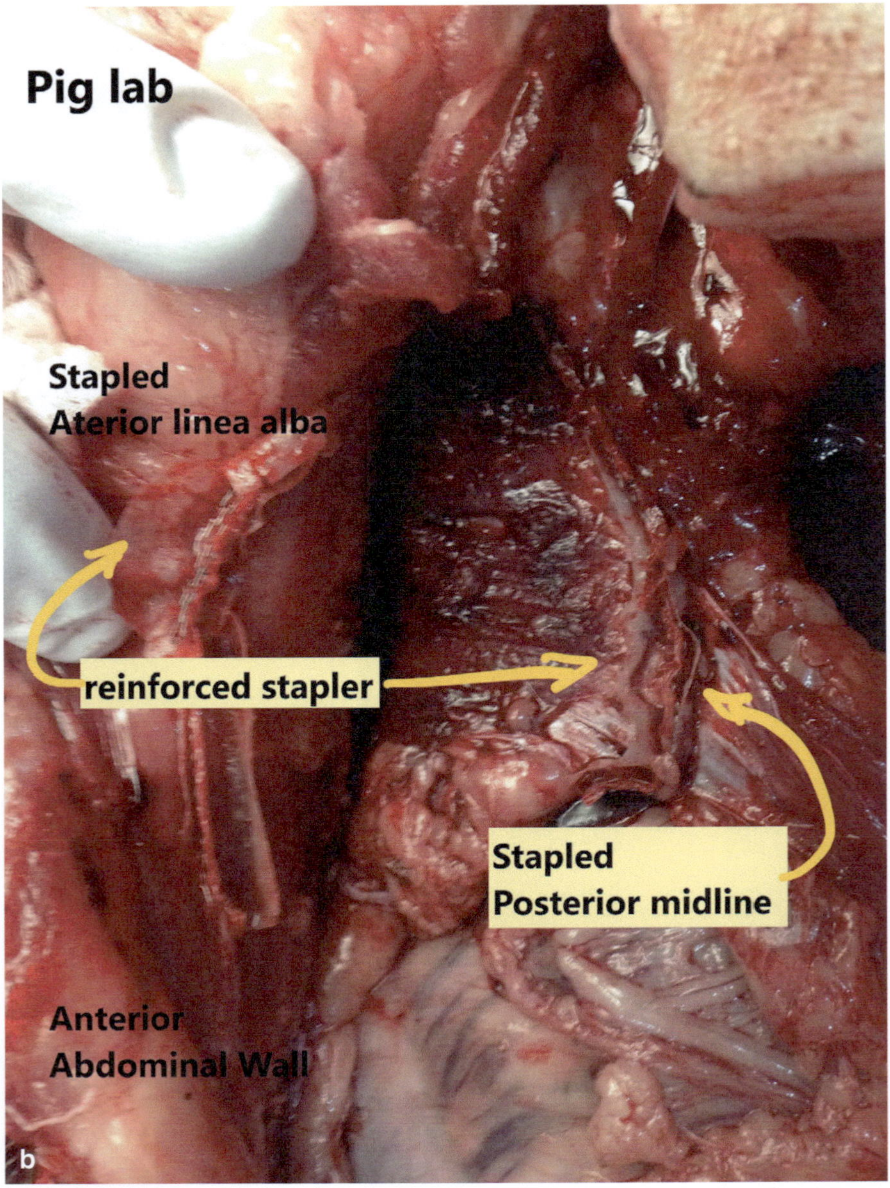

Fig. 19.1 (continued)

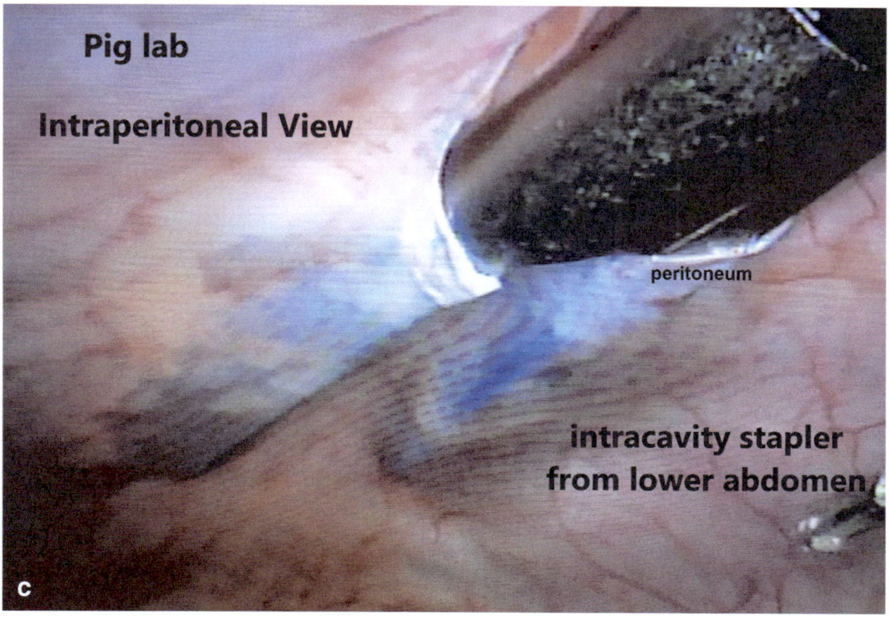

Fig. 19.1 (continued)

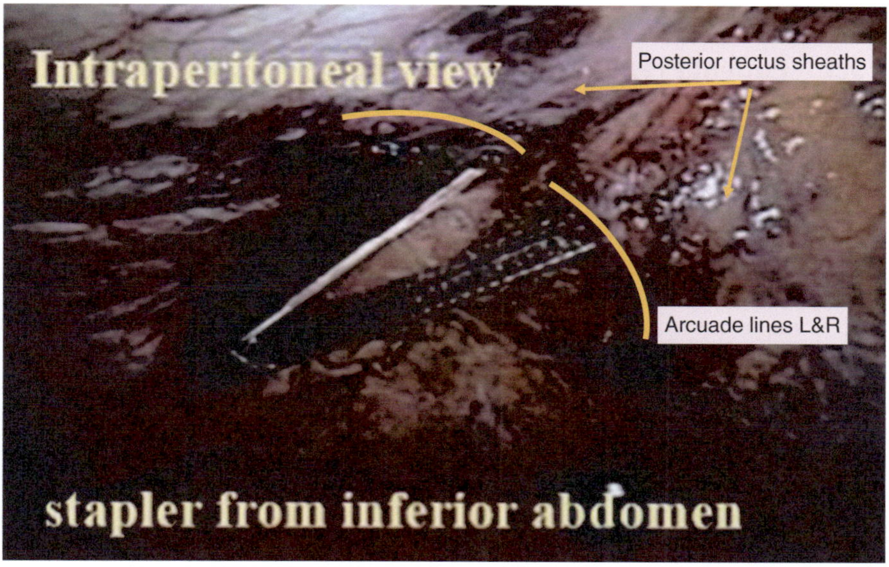

Fig. 19.2 Insertion of the stapler

Table 19.1 Selection/indications

Recti diastasis
Small and medium midline hernias
M2–M3–M4
Limitations:
Large (> 8 cm), location, skin issue

like every new method in technology [23, 24]. However, patient selection, evaluation and preparation of the patient, indications and the use of the various instruments and prosthetics are still undergoing scrutiny to determine the feasibility and results of this new technique.

19.4 Pre-Operative Workup

Before starting the procedure, an evaluation must be made to identify the correct indication and to plan the appropriate surgical repair to be done. While a good physical exam is critical, a CT scan evaluation must be done in order to see assess the defect, identify potential complications and the overall status of the abdominal wall [25, 26].

The indications can be seen in Table 19.1. In general, this technique is most suitable for midline hernias and recti diastasis. Patients with large hernias and skin issues should be carefully evaluated. Any contraindications to the laparoscopic approach and hernias outside of the midline must be considered.

19.5 Patient Preparation and Positioning (Fig. 19.3)

The patient is positioned in a horizontal supine position with the arms close to the body. A slight flex is made on the table so that the staple can be positioned suprapubically (Fig. 19.4a). A urinary catheter is used to empty the bladder and prevent injury to the bladder. All the abdomen must be exposed, especially the midline and the hernia defect(s) (Fig. 19.4b). Patient must be secured to the table and the areas of the body at risk for injury should be protected.

It is important to have in the operative room (OR) all the materials required to complete the procedure (Endostapler, energy devices, cartridges, meshes). It is best if at least two monitors, one at the head of the patient and other one at the right side to allow excellent visualization of the procedure at all times.

19.6 Surgical Technique

The surgical technique can be divided into the respective steps for better comprehension of the procedure. Hence, it will be separated into the following: access, port placement, dissection/adhesiolysis, access to the arcuate line, reconstruction of the midline, mesh placement and fixation.

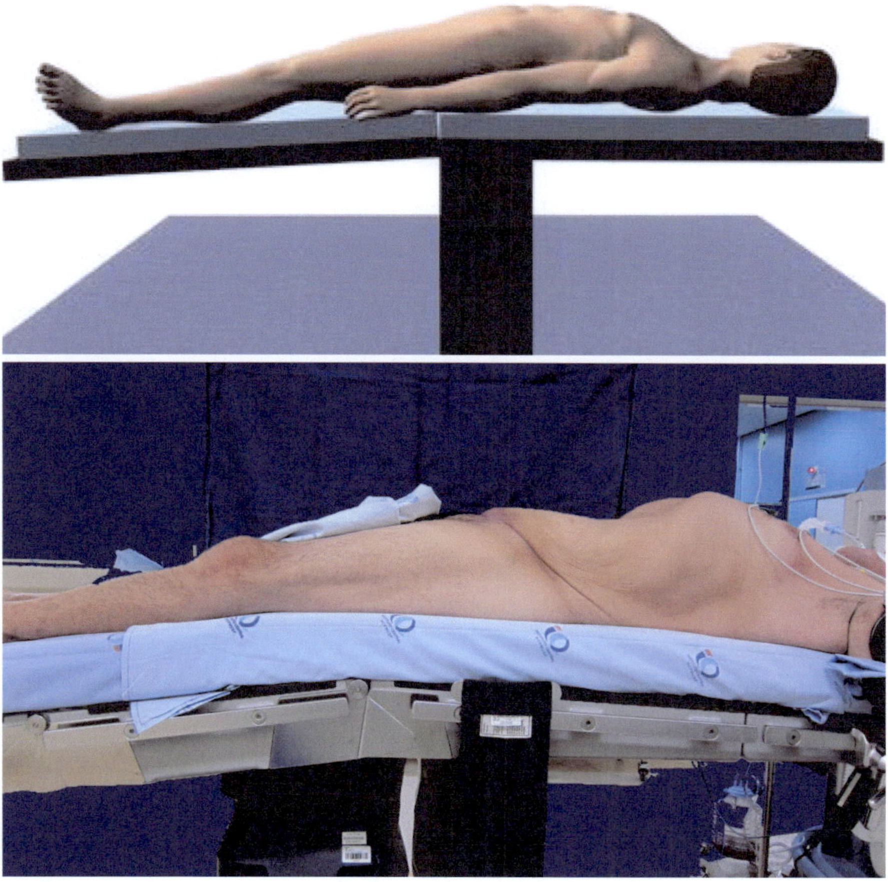

Fig. 19.3 Patient preparation and positioning

19.6.1 Access

The peritoneal cavity is accessed by placement of an optical view cannula at the superior left quadrant, 2 cm below the costal margin, at anterior axillary line. This approach can be done using a Veress needle or with an open access method (Hasson technique).

19.6.2 Port Placement

After the access to the abdominal cavity has been achieved a suprapubic 12 mm trocar is placed either in the intraperitoneal or extraperitoneal space. Two additional 3 or 5 mm trocars are inserted under direct vision in the left and right lower quadrants (Fig. 19.5).

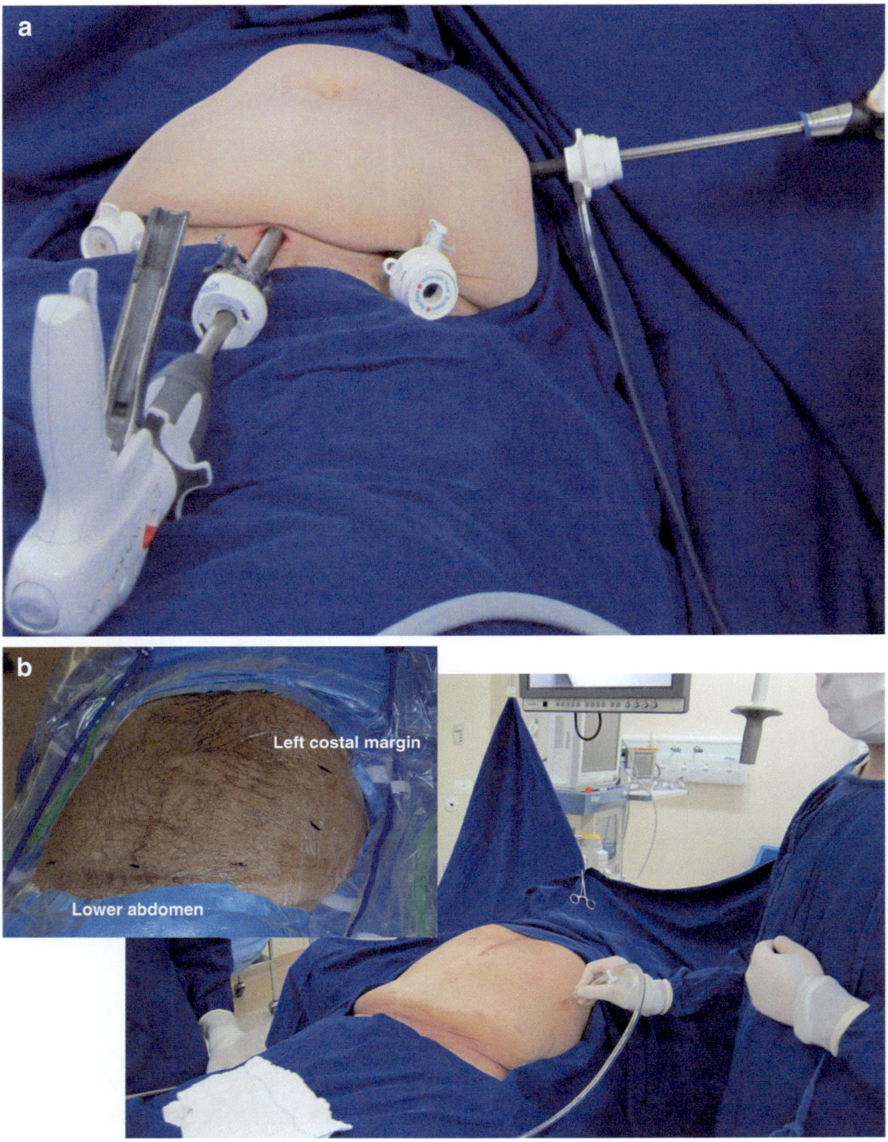

Fig. 19.4 Port placement. (**a**) Trocar positions, (**b**) exposure of the abdomen

19.6.3 Dissection/Adhesiolysis

This is a very important step in minimally invasive hernia repair. The adhesiolysis of all organs from the hernia sac is done to assure that they are freely inside the abdominal cavity. In this manner the complete exposure of the fascial defect borders and recognition of the position of the rectus abdominal muscles is achieved. All the

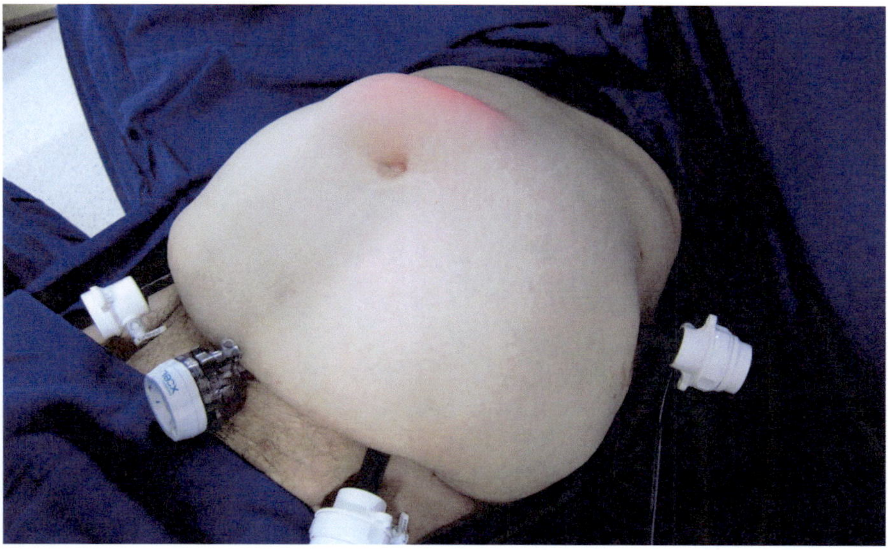

Fig. 19.5 Access to the arcuate line

abdominal wall must be exposed in order to have a clean view of the defect to be repaired.

19.6.4 Access to the Arcuate Line (Fig. 19.6)

After the complete exposure of the abdominal wall the arcuate line is accessed either from a Trans-peritoneal (TAPP) or Extra-peritoneal (TEP) approach.

Similar to the laparoscopic TAPP inguinal hernia repair, the access to the arcuate line can be done by opening the peritoneum to the level of the arcuate line and then accessed.

The other method of approach is by an extra-peritoneal approach (TEP) in which the trocars are inserted directly into the pre-peritoneal space. With this method the arcuate line is accessed above the peritoneum. The main advantage of this approach is to the ability to achieve this working space without the need to open into the peritoneal cavity.

19.6.5 Midline Reconstruction

Once the arcuate line is exposed, the approximation of the dissected posterior sheaths of each side is done using a grasper to observe the retromuscular space formation. This is done by moving the to the lower quadrant trocar. The linear endostapler will be inserted via the supra pubic trocar. This is placed into the dissected

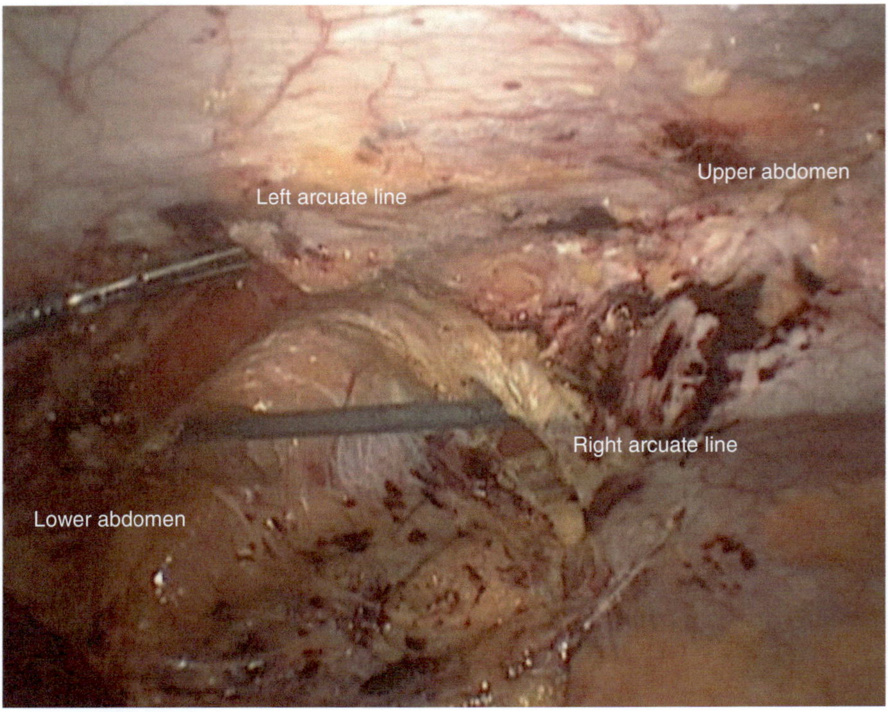

Fig. 19.6 Reconstruction of the midline

space with one of the arms on the left and the other on the right retromuscular spaces. Closure of the jaws of the device with result in the approximation of either side of the posterior sheaths. One must avoid any inclusion of muscular fibers between them these sheaths which can be a source of staple-line dehiscence. With this procedure there is the construction of one retro muscular space which will in turn result in an anterior reconstruction of the midline concomitantly with the closure of the peritoneal cavity by the act of stapling of the posterior sheaths together (Fig. 19.7).

19.6.6 Mesh Placement and Fixation (Fig. 19.8) [27]

Next, the surgeon will insert a lightweight monofilament macroporous mesh into the newly created common retromuscular space. This mesh can then be fixed with either a fibrin sealant or stapled from the inside.

If the TAPP approach was used, the opening in the arcuate line should be completely closed by any preferred method such as closure with sutures, staples or fibrin glue.

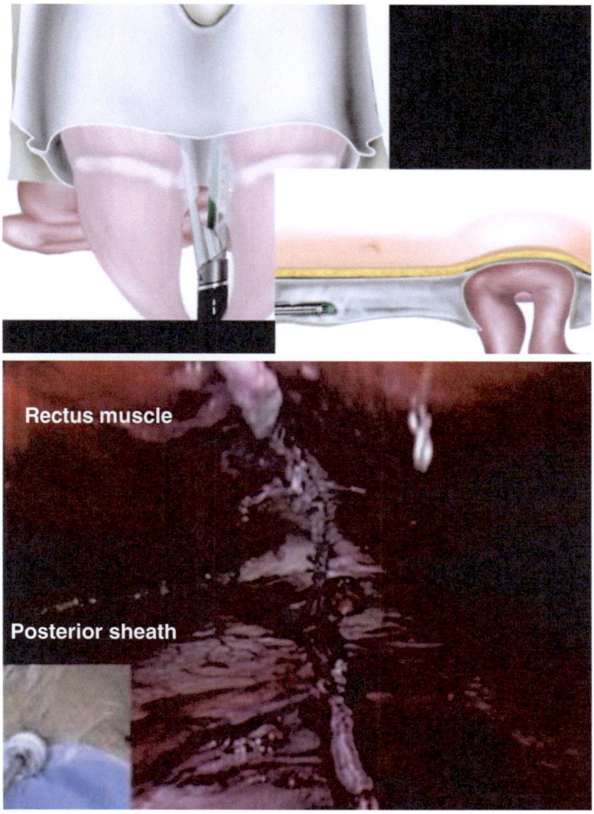

Fig. 19.7 Mesh placement and fixation

19.7 Complications

All types of surgery have possible complications. In the hernia field, those complications can impact in the quality of life (QOL), return to normal activities and recurrence.

The main complications of this procedure are similar to other techniques that place the mesh in a sublay position. Hematoma, seroma and infection are the majority of the problems. Other issues related to any laparoscopic treatment of hernias such as bowel injury or clinical complications can also been seen (Table 19.2).

19.8 Results and Perspectives

Since it is a new technique, there are only a few only case series [22–25], that have shown safety and feasibility. Larger studies are needed to identify the most appropriate indications and outcomes. Nevertheless, the current studies have verified the technical feasibility of the procedure and the low rate of recurrence.

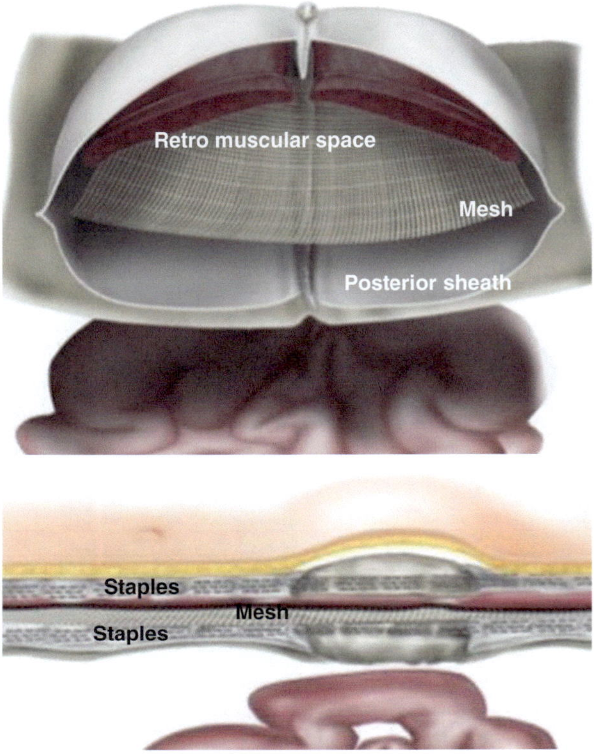

Fig. 19.8 Perspectives—L-TAR

Table 19.2 Complications

Seroma
Hematoma
Skin infection
Mesh infection
Bowel injury
Clinical complications

CT scan and QOL follow up evaluations done before and after the procedure demonstrated adequate abdominal wall reconstruction and improvement in both pain scores and functional activity (Fig. 19.9) [21].

Moreover, the technique can be added to the surgical options in addition to other procedures such as e-tep and L-TAR (Fig. 19.10) [24]. There is potential to perhaps show improvement in the safety profile and speed of the robotic hernia repair.

To further enhance this surgical option, there is the need for the development of new products such as a specific stapler for the abdominal wall or technological devices that can add energy or other substance to the hernia repair.

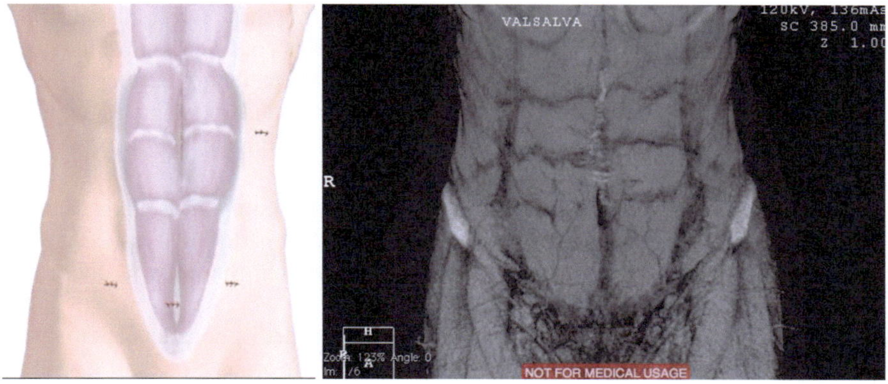

Fig. 19.9 Midline closure after 2 years under Valsalva

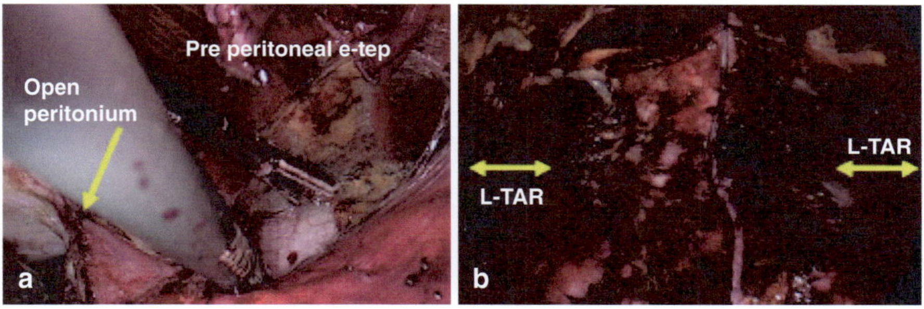

Fig. 19.10 Laparoscopic view of e-tep and L-TAR procedures

19.9 Discussion

Laparoscopic and robotic surgical approaches to hernia repair have an important appeal for causing less tissue damage while improving recovery. There is no need for a large incision and the area to be reconstructed can be well visualized by the intraperitoneal camera. The prosthesis is clearly placed in the right position and its fixation is done with suitable options of stapling, gluing or suturing, as preferred by the surgeon. Another important fact is the lower incidence of wound complications, such as infection or dehiscence when compared to an open procedure.

This procedure is able to achieve better rectus muscular function with approximation of the muscle tissue compared to the laparoscopic bridging maneuver. The use of liner stapling is more appealing than endoscopic suture, due to a safer approach for the patient and better management of time for the surgeon.

This procedure was developed previously by this group through the robotic reconstruction of the midline using single sutures [7]. Afterwards, the linear endo-stapling closure was tested in the laboratory. During these studies the potential benefits of this procedure were identified. Following this confirmation we felt comfortable offering this as a new option of treatment for the patient. The anterior suturing of the midline through the robotic arms from inside the abdominal cavity was able return to the patient the sensation of a normal abdominal wall function and movement.

After linear stapling of the midline, the patient often complained about a bulge that was considered to be the resolution of hernia sac. It is different issue that that noted from the classical laparoscopic approach in which, the bulge is loose and covered by the mesh.

We now believe that this procedure should be another option for patients with multiple or smaller defects of the midline, cranial to the arcuate lines. It is also an option in some patients with some diastasis of the rectus muscles who could be treated without the midline xyphoid to umbilical incision.

19.10 Concluding Remarks

- Indications are mainly midline hernias and recti diastasis.
- The correct indication and preparation must be done for the success of the procedure.
- Although there are few studies, the results show low recurrence and good impact on the QOL.
- Current perspectives are beginning to be considers such as application as an adjunct to other techniques and development of new materials and devices may make more options feasible.

Glossary

Transabdominal Midline Reconstruction (TMR) Surgical procedure to treat midline hernias and rectus diastasis with the use of a linear stapler and sublay mesh repair.

Laparoscopic Transversus Abdominis Release (L-TAR) Minimally invasive surgical procedure proposed as a posterior component separation with transversus abdominis muscle release.

References

1. Tobler WD Jr, Itani KM. Current status and challenges of laparoscopy in ventral hernia repair. J Laparoendosc Adv Surg Tech A. 2016;26(4):281–9.
2. LeBlanc KA, Booth WV. Laparoscopic repair of incisional abdominal hernias using expanded polytetrafluoroethylene: preliminary findings. Surg Laparosc Endosc. 1993;3(1):39–41.
3. Misiakos EP, Machairas A, Patapis P, Liakakos T. Laparoscopic ventral hernia repair: pros and cons compared with open hernia repair. JSLS. 2008;12(2):117–25.

4. Guba PM. A novel surgical mesh suitable for laparoscopy, studied on animal model. Orv Hetil. 2016;157(5):180–4.
5. Cox TC, Huntington CR, Blair LJ, Prasad T, Heniford BT, Augenstein VA. Quality of life and outcomes for femoral hernia repair: does laparoscopy have an advantage? Hernia. 2017;21(1):79–88.
6. Grau-Talens EJ, Ibanez CD, Motos-Mico J, Garcia-Olives F, Arribas-Jurado M, Jordan-Chaves C, et al. Rives technique for the primary larger inguinal hernia repair: a prospective study of 1000 repairs. World J Surg. 2017;41(10):2480–7.
7. Sajid MS, Bokhari SA, Mallick AS, Cheek E, Baig MK. Laparoscopic versus open repair of incisional/ventral hernia: a meta-analysis. Am J Surg. 2009;197(1):64–72.
8. Moreau PE, Helmy N, Vons C. Laparoscopic treatment of incisional hernia. State of the art in 2012. J Visc Surg. 2012;149(5 Suppl):e40–8.
9. Cobb WS, Kercher KW, Heniford BT. Laparoscopic repair of incisional hernias. Surg Clin North Am. 2005;85(1):91–103, ix.
10. Jin J, Rosen MJ. Laparoscopic versus open ventral hernia repair. Surg Clin North Am. 2008;88(5):1083–100, viii.
11. Raftopoulos I, Courcoulas AP. Outcome of laparoscopic ventral hernia repair in morbidly obese patients with a body mass index exceeding 35 kg/m2. Surg Endosc. 2007;21(12):2293–7.
12. Millbourn D, Cengiz Y, Israelsson LA. Effect of stitch length on wound complications after closure of midline incisions: a randomized controlled trial. Arch Surg. 2009;144(11):1056–9.
13. Mudge M, Hughes LE. Incisional hernia: a 10 year prospective study of incidence and attitudes. Br J Surg. 1985;72:70–1.
14. Bittner R, Bingener-Casey J, Dietz U, Fabian M, Ferzli GS, Fortelny RH, et al. Guidelines for laparoscopic treatment of ventral and incisional abdominal wall hernias (International Endohernia Society [IEHS])-part 2. Surg Endosc. 2014;28(2):353–79.
15. Timmermans L, de Goede B, van Dijk SM, Kleinrensink GJ, Jeekel J, Lange JF. Meta-analysis of sublay versus onlay mesh repair in incisional hernia surgery. Am J Surg. 2014;207(6):980–8.
16. Iqbal W, Pham TH, Joseph A, Thompson JMGB, Sarr MG. Long-term outcome of 254 complex incisional hernia repairs using the modified rives-Stoppa technique. World J Surg. 2007;31:2398–404.
17. Bauer J, Harris M, Gorfine S, Kreel I. Rives-Stoppa procedure for repair of large incisional hernias: experience with 57 patients. Hernia. 2002;6(3):120–3.
18. Vorst AL, Kaoutzanis C, Carbonell AM, Franz MG. Evolution and advances in laparoscopic ventral and incisional hernia repair. World J Gastrointest Surg. 2015;7(11):293–305.
19. Kudsi OY, Paluvoi N, Bhurtel P, McCabe Z, El-Jabri R. Robotic repair of ventral hernias: preliminary findings of a case series of 106 consecutive cases. Am J Robot Surg. 2015;2(1):22–6.
20. Gonzalez A, Escobar E, Romero R, Walker G, Mejias J, Gallas M, Dickens E, Johnson CJ, Rabaza J, Kudsi OY. Robotic-assisted ventral hernia repair: a multicenter evaluation of clinical outcomes. Surg Endosc. 2017;31(3):1342–9. https://doi.org/10.1007/s00464-016-5118-0.
21. Abdalla RZ, Garcia RB, da Costa RI, Abdalla BM. Treatment of mid-line abdominal wall hernias with the use of endo-stapler for mid-line closure. Arq Bras Cir Dig. 2013;26(4):335–7.
22. Costa TN, Abdalla RZ, Santo MA, Tavares RR, Abdalla BM, Cecconello I. Transabdominal midline reconstruction by minimally invasive surgery: technique and results. Hernia. 2016;20(2):257–65.
23. Moore AM, Anderson LN, Chen DC. Laparoscopic stapled sublay repair with self-gripping mesh: a simplified technique for minimally invasive extraperitoneal ventral hernia repair. Surg Technol Int. 2016;29:131–9.
24. Nguyen DK, Chen DC. Laparoscopic stapled rives stoppa sublay technique for extraperitoneal ventral hernia repair. Eur Surg. 2017;49:175–9.
25. den Hartog D, Dur AH, Kamphuis AG, et al. Comparison of ultrasonography with computed tomography in the diagnosis of incisional hernias. Hernia. 2009;13:45–8.
26. Tonolini M, Ippolito S. Multidetector CT of expected findings and early postoperative complications after current techniques for ventral hernia repair. Insights Imaging. 2016;7(4):541–51.
27. Reynvoet E, Deschepper E, Rogiers X, Troisi R, Berrevoet F. Laparoscopic ventral hernia repair: is there an optimal mesh fixation technique? A systematic review. Langenbeck's Arch Surg. 2014;399(1):55–63. Review.

Endoscopic Component Separation Techniques

20

Jorge Daes

20.1 Endoscopic Component Separation Techniques

The objective of abdominal wall reconstruction (AWR) is to provide a durable structural, functional, and cosmetic repair. The repair of complex ventral hernias remains a vexing problem with successful outcomes requiring a combination of techniques, technologies and tools. A lack of comparative effectiveness data ensures that we are a long way from standardization of hernia repair to any particular technique. Nevertheless, principles exist that should be applied to all repairs irrespective of technique selected. Incorporating these principles into every day practice allows a surgeon to base a complex ventral hernia repair not on a particular technique but on principles that have consistently resulted in improved outcomes.

Primary closure of defects and reestablishment of the integrity of the linea alba with physiologic tension have been the mainstays of open repairs and recently have been considered essential components of minimally invasive (MI) abdominal wall reconstruction (AWR).

Primary repair of ventral hernias is in general possible with defects up to 3–4 cm depending on tissue pliability. For defects greater than that, a form of physiologic-tension reconstruction is advised. This can be accomplished using various muscle relaxation techniques, including surgical, pharmacological, and mechanical methods, with component separation (CS) techniques being the most common. Almost invariably, repair is reinforced with a mesh.

The anterior component separation (ACS) technique described by Ramirez and colleagues [1] in 1991 creates a compound flap composed of the rectus abdominis, internal oblique, and transversus abdominis muscles that can be moved across the abdominal wall to assist in closing defects. The main drawback of the classic open ACS technique is the need for extensive dissection and its unwanted consequences.

J. Daes (✉)
Minimally Invasive Surgery Department, Clínica Porto Azul, Barranquilla, Colombia

K. A. LeBlanc (ed.), *Robotic Assisted Hernia Repair*,
https://doi.org/10.1007/978-3-030-23025-8_20

Studies have reported major wound morbidity in 30–40% of patients treated with this method [2]. Modifications of the classic ACS to spare the periumbilical perforating vessels and to limit the extent of the dissection have reduced the wound complication rates.

The endoscopic (E) approach to CS addresses these issues. Lowe and associates in 2000 reported an open assisted subcutaneous endoscopic ACS [3]. Maas described a laparoscopic balloon-assisted subfascial approach in 2002 consisted of endoscopically performed dissection, with release through a small cutaneous counter incisions [4]. Rosen is credited with popularization of transfascial endoscopic ACS in 2007 as an adjunct to AWR in combination with mesh reinforcement [5]. Chen described a modification that simplified the transfascial approach by making the initial incision medial to the anterior superior spine and working cephalad with the help of an additional port, making it more ergonomic and easier to perform [6]. Finally, Daes described a totally endoscopic subcutaneous approach in 2010. With this technique preoperative skin marking of the semilunar line under ultrasonic guidance precedes the creation of the subcutaneous space. This space is then developed with a balloon dissector with subsequent division and dissection of the external oblique aponeurosis [7]. This modification imitates the Ramirez approach and is ergonomic and familiar to surgeons.

20.2 Indications for ECS as Adjunct to Minimally Invasive Surgery

1. As an adjunct to the robotic-assisted or laparoscopic intraperitoneal onlay mesh (IPOM) repair or transabdominal preperitoneal (TAPP) ventral repair with primary closure of the fascial defect. This has been the main indication of ECS in our group.
2. As part of robotic-assisted or laparoscopic extended-view totally extraperitoneal (eTEP) access Rives-Stoppa or transabdominal Rives-Stoppa repair as long as the need for mesh coverage does not extend beyond the width of the retrorectus space. When greater mesh coverage is necessary a posterior components separation is indicated.

Other indications of the ECS in open surgery or for the management of the abdominal compartment syndrome are not discussed in this chapter.

20.3 Contraindications for ECS

1. Severe skin dystrophy or ulceration requiring extensive resection or the creation of extensive flaps.
2. Fascial defects that can be closed primarily without undue tension.
3. Fascial defects that are disproportionally wider than longer.
4. Patients with noncompliant abdominal walls from multiple previous repairs/meshes. In these cases, a PCS-TAR may be more appropriate.

5. Patients who have undergone previous bilateral PCS-TAR. However, concomitant anterior and posterior separations to avoid a bridged mesh repair may be a relative contraindication and it is possible to use a PCS-TAR approach on one side (for stoma reversal) and an anterior CS on the other side.

20.4 Operative Steps

20.4.1 Preoperative Preparation

Endoscopic component separation should not be considered a stand-alone procedure but is part of an overall operative plan. Other preoperative considerations depend upon the particulars of that operative plan.

Skin preparation extends from the nipples to the upper thighs and should be laterally extended to beyond the posterior axillary lines. For clean operations, a single dose of a first-generation cephalosporin is administered during anesthetic induction. Urinary catheters are used in complex cases or when pelvic dissection is anticipated. Pneumatic compression devices are used in all patients. During clean contaminated or contaminated cases, ECS should be performed first.

20.4.2 Techniques of ECS

The three approaches to anterior ECS create exactly the same myofascial advancement flap. The two most recent modifications are considered more ergonomic and easier to perform because they imitate the traditional open technique. Moreover, they avoid the difficult dissection in the costal area, avoid a parallax operation method, and require only one additional trocar.

20.5 Operative Technique

20.5.1 Transfascial Approach

In this technique, the patient is placed in the supine position with both arms abducted. A 12-mm incision is made just below the tip of the eleventh rib using an S retractor. The subcutaneous tissues are bluntly divided, exposing the external oblique aponeurosis. The external oblique is sharply incised, exposing the internal oblique muscle. The potential space between the external and internal oblique aponeuroses is developed lateral to the semilunar line using a bilateral balloon dissector. A structural 12-mm balloon port is then placed and the space maintained with a CO_2 insufflation pressure of 12 mmHg. The areolar attachments are bluntly dissected under direct vision using a 10-mm 30° laparoscope. Two additional 5-mm ports are created, one at the level of the umbilicus on the posterior axillary line and another just above the inguinal ligament lateral to the rectus. This entire plane between the external and internal oblique muscles is dissected, extending from just

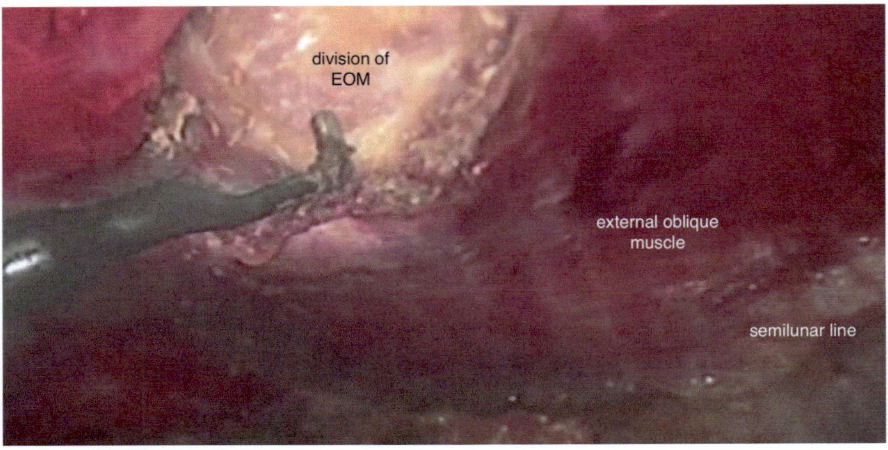

Fig. 20.1 Division of the external oblique muscle takes place at the top of the screen about 2 cm lateral to the semilunar line

above the costal margin to the inguinal ligament and from the semilunar line medially to the posterior axillary line laterally, where the oblique muscles meet the latissimus dorsi. Coagulating scissors are used for component separation, with the division of the external oblique aponeurosis released from the costal margin to the inguinal ligament. The external oblique muscle will be at the top of the screen, the internal oblique muscle at the bottom, and the semilunar line present medially (Fig. 20.1). This process is repeated on the opposite side. Each of the lateral compartments is drained with a closed suction drain. A video of the technique can be found at https://www.youtube.com/watch?v=lKtKXDKIiRM.

20.5.2 Modified Subfascial Approach

The external oblique aponeurosis is accessed 2 cm medially to the anterior superior iliac spine (Fig. 20.2). In this location, the anatomy is easily recognized as the external oblique is less muscular and almost entirely aponeurotic. After making a 1-cm incision in the aponeurosis, a bilateral balloon dissector is used to develop the plane in a similar fashion. A structural 10-mm balloon port is placed, and CO_2 insufflation is initiated, to a pressure of 12 mmHg (Fig. 20.3). A single 5-mm port is inserted at the level of the umbilicus on the posterior axillary line. The areolar attachments between these muscle layers are dissected in similar fashion. Component separation is performed by incising the external oblique aponeurosis 2 cm lateral to the semilunar line. This release is continued well above the costal margin to the insertion of the external oblique on the ninth and tenth ribs (Fig. 20.4). The inferior release from the port site to the inguinal ligament can be easily performed in an open fashion, using shears to divide the aponeurosis 2–3 cm to the inguinal ligament under direct visualization. A closed suction drain is passed through the lateral 5-mm port and

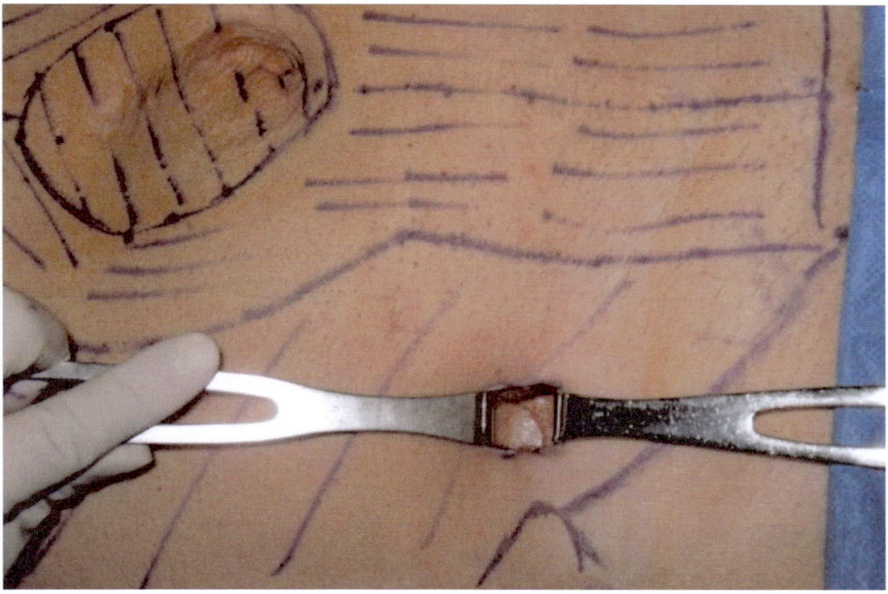

Fig. 20.2 Initial incision 2 cm medial to the anterior superior iliac spine

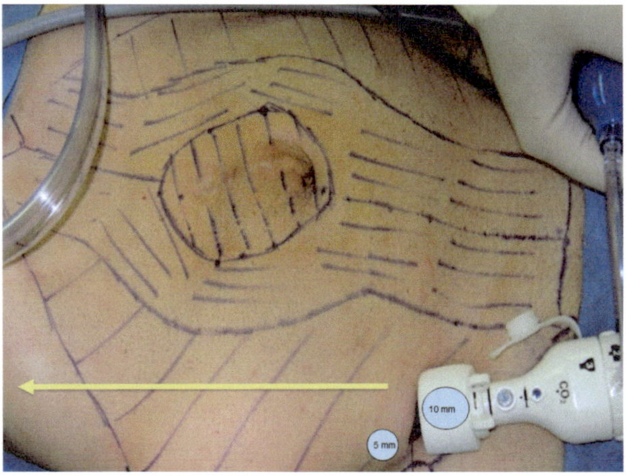

Fig. 20.3 A balloon dissector is introduced between the external and the internal oblique muscles and is directed toward the costal margin

inserted into the intermuscular space. A video of the technique can be found at: https://youtu.be/OXzH_1UQRKE

20.5.3 Endoscopic Subcutaneous CS Approach

The patient is placed in a supine position with both arms tucked and padded at their sides. Under ultrasound guidance, the semilunar lines lateral to the rectus abdominis

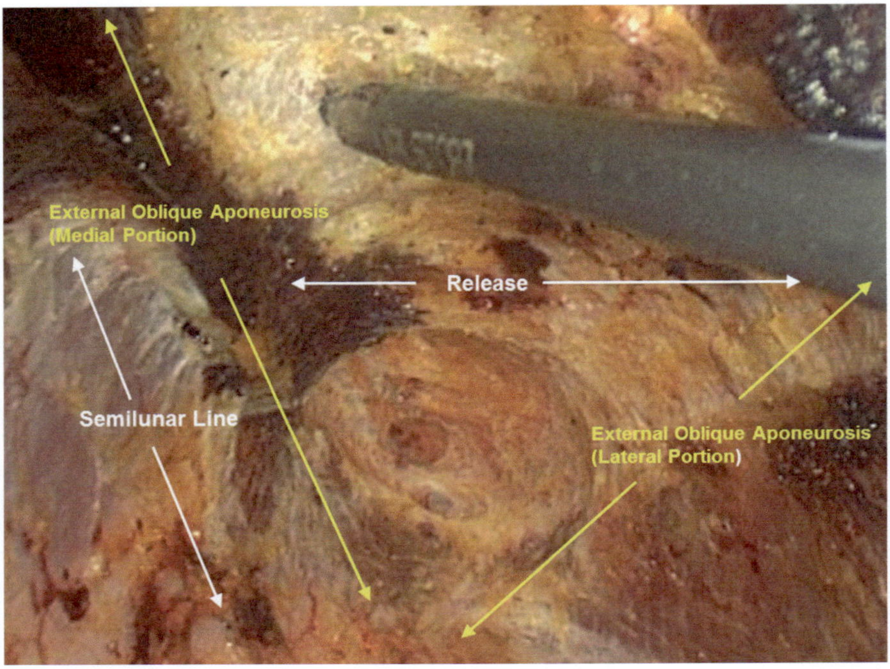

Fig. 20.4 Complete release of the external oblique muscle lateral to the semilunar line

muscle are identified and marked on the skin bilaterally. Marking can be performed by the surgeon using portable ultrasound equipment immediately before skin preparation or can be performed by a radiologist in advance using indelible ink. A 12-mm incision is made in the lower lateral quadrant of the abdomen, lateral to the previously marked semilunar line. A balloon dissector is introduced and advanced over the anterior aponeurosis until the tip reaches the costal margin. The balloon is inflated at two levels using eight to ten pumps (Fig. 20.5). Occasionally, in obese or post-bariatric patients or in patients who have undergone previous abdominoplasty, a blunt rod (trocar interchanger) is used to create a subcutaneous tunnel over the fascia before introducing the balloon dissector. The balloon is then replaced by a simple 10- to 12-mm trocar. The space is maintained with CO_2 insufflation at a pressure of 10 mmHg (Fig. 20.6). An additional 5-mm port is introduced at a position lateral and slightly superior to the camera port (Fig. 20.7). The external oblique aponeurosis is incised laterally to the semilunar line, using the marking on the skin as a guide (Fig. 20.8). Exposure of the fatty tissues without visualization of muscle ensures entry into the correct plane (Fig. 20.9). If muscle can be visualized at this level, either the rectus sheath medially or the muscular part of the external oblique laterally has been divided.

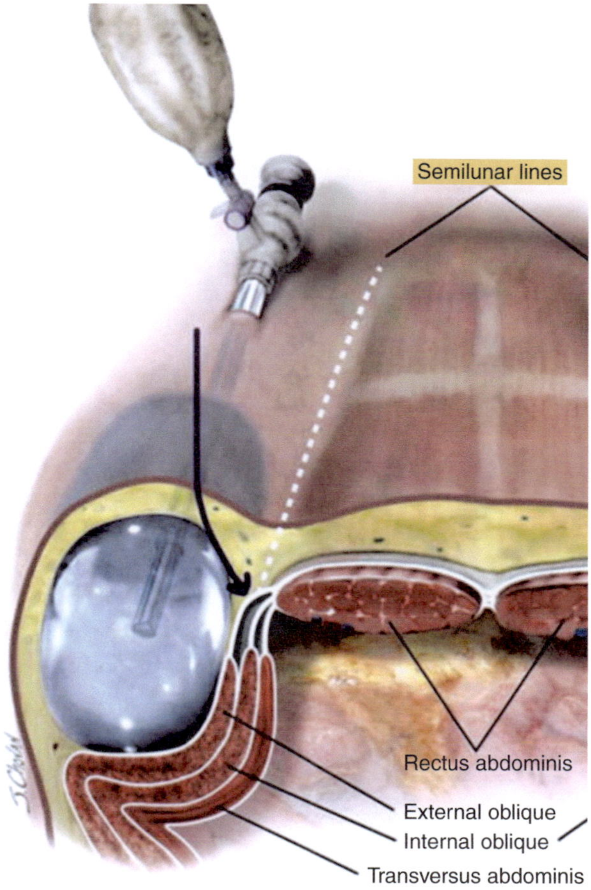

Fig. 20.5 Balloon dissection of the subcutaneous space

The external oblique aponeurosis is incised from this level to 4–6 cm above the costal margin. Above the costal margin, the aponeurosis changes to muscle and division should be performed carefully to avoid bleeding. An ultrasonic device may be useful for this purpose. Scissors and judiciously used cautery can be used to dissect under the external oblique muscle laterally in an avascular plane to provide maximum advancement. With the camera turned downward, the incision in the external oblique muscle is continued below the camera port to include the inguinal ligament. Drains are not used routinely during this technique. The subcutaneous space is re-insufflated at the end of AWR to verify hemostasis. A video of the technique can be found at https://www.youtube.com/edit?video_id=4SpWz7U5uZ0&video_referrer=watch.

A cross-sectional view of the abdomen that shows a comparison of the subcutaneous and subfascial techniques of component separation is provided in Fig. 20.10 for both the balloon dissection and the division of the external oblique fascia (blue arrow).

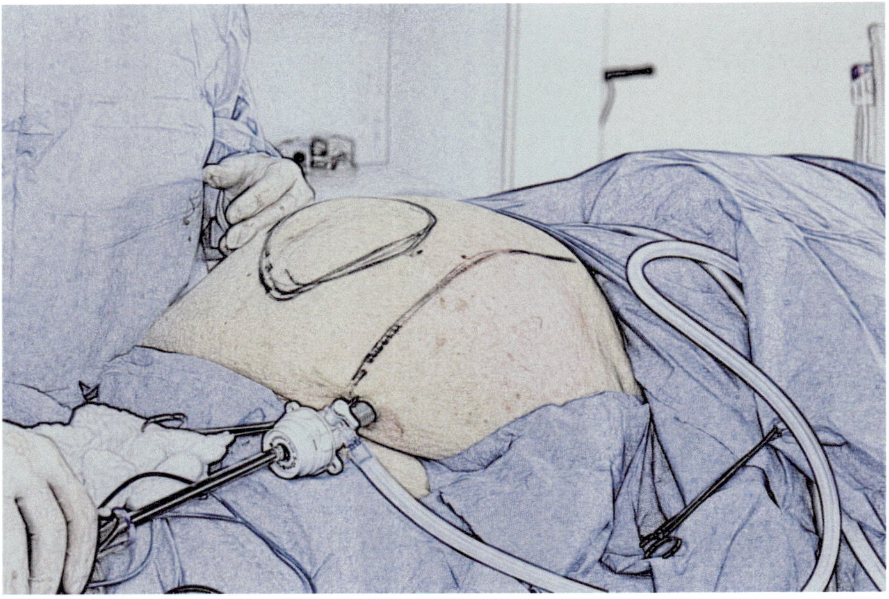

Fig. 20.6 Set up for a unilateral Subcutaneous ECS. A 12 mm camera port has been placed lateral to the previously marked semilunar line in the lower lateral quadrant. The space is maintained with CO_2

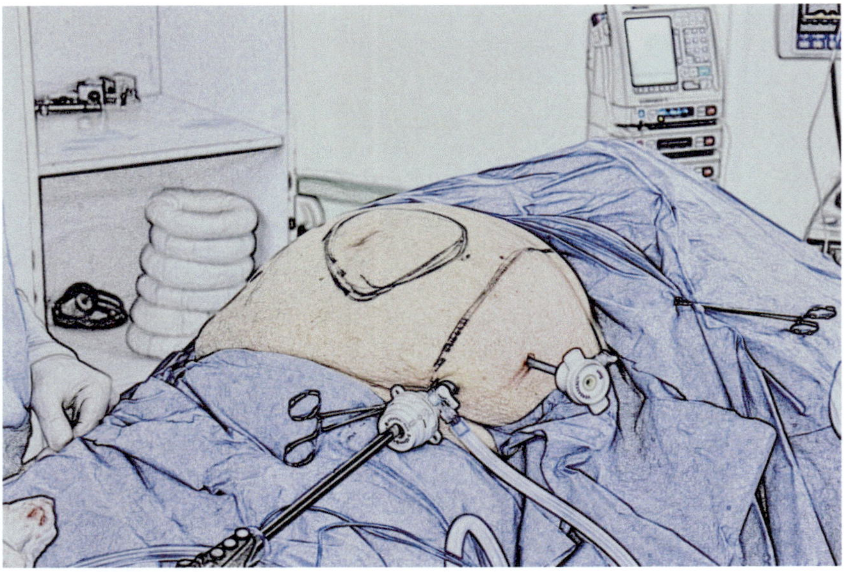

Fig. 20.7 An additional 5 mm working port has been placed laterally and slightly superior to camera port

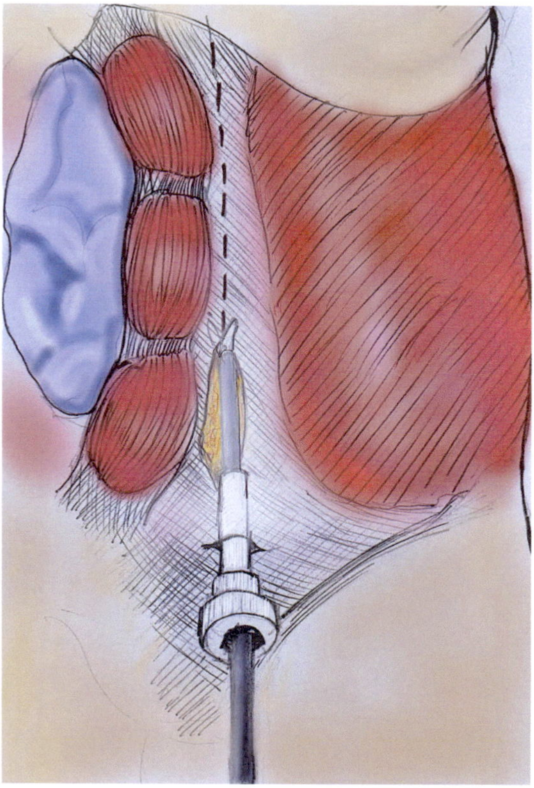

Fig. 20.8 The external oblique aponeurosis is incised laterally to the left semilunar line, using the marking on the skin as a guide

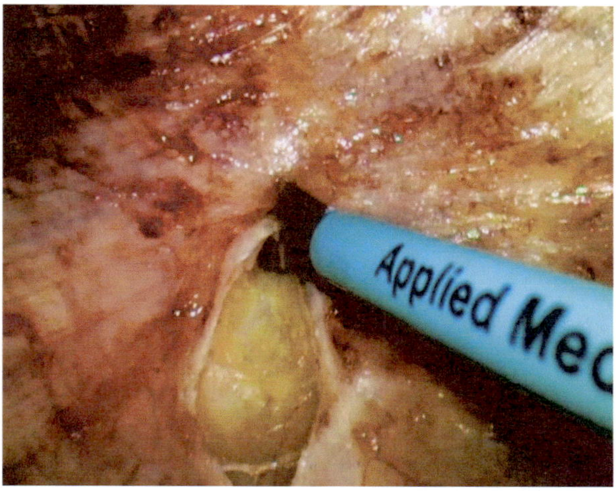

Fig. 20.9 Exposure of the fatty tissues without visualization of muscle ensures entry into the correct plane. In certain cases the external muscle is divided on purpose (presence of ileostomy or defects close to the semilunar line)

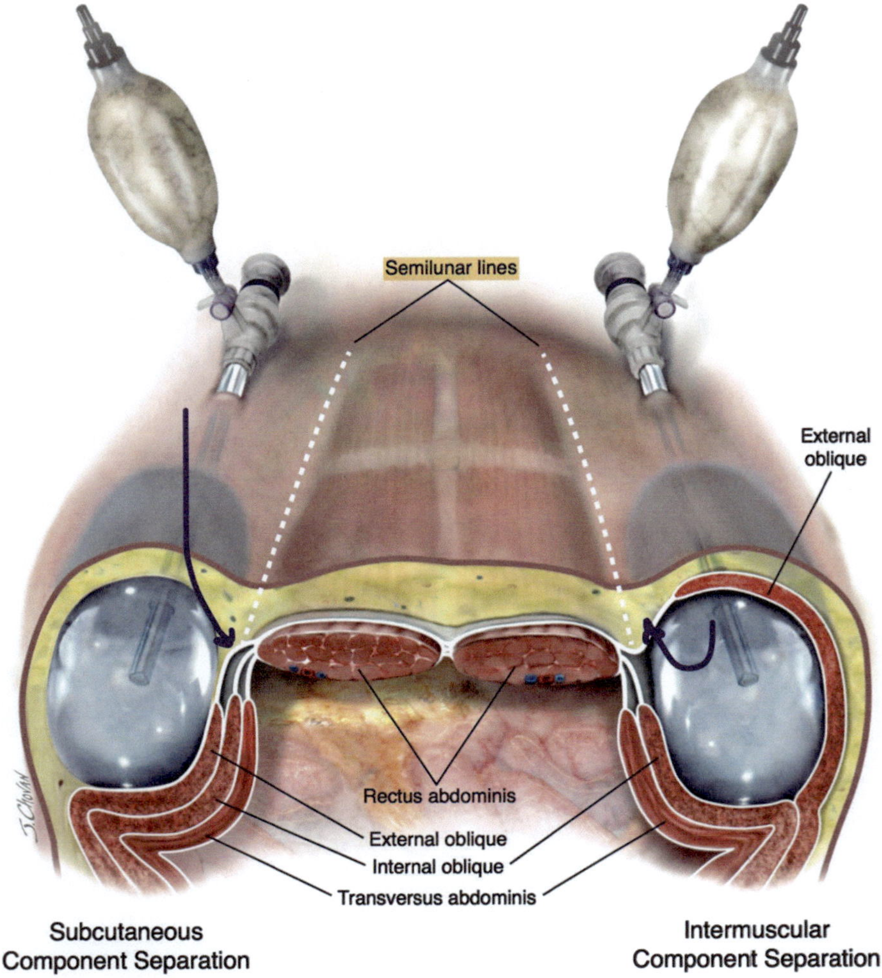

Fig. 20.10 A cross-sectional view of the abdomen that shows a comparison of the subcutaneous and subfascial techniques of component separation for both the balloon dissection and the division of the external oblique fascia (blue arrow)

20.6 Pearls and Pitfalls

1. ECS can be performed first when used as an adjunct to minimally invasive AWR if clinical examination and CT scanning provide thorough information; otherwise, robotic or laparoscopic exploration should precede it.
2. Many times there is no need to perform a bilateral ECS. We have been able to laparoscopically close most defects 6–15 cm in width with a unilateral subcutaneous CS without dehiscence or abdominal wall asymmetry.

3. ECS can be used to repair any suitable lateral defect, not just central defects.
4. When defects are close to the semilunar line, ECS can be performed on the same side by dividing the external oblique muscle more laterally, thus avoiding the division of the semilunar line.
5. A vertical posterior rectus fascia release may be added to an ECS to assist in relieving tension on the closure.
6. Mesh should be used to cover the ECS site during IPOM plus, at least while surgeons are learning the procedure and when in doubt.

20.7 Evaluation of Results

We published a prospective evaluation of endoscopic subcutaneous ACS, with long-term clinical and imaging follow-up [8]. Twenty consecutive patients between 2012 and 2015 were evaluated. These patients had defects 6–15 cm in size, with length greater than width, and without skin dystrophy, loss of domain, or active infection. None of these patients had undergone multiple previous repairs/meshes and there was no reasonable suspicion of severe adhesions. Most ECSs were performed unilaterally as adjuncts to IPOM plus repairs. Primary closure of defects was performed with slowly absorbable barbed sutures. All of the cases were followed clinically and by CT imaging for up to 38 months (mean, 21 months). In 19 of these patients, the repair remained sound clinically and by CT imaging, whereas one patient had a small limited disruption well protected by the underlying mesh. In eight patients, in whom the area was not covered by mesh, there was no defect at the CS site. Morbidity was low, with no development of a surgical site infection (SSI) or mesh-related complication. Cosmetic results were excellent; in particular, despite almost all ECSs being unilateral, we did not observe abdominal wall asymmetry and the degree of patient satisfaction was high.

20.8 Conclusions

Complex ventral hernia repairs remain a frequent and intricate problem with satisfactory results requiring a combination of techniques, technologies and materials. Primary closure of defects as part of the AWR has been an essential part of open repairs and recently also of minimal invasive approaches because it attempts to recreate the anatomy and physiology of the abdominal wall while reducing dead space and its consequences. The posterior component separation owns it present popularity to a natural extension from the Rives-Stoppa technique. However, the anterior endoscopic component separation remains as a safe and effective technique in selected patients as an adjunct to robotic-assisted and laparoscopic AWR as well as for open repairs and other indications.

References

1. Ramirez OM, Ruas E, Dellon AL. "Components separation" method for closure of abdominal-wall defects: an anatomic and clinical study. Plast Reconstr Surg. 1990;86:519–26.
2. Harth KC, Rosen MJ. Endoscopic versus open component separation in complex abdominal wall reconstruction. Am J Surg. 2010;199:342–7.
3. Lowe JB, Garza JR, Bowman JL, Rohrich RJ, Strodel WE. Endoscopically assisted "components separation" for closure of abdominal wall defects. Plast Reconstr Surg. 2000;105:70–729.
4. Maas SM, de Vries RS, can Goor TS, van Goor H, de Jong D, Bleichrodt RP. Endoscopically assisted "components separation technique" for the repair of complicated ventral hernias. J Am Coll Surg. 2002;194:388–90.
5. Rosen M, et al. Laparoscopic component separation in the single-stage treatment of infected abdominal wall prosthetic removal. Hernia. 2007;11:435–40.
6. Daes J, Chen D. Endoscopic components separation techniques. In: Hope W, Cobb W, Adrales G, editors. Textbook of hernia. Basel: Springer; 2017. p. 243–8.
7. Daes J. Endoscopic subcutaneous approach to component separation. J Am Coll Surg. 2014;218:e1–4.
8. Daes J, Dennis RJ. Endoscopic subcutaneous separation as an adjunct to abdominal wall reconstruction. Surg Endosc. 2016;22:1–5.

Robotic Retro-Rectus Repairs

21

Flavio Malcher, Leandro Totti Cavazzola, and Igor Belyansky

21.1 Introduction

Minimally invasive surgery (MIS) ventral repairs were first described by Le Blanc in 1993 with the laparoscopic approach with an intraperitoneal onlay mesh (IPOM) implant. The use of IPOM was never a gold standard in open ventral repairs because of the fear of using uncoated polypropylene and other materials directly in contact with viscera [1]. For the development of laparoscopic techniques to the abdomen wall, several modifications were done, such as the use of new meshes with coated barriers, new fixation devices and mainly changes in surgical techniques, abandoning the traditional onlay and retromuscular/preperitonial options. The intraperitoneal era was inaugurated. Laparoscopic techniques have proven themselves in the last 20 years as safe and efficient in the cure of ventral hernias, despite the increased incidence of adhesions and enterotomies following intraperitoneal surgeries [2].

Despite the advantage of important decrease in wound morbidity and the safeness of the laparoscopic ventral hernia repair, its adoption rate reached a plateau of around 20%. Several reasons have been postulated as explanation for this, as increased costs (IPOM and fixation devices) and difficult learning curve (surgery performed in the "roof" of the cavity with straight instruments) [3, 4].

The implementation of advances in MIS such as the robotic platform, shown us enhanced skills to operate the abdomen wall, as articulated and strong instruments,

F. Malcher (✉)
Abdominal Wall Program, Montefiore Medical Center, Albert Einstein College of Medicine, Bronx, NY, USA

L. T. Cavazzola
Robotic Surgery Program, General Surgery, Hospital de Clínicas de Porto Alegre, Porto Alegre, RS, Brazil

I. Belyansky
Abdominal Wall Reconstruction Program, General Surgery, Anne Arundel Medical Center, Annapolis, MD, USA

K. A. LeBlanc (ed.), *Robotic Assisted Hernia Repair*,
https://doi.org/10.1007/978-3-030-23025-8_21

better visualization and steady and 3D optics. It did not take long to surgeons start to perform surgeries by MIS approach without IPOM, coming back to the traditional open techniques as onlay and sublay, avoiding IPOM and expensive fixation devices (using sutures instead). After robotics shown the way, several skilled surgeons without access to robotics, tried and developed MIS techniques without the robot, using classic endoscopic instruments and resources [3].

While the optimal surgical approach for the repair of ventral incisional hernias remains a subject of considerable debate [3]. In this chapter, we are going to explore several of these techniques, all them designed to keep the mesh outside the peritoneal cavity, as intended in open surgery.

21.2 Robotic Rives: Retromuscular Repairs

Intraperitoneal anatomy is far more familiar for the average surgeon. That's why this approach is more frequently adopted by surgeons when they start using the robot to do MIS abdominal wall reconstruction. There are a lot of options to access the retromuscular space from inside abdominal cavity, and the choice will be based mainly in the location and size of the defect. For example: for suprapubic defects, a caudal single docking approach can be used. This approach will be discussed elsewhere in this book. On the opposite side, defects above the umbilicus can be easily addressed by a cranial docking. For the vast majority of cases, a double docking technique, coming from patient side will be preferable because allows easy recognition of the anatomical landmarks and it's suitable for defects in almost all midline from the xiphoid through the pubic bone. This alternative has the inconvenient that it's obligatory the docking in the contralateral side, which takes additional time. Alternatively, in patients with small defects and large retrorectus space (which can be addressed preoperatively by CT scans), a single lateral docking can be used with good exposure and providing adequate overlap for a large mesh after completion of the procedure. These alternatives will be discussed along this chapter.

21.2.1 Patient Selection

There are some limitations for the robotic approach. Patients with poor skin and soft tissue integrity (ex. prior skin graft), a widened scar from previous wound complications that will require surgical excision, chronic wounds, or poor hernia cosmesis are not good candidates since they probably will need an open approach (or at least an hybrid procedure).

There are no consensus about the best robotic technique to be used. Normally, defects larger than 8 cm will require a double-dock approach, even with bilateral transversus abdominis release (TAR). Mid-sized defects, typically up to 8 cm, are approached with a single-dock retromuscular technique. For smaller defects (less than 5 cm), a single-dock preperitoneal approach (ventral TAPP) is usually preferred by several surgeons, as there is less tension on the defect closure and myofascial release is not usually required and the procedure can be done quickly. This technique will be described elsewhere in this book.

21.2.2 General Measures

All patients are positioned supine with both arms tucked, and a foley catheter is inserted if the defect is infra-umbilical. Antibiotic dosing, body hair clipping, and placement of sequential compression devices are used according to institutional protocols. In the lateral docking options, it's useful to flex the operation table, maintaining the legs extend downward at a minimum of 30° to afford the surgeon and assistant greater instrument range of motion (Fig. 21.1).

21.2.3 Single Docking: Cranial Approach

To deal with hernias located in the supra-umbilical position, the robot can be docked in the cranial position (same as for foregut and bariatric surgery) and approached from a midline position. A two arm configuration is used (one can add the use of an auxiliary portal depending on the will of the surgeon). Camera trocar is inserted

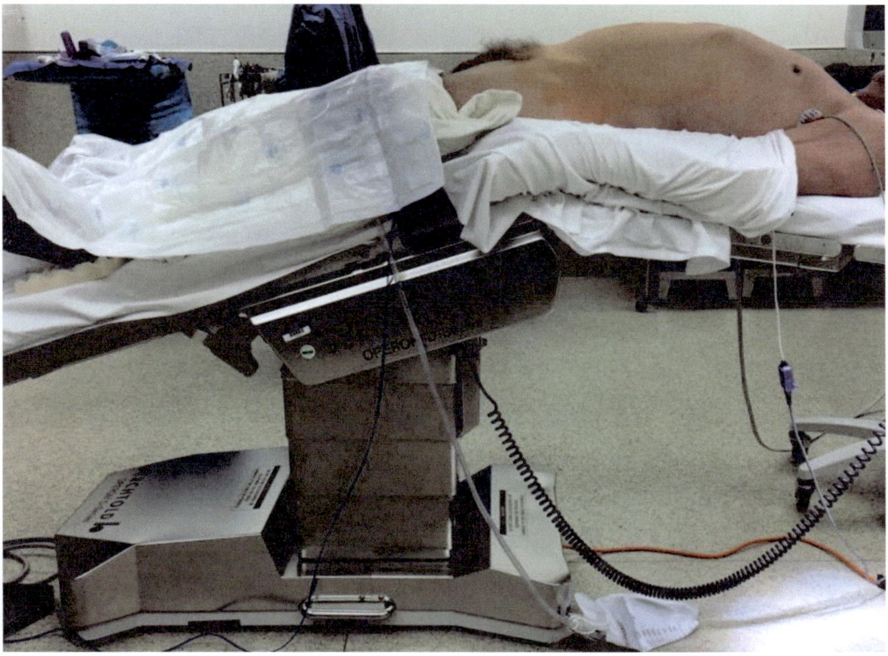

Fig. 21.1 Positioning of the patient for robotic ventral repair. Trendelenburg position with hips extended allows the wider space for ports in the abdominal wall

below the umbilicus, after insufflation and abdominal access is achieved under surgeons preference. Long trocars are used to achieve extra room and avoid arms collision. For this approach, patient is positioned preferable on a split leg table, in moderate reverse Trendelenburg position to allow more room to work upward the abdomen. An initial posterior sheath incision is made transversely, opening from one semilunar line to the other, with division of the posterior sheath on his medial aspect each side to preserve the midline linea alba above and below the hernia defect. After dissecting the defect, hernia repair starts with anterior defect closure, followed by mesh placement and posterior sheath closure as the last part of the procedure (Fig. 21.2).

21.2.4 Double Docking: Lateral Approach

Since this approach can handle most of midline hernia defects, despite their location in the linea alba, it will be described in details. The patient is placed as showed in Fig. 21.1, Pneumoperitoneum is established at surgeon's preference, and a long 12 mm optical trocar is placed midway between the costal margin and iliac crest. This should be done as laterally as possible, to allow adequate distance between trocars and defect. Two long robotic trocars are placed near costal margin close to the iliac crest. The use of long trocars help to get additional clearance of the robotic arms away from the patient. This also allows greater flexibility for advancing the robotic instruments into the extremes of the abdominal cavity. After placing the trocars as described, the robot can be docked with the center column of the patient side cart aligned with the hip or upper thigh, in order to allow more space between the robot and the patient arm for the bedside assistant (Fig. 21.3).

Adhesiolysis is performed either robotically or laparoscopically, and the retromuscular dissection is initiated by incising the posterior rectus sheath close to the linea alba. The retromuscular plane is developed laterally to the linea semilunaris and vertically at least 5 cm above and below the hernia defect, so an adequate mesh overlap will be achieved after defect closure (Fig. 21.4).

At this point the surgeon decides if a transversus abdominis myofascial release (TAR) is necessary. This will be addressed elsewhere in this book. After adequate dissection is performed (either if a TAR is necessary or no), three additional trocars are placed into the dissected space in the contralateral abdomen in a mirror image (Fig. 21.5).

A ruler is used to intracorporeally measure both the hernia defect height and width, and the extent of the dissected space. The height of the dissected space will correspond to the length of mesh required for repair. The half of the dissected space is measured and assumed to be equal to half of the needed mesh width, because a mirror dissection will be performed after redocking. After adequate sizing, the mesh

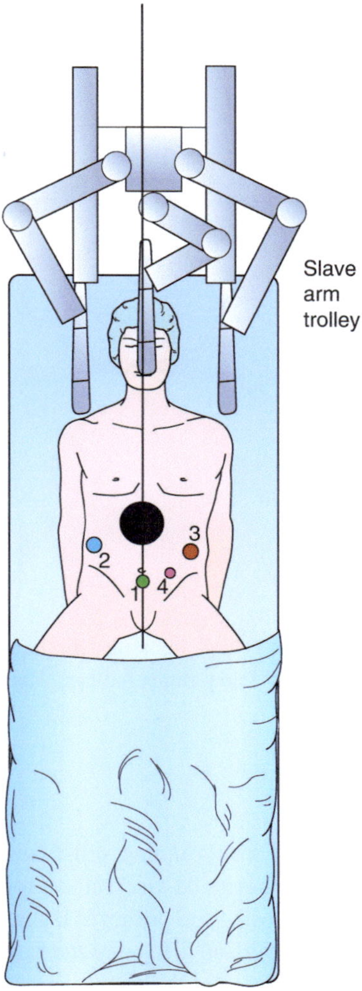

Fig. 21.2 Trocar placement for single docking cranial approach. (1). Camera, (2, 3). Robotic ports. (4). Accessory port (not obligatory)

is rolled and secured with a loosely tied suture. After being deployed in the retromuscular space, it's sutured to the contralateral side (Fig. 21.6).

Patient is then repositioned and the robot docked on the opposite side. When using the Xi plataform, repositioning of the patient may not be necessary, once the boom feature of Xi allows rotation of the arms. That feature facilitates enormously the double doking process. Dissection is carried out in the same fashion to complete the bilateral retromuscular (or transversus abdominis if necessary) flaps. After adequate retromuscular dissection on the contralateral side, posterior fascial defect is

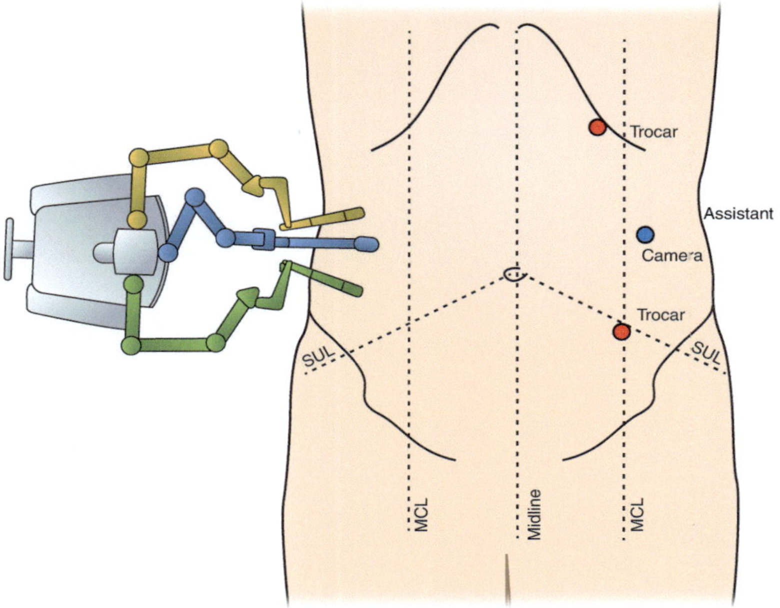

Fig. 21.3 Port position for lateral docking technique

closed with a running self-fixating, slowly absorbable 2-0 suture. This will completely isolate de visceral sac form the retromuscular pocket created for the mesh. After closing the posterior layer, than the mesh is unrolled across the closed posterior sheath and affixed to the right lateral abdominal wall (Fig. 21.7).

At this point the pneumoperitoneum is decreased, and the anterior fascial defect is closed using a self-fixating, nonabsorbable number 1 suture in a running fashion, trying to include intermittent bites of the overlying hernia sac imbricating the hernia sac and thus obliterating the dead space (Fig. 21.8).

21.2.5 Single Docking: Lateral Approach

Small hernias and even mid-sized defects can often be approached using a lateral single-dock approach. It's very important that the preoperative evaluation of the patient showed that a large retrorectus space is available, so adequate overlap will be achieved after dissection. Patient is positioned as described in Sect. 21.2.2. Docking is achieved as describe in the previous section. The main difference

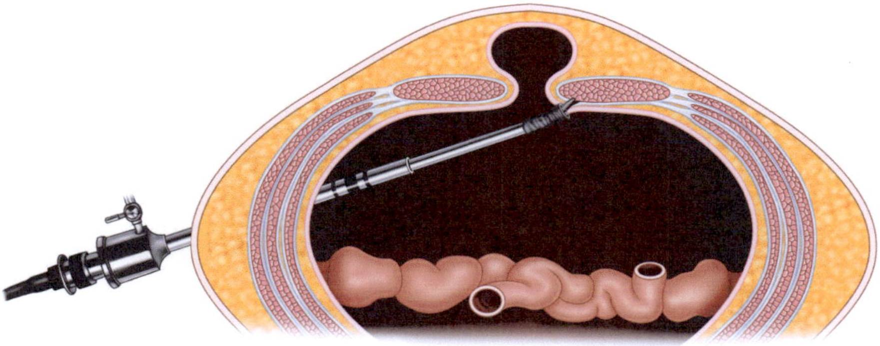

a

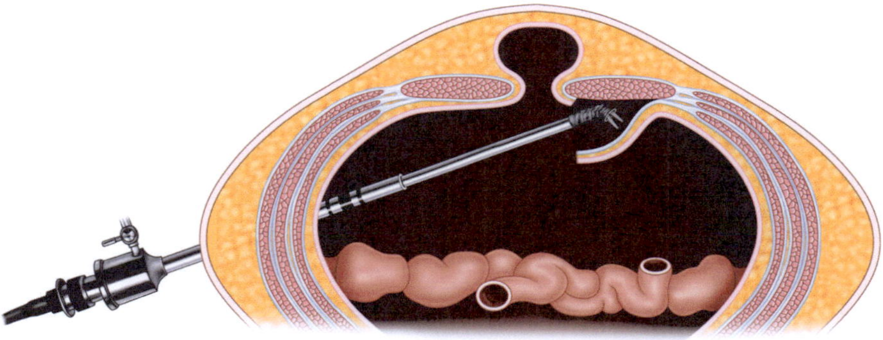

b

Fig. 21.4 Retromuscular dissection in lateral double docking technique. (**a**). Begining of dissection close to hernia defect. (**b**). End of lateral dissection close to semilunaris line, preserving the neurovascular bundles

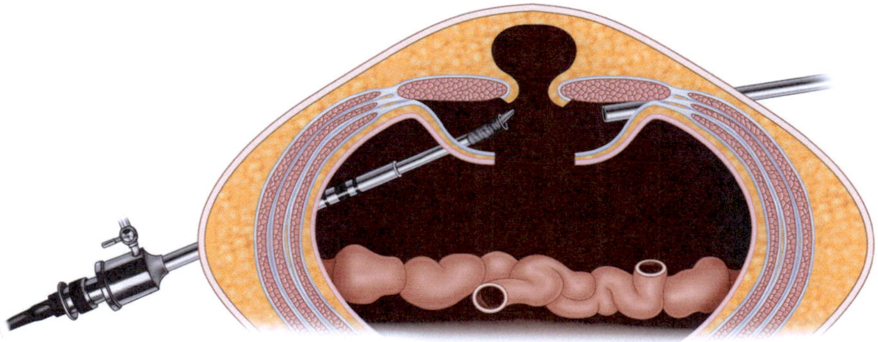

Fig. 21.5 Contralateral mirror positioning of the trocars

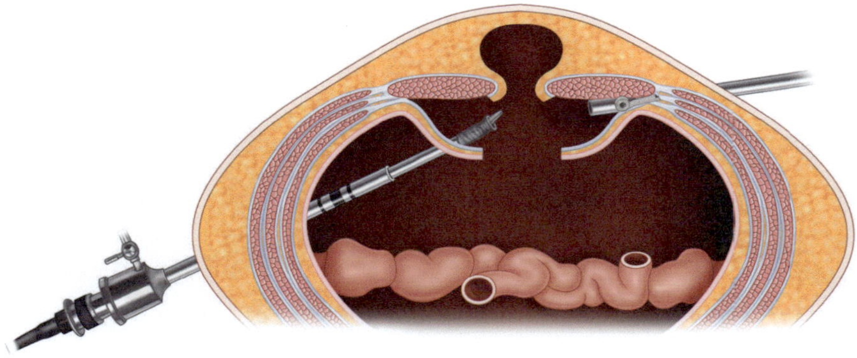

Fig. 21.6 Contralateral mesh fixation

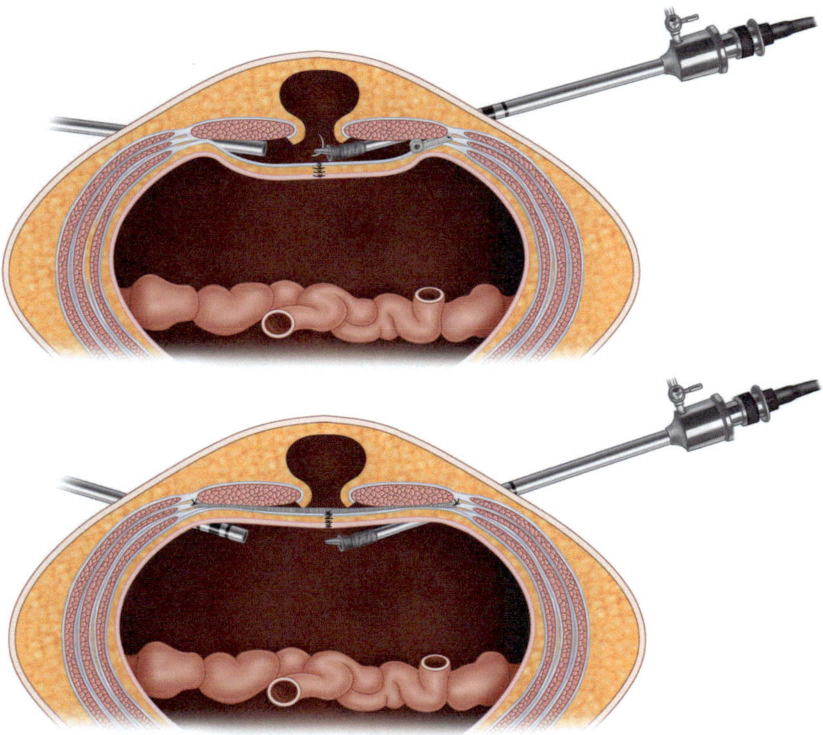

Fig. 21.7 Posterior layer closure and fixation of the mesh

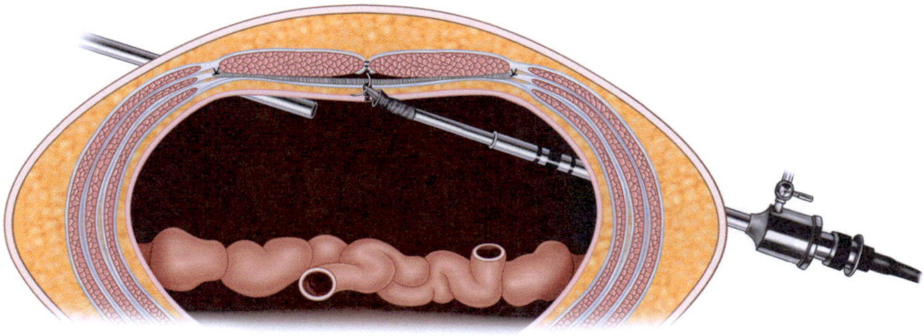

Fig. 21.8 Anterior layer closure

between this approach is the lateral aspect of the ipsilateral rectus sheath is incised to gain access to the retrorectus space. Dissection is continued from lateral to medial until the linea alba (or lateral edge of the hernia defect) is encountered. Then the posterior sheath is incised to enter into the preperitoneal space along the midline, including dissection around and reduction of the midline hernia sac. Once across the midline, the contralateral posterior sheath is incised in it's medial aspect, and dissection completed to the semilunar line, creating a unique flap that is formed by both posterior rectus sheat connected by peritoneum (including hernia sac) at midline. The anterior fascial defect is closed first. The retromuscular space that is available after closure, followed by placement of the proper sized mesh. After fixation of the mesh, the posterior sheath is closed to completely cover the mesh (Fig. 21.9).

21.3 e-TEP

21.3.1 Pre-Operative Planning and Considerations

All potential minimally invasive abdominal wall reconstruction candidates must undergo a comprehensive workup to ensure they are appropriately selected for surgery. There are absolute and relative contraindications to the eTEP approach for hernioplasty (Table 21.1). An up-to-date computed tomography study of the abdomen and pelvis is recommended for effective preoperative planning [5].

21.3.2 Operating Room Setup and Patient Positioning

After induction of general endotracheal anesthesia, all patients are positioned supine with both arms tucked to their sides. Institutional protocols of antibiotics, venous

a
b
c
d

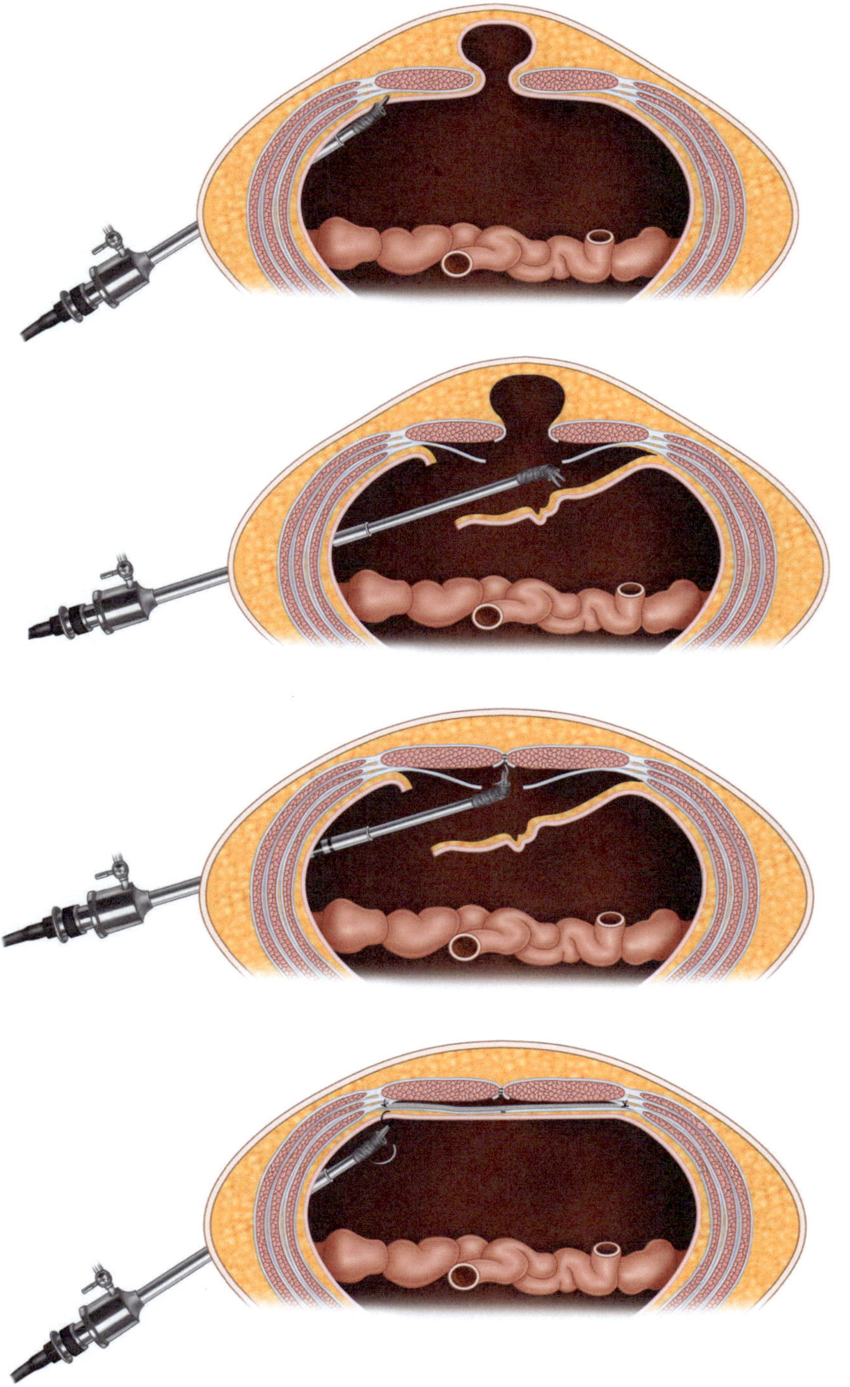

Fig. 21.9 Single docking—lateral approach. (**a**) Incision of posterior rectus sheat—lateral, close to semilunar line. (**b**) Crossover the midline (includes) reduction of the hernia sac, reaching contralateral semilunar line. (**c**) Hernia defect closure. (**d**) Mesh placement against and closure of the posterior sheath

Table 21.1 Absolute and relative contraindications to eTEP approach

Relative	Absolute
Previous incision extending from xiphoid process to the pubic bone	Active mesh infection
Loss of domain	Presence of fistula
Dystrophic or ulcerated skin	
Extensive intraabdominal adhesions	

thrombosis prophylaxis are used [6–8]. A foley catheter is placed in order to decompress the bladder. The operating table is flexed with the legs extend downward at a minimum of 30° to afford the surgeon and assistant greater instrument range of motion (Fig. 21.1). Failure to sufficiently flex the operating table will result in arm's hand collision with the patient's body while dissecting and suturing the defects.

The enhanced-view totally extraperitoneal (eTEP) access approach was previously described for laparoscopic inguinal hernia repair by Daes in 2012 [9]. This approach introduced the notion that the extraperitoneal domain is a limitless space once the confluence of arcuate line and semilunar line are taken down, relying on proper anatomic identification and dissection in the naturally occurring retromuscular spaces. Typically, dissection is initiated in one of the retrorectus spaces and then crosses over to the contralateral side, thus joining the two spaces into one large operative field. Since Daes' initial description, we have adopted this technique for ventral and incisional hernia repair [10–12].

Docking is dependent on the system available (Si vs Xi), the location of the hernia defect and decision where to crossover. Lateral docking with the Si is possible in patients with wide rectus sheet (>7to 8 cm) to a complete lateral approach. Oblique docking may be accomplished for cases where the crossover would be done laparoscopically, before the robotic docking.

21.3.3 Upper Midline Defect

Figure 21.10 demonstrates the port position for upper midline defects. The first incision is made 2 cm bellow a horizontal line drawn through umbilicus just medial to the right linea semilunaris. The anterior rectus sheath is identified and incised sharply. Single site balloon dissector is used to develop the right retrorectus space in cephalad and caudal directions. It is critical to avoid over-inflation which may rupture the linea semilunaris and consequently injure the rectus abdominis muscle. In addition, special care should be given to appreciating the inferior epigastric vessels that travel parallel and medial to linea semilunaris in the vicinity of the #1 port. The telescope dissection without the use of the balloon is an option and allows a cost reduction to the procedure. For robotics procedures, this may be a better option, once the balloon uses a 10/12 mm trocars and the robotic system uses 8 mm trocars. The use 5 mm trocars to create the space may facilitate the change of those to 8 mm ones to be used for the robotic procedure. Once the space of Retzius is developed, ports #2 and #3 are placed under direct vision in the lower abdomen. Thus, even

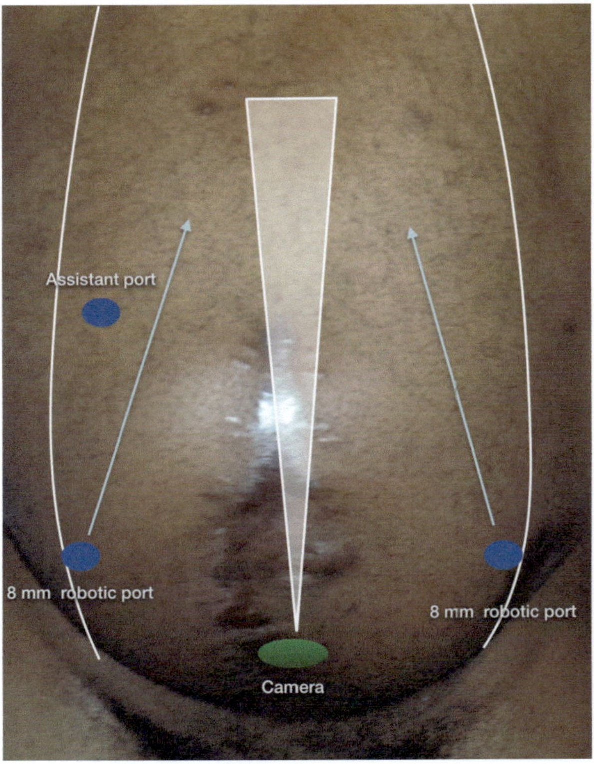

Fig. 21.10 Port positioning for upper midline defects. The balloon dissector is placed in port #1, green ellipse. Ports #2 and #3 are marked with blue circles. The assistant port is located higher, usually on the right side of the patient

before any initiation of sharp dissection the retromuscular space surrounding the hernia defect is completely dissected bluntly with the balloon space-maker.

The timing of docking may vary. One may prefer create a bigger preperitonial space before docking to avoid difficulties due the small working space for the robotic instruments. We prefer to perform the crossover below the level of the umbilicus, developing preperitoneal and retromuscular spaces that have not been previously violated. In the middle we try to preserve the preperitoneal contributions to the posterior layer which are made up of the falciform and umbilical ligaments. In such a fashion the division of posterior rectus sheath and preservation of falciform ligament and umbilical ligaments allows us to join the right and the left retrorectus spaces together with the midline preperitoneal space (Fig. 21.11).

Following the dissection in these planes we then anticipate to encounter the neck of the hernia sac. In an incisional hernia, these layers surrounding the neck of the sack can be thoroughly fused together and difficult to differentiate. An attempt may be made in some cases to reduce the entirety of the sac by separating it from its distal attachments, however this is not often attempted. We frequently give consideration to sharply opening the peritoneal layer just proximal to the neck of the sac to reduce visceral contents under direct visualization and perform limited adhesiolysis (Fig. 21.12). Any defects in the posterior layer can be fixed with 3-0 suture.

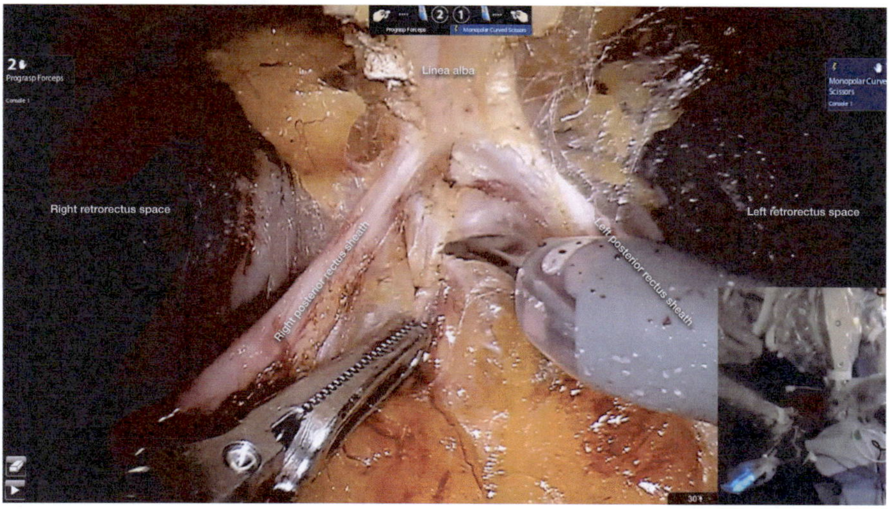

Fig. 21.11 View of the retrorectus space. After crossing over and dissection, the retrorectus spaces on both sides are combined into one large retrorectus space. The pre-peritoneal fat can be seen below

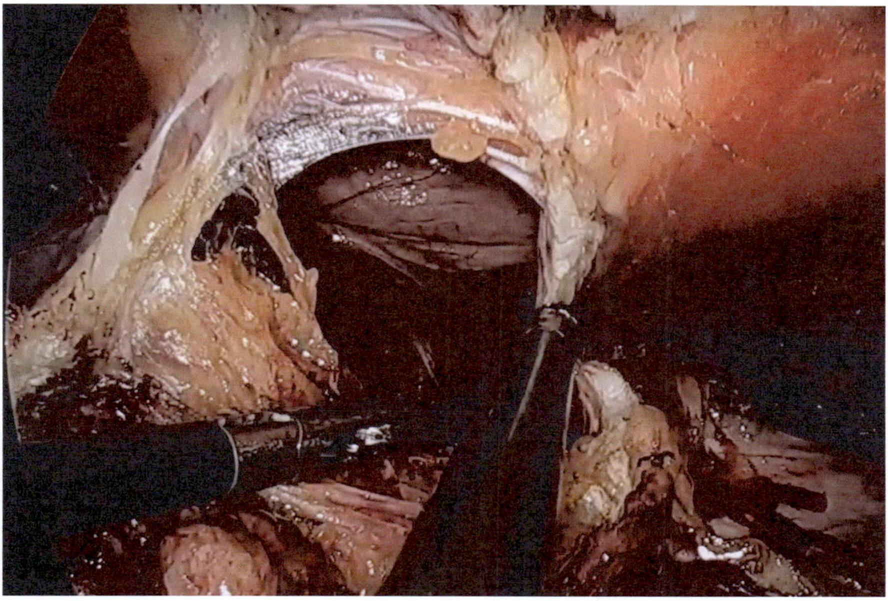

Fig. 21.12 Sharp opening of the peritoneal layer proximal to the neck of the hernia sac, allowing for reducing visceral contents under direct visualization and limited adhesiolysis

Once the hernia contents are reduced, retromuscular dissection commences with release of the medial aspect of the posterior rectus sheath and concludes just below the level of the xiphoid process.

Closure The edges of the PRS are sutured together in the midline with 2-0 absorbable or barbed suture starting near the xiphoid process running caudally. Starting at the dome of the bladder the surgeon and assistant switch positions and suture is run cranially, meeting in the middle where the two sutures are tied together. On the anterior layer closure, the pneumoperitoneum is dropped to 8–10 mm Hg to decrease the tension placed on the anterior layer closure. The defect being closed is at the top of the monitor and is sutured "upside down" with back handed needle driving. A 0 barbed suture is used for this closure due to technical ease of use afforded in this situation. If a large subcutaneous sac is present, one or more bites of the sac are included in the suture line for plication in order to reduce the likelihood of developing a postoperative seroma (Fig. 21.13). With the previously performed posterior CS, the defect edges should come together in a tension-free fashion. The defect is closed with v-lock suture, completed with four or five throws run in a backwards fashion (Fig. 21.13). Once both anterior and posterior fascial layers are closed, the mesh is deployed in the retromuscular sublay position. The developed retromuscular space is measured for appropriate mesh size selection. Our preference is medium weight macroporous polypropylene mesh which is deployed through our 12 mm trocar (Fig. 21.14). There is no need for antiadhesion barriers as there now exists an autologous barrier between the mesh and viscera; a significant advantage of the sublay position. Mesh placement in the retromuscular space has allowed for the discontinuation of aggressive penetrating fixation techniques with transfascial

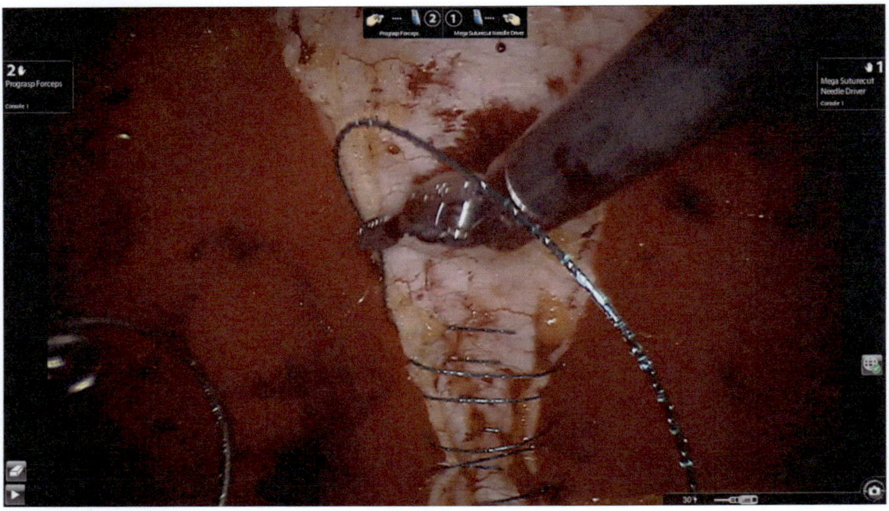

Fig. 21.13 Closure of the anterior layer. A 0 barbed suture is used in a back-handed fashion with an "upside down" view to take bites of the edges of the defect while including the sac (if a large subcutaneous portion is present) in between to reduce the chance of postoperative seroma

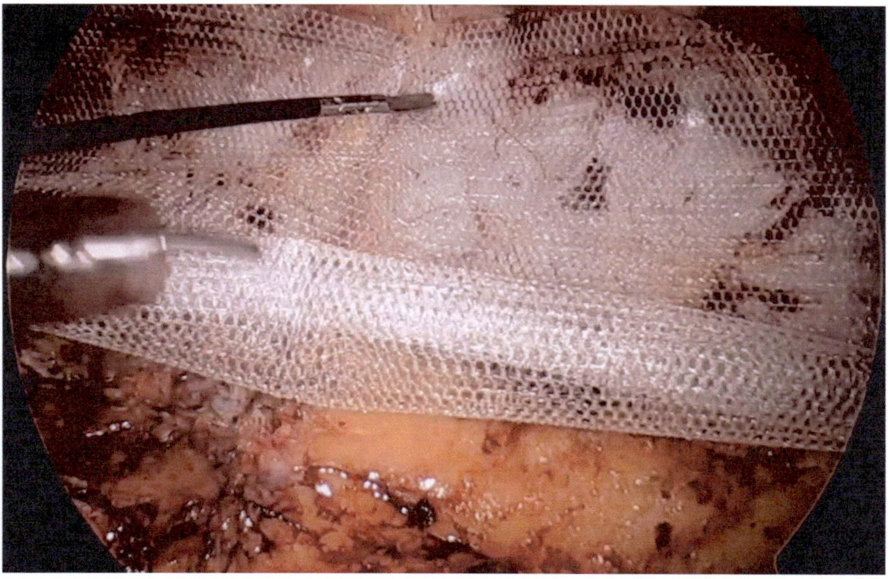

Fig. 21.14 Placement of a medium weight macroporous polypropylene mesh deployed through the 12 mm trocar. There is no need for antiadhesion barriers as there now exists an autologous barrier between the mesh and viscera

sutures, transitioning first to fibrin glue and, more recently, to complete cessation of mesh fixation as our data illustrates penetrating fixation is associated with higher incidence of chronic pain without the added benefit of lowered rates of recurrence. Pneumoperitoneum is released under direct vision, assuring the mesh is lying flat and wrinkle-free between the posterior and anterior layers (Fig. 21.14).

Formerly, we once placed drains just superficial to the mesh in all hernia repair cases. We are now more selective with drain placement and do not utilize it for most patients. To date we have not observed an increase in wound morbidity as a result.

21.3.4 Lower Midline Defects

For a right-handed surgeon, we found that lower midline defects are easier to address by initiating the dissection in the upper portion of left retrorectus space. Figure 21.15 demonstrates the typical port position that we chose to use for this approach. Balloon dissector is used at port position #1 to develop the left retrorectus space, followed by direct visualization for placement of port #2 into the developed space with an optional port #3. Blunt dissection in the left retrorectus space is performed in a caudal direction and the pubis is identified. As the upper midline has not previously been violated above the level of umbilicus, the medial aspect of the left posterior rectus sheath is incised and the preperitoneal space entered just superficial to falciform ligament (Fig. 21.16). The right posterior rectus sheath is identified and

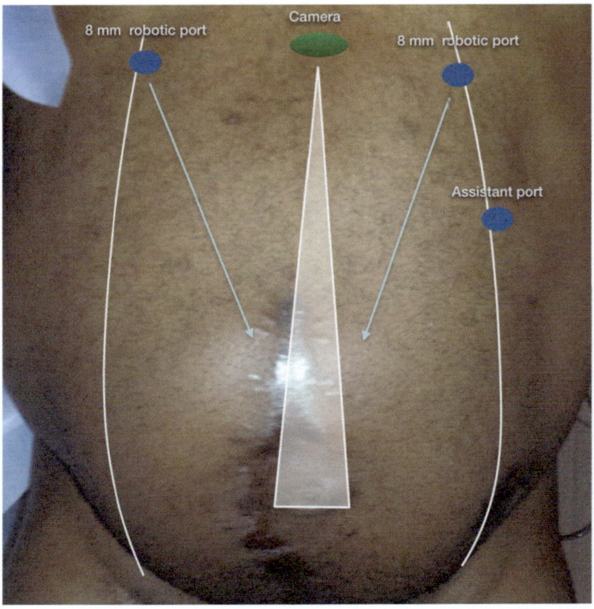

Fig. 21.15 Port placement for a right-handed surgeon addressing a lower midline defects. We initiate the dissection in the upper portion of left retrorectus space. Balloon dissector is used at port position #1 (green elipse) to develop the left retrorectus space, followed by direct visualization for placement of port #2 (blue circle)into the developed space with an optional port #3 for assistant. The left side port is positioned after the cross-over

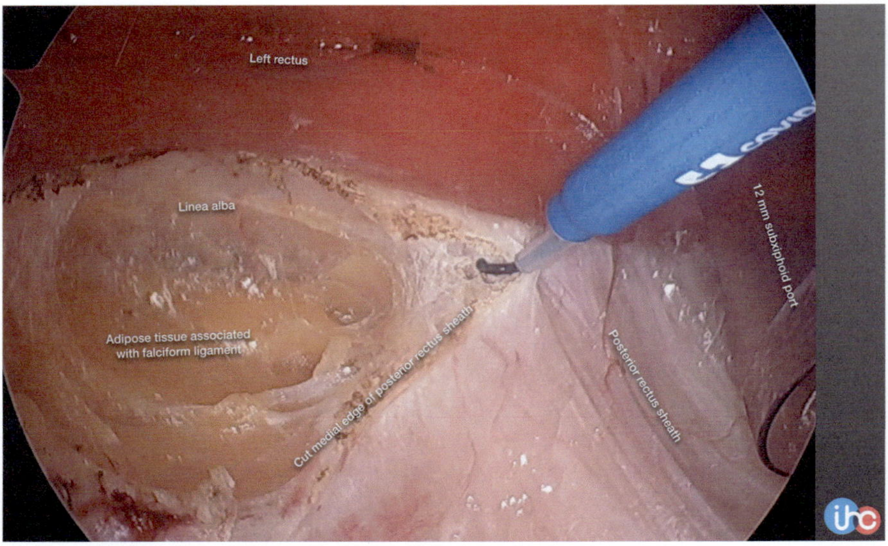

Fig. 21.16 Medial aspect of the left posterior rectus sheath is incised and the preperitoneal space entered just superficial to falciform ligament

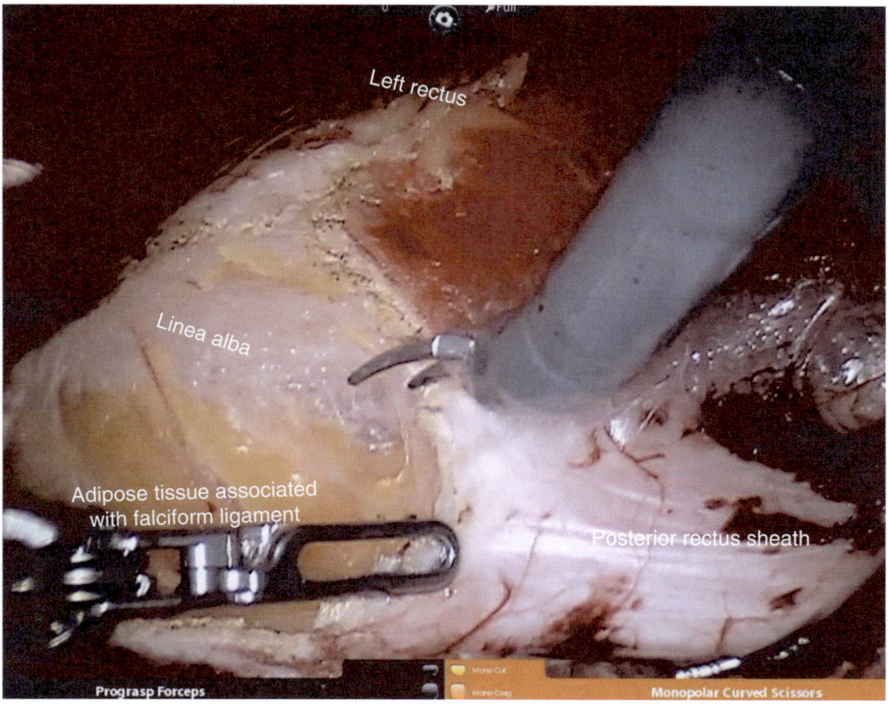

Fig. 21.17 The right posterior rectus sheath is identified and its medial aspect incised then released in a cephalad to caudal direction followed by blunt dissection in the right retrorectus space

its medial aspect incised and released in a cephalad to caudal direction followed by blunt dissection in the right retrorectus space (Fig. 21.17). Port #4 is then placed under direct vision through the upper aspect of right rectus abdominis muscle which is then used as the camera port. The retrorectus dissection is carried out in the caudal direction completing bilateral release of the posterior rectus sheathes. When encountering the hernia sac we try to sharply dissect the distal attachments, thus mobilizing it downward. Alternatively, the sac can be sharply entered and laparoscopic adhesiolysis performed as needed. The closure of the posterior and anterior fascias are performed as similar manner as described previously, as well the mesh positioning.

21.3.5 Side-Docking

For patients with xipho-pubic defects, a side-docking is prefered, once no virgin regions are available for a easier cross-over. The ports set-up are illustrated on Fig. 21.18. We initiate with the superior trocar to create bluntly the retro-rectus

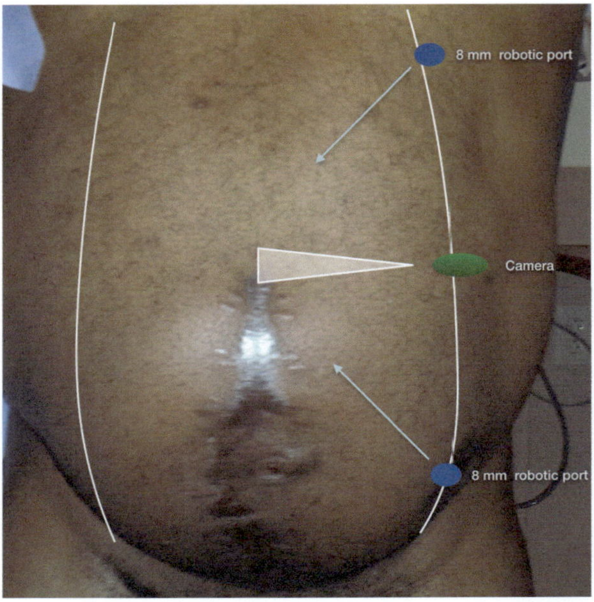

Fig. 21.18 Port set-up for side docking. First superior trocar is positioned high on the left rectus sheet and the retro-rectus space created to position the 12 mm camera port (green ellipse) and the second working trocar

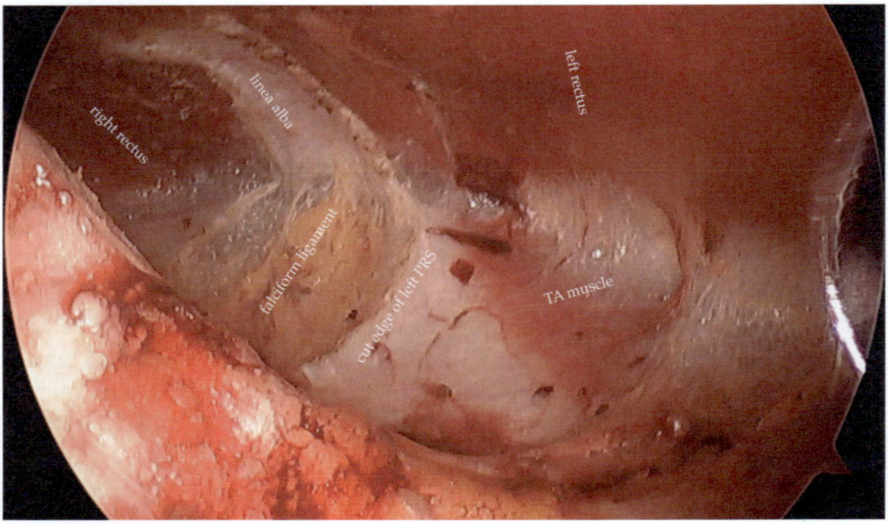

Fig. 21.19 Cross-over view on top of the facilform from the left side

space, following the positioning of the other lateral ports. The cross-over is done with the robotic instruments (Fig. 21.19). Once both retro-rectus spaces are created, the closure and mesh positioning follow the previous described techniques.

21.4 Conclusion

MIS for ventral hernias have been changing for the last few years, with a clear trend to reproduce traditional open techniques and avoiding IPOM meshes. As happens with the open techniques, there is no one gold standard, but each different approach described in this chapter has its own indications and contra-indications. The role of the surgeons is to analyze and decide the best technique for each patient.

References

1. Halm JA, de Wall LL, Steyerberg EW, Jeekel J, Lange JF. Intraperitoneal polypropylene mesh hernia repair complicates subsequent abdominal surgery. World J Surg. 2007;31(2):423–9.
2. Patel PP, Love MW, Ewing JA, Warren JA, Cobb WS, Carbonell A. Risks of subsequent abdominal operations after laparoscopic ventral hernia repair. Surg Endosc. 2017;31(2): 823–8.
3. Warren JA, Carbonel AM. Robotic ventral hernia repair. In: Hope W, Cobb W, Adrales G, editors. Textbook of hernia. Cham: Springer International; 2017. p. 381–94.
4. Warren JA, Cobb WS, Ewing JA, Carbonell AM. Standard laparoscopic versus robotic retromuscular ventral hernia repair. Surg Endosc. 2017;31(1):324–32.
5. Earle D, Roth JS, Saber A, et al. SAGES guidelines for laparoscopic ventral hernia repair. Surg Endosc. 2016;30(8):3163–83.
6. Sanchez-Manuel FJ, Lozano-Garcia J, Seco-Gil JL. Antibiotic prophylaxis for hernia repair. Cochrane Database Syst Rev. 2012;(2):CD003769.
7. Hull RD, Brant RF, Pineo GF, Stein PD, Raskob GE, Valentine KA. Preoperative vs postoperative initiation of low-molecular-weight heparin prophylaxis against venous thromboembolism in patients undergoing elective hip replacement. Arch Intern Med. 1999;159(2):137–41.
8. Venturi ML, Davison SP, Caprini JA. Prevention of venous thromboembolism in the plastic surgery patient: current guidelines and recommendations. Aesthet Surg J. 2009;29(5):421–8.
9. Daes J. The enhanced view-totally extraperitoneal technique for repair of inguinal hernia. Surg Endosc. 2012;26(4):1187–9.
10. Belyansky I, Radu VG, Balasubra-manian R, Zahiri HR, Weltz AS. A novel approach using the enhanced-view totally extraperitoneal (eTEP) technique for laparoscopic retromuscular hernia repair. Surg Endosc. 2018;32(3):1525–32.
11. Ghali S, Turza KC, Baumann DP, Butler CE. Minimally invasive component separation results in fewer wound-healing complications than open component separation for large ventral hernia repairs. J Am Coll Surg. 2012;214(6):981–9.
12. Belyansky I, Zahiri HR, Park A. Laparoscopic transversus abdominis release, a novel minimally invasive approach to complex abdominal wall reconstruction. Surg Innov. 2016;23(2):134–41.

Robotic Transversus Abdominus Release 22

David Bernstein and Garth R. Jacobsen

22.1 Introduction

Advanced abdominal wall reconstruction has seen a great evolution in recent decades. It is a burgeoning field, growing rapidly in breadth and procedural complexity, and with it, a growing evidence-based foundation. However, as with any surgical field where a major consideration for success or failure is largely determined by the incidence or absence of recurrence, and where this determination is made on the order of years to decades, we find ourselves advancing at a speed far greater than our evidence can keep pace. As a result, much of our clinical and operative decision-making is based on theoretical, albeit increasingly well understood principals of anatomy, physiology and biomechanics.

The adoption of minimally invasive techniques in hernia surgery has had more of an impact on operative design than arguably any other general surgery discipline. The advancement and popularization of minimally invasive inguinal and ventral hernia repairs has been achieved via novel approaches that do not merely decrease the length of incisions, but employ unique reconstructive principals, and as such have the potential for far greater impact on outcomes.

The adoption and advancement of robotic surgery represents a continuation of this trend and is poised to have a remarkable impact on this evolution. The employment of robotics in hernia surgery has the potential to further the progression of the field perhaps more than any other area of general surgery.

The robotic transversus abdominus release (rTAR) is a relatively novel procedure that has rapidly gained popularity in the field of hernia surgery and abdominal wall reconstruction. The procedure as a whole represents the culmination of a number of fundamental advancements made in the field through the last century; this

D. Bernstein · G. R. Jacobsen (✉)
Department of Surgery, Division of Minimally Invasive Surgery, UC San Diego Medical Center, San Diego, CA, USA
e-mail: Gjacobsen@ucsd.edu

K. A. LeBlanc (ed.), *Robotic Assisted Hernia Repair*,
https://doi.org/10.1007/978-3-030-23025-8_22

includes the advent of the robotic platform in general, as well as each elemental shift in our understanding of just how far it is possible to manipulate the structure of the abdominal wall.

In this chapter, we describe the historical context that brought about the emergence of this procedure, as well as the details surrounding the perioperative care and surgical technique.

22.2 Historical Context

22.2.1 Development of the Component Separation

To understand the recent popularization of the TAR technique one needs to view it in the context of the historical advancement of complex abdominal wall reconstruction. Arguably one of the most important breakthroughs in abdominal wall reconstructive techniques came about in the early twentieth century with the conceptual development of the relaxing incision and component separation. First described by Gibson in 1916 [1] as an external oblique relaxing incision, and then further modified by Young [2] in the 1960s by expounding on the concept of the myofascial release. In the early 1990s, Ramirez et al. [3] introduced the practice of undermining the plane between the external and internal oblique fascia to create additional abdominal wall laxity and coined the term "component separation". This technique, now commonly described as an anterior component separation (ACS), allowed for the restoration of abdominal wall function through medialization and re-establishment of the midline fascia in patients with large hernias defects that could not otherwise be approximated. This technique served to help mitigate the difficult burden—born by patients and surgeons alike—of managing an open abdomen after major abdominal trauma or emergency laparotomy.

22.2.2 Limitations of the Anterior Component Separation

The ACS, however, was not without its drawbacks. Due to the requisite subcutaneous dissection, wound complications represent a major source of morbidity, with reported infection rates ranging between 25% and 57% [4], and a similar overall complication rate [5, 6]. The ACS technique is also limited in its utility in treating larger subxiphoid and suprapubic defects as their proximity and fascial attachment to the costal margin and pelvic bones, respectively, limit the extent to which the fascia can be medialized. These shortcomings were tempered with the development of minimally invasive techniques such as endoscopic, or perforator-sparing ACS, however overall complication rates remain high [4, 7].

22.2.3 The Rives-Stoppa Repair

In the 1960s, the contributions of Jean Rives and Rene Stoppa led to the development of what is now often considered the gold standard of mesh-reinforced autologous tissue repair. The Rives-Stoppa (RS) technique employs the principle of component separation introduced by Ramirez but does so in the retrorectus space [8, 9]. This innovation allowed for significant medialization of the midline fascia—up to 10 cm at the mid-abdomen—and a plane for mesh placement that is protected from both the abdominal viscera and the external environment. Mesh placement in the retro-rectus space also obviates the need for wide subcutaneous tunneling, a likely benefit with regards to wound complications [7, 10–13]. While RS repair and other sublay mesh techniques are generally preferred over an onlay mesh placement used with ACS, the literature comparing the RS repair and ACS is limited and without definitive consensus. It is generally agreed that each technique has legitimate indications and should be called upon when appropriate [10–13].

While the RS repair remains a mainstay in the hernia surgeon's armamentarium, it too has its limitations. Despite the significant improvement in the ability to medialize the fascia, wider defects that do not lend themselves to midline closure with a RS repair alone would require a bridging prosthesis, a less than ideal scenario in terms of both wound complication and abdominal wall function [12]. Additionally, for hernias with lateral margins close to the linea semilunaris, sufficient lateral mesh overlap becomes limited.

22.2.4 Posterior Component Separation

To combat this shortcoming, lateral dissection techniques were developed to facilitate additional laxity and medial mobilization. This involved creating pre-peritoneal planes, or by extending the component separation dissection beyond the linea semilunaris to include the plane between the internal oblique and transversus abdominis musculature [14]. These techniques were limited by the presence of scarring or inflammation in the case of the former, or by concern for potential damage to the neurovascular (NV) bundles in the latter [15].

22.2.5 Posterior Component with Transverse Abdominus Release

In 2012, Novitsky et al. published their experience with a novel technique that utilized the RS repair with a transversus abdominus releasing incision [16]. This clever modification allowed for wide extension of the retrorectus dissection that could be taken as far lateral as the psoas muscles without risking injury to the NV bundle, and providing a more robust posterior fascial layer in which to lay a prosthesis. This dissection could also extend further cranio-caudally than an ACS and is therefore more useful for hernias with subxiphoid and/or suprapubic components. This technique which came to be known as the posterior component separation with transversus abdominus release (TAR) proved highly useful, quickly becoming a mainstay of complex abdominal wall reconstructive techniques.

In their 2012 case series of 42 patients, Novitsky et al., reported a 24% wound complication rate with 7% of these cases required operative intervention. Their recurrence rate was 4.7%, with a median follow-up of 26 months; 86% percent of patients were followed beyond 1 year [16].

In 2016, Novitsky et al. reported subsequent outcome data for TARs performed on 428 patients with an average BMI of 34.4, the majority of whom had recurrent hernias. For patients with at least 12 months follow-up (mean 31.5 months) the recurrence rate was 3.7%. Surgical site events (SSE) occurred in 18.7% of patients; surgical site infections (SSI) occurred in 9.1%; approximately 7% required intervention beyond antibiotics [17].

Comparative analysis of reconstructive techniques is difficult to perform. The results of systematic reviews, meta-analyses, and expert consensus panels are often bridled with the caveat that study heterogeneity limits the ability to draw definitive conclusions. This heterogeneity often relates to differences in technical nuance, mesh type, follow-up period, and definition of recurrence (i.e. imaging-based, patient reported, physical exam, etc.). With that in mind, these studies may still provide some insight into the values and shortcomings associated with different reconstructive options.

Cornette et al., published a systematic review comparing open ACS, endoscopic/laparoscopic ACS, perforator preserving ACS, and TAR. They found no significant different in rates of SSE between procedures, with means ranging from 16% to 23.7%. The only significant difference in recurrence rates were found between open ACS and TAR (11.9% vs. 5.3%, $p < 0.001$), with mean follow-up ranging from 17 to 22 months [18].

Hodgkinson et al., published a meta-analysis comparing open ACS and TAR for midline ventral hernias. Pooled analysis of recurrence rates was 9.5% for open ACS and 5.7% for TAR; however, on comparative analysis these differences were not statistically significant. Similar results were found regarding wound complications, re-operation rates, placement of bridging mesh, and length of stay (LOS) [19]. Again, the authors of both reports cite lack of randomized control trials, and significant heterogeneity amongst pooled studies as considerable limitations.

22.2.6 Minimally Invasive Approaches

The value of minimally invasive approaches to ventral hernia repair has been well-established offering improved recovery times, fewer wound complications, and comparable recurrence rates [20–24]. It is therefore no surprise that within only a few years a minimally invasive (MIS) TAR technique was sought after. In 2016 Belyansky et al., published the first report of an MIS approach to the PCS-TAR procedure. In this case series of 3 patients there were no major intraoperative or early post-operative complications, mean operative time was 329 min and there were no reported wound complications. While this demonstrated the technical feasibility of an MIS approach, the laparoscopic repair may pose a significant technical challenge for surgeons who lack advanced MIS training.

A robotic platform was the obvious contender as the preferred minimally invasive approach to the TAR procedure. Robotic surgery provides improved visualization and dexterity allowing for more precise dissection, easier and more efficient intracorporeal suturing, and superior ergonomics.

Given the relatively recent incorporation of the robotic platform amongst hernia surgeons, outcomes have been reported in only a handful of studies. One of the first studies looking at robotic ventral hernia repair was by Warren et al., comparing laparoscopic and robotic ventral hernia repairs (VHR) using data collected from the Americas Hernia Society Quality Collaborative (AHSQC), a prospectively maintained database. In the laparoscopic group(n = 103), mesh was placed intraperitoneally in 90.3% of cases, the remainder were preperitoneal or retromuscular. In the robotic arm(n = 53), mesh was placed in an extraperitoneal position in 96% of cases, ~70% retromuscular, 26.4% pre-peritoneal and a TAR procedure was performed in 43.4% of cases. Average defect size was similar between laparoscopic VHR and Robotic VHR (6.9 cm vs. 6.5 cm, $p = 0.508$). Patient demographics were otherwise similar between the two groups with the exception of age, in that patients in the laparoscopic group were slightly older (60 vs. 53 years, $p = 0.001$). When comparing outcomes, robotic VHRs had a longer operative time (245.6 ± 98.5 vs. 121.5 ± 57.2 min, $p < 0.001$), decreased LOS (1 vs. 2 days, $p = 0.004$), and a higher rate of fascial closure (96% vs. 50.5%, $p < 0.001$). SSEs were more common in the robotic group (53% vs 18.5%, $p < 0.001$); however, the vast majority of these were seromas that did not require intervention. There was no difference in SSI rates, perioperative complications, narcotic use, readmissions, or re-operations [25].

Carbonell et al., utilizing data from the AHSQC, compared open(n = 111) vs. robotic(n = 222) retromuscular ventral hernia repair (RVHR), with LOS as a primary outcome. TAR procedures were performed in 83% and 85% of open and robotic groups, respectively. They reported a decreased LOS in the robotic group (2 days vs 3 days, $p < 0.001$). Analysis of secondary outcomes showed no difference in SSI rate, intraoperative complications, or 30-day re-admissions. SSEs were more common in the robotic group, the majority of which were seromas that did not require intervention [26].

In a retrospective review by Bittner et al., outcomes of a single surgeon's experience comparing open(oTAR) vs. robotic TAR(rTAR) were reported. Patient demographics were similar between groups except for diabetes, being significantly greater in the oTAR group (29% vs. 0%, $p = 0.04$). There was no significant difference in SSI or SSE rates between cohorts. Operative time was longer in the robotic arm (287 ± 121 vs. 365 ± 78 min, $p < 0.01$), and LOS was shorter (6.7 ± 4.3 vs. 3.5 ± 0.9 days, $p < 0.01$). oTAR trended toward higher overall morbidity, without reaching statistical significance (39.2 vs. 19.2%, $P = 0.09$) [27].

Martin-del-campo et al., performed a comparison of 38 consecutively performed rTARs with a case-matched historic cohort of oTARs performed at two specialized hernia surgery centers. Cohort demographics were similar with two notable exceptions, patients in the oTAR group had a greater proportion of recurrent hernias, and ASA class III patients. Similar to other comparisons, they found longer operative times (299 ± 95 vs. 211 ± 63 min, $p < 0.001$) and a shorter LOS (1.3 ± 1.3 vs. 6.0 ± 3.4 days, $p < 0.001$) in the rTAR group. There was no difference in SSE or SSI rate between groups. Blood loss was significantly reduced in the rTAR group (49 ± 60 vs. 139 ± 149 mL, $p < 0.001$). The rTAR group had no reported postoperative complications (excluding SSEs) compared to a 17.1% complication rate in the oTAR group (p = 0.007). Complications included urinary tract infections, ileus, venous thromboembolism, and pneumonia.

22.2.7 Operative Considerations

Surgeons who elect to perform major abdominal wall reconstruction need to be flexible in their approach, given that the presence of scarring or poor tissue quality, accidental bowel injury, and/or newly discovered pathology may alter the initial operative plan. The surgeon will need to be familiar with varying techniques and be able to call upon them when clinically indicated.

22.2.8 Patient Selection

Proper patient selection is of crucial importance when performing any major abdominal wall reconstruction; perhaps more so when considering a robotic approach. Considerations include defect size, overlying skin condition, loss of domain, and myofascial anatomy as identified by cross sectional imaging.

Generally, patients with moderate-to-large sized defects not suitable for a laparoscopic intraperitoneal onlay mesh(IPOM) approach, and without significant loss of domain that would necessitate an open repair are considered candidates for rTAR. Relative contraindications include the likelihood of severe intra-abdominal adhesions, complete loss of domain, need for panniculectomy, and extensive prior disruption of the retromuscular and/or TAR planes. In patients with a history of prior anterior myofascial release, rTAR as well as open TAR should be carefully considered as this may lead to lateral abdominal wall laxity as the only remaining lateral abdominal muscular group would be the internal oblique. Patients should be made aware of this possibility, and that they may experience lateral bulging and abdominal wall disfunction. With that in mind, patients with recurrent hernias after ACS may have limited reconstructive options and the TAR has been shown to be an effective option [28], though long-term data is not yet available. Absolute contraindications include inability to tolerate laparoscopy, and the presence of any comorbidities which would inhibit the patient from tolerating a major operation under general anesthesia.

22.3 Pre-Operative Planning

Appropriate pre-operative planning is perhaps the most important—and often neglected—aspect of any type of major abdominal wall reconstruction. We begin our work-up with a detailed history focusing on prior surgical procedures, relevant comorbidities such as diabetes mellitus (DM), obstructive sleep apnea (OSA), smoking history, steroid use. Physical exam focuses on assessing abdominal wall function, skin condition, evaluation for significant diastasis recti, previous surgical incisions, and additional hernias. It is important to identify and document any evidence of pre-operative muscular dysfunction commonly seen in post-spinal or kidney surgery patients. If evident, patients should be made aware of the possibility of worsening lateral dysfunction and/or bulging after surgery.

It is our practice to obtain axial imaging on all patients who may require a rTAR. Our preference is CT abdomen and pelvis, and unless looking for other intra-abdominal pathology, contrast is unnecessary. Imaging allows us to determine the condition of the relevant abdominal wall components, to identify anatomical concerns regarding access to the intraperitoneal space, and to get a sense of the amount of pre-operative weight loss to recommend to patients based on the perceived intra-abdominal volume relative to the volume of the hernia sac. It also allows us to identify potentially unrelated pathology that may warrant additional workup, and possibly treatment prior to, or during, the time of surgery.

We generally do not operate on patients who are actively smoking unless there is concern for imminent incarceration. Patients are advised to quit smoking at least 6 weeks prior to surgery and routinely undergo nicotine testing. Though there is little evidence addressing the effect of marijuana use prior to surgery, we do recommend cessation of all inhaled forms of marijuana for at least 6 weeks pre-operatively. Patients with ongoing or recent history of drug abuse undergo pre-operative testing the day of surgery.

Generally speaking, all patients who are considered overweight are advised to lose weight prior to surgery. Obese patients are given a goal BMI of <30 to 32. Morbidly obese patients who are unable to lose significant weight pre-operatively, and who are not severely symptomatic or have concerns for imminent incarceration are referred to our weight management team and, when appropriate, bariatric surgery.

Patients with uncontrolled diabetes are referred to their primary care physician, and in severe cases to an endocrinologist to assist in their glucose management. Malnutrition is a risk factor for mortality and incisional hernia after major abdominal surgery. Measures should be taken to evaluate and treat at-risk patients prior to undergoing a major reconstruction. Referral to a nutrition specialist should be considered in select patients [29, 30].

22.4 Technique

While there are several techniques which can be employed robotically to undertake a robotic transversus abdominus release, this chapter will focus on a transabdominal approach. It will also be very helpful for the surgeon embarking on the below techniques to be very familiar with the performance of the open transversus abdominus releases.

22.4.1 Patient Preparation and Positioning

1. The patient is laid supine on the operating table. After induction of general anesthesia, a urinary catheter is placed. The patient is positioned with the bed slightly flexed to increase the distance between the anterior superior iliac spine

(ASIS) and the costal margin to allow for additional space for trocar placement. Both arms are tucked, and padding is placed over the hands to protect against contact with the robotic arms. In this regard, the bedside assistant plays an important role in ensuring the patient is protected and not incurring any injury during the procedure. It can also be helpful to drop the arms below the level of the table to minimize contact between the robot and the extremities. Care should be taken to support the elbows and the wrists appropriately. Straps are placed across the hips and chest. We also make sure the face is padded with either a Mayo stand placed directly above the face or with the use of a specialized face pad.

2. The patient is prepped and draped from the nipples to the upper thigh, and laterally beyond the midaxillary line.
3. Pre-operative antibiotics are administered, usually a first generation cephalosporin.

22.4.2 Abdominal Access and Adhesiolysis

4. The method of abdominal access should be based on surgeon experience and comfort. The access site is determined again by surgeon comfort and prior incisions if present. With the use of the Si robotic platform, we prefer a left upper quadrant (LUQ) 5 mm optical trocar entry with a laparoscope. For the Xi platform, we use the 8 mm robotic camera with the corresponding optical trocar. Preoperative CT imaging can be particularly helpful in the determination of the initial access location, favoring areas that do not have bowel directly abutting the access site. If the access site is to be used as the right or left arm access port, consideration should be made to have this incision as lateral as the surgeon is comfortable with. This is usually at or about the anterior axillary line. Safe access is always the best access, so the site should be selected on this principle with additional ports placed later for the robotic system.
5. Once abdominal access is achieved the intraperitoneal space is assessed and adhesiolysis is performed to allow for additional trocar placement. The robotic platform allows for an incredible advantage in regard to adhesiolysis when compared to traditional laparoscopy and may even rival the open approach.

22.4.3 Trocar Placement

6. Additional trocars are placed equidistant from one another along the mid- and anterior axillary lines triangulated towards the center of the hernia sac. Trocars should be placed as lateral as possible while allowing for clearance of the robotic arm to avoid contact with the patient or the edge of the operating table (Fig. 22.1).
7. When using the Xi platform, one must keep in mind that at least one 12–15 mm trocar must be placed to allow for mesh insertion, this can be done by nesting an 8 mm port into a large diameter trocar or by placing an accessory/assist port. The latter provides the additional benefit of quick and easy insertion and

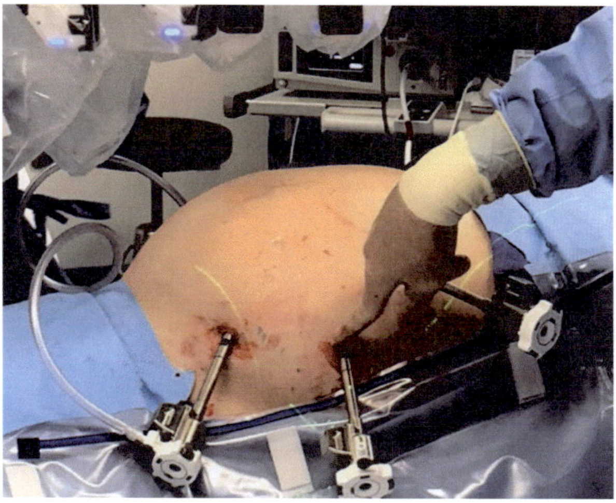

Fig. 22.1 Trocars are placed equidistant from each other along the mid- and anterior axillary lines, triangulated towards the center of the hernia defect

removal of sutures, suctioning devices, assistant retraction, etc. The Si robot requires a 12 mm camera port which can be used for mesh placement, however it is still our practice to place an assist port for the above listed benefits.

22.4.4 Docking

8. rTARs are most commonly performed using a double-dock technique. There are multiple docking orientations that can be used depending on the robotic platform, the available operating room space, and surgeon preference. Our preference when using the Si platform is for the robot to be positioned at a 90° angle to the operating table. The contralateral dock can be accomplished by maneuvering the robot, or by turning the patient. In either case, it is important to discuss the docking plan with the operating room staff and anesthesia team to allow for appropriate preparation.

   A primary advantage of the Xi platform is the incorporation of a rotating boom. This allows for re-docking without having to reposition the surgical cart. When the Xi platform is available, we prefer a low-lateral dock whereby the robot is positioned towards the foot of the bed lateral to, and in-line with the patient. This allows for appropriate positioning while providing the bedside assistant and operating technicians additional space to maneuver.

22.4.5 Retromuscular Dissection

9. Once trocar placement and docking are completed, additional adhesiolysis and sac reduction are performed robotically.
10. There are several useful robotic instruments commonly used to facilitate retromuscular dissection and component separation. We prefer a Prograsp forceps

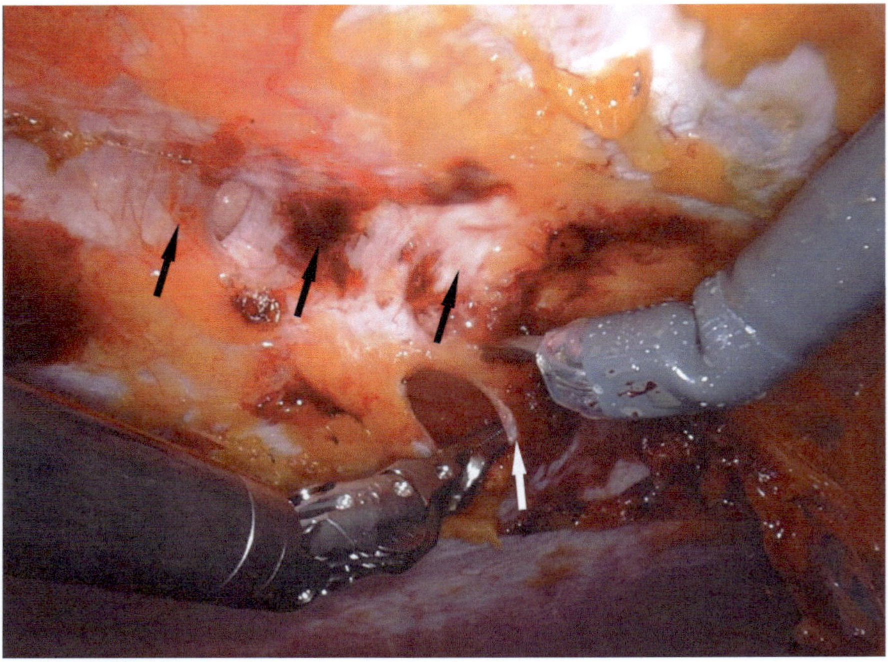

Fig. 22.2 The retromuscular dissection is initiated by incising the posterior sheath (white arrow) just lateral to the linea alba (black arrows) and ~5 to 10 cm superior to the hernia defect (not shown)

and a monopolar curved scissors for the left and right arms, respectively. Recently released is the Force Bipolar grasper which allows the surgeon to modulate the grasping strength from once which it would be safe to grab bowel, and a more aggressive grip useful for pulling on fascia or peritoneum. If available, this is the instrument of choice opposite the scissors.

11. The right sided retromuscular dissection is initiated by incising the posterior rectus sheath approximately 5–10 cm superior to the hernia defect and about 1 cm lateral to the linea alba (Fig. 22.2). In cases involving significant diastasis or an attenuated linea alba the surgeon may elect to initiate the dissection more superiorly. This "top-down" approach is then continued inferiorly beyond the caudal margin of the defect.
12. As the dissection proceeds inferiorly the arcuate line is encountered and incised from its connection to the linea alba (Fig. 22.3). Care should be taken to maintain a preperitoneal dissection plane in this region to avoid injury to the inferior epigastric vessels which travel along the posterior aspect of the rectus muscle in the pre-transversalis plane.
13. The retromuscular plane is then dissected out laterally using mostly blunt dissection until the medial edge of the linea semilunaris is encountered. Care should be taken not to injure the neurovascular bundles as they are encountered as this may result in denervation and ischemia of the rectus muscle (Fig. 22.4).

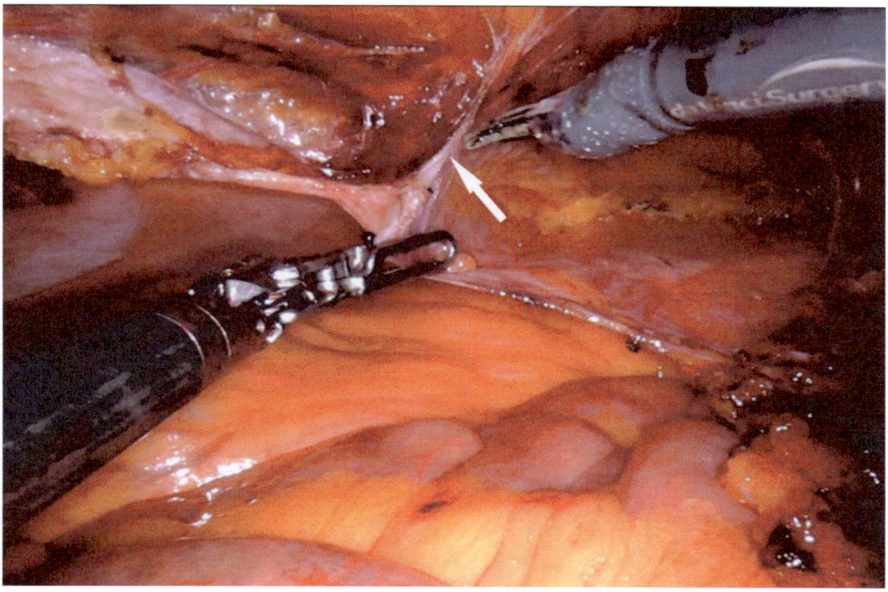

Fig. 22.3 Incision of the medial attachments of the arcuate line (arrow) as they are encountered in the "top-down" and "Bottom-up" (depicted here) dissection

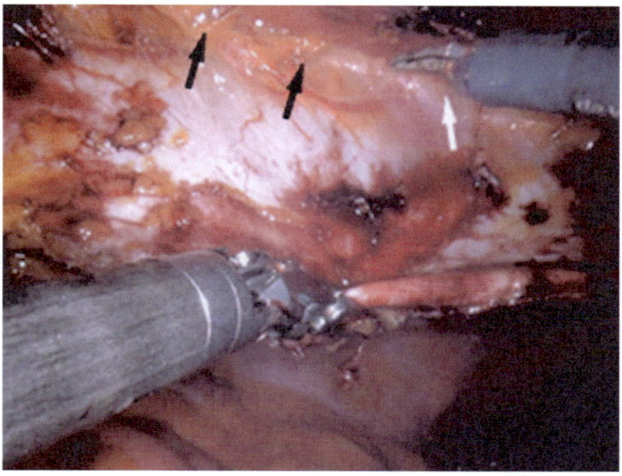

Fig. 22.4 Completed retromuscular dissection, showing medial border of the linea semilunaris (white arrow) with neurovascular bundles (black arrows)

22.4.6 Transversus Abdominis Release

14. The transversus abdominis release is then performed. As described by Novitsky et al. [16], the transversus abdominis (TA) muscle fibers extend medially beyond the linea semilunaris; this overlap is most pronounced in the upper third of the abdomen. This key anatomic distinction allows for entry into the lateral pre-peritoneal plane without disrupting the linea semilunaris or the neurovascular supply to the rectus muscle.

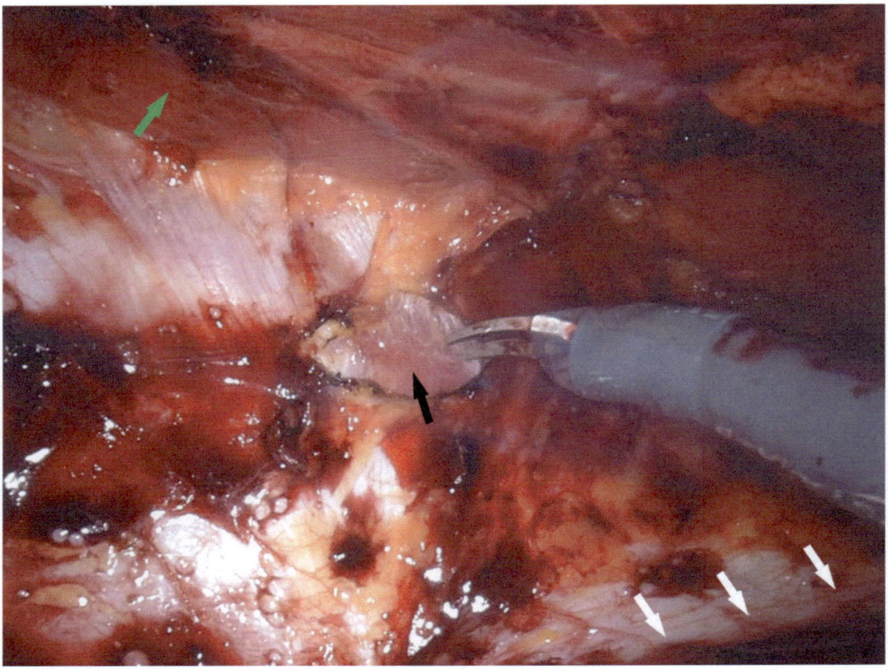

Fig. 22.5 Initiation of the TA release. The TA fascia is incised just medial to the NV bundles, exposing the TA muscle (black arrow) beneath. White arrows depicting the medial border of the posterior rectus sheath

The dissection is initiated by incising the TA fascia just medial to the neurovascular bundles in the upper third of the abdomen (Fig. 22.5). This will expose the underlying TA muscle fibers which are also incised, taking care not to violate the peritoneum beneath.

The pre-peritoneal plane can be developed as far lateral as the psoas muscle to achieve midline closure. Once the preperitoneal plane is developed at this level, it is often easier to extend the plane inferiorly by first creating a lateral pre-peritoneal tunnel, and then simply incising the medially connecting fascia. This same concept is utilized on the contralateral side in the opposing direction i.e. "bottom-up" dissection (Fig. 22.6).

To ensure an adequate dissection has been performed the posterior sheath should be seen to lay slack over the abdominal viscera.

22.4.7 Mesh Sizing and Contralateral Trocar Insertion

15. Once the dissection on the right is completed, contralateral trocars are placed in an opposing orientation. These trocars are inserted directly into the newly created pre-peritoneal space. Some surgeons also prefer to insert the mesh at this time.

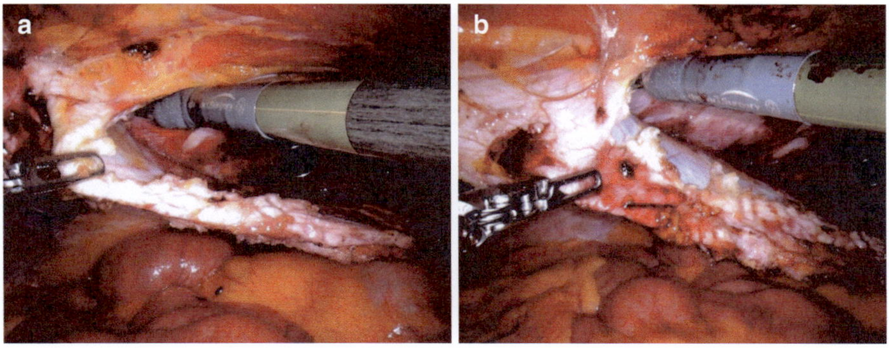

Fig. 22.6 (**a**) Creation of a lateral pre-peritoneal tunnel prior to incising the adjacent TA fascia and muscle. (**b**) After tunneling, the incision of TA fascia and muscle fibers is easily achieved

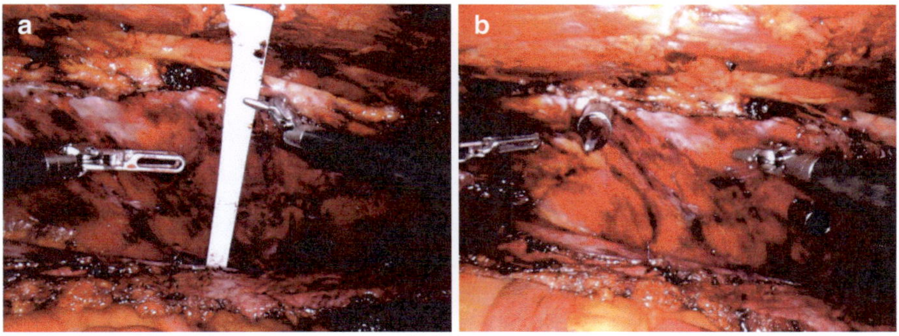

Fig. 22.7 (**a**) The mesh width is determined by measuring the distance from the lateral edge of the dissection plane to the midline. (**b**) Contralateral trocars are placed directly into the pre-peritoneal plane

16. The cranio-caudal dimension of the hernia defect is measured to ensure adequate superior and inferior overlap. The width of the mesh is determined by doubling the distance between the lateral border of dissection plane and the patient's midline (Fig. 22.7).

22.4.8 Contralateral Dissection

17. After the robot is docked on the patient's right side, contralateral dissection proceeds according to the same basic principles. We prefer to use the "bottom-up" approach for the left sided dissection however a "top-down" approach can also be utilized. As the TAR dissection proceeds the original trocars are encountered and need to be retracted and then advanced into the pre-peritoneal plane. We routinely suture the peritoneal defects closed, as well as any other defects in the posterior lamella that may have occurred during the procedure (Fig. 22.8).

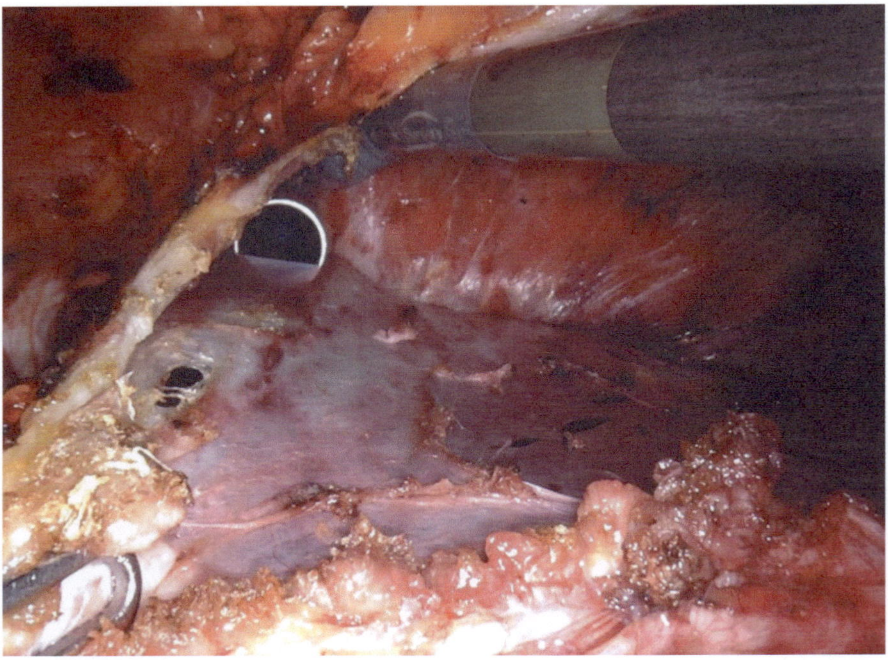

Fig. 22.8 Contralateral trocars encountered during TAR dissection are re-positioned

22.4.9 Fascial Closure

18. After completion of the TAR on the left, we attempt closure of the hernia defect, as well as any significant diastasis, using a 0-PDS barbed suture (Fig. 22.9). This is followed by closure of the posterior sheath using a 2-0 absorbable barbed suture (Fig. 22.10).

22.4.10 Mesh and Drain Placement

19. Once the posterior sheath is closed the mesh is positioned to lay flat and even over the posterior sheath. The mesh can be left as is or can be fixated using a tacking device, sutures, or glue, depending on surgeon preference (Fig. 22.11).
20. Once the mesh is positioned, a drain is routinely placed to prevent fluid accumulation and subsequent seroma formation. We prefer to use a single 19Fr Blake Drain (Ethicon, Inc., Somerville, NJ). Once the drain is positioned and secured to the skin, insufflation is released, trocars are removed, and the procedure is concluded.

22.4.11 Post-Operative Care

The care pathways for robotic component separation at our institution are very similar if not identical to those involved in our open component separation pathway.

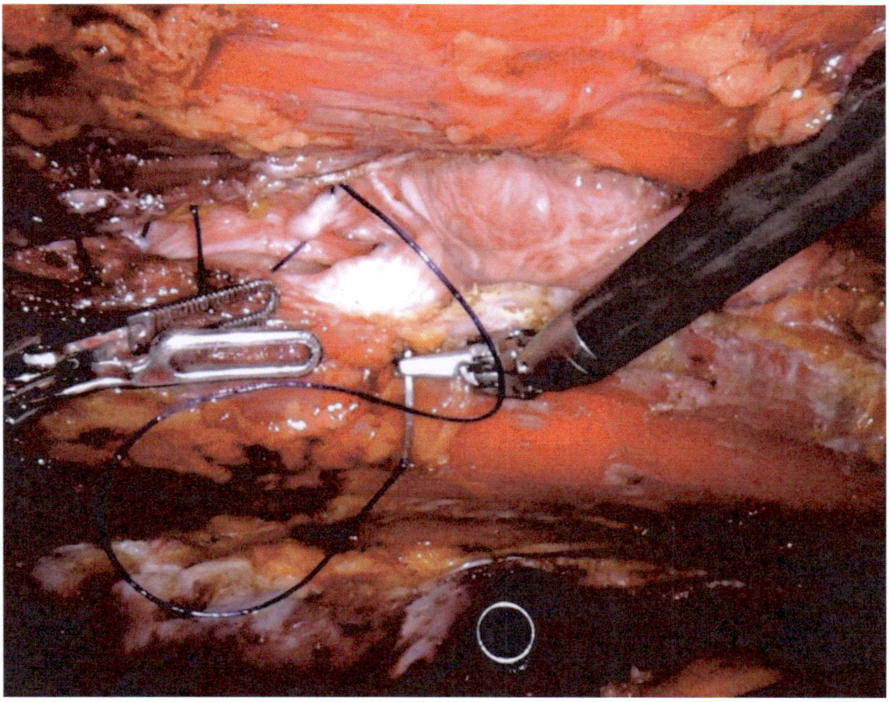

Fig. 22.9 Closure of the hernia defect

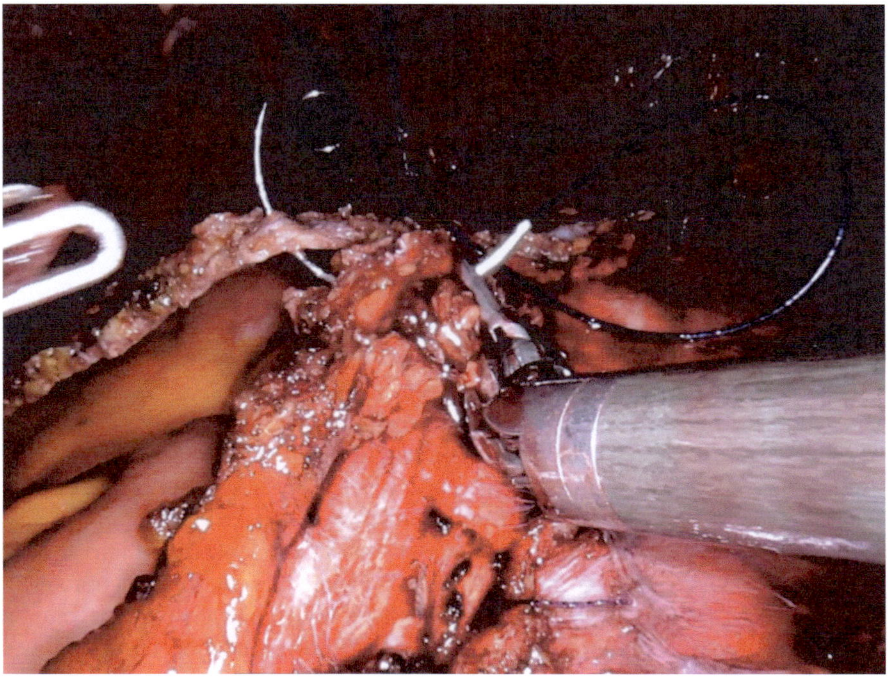

Fig. 22.10 Closure of the posterior sheath

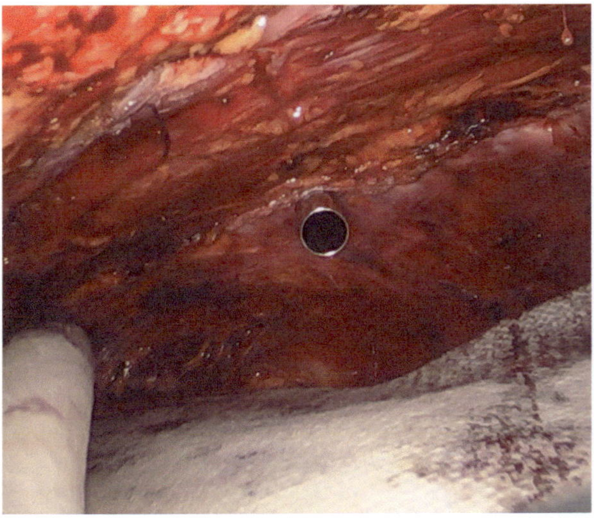

Fig. 22.11 Mesh placement above the closed posterior sheet, Pictured GORE® SYNECOR Preperitoneal Biomaterial

However, we have noted that setting expectations in the clinic preoperatively is an essential component of any enhanced recovery pathway. For open component separations we have traditionally informed the patients that their stay will be between 3 and 5 days on average. We have noted a significant decrease in the length of stay for our robotic group and inform them that we are currently averaging two to three days.

As with any component separation it is critical to monitor patients for sign of abdominal compartment syndrome. This is more likely in patients with massive loss of domain, whom likely would not have been placed into the robotic pathway in the first place, but it is certainly possible with larger defects. These patients will develop evidence of decreased end organ perfusion which is usually hallmarked by a decrease in urine output and culminates in respiratory failure if not recognized. We do prefer to remove any drain placed directly in contact with the mesh before discharge.

22.5 Conclusions

Over the last two decades the techniques employed in abdominal wall reconstruction have evolved at a rapid pace. Surgeons inclined to harness the power of laparoscopy immediately set upon the repair of larger and larger defects with the goal of decreasing the overall morbidity of these repairs. The technique of the intraperitoneal onlay was perfected, and devices were developed to aid in mesh fixation (tackers) and biomaterials evolved for intra-abdominal placement. The robot, while available since the early part of the century, was largely ignored. The reasons are unclear but were likely secondary to access and cost. While the laparoscopic repairs did offer a satisfactory solution in most cases, many have looked to improve upon the bridging nature of these repairs and provide a more reconstructive option.

The techniques of component separation have undergone their own evolution and the transversus abdominus release emerged as a powerful adjunct to component separation. This technique allowed for reconstruction of the linea alba with massive overlap of mesh resulting in a durable repair. However, these repairs are far from minimally invasive and carry with them all of the problems which minimally invasive surgeons have sought to minimize (wound complications, pain, long hospital stays etc.)

Recently there is increasing data that we can accomplish complex abdominal wall reconstructions utilizing the robot as an enabling technology. Certainly, the robotic transversus abdominus release as described above is technically feasible, and there are increasing data that patients at the very least have decreased lengths of stay when compared to their open counterparts. We find that our patients are also requiring less pain medications, and seem to have a lower wound complication rate, though definitive study of all of these issues is ongoing. Patient selection is however important, and those with massive loss of domain, or those with large amounts of skin which will likely need resection upon reapproximation of the muscles are likely better served by an open technique.

Finally, as a minimally invasive surgeons it is certainly exciting to see the robot allow for these complex reconstructions in a less invasive manner, and we look forward to continuing refinement and evolution of technique, as well as robust outcomes analysis to validate the true value of these efforts.

Acknowledgements Dr. Jacobsen has received honoraria from W. L. Gore and Associates to provide educational training of their products. Additionally, W. L. Gore and Associates provides financial support for the Minimally Invasive Surgery Fellowship that Dr. Jacobsen is an instructor. One of the products made by W. L. Gore and Associates was reviewed in this invited article. Dr. Bernstein has no financial interest in any of the products, devices, or drugs mentioned in this manuscript.

References

1. Gibson CL. Post-operative intestinal obstruction. Ann Surg. 1916;63:442–51.
2. Halvorson EG. On the origins of components separation. Plast Reconstr Surg. 2009;124(5):1545–9. https://doi.org/10.1097/PRS.0b013e3181b98ab8.
3. Ramirez OM, Ruas E, Dellon AL. "Components separation" method for closure of abdominal-wall defects: an anatomic and clinical study. Plast Reconstr Surg. 1990;86(3):519–26.
4. Switzer NJ, Dykstra MA, Gill RS, Lim S, Lester E, de Gara C, Shi X, Birch DW, Karmali S. Endoscopic versus open component separation: systematic review and meta-analysis. Surg Endosc. 2015;29(4):787–95. https://doi.org/10.1007/s00464-014-3741-1.
5. Tong WM, Hope W, Overby DW, Hultman CS. Comparison of outcome after mesh-only repair, laparoscopic component separation, *and open component* separation. Ann Plast Surg. 2011;66(5):551–6. https://doi.org/10.1097/SAP.0b013e31820b3c91.
6. Deerenberg EB, Timmermans L, Hogerzeil DP, Slieker JC, Eilers PH, Jeekel J, et al. A systematic review of the surgical treatment of large incisional hernia. Hernia. 2015;19(1):89–101. https://doi.org/10.1007/s10029-014-1321-x.
7. Holihan JL, Askenasy EP, Greenberg JA, Keith JN, Martindale RG, Roth JS, Mo J, Ko TC, Kao LS, Liang MK, Ventral Hernia Outcome Collaboration Writing Group. Component separation vs. bridged repair for large ventral hernias: a multi-institutional risk-adjusted comparison, systematic review, and meta-analysis. Surg Infect. 2016;17(1):17–26. https://doi.org/10.1089/sur.2015.124.

8. Rives J, Lardennois B, Pire JC, Hibon J. Large incisional hernias. The importance of flail abdomen and of subsequent respiratory disorders. Chirurgie. 1973;99(8):547–63.
9. Stoppa RE. The treatment of complicated groin and incisional hernias. World J Surg. 1989;13(5):545–54.
10. Timmermans L, de Goede B, van Dijk SM, Kleinrensink GJ, Jeekel J, Lange JF. Meta-analysis of sublay versus onlay mesh repair in incisional hernia surgery. Am J Surg. 2014;207(6):980–8. https://doi.org/10.1016/j.amjsurg.2013.08.030.
11. Muse TO, Zwischenberger BA, Miller MT, Borman DA, Davenport DL, Roth JS. Outcomes after ventral hernia repair using the Rives-Stoppa, endoscopic, and open component separation techniques. Am Surg. 2018;84(3):433–7.
12. Liang MK, Holihan JL, Itani K, Alawadi ZM, Gonzalez JR, Askenasy EP, Ballecer C, Chong HS, Goldblatt MI, Greenberg JA, Harvin JA, Keith JN, Martindale RG, Orenstein S, Richmond B, Roth JS, Szotek P, Towfigh S, Tsuda S, Vaziri K, Berger DH. Ventral hernia management: expert consensus guided by systematic review. Ann Surg. 2017;265(1):80–9. https://doi.org/10.1097/SLA.0000000000001701.
13. Albino FP, Patel KM, Nahabedian MY, Sosin M, Attinger CE, Bhanot P. Does mesh location matter in abdominal wall reconstruction? A systematic review of the literature and a summary of recommendations. Plast Reconstr Surg. 2013;132(5):1295–304. https://doi.org/10.1097/PRS.0b013e3182a4c393. Review.
14. Carbonell AM, Cobb WS, Chen SM. Posterior components separation during retromuscular hernia repair. Hernia. 2008;12(4):359–62. https://doi.org/10.1007/s10029-008-0356-2.
15. Novitsky YW. Posterior component separation via transversus abdominis muscle release: the TAR procedure. In: Novitsky YW, editor. Hernia surgery: current principles. New York: Springer; 2016. p. 15–22.
16. Novitsky YW, Elliott HL, Orenstein SB, Rosen MJ. Transversus abdominis muscle release: a novel approach to posterior component separation during complex abdominal wall reconstruction. Am J Surg. 2012;204(5):709–16. https://doi.org/10.1016/j.amjsurg.2012.02.008.
17. Novitsky YW, Fayezizadeh M, Majumder A, Neupane R, Elliott HL, Orenstein SB. Outcomes of posterior component separation with transversus abdominis muscle release and synthetic mesh sublay reinforcement. Ann Surg. 2016;264(2):226–32. https://doi.org/10.1097/SLA.0000000000001673.
18. Cornette B, De Bacquer D, Berrevoet F. Component separation technique for giant incisional hernia: a systematic review. Am J Surg. 2018;215(4):719–26. https://doi.org/10.1016/j.amjsurg.2017.07.032.
19. Hodgkinson JD, Leo CA, Maeda Y, Bassett P, Oke SM, Vaizey CJ, Warusavitarne J. A meta-analysis comparing open anterior component separation with posterior component separation and transversus abdominis release in the repair of midline ventral hernias. Hernia. 2018;22(4):617–26. https://doi.org/10.1007/s10029-018-1757-5.
20. Sauerland S, Walgenbach M, Habermalz B, Seiler CM, Miserez M. Laparoscopic versus open surgical techniques for ventral or incisional hernia repair. Cochrane Database Syst Rev. 2011;(3):CD007781. https://doi.org/10.1002/14651858.CD007781.pub2. Review.
21. DeMaria EJ, Moss JM, Sugerman HJ. Laparoscopic intraperitoneal polytetrafluoroethylene (PTFE) prosthetic patch repair of ventral hernia. Prospective comparison to open prefascial polypropylene mesh repair. Surg Endosc. 2000;14(4):326–9.
22. Carbajo MA, Martín del Olmo JC, Blanco JI, de la Cuesta C, Toledano M, Martin F, Vaquero C, Inglada L. Laparoscopic treatment vs open surgery in the solution of major incisional and abdominal wall hernias with mesh. Surg Endosc. 1999;13(3):250–2.
23. Bingener J, Buck L, Richards M, Michalek J, Schwesinger W, Sirinek K. Long-term outcomes in laparoscopic vs open ventral hernia repair. Arch Surg. 2007;142(6):562–7.
24. Pierce RA, Spitler JA, Frisella MM, Matthews BD, Brunt LM. Pooled data analysis of laparoscopic vs. open ventral hernia repair: 14 years of patient data accrual. Surg Endosc. 2007;21(3):378–86.

25. Warren JA, Cobb WS, Ewing JA, Carbonell AM. Standard laparoscopic versus robotic retromuscular ventral hernia repair. Surg Endosc. 2017;31(1):324–32. https://doi.org/10.1007/s00464-016-4975-x.
26. Carbonell AM, Warren JA, Prabhu AS, Ballecer CD, Janczyk RJ, Herrera J, Huang LC, Phillips S, Rosen MJ, Poulose BK. Reducing length of stay using a robotic-assisted approach for retromuscular ventral hernia repair: a comparative analysis from the Americas Hernia Society Quality Collaborative. Ann Surg. 2018;267(2):210–7. https://doi.org/10.1097/SLA.0000000000002244.
27. Bittner JG 4th, Alrefai S, Vy M, Mabe M, Del Prado PAR, Clingempeel NL. Comparative analysis of open and robotic transversus abdominis release for ventral hernia repair. Surg Endosc. 2018;32(2):727–34. https://doi.org/10.1007/s00464-017-5729-0.
28. Pauli EM, Wang J, Petro CC, Juza RM, Novitsky YW, Rosen MJ. Posterior component separation with transversus abdominis release successfully addresses recurrent ventral hernias following anterior component separation. Hernia. 2015;19(2):285–91. https://doi.org/10.1007/s10029-014-1331-8.
29. Nakayama M, Yoshimatsu K, Yokomizo H, Yano Y, Okayama S, Satake M, Matsumoto A, Fujimoto T, Usui T, Yamaguchi K, Shiozawa S, Shimakawa T, Katsube T, Naritaka Y. Incidence and risk factors for incisional hernia after open surgery for colorectal cancer. Hepato-Gastroenterology. 2014;61(133):1220–3.
30. Basta MN, Fischer JP, Wink JD, Kovach SJ. Mortality after inpatient open ventral hernia repair: developing a risk stratification tool based on 55,760 operations. Am J Surg. 2016;211(6):1047–57. https://doi.org/10.1016/j.amjsurg.2015.03.009.

23 Subxiphoid and Suprapubic Hernia Repair

Karl A. LeBlanc

23.1 Introduction

Subxiphoid and suprapubic hernias represent an especially difficult subset of incisional hernias to repair. This is because they are located in anatomically challenging areas of the abdominal wall that make surgical repair very difficult. The bony structures that are associated with them and the tissues associated make the repair somewhat different to that of the traditional incisional hernias in the midline of the abdominal wall. It is oftentimes difficult or impossible to achieve fascial closure of the hernia in these locations as well. The use of the robot has represented an advance that makes this more feasible than with traditional laparoscopic methods.

The subxiphoid hernias can develop after median sternotomy or the use of a mediastinal tube during cardiac surgery or laparoscopic surgical trocar placement such as during laparoscopic cholecystectomy [1, 2]. Poststernotomy hernias are uncommon but do occur in approximately 1–4.2% of these procedures [3–5]. Rarely they can occur spontaneously or associated with diastasis recti. Most of these are asymptomatic and/or are identified during an unrelated operative procedure. They generally do not contain any intra-abdominal contents other than the omentum and/or the falciform ligament, but they can occasionally contain intestine or stomach. Preoperative testing with CT scanning is recommended to evaluate the size and contents of the hernia. Open repair with sutures alone has a recurrence rate as high as 80%; the use of a mesh lowers this rate to up to 33% [3]. The laparoscopic approach has a failure rate of approximately 10%. In my experience, this type of hernia represents approximately 4% of my incisional hernia repairs. I have had success with the laparoscopic repair but feel the robotic repair will be the best repair, but this is anecdotal opinion. There is no literature to report at this time.

K. A. LeBlanc (✉)
Our Lady of the Lake Physician Group, Baton Rouge, LA, USA

Louisiana State University Health Sciences Center, New Orleans, LA, USA

K. A. LeBlanc (ed.), *Robotic Assisted Hernia Repair*,
https://doi.org/10.1007/978-3-030-23025-8_23

Suprapubic hernias are nearly always the result of a midline incision from prior surgery in the lower abdomen but can also occur after Pfannenstiel incisions and even after the placement of a suprapubic catheter. Most often they are an extension of a larger incisional hernia. Here, too, preoperative CT imaging will be very helpful to delineate the presence and extent of the hernia borders. The true incidence of these defects is poorly known as most of them are not reported separately from an incisional hernia. These types of hernias are generally defined as a hernia less than 4 cm from the pelvic rim in the midline of the abdomen [6, 7]. The open repair of this hernia is well described and reproducible [8]. Some authors have used bone anchors to insure a sound repair [9]. The laparoscopic repair is also very effective and is nearly identical to some of the open repairs [1, 2, 10–13]. It has been demonstrated that the presence of such a hernia increases the complexity and consequently the operative time to repair such a defect laparoscopically [14]. Bone anchors have also been applied in the laparoscopic repair as well [15]. To date, there are no reports of robotic assisted repair of suprapubic hernia although it is known to have been used for this hernia multiple times. In my practice, the incidence of a suprapubic hernia associated with an incisional hernia is 8%. I have repaired these with the robotic assisted repair since early 2014.

The methods described below will use the intraperitoneal placement of the mesh material. There are a variety of other methods such as the retrorectus repair, the transversus abdominis release and others that are described elsewhere in this textbook. While those chapters focus on the incisional hernias for the most part, the principles also can be applied to these types of hernias as well.

23.2 Operating Room Set Up

The overall operating room set up is discussed in another chapter in this book. The use of either the Intuitive Surgical Si, X, or Xi will be adequate to repair all of these hernias. At the time of this writing, I am unaware of the use of any other robot to repair these hernias. As with my incisional hernias, I prefer the use of three robotic trocars plus a fourth 12 mm accessory trocar (Figs. 23.1, 23.2, 23.3, and 23.4). As noted in three of these figures, there is that additional trocar in the subcostal region. I most often use this location as my initial point of entry into the abdomen. The 5 mm optical trocar will be replaced with a 12 mm trocar after insertion of the robotic trocars. This initial site will allow the assessment of the location of adhesions and the location of the robotic trocars. This method also allows the insufflation of the abdominal cavity prior to introduction of the additional trocars. This will elevate the abdominal wall and allow an increase in the lateral distance of the intestine and the abdominal wall. The effect of this is to allow a more lateral location of the robotic trocars if needed to treat the hernia. It is not used to dock the fourth arm of the robot but is instead used to insert sutures and mesh and then to remove the needles or any excised mesh from prior operations.

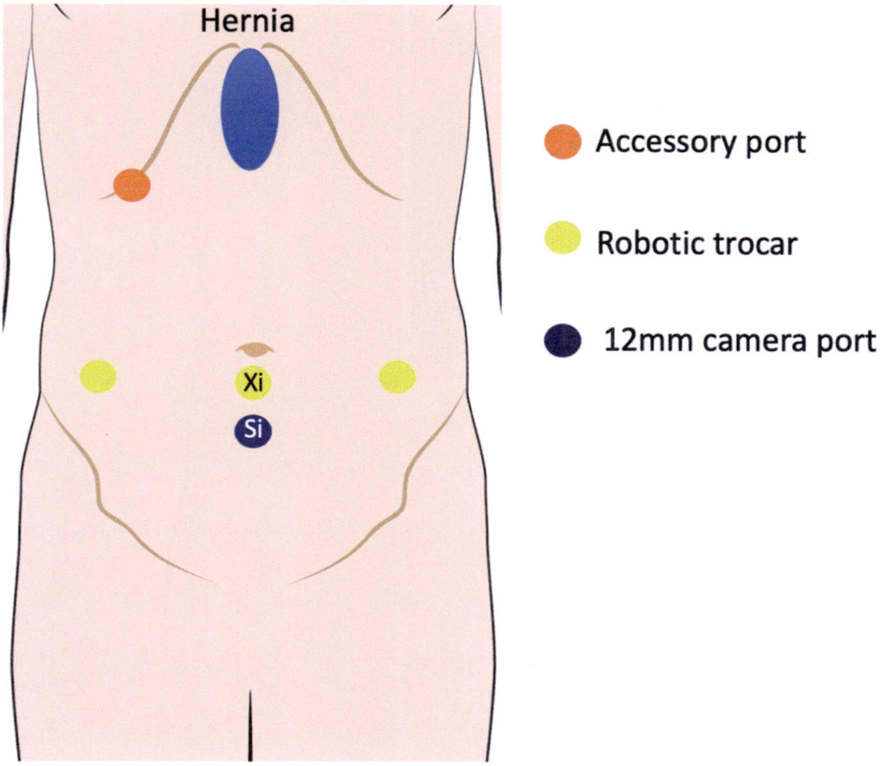

Fig. 23.1 Port placement—subxiphoid hernia (legend applies to Figs. 23.1, 23.2, 23.3, and 23.4)

For ease of use by the scrub assistant, it is preferred to locate this trocar on that side of the table. Figures 23.1 and 23.3 exemplify the preferred locations of the trocars for the "simpler" defects. Figures 23.2 and 23.4 represent the trocar locations with hernias that are larger and/or associated with midline incisional hernias beyond the subxiphoid and suprapubic locations. The Xi and X cameras will be placed in identical locations. The Si camera is placed less in a straight line but more in a triangle type configuration as noted in these figures.

23.3 Surgical Technique

Prophylactic antibiotics and anticoagulation are given to all patients. A two-way urinary catheter is used for either hernia repair. On occasion, a three-way urinary catheter is used during the repair of the suprapubic hernias if there has been extensive prior surgical dissection in this area. This will allow the surgeon to fill the bladder with fluid to aid in identification of the organ if needed. Orogastric tubes

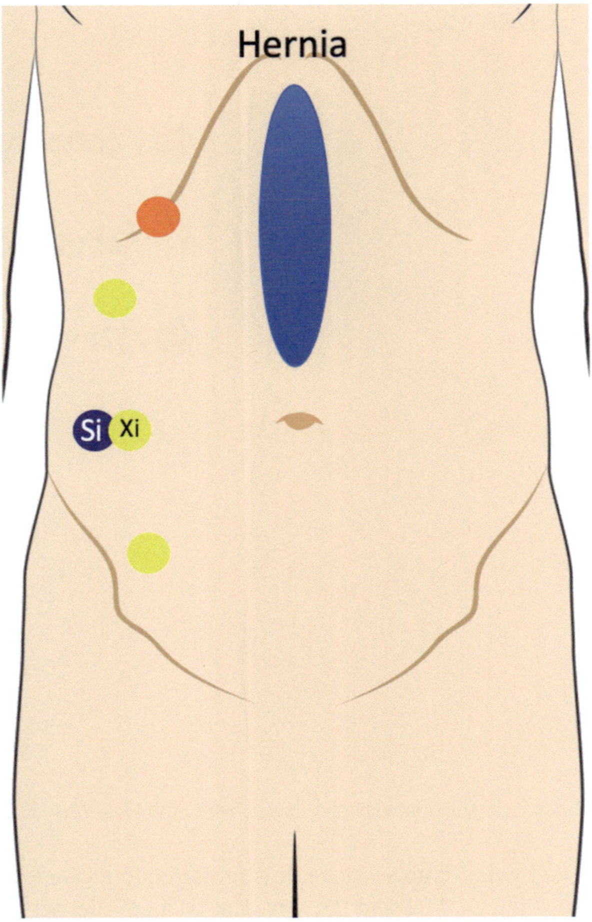

Fig. 23.2 Alternate port placement—subxiphoid hernia

are also used prior to the introduction of the first trocar to decompress the stomach.

For both of these hernia types, as all ventral and incisional hernias, adhesiolysis will initiate the procedure. I prefer to use the robotic fenestrated bipolar and the robotic electrocautery scissors for the dissection. Upon completion of this step it is imperative to separate as much of the preperitoneal fat from the tissues to allow for good approximation of the intraperitoneal mesh with the abdominal wall. In the upper abdomen, this will require the dissection of the falciform ligament as much as possible. In the lower abdomen, the preperitoneal space must be entered and the bladder dissected away until the exposure of Cooper's ligament has been realized. This latter dissection will mimic that performed for the robotic assisted transabdominal preperitoneal (TAPP) inguinal hernia repair.

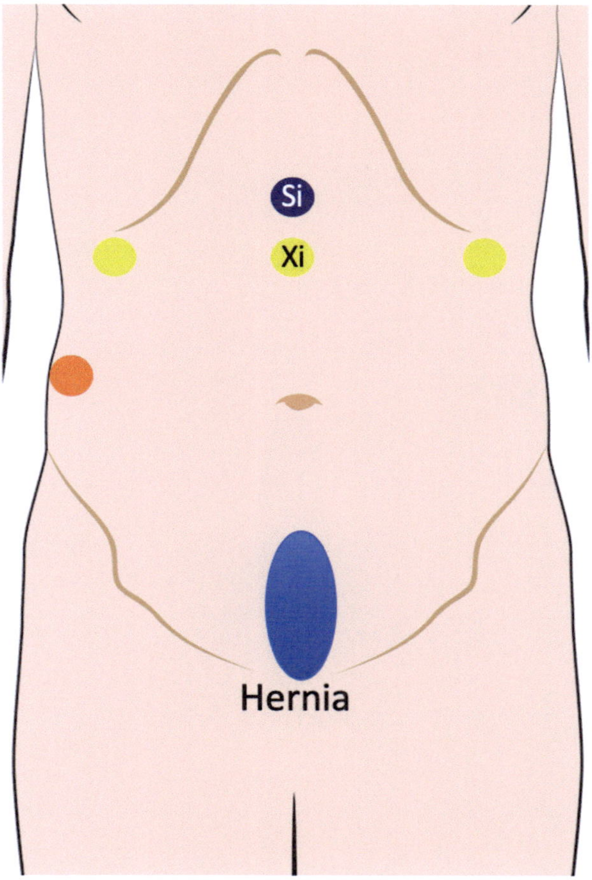

Fig. 23.3 Port placement—suprapubic hernia

All dissection is done with the intra-abdominal pressure set at 15 mm Hg. A ruler is then inserted into the abdomen and used to measure the defect at its greatest dimensions. This should be done in transverse and vertical directions. If there are multiple defects rather than a single defect, the largest distance of all of the defects are used as a single measurement. It is important to emphasize that this measurement is performed *prior* to the closure of the fascial defect. In only this manner, will adequate overlap be assured in the event that the fascial closure does not remain intact at any point postoperatively. The mesh and the mesh size are then selected. As a general rule of thumb, a minimum of 5 cm overlap is used for the usual incisional hernias. Due to the complexity of the location of these hernias, these overlap considerations are modified as noted below.

To accomplish the suture placement, the instruments are changed to a MegaSuture Cut and a MegaSuture device. During closure of the fascia, the intra-abdominal pressure will be reduced to 6–8 mm Hg to reduce the tension on the re-approximated tissue. As noted earlier, it is not always possible to re-approximate the fascia in these hernias.

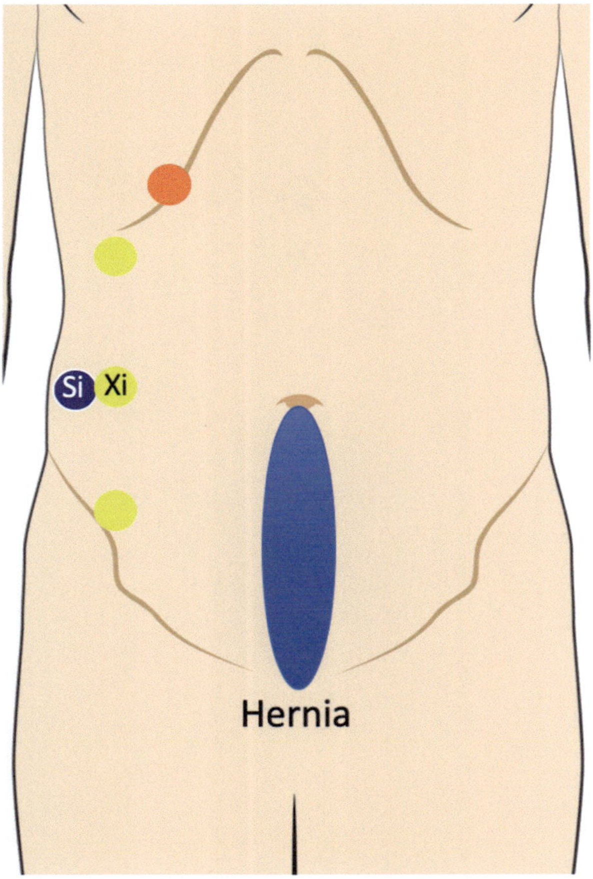

Fig. 23.4 Alternate port placement—suprapubic hernia

Consideration at that time to conversion to the posterior component separation procedure can facilitate this closure if deemed necessary. Alternatively, the mesh can be "bridged" across the defect as one does during the traditional laparoscopic repair.

Once the closure of the fascial defect is completed, the pressure will be brought back to 15 mm Hg. to make suturing of the mesh easier to accomplish. For all of my incisional hernia repairs and certainly for these hernias, I will place four rows of sutures (Fig. 23.5). I use two double armed polypropylene barbed sutures (#2). These are started in the middle of the mesh on either side as the starting point (A & B). As noted in the figure, there is a row at the periphery of the mesh. I continue to use these sutures from this line to place a row on either side of the closed fascia. This will bolster the fascial closure, perhaps minimizing the chance of separation of the closure, which will reduce the risk of recurrence. Additionally, the mesh will instantly contact the tissue to reduce the chance of seroma formation and increase the rapidity of ingrowth into the mesh material. A difference that will be noted below is that additional fixation will be needed to attach the mesh in the suprapubic hernia repair.

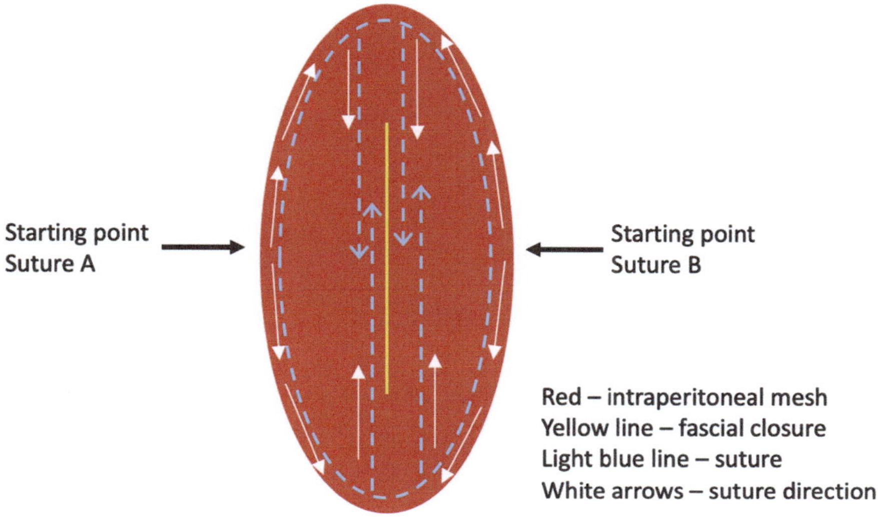

Fig. 23.5 Typical suture pattern of subxiphoid and suprapubic hernia

Fig. 23.6 Undissected subxiphoid hernia

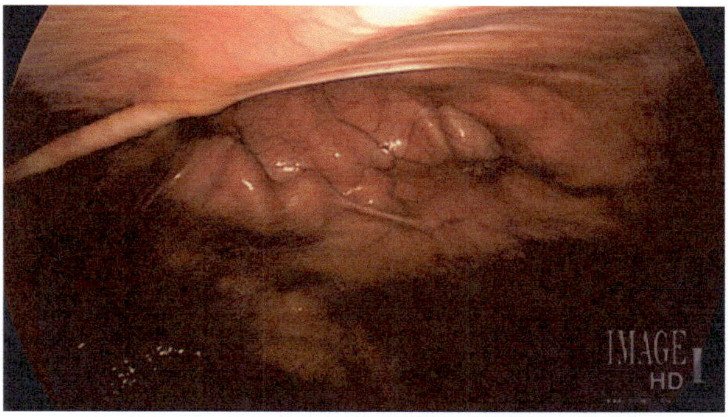

For subxiphoid hernias, the ribs and sternum are usually very near or at the borders of this hernia making fascial closure especially challenging (Figs. 23.6 and 23.7). Consequently, a larger overlap is recommended; up to 8 cm will be best during repair of these hernias. Due to the fact that surgical closure of the fascial defect is not always feasible it is especially important to adhere to this recommendation (Fig. 23.8).[1] Although not demonstrated in this figure, I currently prefer to insert the mesh prior to closure of the defect so that a centrally placed suture on the mesh can be used to assure the correct location of the mesh. If the ECHO or ECHO2 positioning device is used, the tubing or suture will likewise be used to locate the mesh. This can be difficult but usually there is enough room to allow for this to occur. If one pulls the central suture through the abdominal wall after closure of the fascial defect, there is a real possibility of losing the center of the fascial defect resulting in an

[1] The hernia in Figs. 23.6 and 23.7 are not the same as the hernia repaired in Figs. 23.8 and 23.9.

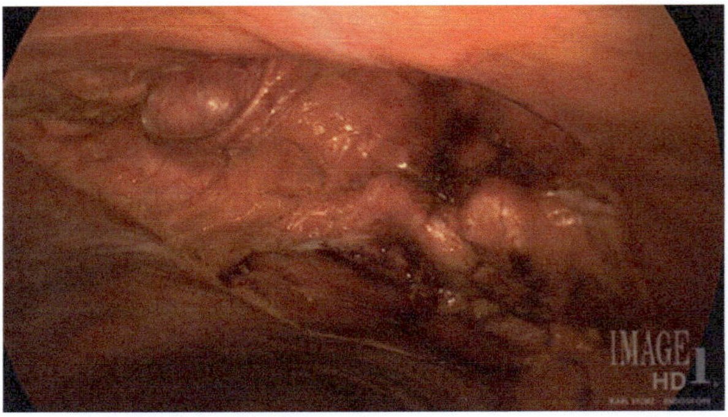

Fig. 23.7 Fully dissected subxiphoid hernia

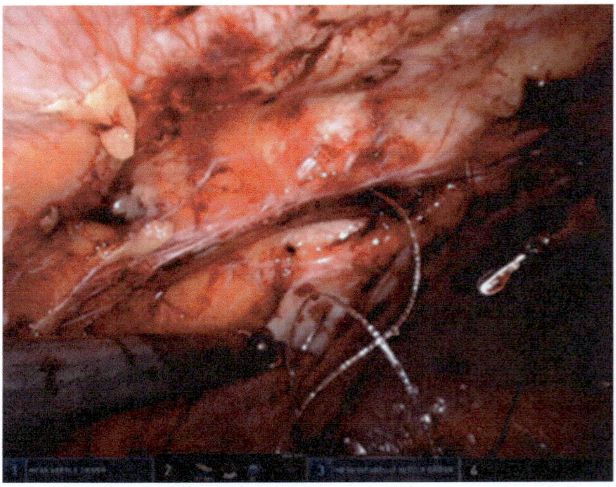

Fig. 23.8 Closure of the defect (view is from the right side of the patient)

incorrect (off center) position of the mesh. The defect will then be closed with permanent barbed suture (polypropylene) when possible.

Fixation of the prosthetic material is critically important here. The significant advantage of the robotic technology is the ability to sew very effectively compared to the traditional laparoscopic technique. The prosthetic chosen should be sewn with the sutures of surgeon preference, but I prefer the use of barbed permanent sutures. The superior portion of the mesh should be sewn to the diaphragm taking care to avoid penetration into the mediastinum or chest cavity. One should assure that the mesh is taut and without any laxity (Fig. 23.9) (see footnote 1).

Similar considerations apply to the suprapubic hernias. If the definition of this hernia is the location at 4 cm or less from the pubic bone, then it is impossible to obtain a 5 cm overlap of the prosthetic to just tissue. The most common cause of recurrence in the repair of suprapubic hernias is inadequate dissection in the pelvis which results in inadequate overlap and inadequate fixation. To avoid this fact, the dissection should be performed similar to that of TAPP inguinal hernia repair.

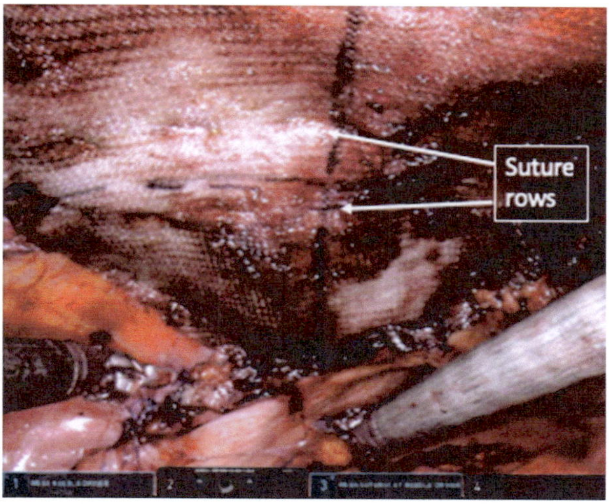

Fig. 23.9 Mesh in place to cover the defect (view is from right side of the patient)

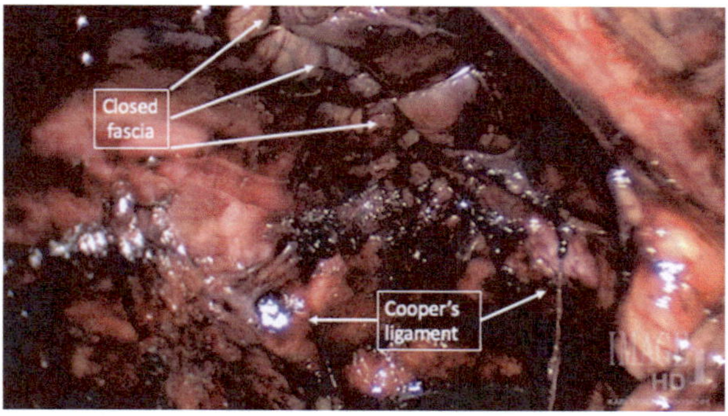

Fig. 23.10 Closed fascial defect of suprapubic hernia

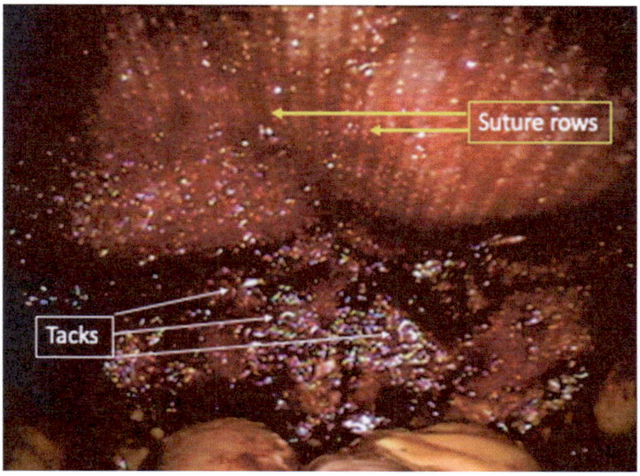

Fig. 23.11 Mesh fixation with sutures and tacks to Cooper's ligament

The exposure down to Cooper's ligament will allow excellent fixation the mesh onto that structure. The fascial defect of the hernia will be closed first (Fig. 23.10). One may sew the material to this ligament and/or use permanent tacks (Fig. 23.11). If there is any remnant of tissue above the pubic bone, I will also sew this to the mesh with permanent barbed sutures. The remaining portion of the prosthetic will be sutured in place as well as described above (Fig. 23.5). It is recommended that any positioning aid such as the suture or positioning device be pulled through the abdominal wall prior to the closure of the fascia as discussed for the subxiphoid hernia.

23.4 Postoperative Care

An immediate postoperative chest radiograph after subxiphoid hernia repair is frequently performed if there is concern of passage of the suture through the diaphragm. Occasionally one will see a small pneumothorax, but this is merely observed as the carbon dioxide in the chest will resorb quickly. If the patient develops symptoms from this, then appropriate measures should be undertaken, although I have never had to act on any of them.

Most of these have been performed on an outpatient basis. If there are multiple co-morbidities or extensive dissection resulting in potential medical or postsurgical adverse events, then the patients will remain in the hospital. Activities are limited for 2–4 weeks to allow sufficient time for the fascial closure to become secure and ingrowth of tissue into the mesh. These are very tenuous tissues in some cases, so caution is preferred. Higher risk patients, such as those that are diabetic, overweight or with compromised immune systems, etc., will take a much longer period of time to heal these tissues. In these cases, I will limit activities for even longer periods of time.

In these locations of the body it is virtually impossible to insure a good fit of an abdominal binder. Therefore, these are rarely used. Most individuals will not develop a seroma. Even those that do, these will resolve in nearly all cases.

23.5 Conclusion

The use of the robot to repair these infrequent yet difficult hernias has allowed the opportunity to perform these repairs with more secure fixation. While more data is needed, the perception that these techniques will improve outcomes. Due to the infrequent development of these defects, more time is needed to establish the best methods of repair. In my practice, I am unaware of any recurrence of these hernias to date.

References

1. Charles A, Shaikh AA, Domingo S, Kreske E. Falciform ligament hernia after laparoscopic cholecystectomy: a rare case and review of the literature. Am Surg. 2005;71(4):359–61.
2. Dusu K, Dindyal S, Gadhvi V. Small bowel obstruction via herniation through an iatrogenic defect of the falciform ligament following laparoscopic cholecystectomy. Ann R Coll Surg Engl. 2015;97(6):e93–5.
3. Landau O, Raziel A, Matz A, Kyzer S, Haruzi I. Laparoscopic repair of poststernotomy subxiphoid epigastric hernia. Surg Endosc. 2001;15(11):1313–4.
4. Davidson BR, Bailey JS. Incisional herniae following median sternotomy incisions: their incidence and aetiology. Br J Surg. 1986;73:995–6.
5. Losanoff JE, Basson MD, Laker S, Weiner M, Webber JD, Gruber SA. Subxiphoid incisional hernias after median sternotomy. Hernia. 2007;11:473–9.
6. Sharma A, Dey A, Khullar R, et al. Laparoscopic repair of suprapubic hernias: transabdominal partial extraperitoneal (TAPE) technique. Surg Endosc. 2011;25:2147–52.
7. Palanivelu C, Rangarajan M, Parthasarathi R, et al. Laparoscopic repair of suprapubic incisional hernias: suturing and intraperitoneal composite mesh onlay. A retrospective study. Hernia. 2008;12:251–6.
8. Renard Y, Simonneau AC, de Mestier L, Teuma L, Meffert JL, Palot JP, Kianmanesh R. Standard of open surgical repair of suprapubic incisional hernias. World J Surg. 2017;41(6):1466–74.
9. Blair LJ, Cox TC, Huntington CR, Ross SW, Kneisl JS, Augenstein VA, Heniford BT. Bone anchor fixation in abdominal wall reconstruction: a useful adjunct in suprapubic and para-iliac hernia repair. Am Surg. 2015;81(7):693–7.
10. Carbonell AM, Kercher KW, Matthews BD, et al. The laparoscopic repair of suprapubic ventral hernias. Surg Endosc. 2005;19:174–7.
11. Varnell B, Bachman S, Quick J, et al. Morbidity associated with laparoscopic repair of suprapubic hernias. Am J Surg. 2008;196:983–7.
12. Hope WW, Hooks WB 3rd. Atypical hernias: suprapubic, subxiphoid and flank. Surg Clin North Am. 2013;93:1135–62.
13. Sikar HE, Çetin K, Eyvaz K, Kaptanoglu L, KüÇük HF. Laparoscopic repair of large suprapubic hernias. Wideochir Inne Tech Maloinwazyjne. 2017;12(3):244–50.
14. Jenkins ED, Yom VH, Melman L, Pierce RA, Schuessler RB, Frisella MM, Christopher Eagon J, Michael Brunt L, Matthews BD. Clinical predictors of operative complexity in laparoscopic ventral hernia repair: a prospective study. Surg Endosc. 2010;24(8):1872–7.
15. Yee JA, Harold KL, Cobb WS, Carbonell AM. Bone anchor mesh fixation for complex laparoscopic ventral hernia repair. Surg Innov. 2008;15(4):292–6.

Lumbar Hernia

24

Maamoun Harmouch and Karl A. LeBlanc

24.1 Introduction

24.1.1 Historical Background

Lumbar hernia was first noted in the sixteenth century by P. Barbette. It was not until 1731 when Garangeot published the first case of an incarcerated lumbar hernia found at autopsy [1]. In 1750, Ravaton performed the first surgical repair on a strangulated lumbar hernia in a pregnant woman. In 1783, the French surgeon Jean Petit described the anatomical boundaries of what is known as the inferior lumbar triangle [2]. In 1866, Grynfeltt described the superior lumbar space [3]. This was also confirmed by Lesshaft in 1870 when he described another case of lumbar hernia through the superior lumbar space. Hence, the superior lumbar space is often called the Grynfeltt-Lesshaft triangle. In 1906, Selby described the first case of traumatically acquired lumbar hernia after a fall [4]. In 1939, Kelton described iatrogenic post-incisional lumbar hernias [5] and in 1951 Kretchmer published a case series of acquired lumbar hernias after renal surgery [6].

24.1.2 Classifications

Lumbar hernias are uncommon and represent a reported incidence of 1.5% of all hernias. Consequently these are rarely encountered by the average surgeon. Certainly, there are controversies and overlap when classifying these defects. Often, they are described as congenital or acquired. Congenital lumbar defects consist of

M. Harmouch
Fellow, Minimally Invasive Surgery Institute, Our Lady of the Lake Physician Group, Baton Rouge, LA, USA

K. A. LeBlanc (✉)
Our Lady of the Lake Physician Group, Baton Rouge, LA, USA

K. A. LeBlanc (ed.), *Robotic Assisted Hernia Repair*,
https://doi.org/10.1007/978-3-030-23025-8_24

approximately 20% of cases and are classically described as Grynfeltt and Petit which arise in the superior and inferior lumbar triangle; respectively. Acquired lumbar defects consist of approximately 80% of cases [7]. These are further classified as primary or spontaneous and secondary which occur as a result of trauma, surgical procedures, and infections. Some of the risk factors that have been shown to contribute to the development of spontaneous herniation include older age, obesity, COPD, extreme leanness, and/or chronic debilitating illness [5]. Secondary defects are further divided into "true hernia" with a fascial defect and "pseudo-hernia" with intact fascia but denervated and paralyzed lateral abdominal wall musculature. Pseudo-hernia results from injury to the intercostal nerves which result in muscle paralysis and subsequent atrophy. The end result of which is a flank bulge that is accentuated with the Valsalva maneuver. This entity presents a challenge to the treating surgeon, as they are often difficult to affect a permanent and cosmetically acceptable repair.

24.1.3 Surgical Anatomy

Lumbar hernia is a broad term that encompasses defects that arise in the posterolateral abdominal wall. The abdominal wall in this region is made up of the skin, Camper's and Scarpa's fascia, three muscular layers (superficial, middle, and deep), lumbodorsal fascia, transversalis fascia, and the extraperitoneal tissue [8]. The superficial muscle layer consists of latissimus dorsi and external oblique muscles. The middle muscular layer consists of the sacrospinalis, internal oblique, and the serratus inferior muscles. The deep muscular layer consists of quadratus lamborum and psoas muscles [7].

Anatomically, the lumbar region spans the area bounded by the 12th rib cephalad, the iliac crest caudad, the erector spinae muscles posterolaterally, and the linea semilunaris anterolaterally [5, 7]. There are two anatomical spaces in the lumbar region known as the superior and inferior lumbar triangles. The superior lumbar triangle tends to be larger, deeper, and of variable morphology [9]. This inverted triangle is bordered by the 12th rib and the inferior edge of the serratus muscle as its base, the posterior edge of the internal oblique muscle anteriorly, and the anterior edge of the sacrospinalis muscle posteriorly. The roof and floor are bounded by the external oblique/latissimus dorsi and the aponeurosis of the transverses abdominis, respectively. It is believed that this is the most common site of lumbar hernias [9, 10]. On the other hand, the inferior triangle is often consistently triangular and is bordered by external oblique laterally, latissimus dorsi medially, iliac crest inferiorly, with the internal oblique muscle as its floor [9, 10]. Lumbar hernias that do not respect the anatomical boundaries are often termed "diffuse". These often surpass the boundaries of the lumbar space and can encompass both triangles [5, 11] (Fig. 24.1).

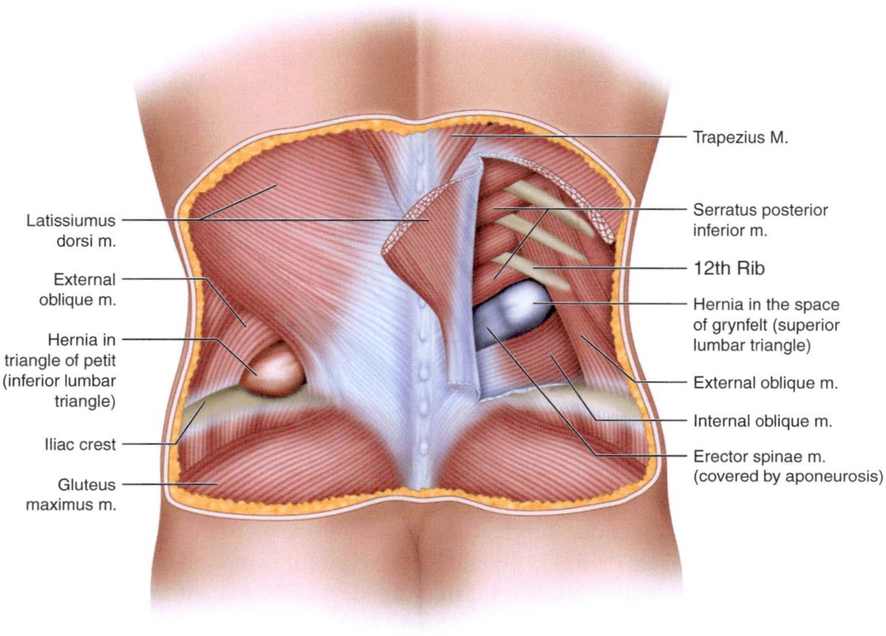

Fig. 24.1 Anatomy of superior and inferior lumbar hernias

24.1.4 Pathogenesis

It has been theorized that the combination of increased intraabdominal pressure, anatomical alteration of muscles, and the presence of a natural orifice in the lumbodorsal fascia predispose certain individuals to acquire this defect [5]. In contrast, secondary herniation can result from direct injury to one or more of the musculature, lumbodorsal fascia, and intercostal nerves. This is often the result of a surgical incision or trauma [4, 6, 12]. The abdominal wall muscles are segmentally innervated by spinal roots T7–T12 [13]. Violation of these nerves, which can occur with certain surgical procedures, will cause atrophy of the abdominal wall musculature [9, 14]. This can ultimately result in either a "denervation" bulge and/or a true fascial defect. Common surgical procedures that yield this pathology include nephrectomies, aortic surgery, and lateral approaches to lumbar disc fusion, resection of abdominal wall tumors, iliac bone harvest, and the latissimus dorsi flap used for reconstruction of a tissue defect [5]. It has been noted that up to 50% of patients that undergo radical nephrectomy through a lumber incision will develop a permanent bulge [15].

24.1.5 Clinical Presentation

Clinically, a lumbar hernia can present as an incidental finding on an imaging study or as an asymptomatic bulge that increases in size with the Valsalva maneuver. There can be significant asymmetry of the abdominal wall in the instance of the "denervation hernia" (Fig. 24.2). When symptomatic, it typically presents with vague lower back pain. In extreme cases, it can cause bowel or urinary obstruction. Diagnosis is often made by history and physical examination. The CT scan can be a helpful tool in not only confirming the diagnosis, but more importantly it can provide valuable information that will guide the surgical approach [5, 8, 9, 11, 14].

24.2 Preoperative Planning

Similar to other types of abdominal wall hernias, surgical planning for flank hernias can be quite challenging especially when faced with a complex defect and a patient with multiple co-morbidities. Therefore, patient selection, pre-operative medical optimization, and meticulous surgical techniques are keys to desirable outcomes. Due to its elective nature, surgery should be reserved for symptomatic patients with a favorable risk profile. It is prudent for the surgeon and the patient to work together to identify modifiable risk factors. This should be followed by a plan to implement

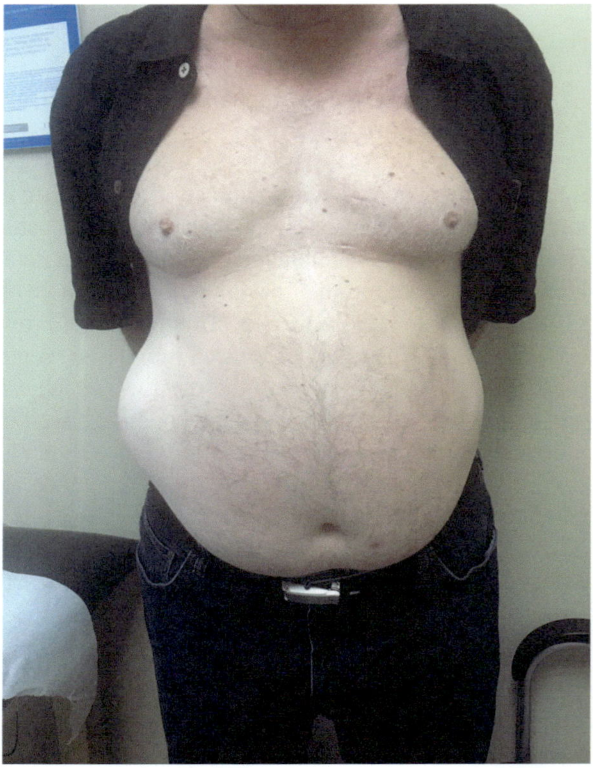

Fig. 24.2 Right sided denervation defect in a patient after a right nephrectomy

an effective pre- operative multidisciplinary counseling and therapy. The patient must show motivation and comply with any dietary, exercise, and smoking session programs when applicable [16, 17].

Factors that play an important role in surgical decision making can be divided into patient specific and hernia specific factors. These include obesity, smoking status, poorly controlled diabetes, size of the hernia, status of abdominal wall domain, presence of overlaying redundant and atrophic skin, and lastly whether the hernia represents a true defect versus a denervation injury [16, 17]. Owing to the rarity of the condition and the poor quality of the available evidence, recommendations regarding the optimal surgical approach are still ambiguous. Based on the current evidence, the laparoscopic approach appears to have fewer complications, less post operative pain, and a decreased length of hospital stay when compared to open surgery [17–19]. In general, the inherent advantages seen with minimally invasive surgery are often translated to the management of lumbar hernias. Although, one must take all factors into consideration to help guide the surgical decision making. For example, patients that have multiple risk factors for poor wound healing and a small to moderate sized hernia will be better served with a minimally invasive approach. On the other hand, patients with large defects, redundant overlaying skin and soft tissue or a "denervation" hernia might have better outcomes with an open or hybrid approach. More recently, there has been an increase utilization of robotic technology in the management of abdominal wall hernias. This stems from the multiple features that it offers which enable the surgeon to perform more complex repair in a minimal invasive fashion that was once considered to be too difficult or impossible laparoscopically. It is therefore not surprising that there seems to be a trend in the treatment of these large flank hernias utilizing a minimally invasive fashion with the robotic platform [20].

24.3 Operative Technique

The surgical approach to lumbar hernia repair is inherently similar to other types of abdominal wall hernia repair. These include open, laparoscopic, robotic, and hybrid techniques. In addition, the surgical techniques and intraoperative pearls that deal with abdominal wall hernia repair are quite similar to the management of these uncommon fascial defects. These include dissection of hernia sac to the fascial edges and development of a preperitoneal pocket if mesh placement will be in that location. Additional important considerations are the primary closure of fascial defect, allowance for 5 cm or greater overlap of mesh, appropriate mesh fixation, and layered closure of soft tissue and skin. Unlike other forms of abdominal wall hernias, the presence of two bony landmarks (ribs and iliac wing) can make repair and mesh fixation a challenging task for the surgeon dealing with flank hernias. This is especially challenging in those situations where traumatic events have disrupted the anatomic muscular attachments to these bony structures.

Irrespective of the approach employed, the patient is positioned similarly whether a minimally invasive or an open approach is utilized. After induction of general anesthesia, a urinary drainage catheter and an orogastric tube should be placed. The patient is then placed in the lateral decubitus position with the involved side up. All areas must be padded appropriately. One must ensure that the surgical field spans the 4 to 5th intercostal space cephalad, below the iliac crest caudad, the spinous process medially and the contralateral midclavicular line laterally. For excellent exposure the operating room table is flexed in order to stretch the lumbar space. While this flexion will aid in exposure of the operative field, it can compromise the laxity of the final repair and mesh tautness so this must be restricted as much as possible. In general, we prefer to avoid flexion of the bed completely.

24.3.1 Open Approach

The open technique is often used with very large flank hernias. The incision is typically made over the old incision or directly over the primary hernia. Dissection is carried down to the hernia sac which is then freed circumferentially. Musculocutaneous flaps are then developed. The preperitoneal space entered and a space is then developed to allow a minimum 5 cm of mesh overlap in all directions. The mesh that is selected will be based upon surgeon preference but a lightweight material is not recommended.

24.3.2 Mimimally Invasive Approach

24.3.2.1 Conventional Laparoscopy

These hernias can be repaired with either the preperitoneal placement or intraperitoneal placement of mesh (IPOM). It has been shown that the main consideration in the repair of lumbar hernias is the placement of a prosthetic material, whether open or laparoscopically repaired [21]. The choice of mesh will be influenced by the location of its final placement. The preperitoneal dissection will expose the fascia as part of the procedure and covers it once the repair is complete. In that method, a "non-coated" product may be used. A "coated" (i.e. tissue separating) product is required if the IPOM is performed. If the latter technique is utilized, it is important to dissect the preperitoneal fat away from the fascia so that the uncoated surface of the mesh contacts as little of the adipose tissue as possible to ensure an effective repair. This is the fundamental difference between these methods. In many patients, this extraperitoneal fat will be so extensive that the use of the preperitoneal space for placement of an uncoated mesh will be most appropriate. The following procedure description will apply to both.

This repair will be similar to the traditional incisional hernia repair. If possible, the fascial defect can be closed with either transfascial or intracorporeal sutures. The latter option seems easiest if barbed sutures are utilized in the closure. If transfascial sutures are to be placed, one must be careful not to inadvertently place them through the chest cavity if the hernia is adjacent to the thoracic cavity. Closure of the defect becomes more difficult with larger defects.

The mesh will be placed to cover the defect with at least a five-centimeter overlap of the fascial defect. It is preferred that the size be selected on the measurement of the unclosed defect as one cannot be assured that the closed defect will remain permanently closed [22] If a bridged repair is chosen, then an even greater attention to the amount of mesh overlap is required. The mesh:defect ratio will be a factor [23]. If fixation to the diaphragm is necessary, this can be sutured with either interrupted or running permanent sutures. If additional fixation with a device other than sutures is needed, one should only place them below the diaphragm

24.3.2.2 Robotic Assisted

Minimal invasive lumbar hernia repair can be performed via different approaches. We describe a technique for robotic-assisted transabdominal laparoscopic repair

1. *Trocar placement*

   Access to the abdominal cavity can be done via the Hassan method, a Veress needle, and optical trocar techniques. We prefer using a 5 mm optical trocar at the ipsilateral subcostal space. Pneumoperitoneum is established and pressure set to 15 mm Hg. A 30-degree scope is used to explore the abdominal cavity to ensure no adhesions that will prohibit the placement of the remaining reusable trocars. The 8.5 mm robotic trocars will then be placed at appropriate locations. Two additional trocars are placed to allow sufficient distance from the working site, including both the fascial defect and the desired 5 cm overlap of the mesh. Most often, these will be placed in the midclavicular line. Consideration must be given to the laxity of the abdominal wall especially in morbidly obese individuals. Insufflation can result in a significant increase in the distance away from the hernia defect making the performance of the operation more challenging. The trocars are placed in a linear or "C" shaped fashion if the Xi or Si platforms are used, respectively. After the robotic trocars are positioned the 5 mm trocar will be replaced with a 12 mm trocar to allow the introduction of needles, suture and mesh (Fig. 24.3). The robotic scissors, bipolar grasper and needle holder are the instruments of choice for the authors. The use of three arms of the robot is all that is usually required.

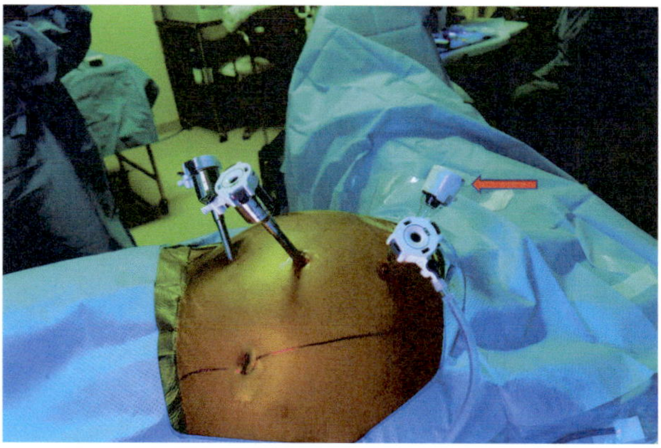

Fig. 24.3 Robotic trocar placement for a "true" right lumbar hernia repair (red arrow denotes the 12 mm trocar)

2. *Docking the robot*

   The robot is brought in from the flank. Fine adjustment should be made to bring the robotic arms in line with the dissection. Sufficiently distant trocar placement is essential prior to docking to limit the collision of the robotic arms (Fig. 24.4). It is important to ensure that all arms are "bumped up" to ensure both that there is no tension on abdominal wall and that the range of movement for each arm is sufficient. Proper port placement and docking of the robot entails a learning curve; ensuring proper port placement and arm docking will limit an increase in the operative time for needed trouble shooting during the case.

3. *Identification of the lumbar hernia*

   The peritoneum is incised from the 10th rib to the iliac crest. The peritoneum and retroperitoneal tissues are dissected at least 6–8 cm away from the hernia defect to ensure proper mesh coverage. In general, however, more dissection is required to allow for ample manipulation of the mesh and the proper placement of sutures. Reduction of all hernia contents is performed to identify the exact dimensions of the hernia defect (Fig. 24.5a, b).

4. *Defect closure*

   The hernia defect is closed primarily using a double armed 0 barbed non-absorbable suture. Barbed sutures facilitate closure as they more evenly distribute the tension of the closure itself. However, other suture types can be used according to surgeon preference. Decreasing the pneumoperitoneum to 6–8 mm Hg and utilizing the shoelace concept by taking all fascial bites and then tightening each one separately to decrease defect size will facilitate fascial closure in larger defects. The authors find it best to insert the mesh and pull out a centrally placed suture to accurately locate the material. Once the defect itself is closed, the exact location of the central portion of the fascial defect may be difficult. This could cause an inadvertent shift of mesh placement resulting in an improper overlap and increase the likelihood of recurrence. Closure of the defect is nearly always possible but occasionally the defect must be bridged with very large

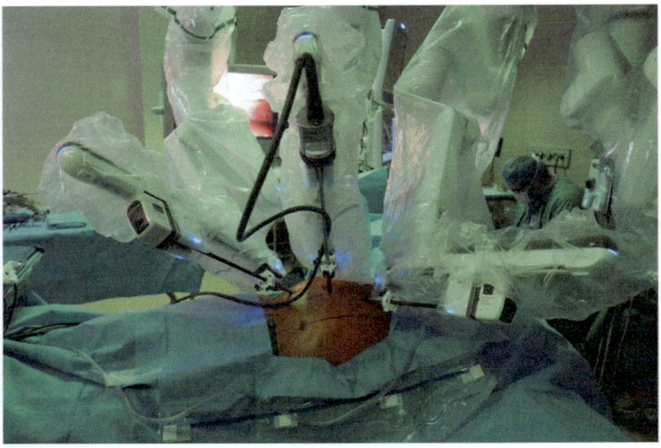

Fig. 24.4 Typical spatial relationship between the robotic arms

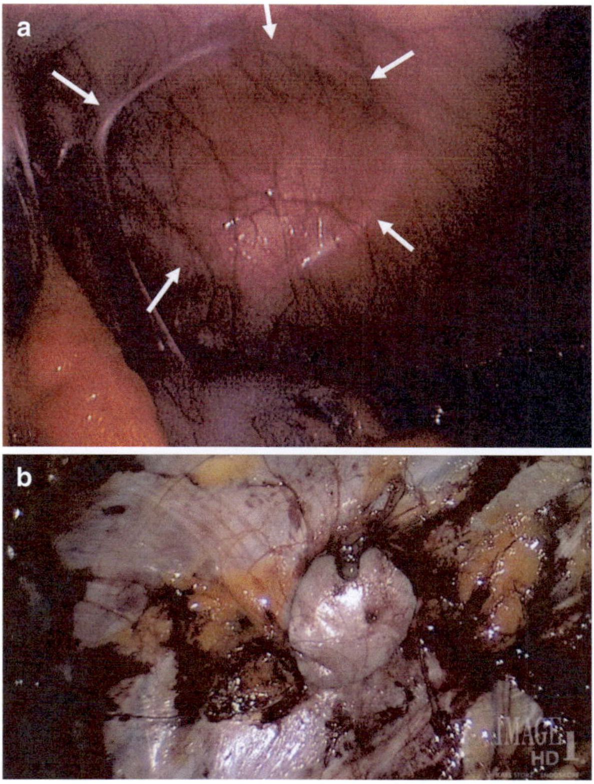

Fig. 24.5 (**a**) Left lumbar hernia prior to dissection (arrows delineate the border). (**b**). Left lumbar hernia after full dissection (from Fig. 24.5a)

hernias. An attempt is always made a defect closure because the sutures can also act as a "backstop" for the mesh in such situations.

5. *Mesh placement and fixation*

   It is important to size the mesh based on the defect prior to closure of the fascial defect. Mesh should be sized with minimum of 5 cm overlap in mind. As noted above, if the mesh is entirely within the preperitoneal space, a non-coated material can be used. If there is exposure to the internal organs, then a tissue separating product should be used. There are many products available and are discussed extensively in Chap. 4. The authors prefer either a polypropylene or polytetrafluoroethylene hybrid material. Although the mesh could be tacked with a few sutures or a fixation device of some type, we prefer to use the same permanent suture described above using in two rows on either side of the closed defect (Fig. 24.6). This allows the suture line to bolster the fascial closure while approximating the mesh to the abdominal wall, which will increase the rapidity of ingrowth into the material. All techniques utilizing fixation with either suture or tacks should respect the path of the nerves that arise from the anterior rami of the T12/L1 nerve roots (ilioinguinal, iliohypogastric, and genitofemoral nerves).

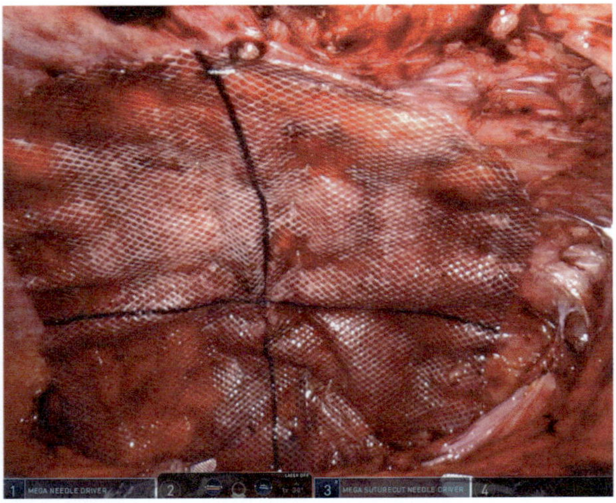

Fig. 24.6 Intracorporeal sutured mesh using barbed polypropylene suture

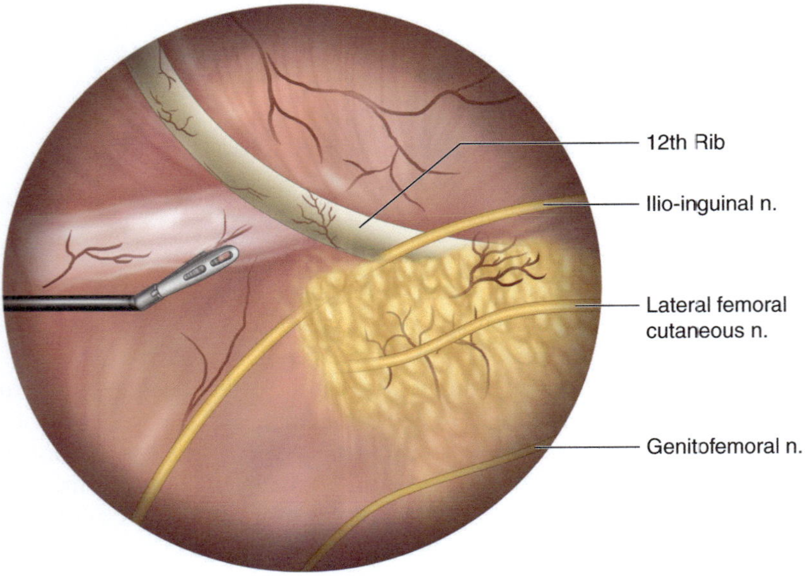

Fig. 24.7 Anatomic course of the nerves near the 12th rib

This path will not be consistent and will splay out over the psoas muscle. Consequently, the course of these nerves can be difficult to identify (Fig. 24.7). Biosynthetic glue has been described as a method for mesh fixation as well but we have no experience in this application.

6. *Peritoneal closure*

   The peritoneal flap is then closed using an 18-inch double armed long lasting absorbable suture. During the suturing to close the peritoneal pocket it is crucial to assess the peritoneal flap at the end to identify and close any significant tears with interrupted absorbable sutures.

24.3.3 Hybrid Approach

Due to the inherent anatomic issues due to the paralysis of these muscles, the authors prefer this approach for the "denervation" hernia. It typically consists of both an initial open followed by a robotic assisted approach. The skin incision of the prior procedure is utilized and in most cases, this must be extended. The initial dissection will require the development of significant skin flaps in all directions to accommodate an onlay mesh overlap that extend above the ribs superiorly, below the iliac crest inferiorly, onto the rectus sheath medially, and near the spine posteriorly. This will provide coverage of the entire area of denervation injury.

At that point, the muscles are incised to enter the abdominal cavity. Adhesiolysis is performed as necessary. Again, this dissection must extend above the diaphragm superiorly, into the pelvis inferiorly, to the midline medially, and to the paraspinus muscles posteriorly. The mesh should be large enough to cover all of these areas. This is required whether the mesh is to be placed in the extraperitoneal space or intra-abdominally. Generally the intraperitoneal onlay approach is selected as this combined method is best completed in this fashion.

Preplaced sutures will allow for transfascial suture fixation as described above (Fig. 24.8). The mesh material will be inserted and sutured to the paraspinus muscles initially. One to three posteriorly placed transfascial sutures are also utilized. The superior portion of the mesh will then be sutured to the diaphragm with

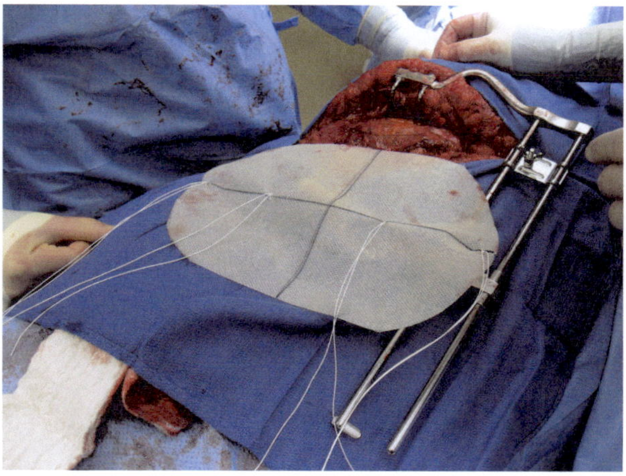

Fig. 24.8 Preplaced transfascial suture to help with mesh fixation

interrupted sutures. Occasionally, transfascial sutures are added below the costal margin. However, a medially placed transfacial suture will allow this portion of the mesh to be identified and fixed. Usually, two sutures that are preplaced on the mesh will allow the transfascial sutures to assure that the mesh is apposed against the closed muscles and fascia, which greatly aids in the robotic fixation. The inferior location of the mesh will be determined during the robotic portion of the procedure so no fixation will occur at this time. This fact is the reason that the hybrid approach is so beneficial as this allows us to fix the mesh with minimal laxity.

Prior to the medial fixation of the mesh, three robotic trocars are placed where best located. Usually these are to the contralateral side of the midline. At this point the divided muscles will be plicated in a "vest over pants" configuration and these should be pulled as tight as feasible. One must account for this portion of the procedure during placement of the subcostal transfascial sutures, if used. We usually elect to place the onlay mesh at this time (Fig. 24.9). This mesh will cover all of the previously dissected areas below the skin flaps. We generally do this at this time but one might occasionally need to reopen the closed muscles for additional fixation should these become dislodged during the robotic portion. This is so seldom necessary that we will place the selected mesh and quilt the subcutaneous tissue using barbed absorbable sutures to the underlying mesh and fascia to close the dead space and thereby eliminate the need for any drains (Fig. 24.10). Frequently, fibrin tissue glue is used to fixate the product in its entirety.

The robot will then be docked and the laparoscopic portion will commence. The goal here is to pull the inferior portion of the mesh taut and fixate it firmly. This will be done with running barbed sutures robotically. The robotically placed sutures will also be run over the interior of the mesh to firmly fixate all of it to the abdominal wall (Fig. 24.11). This will aid in the prevention of a seroma while assuring firm attachment and early ingrowth of tissue into the prosthesis.

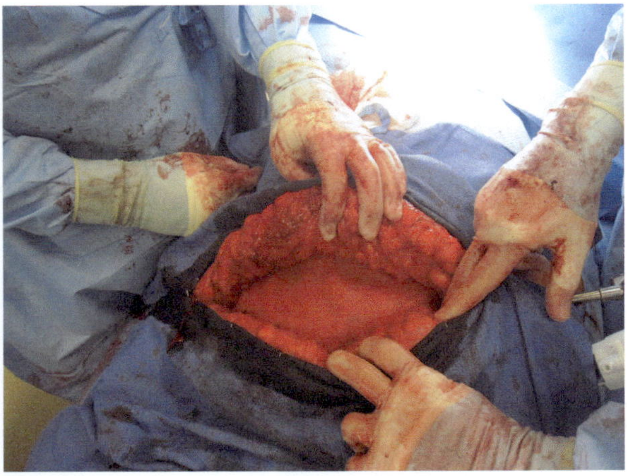

Fig. 24.9 Onlay mesh placement

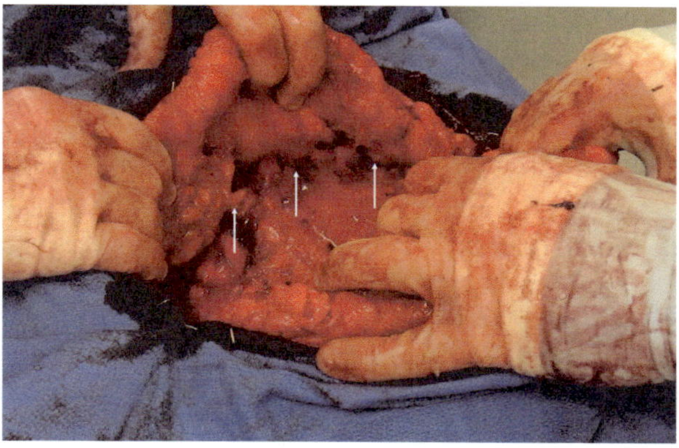

Fig. 24.10 Arrows indicate the quilting of the subcutaneous tissue with barbed absorbable sutures, the process is not completed until the entire layer is done

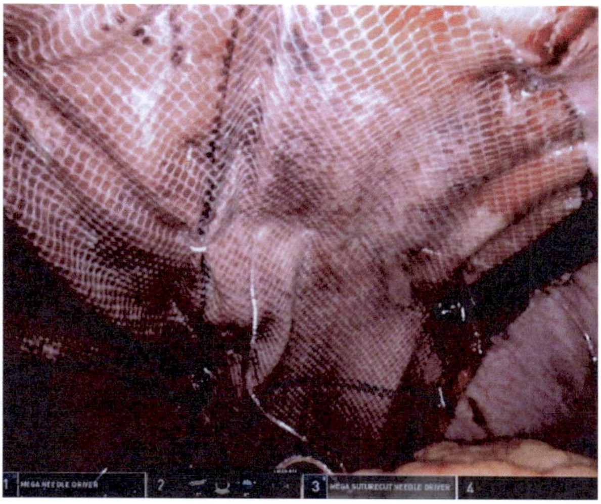

Fig. 24.11 Intracorporeal suturing of the mesh

If the onlay mesh and skin closure has not been done already, the procedure returns to the open portion. A large onlay of the selected mesh is placed to cover the entire area as noted above. Quilting is always performed as noted above. The subcutaneous tissue is closed in layers and the skin closed.

Although not mentioned above, it is extremely beneficial to inject a long acting local anesthetic, liposomal bupivacaine into the tissues and as a TAP or erector spinae block during the open portion of the operation. This is a painful operation and the addition of this drug aids in pain control postoperatively

24.4 Conclusion

Lumbar hernia, although rare, can be a significant cause of chronic lumbar pain, cosmetic deformity, and potential morbidity from incarceration and strangulation of retroperitoneal and intraabdominal contents, and all patients diagnosed with lumbar hernia should be referred for elective repair. The recognition and incidence of these hernias will continue to increase, and knowledge of repair of these hernias is essential to the practice of hernia specialists. The minimally invasive approach lends itself well to repair of circumscribed lumbar hernia defects. Adequate mesh overlap is essential, and repair of these rare hernias can be technically challenging. The increased freedom of laparoscopic articulation provided by robotic technology allows the opportunity for these patients with a traditional lumbar hernia to be treated in the ambulatory setting.

References

1. Garangeot RJ. Colon traite d'operation. Chirurgie. 1731;1:369–70.
2. Petit JL. Traite des Maladies Chirurgicales, et des Operations Qui Leur Conviennent. Paris, France. TF Didot. 1774;2:256–9.
3. Grynfeltt J. Quelque mots sur la hernie lombaire. Montp Med. 1866;16:323.
4. Selby CD. Direct abdominal hernia of traumatic origin. JAMA. 1906;47:1485.
5. Moreno-Egea A, Baena EG, Calle MC, et al. Controversies in the current management of lumbar hernias. Arch Surg. 2007;142:82–8.
6. Kretchmer HL. Hernia of the kidney. J Urol. 1951;65(5):944–9.
7. Stamatiou D, Skandalakis JE, Skandalakis LJ, et al. Lumbar hernia: surgical anatomy, embryology, and technique of repair. Am Surg. 2009;75(3):202–7.
8. Geis WP, Saletta JD. Lumbar hernia. In: Nyhus LM, Condon RE, editors. Hernia. 3rd ed. Philadelphia: J. B. Lippincott; 1989. p. 401–15.
9. Goodman EH, Speese J. Lumbar hernia. Ann Surg. 1916;63:548–60.
10. Skandalakis JE, Colborn GL, Weidman TA, et al. Skandalakis' surgical anatomy: the embryologic and anatomic basis of modern surgery. Athens: Paschalidis Medical Publications; 2004. p. 457–60.
11. Cavallaro G, Sadighi A, Paparelli C, et al. Anatomical and surgical considerations on lumbar hernias. Am Surg. 2009;75(12):1238–41.
12. Burt BM, Afifi HY, Wantz GE, et al. Traumatic lumbar hernia: report of cases and comprehensive review of the literature. J Trauma. 2004;57:1361–70.
13. Sutherland RS, Gerow RR. Hernia after dorsal incision into lumbar region: a case report and review of pathogenesis and treatment. J Urol. 1995;153:382–4.
14. Fulham SB. Lumbar hernia. J R Coll Surg Edinb. 1985;30(5):315–7.
15. Chatterjee S, Nam R, Fleshner N, Klotz L. Permanent flank bulge is a consequence of flank incision for radical nephrectomy in one half of patients. Urol Oncol. 2004;22:36–9.
16. Pezeshk RA, Pulikkottil BJ, Bailey SH. An evidence-based model for the successful treatment of flank and lateral abdominal wall hernias. Plast Reconstr Surg. 2015;136(2):377–85.
17. Beffa LR, Margiotta AL, Carbonell AM. Flank and lumbar hernia repair. Surg Clin North Am. 2018;98(3):593–605.
18. Moreno-Egea A, Alcaraz AC, Cuervo MC. Surgical options in lumbar hernia: laparoscopic versus open repair. A long-term prospective study. Surg Innov. 2013;20(4):331–44.
19. Edwards C, Geiger T, Bartow K, et al. Laparoscopic transperitoneal repair of flank hernias: a retrospective review of 27 patients. Surg Endosc. 2009;23(12):2692–6.

20. Kirkpatrick T, Zimmerman B, LeBlanc K. Initial experience with robotic hernia repairs: a review of 150 cases. Surg Technol Int. 2018;33:139.
21. Bittner R, Bingener-Casey J, Dietz U, Fabian M, Ferzli G, Fortelny R, Köckerling F, Kukleta J, LeBlanc K, Lomanto D, Misra M, Morales-Conde S, Ramshaw B, Reinpold W, Rim S, Rohr M, Schrittwieser R, Simon T, Smietanski M, Stechemesser B, Timoney M, Chowbey P. Guidelines for laparoscopic treatment of ventral and incisional abdominal wall hernias (International Endohernia Society (IEHS)) - part III. Surg Endosc. 2014;28:380–404.
22. LeBlanc KA. Proper mesh overlap is a key determinant in hernia recurrence following laparoscopic ventral and incisional hernia repair. Hernia. 2016;20(1):85–9.
23. Hauters P, Desmet J, Gherardi D, Dewaele S, Poilvache H, Malvaux P. Assessment of predictive factors for recurrence in laparoscopic ventral hernia repair using a bridging technique. Surg Endosc. 2017;31:3656–63.

Robotic-Assisted Parastomal Hernia Repair: Sugarbaker Repair (With and Without Component Release)

25

Alex Addo, Richard Lu, Igor Belyansky, and Karl A. LeBlanc

25.1 Background

A parastomal hernia results when there is protrusion of abdominal contents through an abdominal wall defect adjacent to a stoma. The reported incidence is up to 75% [1, 2]. Risk factors for development include diabetes mellitus, chronic pulmonary disease, older age, smoking, malnutrition and chronic steroid use [2]. Obesity also significantly contributes to the risk of parastomal hernia formation through an increase in intraabdominal pressure and altered maturation of collagen leading to tissue laxity [3].

The two most common types of parastomal hernia repairs are the Sugarbaker and the keyhole techniques. The purpose of this chapter is to describe the operative method for the robotic-assisted modified Sugarbaker repair. The original Sugarbaker method, first published in 1985, described repairing parastomal hernias with intraabdominal prosthetic mesh placement and lateralization of the bowel conduit [4]. The mesh was circumferentially secured with interrupted sutures around the defect except laterally for the bowel conduit to pass through. The bowel conduit was then secured to the lateral abdominal wall with sutures. Currently, this procedure can be performed utilizing a minimally invasive approach. Pauli et al. described the Pauli

A. Addo · R. Lu
Department of Surgery, Anne Arundel Medical Center, Annapolis, MD, USA

I. Belyansky (✉)
Department of Surgery, Anne Arundel Medical Center, Annapolis, MD, USA

Abdominal Wall Reconstruction Program, General Surgery, Anne Arundel Medical Center, Annapolis, MD, USA
e-mail: ibelyansky@aahs.org

K. A. LeBlanc
Our Lady of the Lake Physician Group, Baton Rouge, LA, USA

Department of Surgery, Louisiana State University Health Sciences Center, New Orleans, LA, USA

K. A. LeBlanc (ed.), *Robotic Assisted Hernia Repair*,
https://doi.org/10.1007/978-3-030-23025-8_25

modified Sugarbaker technique in 2016, which combined a posterior components release (transversus abdominis release or TAR) with the Sugarbaker repair [5]. We often use this approach as it optimizes lateralization of the bowel conduit and enhances mesh coverage area without the need for penetrating fixation.

25.2 Indications for Repair

The most common indications for surgery are quality of life issues related to the stoma appliance or discomfort related to bulging of the herniated contents and/or a history of bowel obstruction [1, 2]. Due to the high recurrence rate and other postoperative complications, asymptomatic patients can usually be managed non-operatively.

25.3 Preoperative Considerations

An extensive evaluation including a history and physical examination, basic laboratory testing and appropriate imaging, is recommended prior to surgical intervention. A current computed tomography study of the abdomen and pelvis is recommended for accurate diagnosis, assessment of anatomy and effective preoperative planning. An up-to-date screening colonoscopy for patients over the age of 50 years is also recommended. All major comorbid conditions must be addressed by means of a multidisciplinary approach before proceeding to the operating room. Patients with a current smoking history must discontinue smoking for at least 4 weeks before their surgery. It is also important for diabetic patients to have their glycated hemoglobin level below 7.0% and the morbidly obese to achieve a body mass index of <40 kg/m^2.

25.4 Operating Room Set Up

A list of necessary equipment to perform a robotic-assisted Pauli modified Sugarbaker parastomal hernia repair is shown in Table 25.1. This includes a standard laparoscopy set of instrumentation.

Table 25.1 Equipment list

Laparoscopic equipment	• 5-mm 30-degree scope • Laparoscopic needle driver • 5-mm Kii Fios First Entry® (Applied Medical, Rancho Santa Margarita, CA) port
Robotic equipment	• 10-mm 30-degree and 0-degree scopes (Si) or 8 mm (Xi) • Two 8-mm robotic ports • 12-mm bariatric port for robotic camera (Si) or 8 mm (Xi) • Monopolar scissors • ProGrasp™ grasper (Intuitive Surgical, Sunnyvale, CA) • Mega Suture Cut™ needle driver (Intuitive Surgical) • Monopolar cord • Bipolar cord (optional if bipolar fenestrated grasper is used)

25.5 Description of Technique

25.5.1 Initial Access and Retromuscular Dissection

An extended-view totally extraperitoneal (eTEP) approach is preferred in our practice. However, an intraabdominal approach may be considered if the patient has large midline defects necessitating bilateral TAR. The initial steps of this procedure follow an eTEP Rives-Stoppa repair in regard to accessing the retrorectus space (Chap. 20) [6]. The patient is placed in a supine position with both arms tucked to the side and then placed in steep Trendelenburg position with the lower extremities flexed at a 30° downward angle. The contralateral retrorectus space to the stoma is entered directly using a 5-mm optical trocar. The retrorectus space is developed lateral to the linea alba and medially to the neurovascular bundles (Fig. 25.1a). A 12-mm camera and a 8-mm robotic working port are placed medial to the linea semilunaris (Fig. 25.1b).

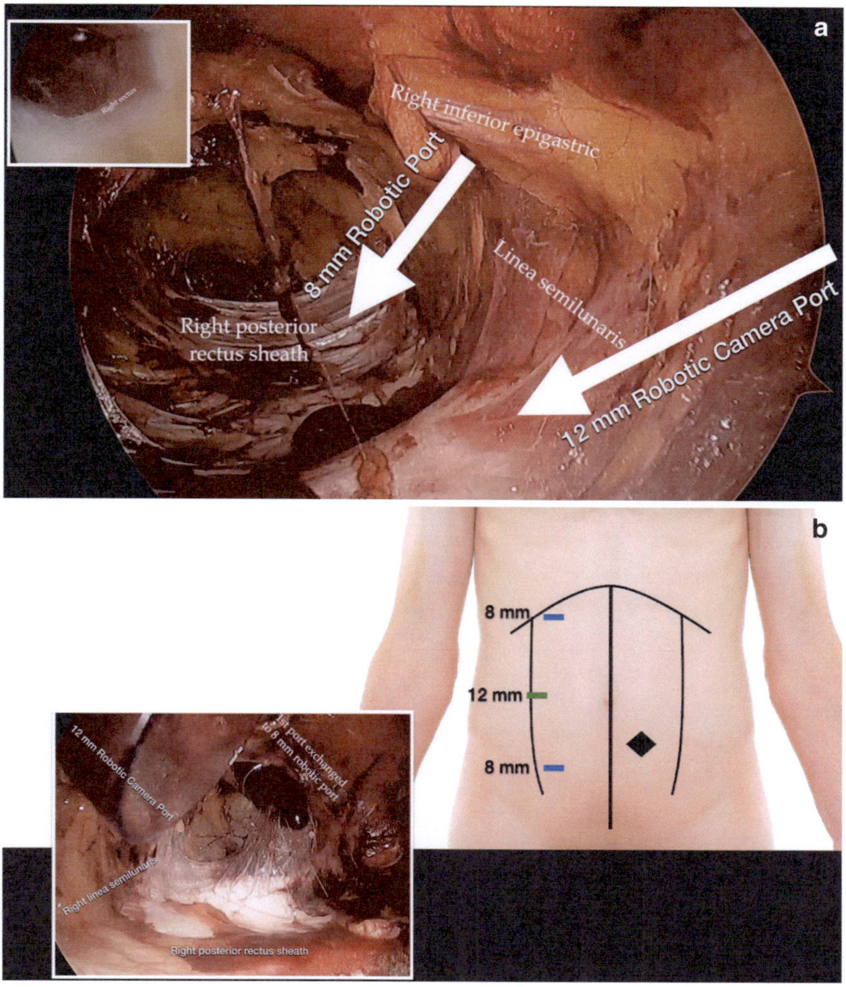

Fig. 25.1 (**a**) Accessing retrorectus space (**b**) Port placement relative to hernia defect. Example of port placement. Blue: robotic working ports, Green: camera port, Diamond: Ostomy site

A crossover maneuver is performed to connect the bilateral retrorectus and preperitoneal spaces (Fig. 25.2). This maneuver is initiated by incising the medial aspect of the posterior rectus sheath in a longitudinal fashion. Once the preperitoneal space is entered, the adipose tissue from the falciform and umbilical ligaments are swept down, exposing the linea alba and the contralateral posterior rectus sheath. A longitudinal incision is made along the contralateral posterior rectus sheath and the retrorectus space to the hernia defect is entered and developed. It is crucial to avoid injury of the linea alba during incision of the posterior rectus sheaths. Once the hernia sac is encountered, it is sharply incised circumferentially creating a defect in the posterior layer (Fig. 25.3).

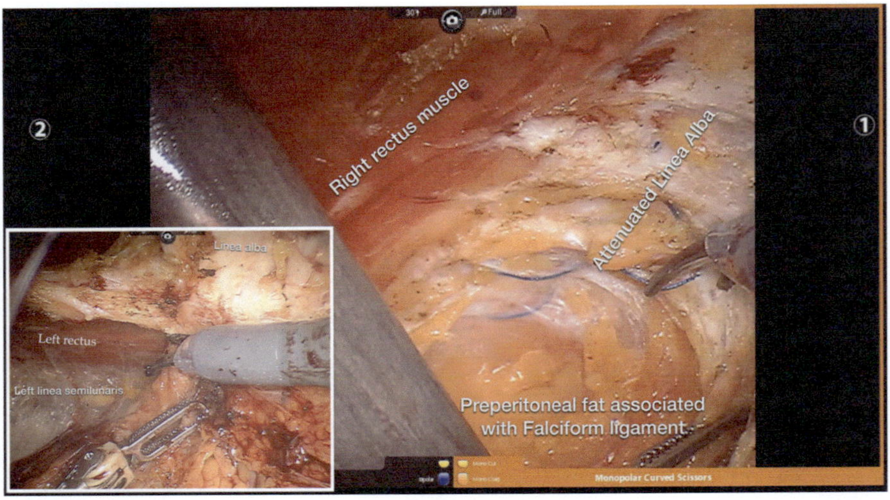

Fig. 25.2 Performing crossover maneuver

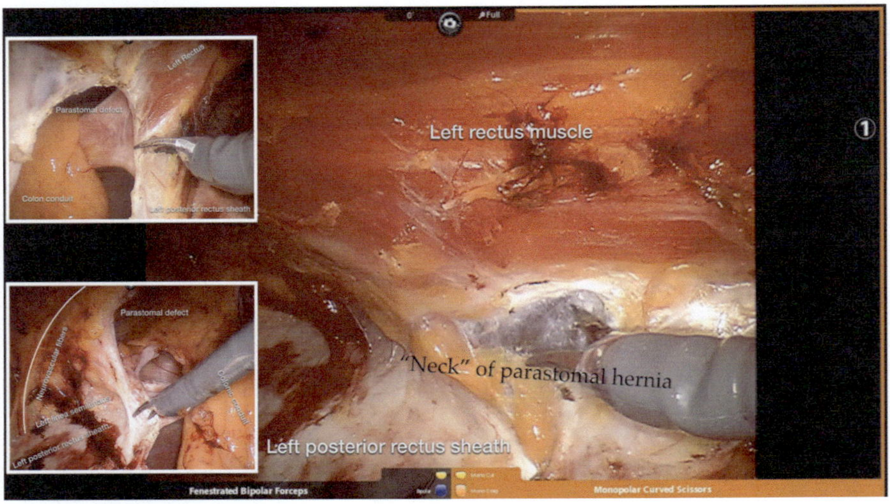

Fig. 25.3 Dissecting around hernia sac

25.5.2 Transversus Abdominis Release (TAR)

After development of the retrorectus space, we typically initiate the TAR by first developing the Space of Bogros (Fig. 25.4). The posterior lamella and contributions from the transversus abdominis muscle are then identified and divided medial to the linea semilunaris (Fig. 25.5), leaving the underlying transversalis fascia intact. The retromuscular space, which now encompasses the retrorectus and pretransversalis spaces, is developed by blunt dissection, which creates a large area for mesh placement and lateralization of the colonic conduit. It is our practice to develop the retromuscular space until the posterior layer lays flat.

Fig. 25.4 Developing the Space of Bogros

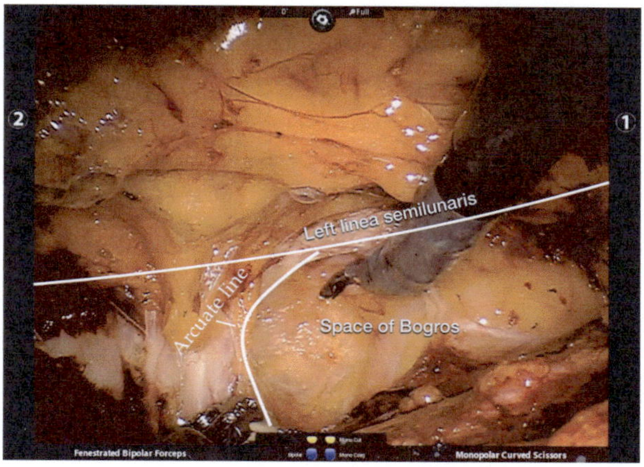

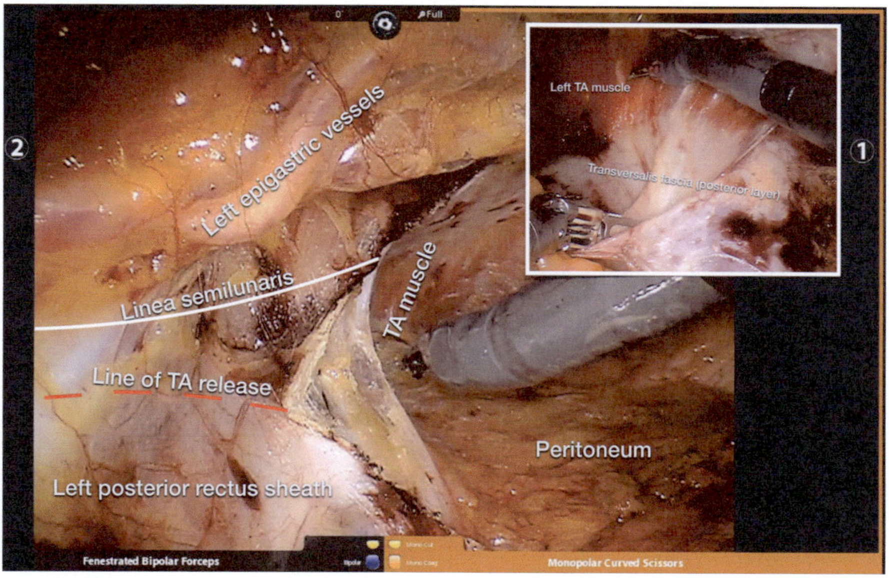

Fig. 25.5 Dividing the posterior lamella of the internal oblique

25.5.3 Lateralization of Conduit and Closure of Posterior Layer and Parastomal Defects

Once the retromuscular space is fully developed, the posterior parastomal hernia defect is extended laterally (Fig. 25.6). This step is important as it aids in lateralization of the colonic conduit by shifting its entry point laterally as it enters the retromuscular space. Lateralization of the conduit is assisted by suturing it to the lateral abdominal wall which is typically the aponeurotic portion of the transversus abdominis muscle (Fig. 25.7). The posterior layer defect is closed with 2–0 barbed

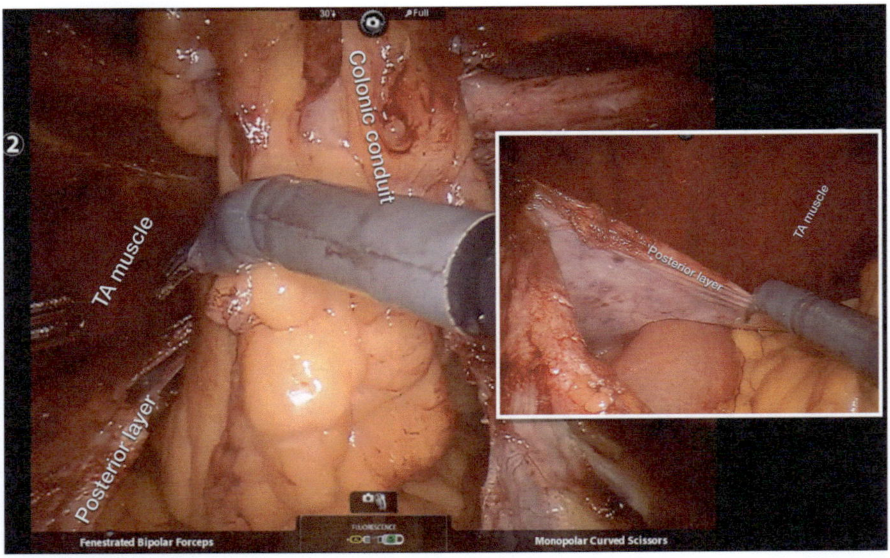

Fig. 25.6 Incising posterior layer and extending hernia defect laterally

Fig. 25.7 Lateralizing bowel conduit

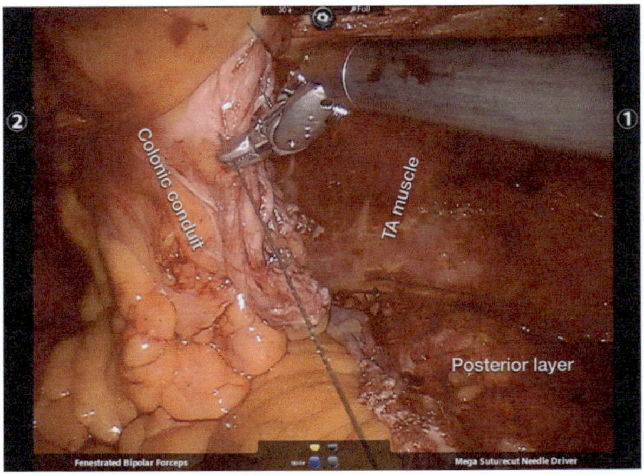

absorbable suture (Fig. 25.8). The conduit should now enter the retromuscular space laterally and exit medially through the rectus abdominis muscle. The goal is to have between 5 and 7 cm of the bowel conduit traversing the retromuscular space. The anterior hernia defect is then closed in a running fashion with 0 barbed absorbable suture (Fig. 25.9).

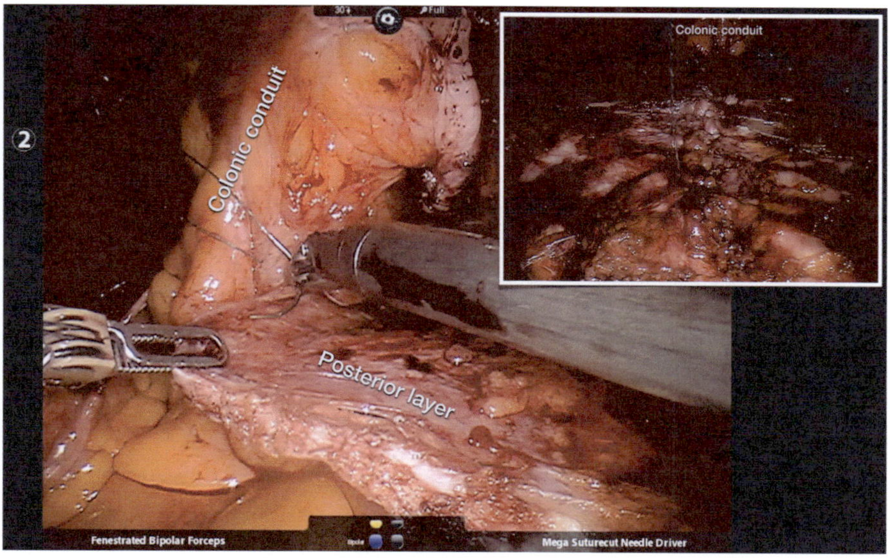

Fig. 25.8 Closing posterior defect

Fig. 25.9 Closing anterior defect

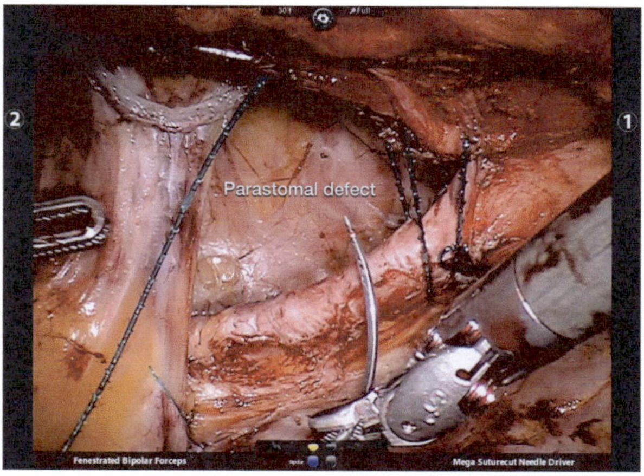

25.5.4 Mesh Placement

A macroporous medium-weight polypropylene mesh is trimmed to provide adequate coverage of the entirety of the developed retromuscular space (Fig. 25.10). A keyhole is used to allow exit of the colon but we recommend that a minimum of 5 cm circumferential overlap around the defect is achieved. In our practice, a closed-suction drain is positioned over the mesh to prevent seroma formation in the early postoperative period which could potentially compromise the integrity of the posterior layer.

25.6 Postoperative Management of Modified Sugarbaker with TAR

Patients are admitted to the floor and started on a clear liquid diet within 24 h of surgery. Postoperative pain is controlled with patient-controlled analgesia (PCA) for the first 24 h. Patients are then transitioned to oral analgesia on the first postoperative day. We prefer to await return of ostomy function prior to discharge which results in a typical hospital stay between 2 and 3 days. The retromuscular drain is removed in clinic within a week.

25.7 Complications

Common complications include subcutaneous seroma formation associated with dead space after reduction of large parastomal hernias. In a cohort of 12 patients who recently underwent this procedure at our institution, one required drain

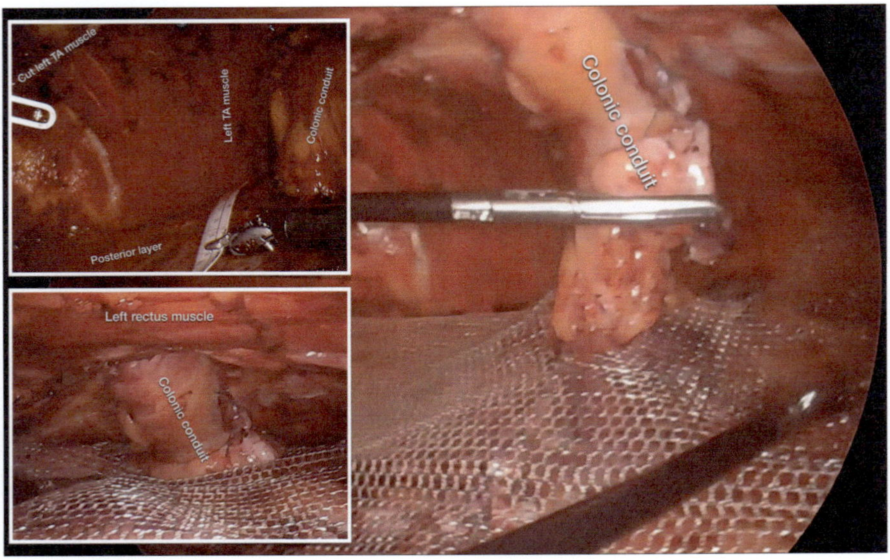

Fig. 25.10 Mesh placement

placement by interventional radiology secondary to seroma formation. In addition, retromuscular dissection performed close to well-vascularized rectus muscles is associated with a higher risk of hematoma formation postoperatively. There is also concern about the placement of mesh against the bowel conduit. However, to date we have not seen any undesired effects associated with this, including mesh erosion or bowel obstruction. One must consider the intimate interaction of the mesh and bowel at the transition point from the intraabdominal cavity into the retromuscular space. If the mesh has increased tightness near the bowel conduit transition point the mesh should be incised to release tension. Otherwise, mesh erosion of bowel may occur. Additionally, attention should be taken intraoperatively to ensure that the mesh is snug but not strangulating the conduit in that area.

25.8 Traditional Sugarbaker Repair

The above technique has recently evolved since the adoption of robotic technology for hernia repair. There have been similar modifications for various hernias that are detailed elsewhere in this textbook. There has also been a prior history of the use of the Sugarbaker with purely laparoscopic methods. This method has a longer history than that described above. This more traditional method is presented below. It is somewhat easier to adopt for the surgeon that is new to the robotically assisted repair of ventral and parastomal hernias and especially those surgeons that are just developing their skill sets with the posterior component separation method of any hernia repair.

The robotic assisted laparoscopic repair does not differ from the laparoscopic repair other than the use of the robot and the efficiencies that it provides. The initial goal is the dissection of all adhesions and identification of the anatomy of the hernia. This dissection can be hampered if there is difficulty ascertaining the different structures such as omentum and mesentery. This can be very difficult in the incarcerated hernias. Occasionally an internal hernia will also be identified, making this separation of tissues especially challenging.

The initial workup should not differ from that noted earlier in the chapter. A significant loss of domain can make the minimally invasive option impossible. The examination of the patient, the clinical status along with a preoperative CT scan will greatly assist the approach to this problem. The latter evaluation is helpful in that it can also identify the presence of additional hernias that are so frequent in the prior midline incision. The surgeon can also assess the contents of the hernia, the size of the defect, and the exact location of the defect(s). The laterally located herniation is more challenging to repair than the more medially located one (resulting in a higher recurrence rate).

25.8.1 Operating Room Set Up

In all cases the trocars will be inserted on the side of the abdomen opposite the location of the parastomal hernia (Fig. 25.11). As noted in the figure, the location of the camera will differ slightly for the two different robots. The location of the trocars for the X robot will be identical to that of the Xi robot. Occasionally it will be helpful to add the fourth arm to the robot to repair these hernias when there is a significant amount of adhesions or the habitus of the patient requires it but this is seldom needed. The instruments that are preferred are not substantially different from that of Table 25.1 (Table 25.2).

25.8.2 Initial Access and Technique

The initial entry can be with the optical trocar noted above or one without the ability to insufflate via the obturator of the trocar itself. As shown in Fig. 25.11, I will use the 5 mm port (not shown) to inspect the abdomen, but this will be replaced with a 12 mm accessory port to allow introduction of suture and mesh and extraction of needles during the operation. The use of the laparoscopic grasper may be needed to dissect adhesions that prevent the safe insertion of the robotic trocars. The ProGrasp™ is not often required with this method unless mesh must be removed as part of the procedure. The need to heavily grasp tissues is not often required.

As with all intra-abdominal procedures for hernia repair, the initial phases of the procedure will center on the lysis of adhesions (Fig. 25.12). The reduction of incarcerated hernia contents will be the next order of business to allow for the delineation of the fascial edges. For the use of the intraperitoneal onlay method that will be described here, all adipose tissue that might be interposed between the mesh and the

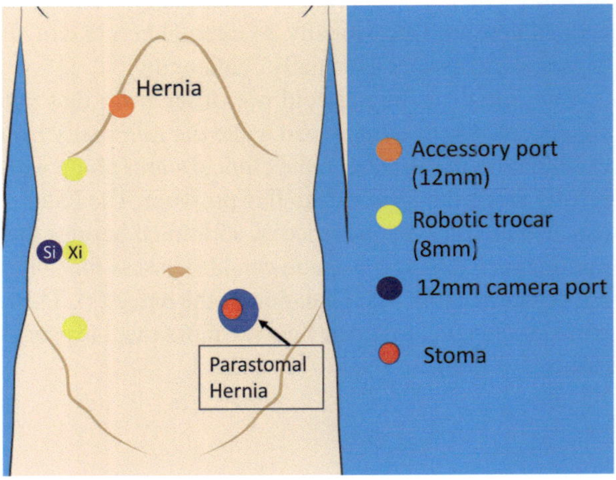

Fig. 25.11 Port placement—parastomal (colostomy) hernia

Table 25.2 Equipment list

Laparoscopic equipment	• 5-mm 0-degree scope • Laparoscopic grasper • Optical viewing trocar (5 mm) • 12 mm trocar • Suture passing device
Robotic equipment	• 8 mm (Xi) or 10-mm (Si) 30-degree camera • Two 8-mm robotic ports • 12-mm port for robotic camera (Si) or 8 mm (Xi) • Monopolar scissors (Intuitive Surgical, Sunnyvale, CA) • Fenestrated Bipolar™ grasper (Intuitive Surgical) • Mega Suture Cut™ needle driver (Intuitive Surgical) • Mega™ Needle driver (Intuitive Surgical)

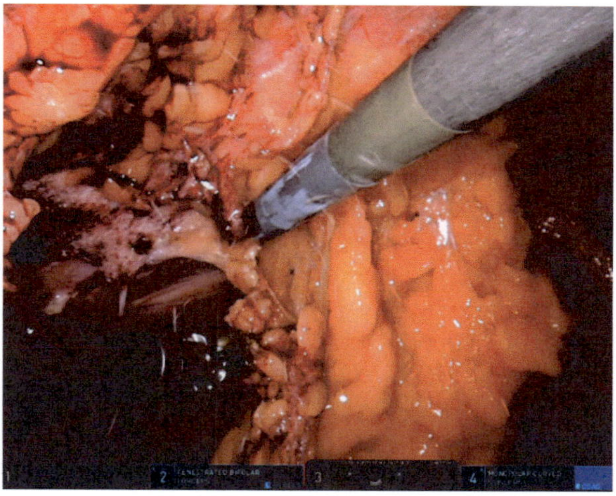

Fig. 25.12 Initial dissection (prior midline incisional and parastomal keyhole hernia repair in all figures)

abdominal wall should be cleared away to allow for ingrowth of the tissues into the selected mesh material.

After this has been accomplished, the defect and the area that will be covered by the mesh will be measured by placing a ruler into the abdomen (Fig. 25.13). The use of the largest dimension is used to size the mesh. It is very important to obtain a minimum of 5 cm overlap (as noted above). in all directions using these measurements (Fig. 25.14). Any additional overlap laterally will be beneficial because this area will most likely be the location of a recurrence. The fascial defect will then be re-approximated with #2 permanent barbed sutures (Fig. 25.15). Care must be taken to avoid any compromise to the opening through which the intestine must pass to avoid an obstruction.

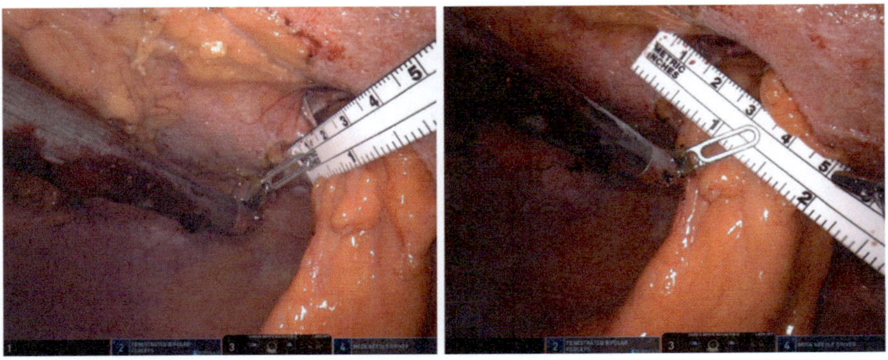

Fig. 25.13 Measurement of the defect in both directions

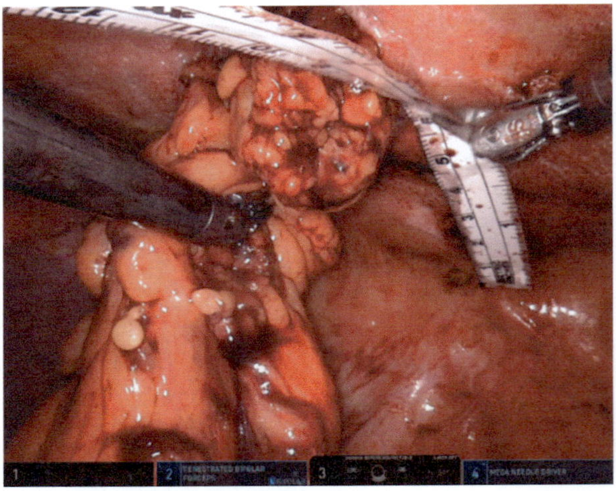

Fig. 25.14 Measurement of the lateral coverage of the mesh (in this case, 6 cm overlap)

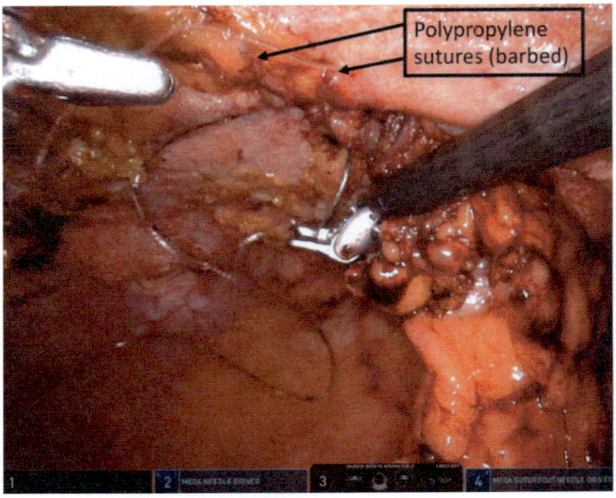

Fig. 25.15 Closure of the defect

As noted above, the mesh selected should allow for a minimum of 5 cm overlap in all directions but if there is an associated incisional hernia, then a larger size will be needed to repair this hernia at the same time. Three polyglactin sutures will be placed onto the mesh prior to introduction into the abdomen to aid in positioning of it. It is recommended that they be placed 8–10 cm apart to allow an adequate orifice for the intestine to pass and avoid compression on the intestine. This material will be inserted into the abdominal cavity via the 12 mm trocar in the right upper quadrant (Fig. 25.16). Generally, it is not necessary to lateralize the intestine with suture as the mesh will assure lateralization. As shown in Fig. 25.17, two white sutures are used and placed 10 cm apart while a third purple suture is placed at the opposite end of the mesh to position the middle of that portion of the mesh to center the hernia. These two different colors help differentiate the sutures during manipulation of the sutures.

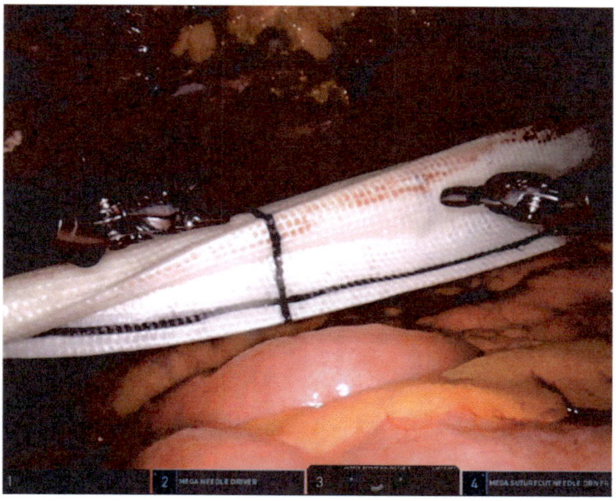

Fig. 25.16 Mesh inserted through 12 mm trocar

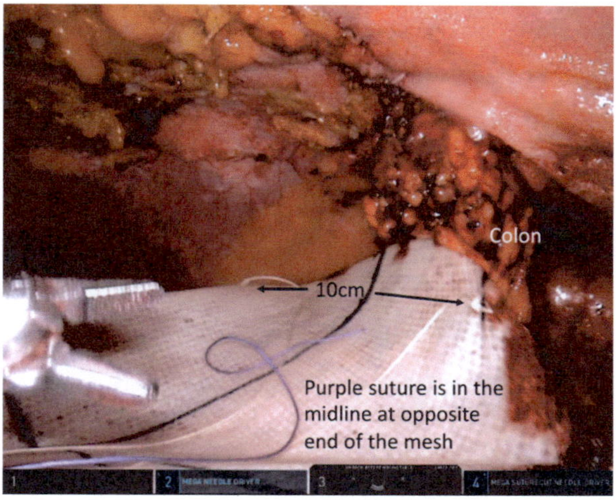

Fig. 25.17 Preplaced sutures to position the mesh

As single 2–3 mm incision lateral to the stoma will be placed through which the two white sutures will be pulled through the abdominal wall (Fig. 25.18). This will insure the adequacy of overlap while positioning the mesh to be sewn into the abdominal with #2 permanent barbed sutures. A double armed suture will make this easier as each limb can be used on one side of the intestine to fixate that side of the mesh material. It is preferred to start suturing on the lower portion of the mesh adjacent to the intestine with the first limb (Fig. 25.19). The second limb will be used to sew the periphery of the mesh on that same side (Fig. 25.20).

The second double armed suture will be started on the opposite (cephalad) side of the intestine. The goal is to create a tube of mesh through which the intestine will

Fig. 25.18 Retrieval of lateral positioning sutures

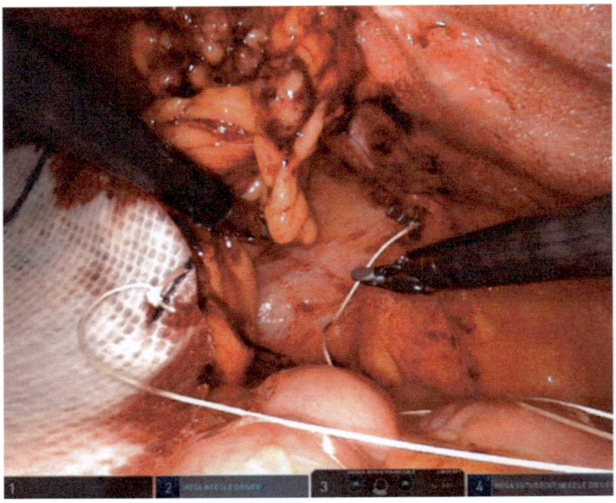

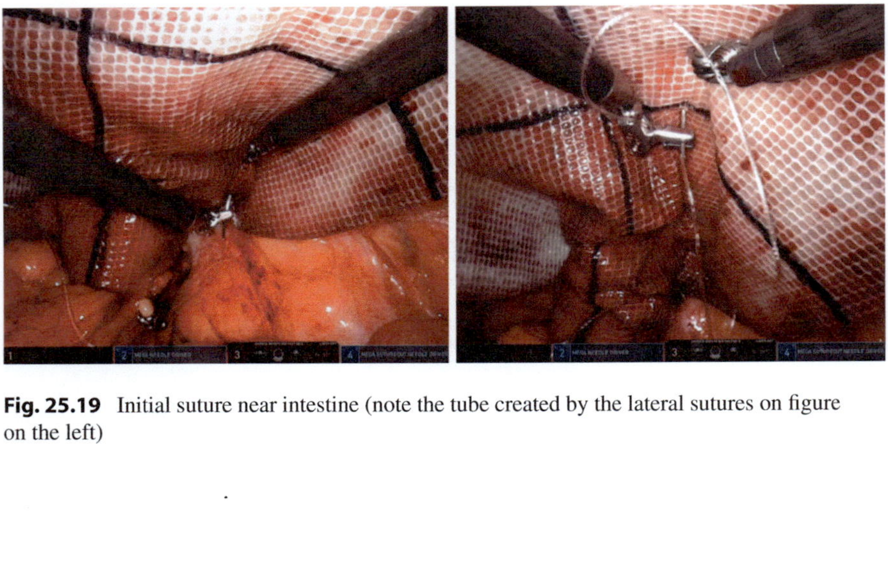

Fig. 25.19 Initial suture near intestine (note the tube created by the lateral sutures on figure on the left)

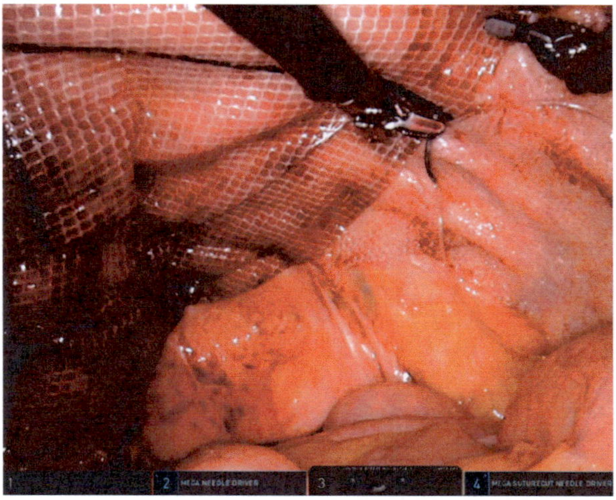

Fig. 25.20 Suture placement at the periphery of the mesh

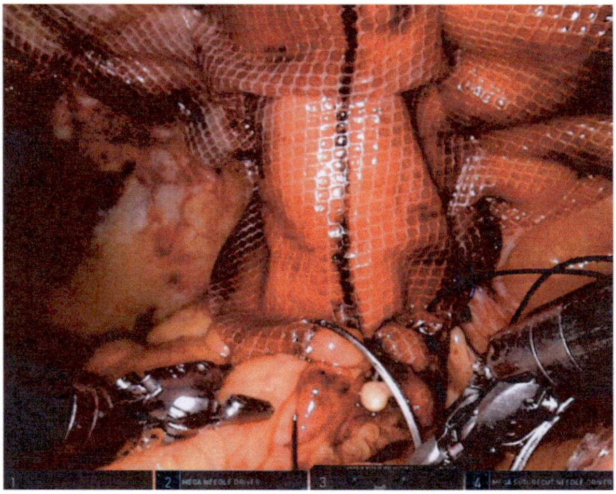

Fig. 25.21 Absorbable suture of colon to mesh

pass. As before, the first pass will be adjacent to the intestine and the second limb will used to fixate the periphery of the prosthetic material. After this has been completed, an absorbable 2-0 barbed suture will be used to sew the intestine to the mesh to close off the potential space that exists between the intestine and the mesh (Fig. 25.21). At the completion of the suturing, the mesh will be fashioned as a tube through which the intestine will pass through and the periphery of the mesh will be sewn with the wide overlap (Fig. 25.22).

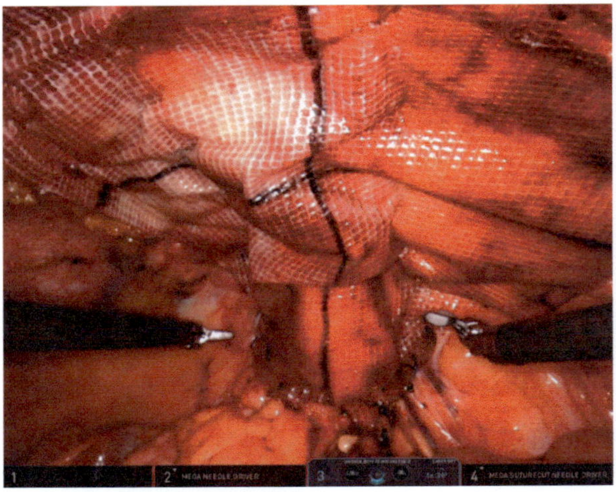

Fig. 25.22 Completed procedure

25.9 Postoperative Management

The majority of patients will have the use of a transversus abdominis plane block. This significantly diminishes opioid use and decreases the length of stay. A regular diet is begun the next day. In the past, we required the patient to have a bowel movement prior to discharge but no longer make this an absolute requirement. This technique has been applied to 22 patients with excellent results. To date only one recurrence has been seen. This was a contracted, debilitated wheelchair bound patient on chronic high dose steroid medication for severe osteoarthritis. It would seem there are multiple possible reasons for recurrence in this patient.

25.10 Conclusion

Two options for repair of parastomal herniation have been presented in this chapter. Of note, no description of the pure keyhole approach has been given because the rate of recurrence is prohibitively high to recommend this procedure. We suggest that the reader explore either of these two options as experience is gained in the robotic incisional repair and the TAR repair.

References

1. Shah N, Craft R, Harold K. Parastomal hernia repair. Surg Clin North Am. 2013;93(5):1185–98.
2. O'Neill C, Borrazzo E, Hyman N. Parastomal hernia repair. J Gastrointest Surg. 2014;19(4):766–9.
3. Liu N, Hackney J, Gellhaus P, Monn F, Masterson T, Bihrle R, Gardner T, House M, Koch M. Incidence and risk factors of parastomal hernia in patients undergoing radical cystectomy and ileal conduit diversion. J Urol. 2014;191(2):1313–8.

4. Sugarbaker P. Peritoneal approach to prosthetic mesh repair of paraostomy hernias. Ann Surg. 1985;201(3):344–6.
5. Pauli E, Juza R, Winder J. How I do it: novel parastomal herniorrhaphy utilizing transversus abdominis release. Hernia. 2016;20(4):547–52.
6. Belyansky I, Zahiri R, Sanford Z, Weltz A, Park A. Early operative outcomes of endoscopic (eTEP access) robotic-assisted retromuscular abdominal wall hernia repair. Hernia. 2018;22(5):837–47.

Robotic Ventral and Incisional Hernia Repair: Management of Adverse Events

26

Anthony M. Gonzalez and Rodolfo J. Oviedo

Ventral and incisional hernia repair remains one of the most common, and sometimes challenging, procedures performed by general surgeons in the United States and around the world. Despite this fact, there is little consensus on the best approach to repair this type of hernia. Due to the rapid advancement of technology, the development of robotic surgery has been applied to simple and complex ventral and incisional hernia repair [1].

The robotic platform has been used for simple fascial closure and intraperitoneal placement and fixation of mesh, and more recently, for minimally invasive retrorectus dissection, closure of the linea alba and extraperitoneal placement of mesh. The most advanced hernia specialists use this technology to release the abdominal wall musculature to allow for primary closure of the midline, which in turn restores and maintains the integrity of the abdominal wall, not only from an anatomic standpoint, but also with respect to its physiology.

As with any surgical procedure, adverse events or complications may occur. The purpose of this chapter is to describe the most common post-operative occurrences during and after robotic ventral and incisional hernia repair, and their appropriate management.

A. M. Gonzalez (✉)
Baptist Hospital of Miami, Miami, FL, USA

Florida International University College of Medicine, Miami, FL, USA

Bariatric Surgery Baptist Health South Florida, Miami, FL, USA

MIS/Bariatric Surgery Fellowship, BHSF, Miami, FL, USA
e-mail: AnthonyG@Baptisthealth.net

R. J. Oviedo
Florida State University College of Medicine, Tallahassee, FL, USA

Winchester Medical Center, Valley Health Metabolic and Bariatric Program, Winchester, VA, USA

K. A. LeBlanc (ed.), *Robotic Assisted Hernia Repair*,
https://doi.org/10.1007/978-3-030-23025-8_26

Intraoperative complications can occur during robotic primary ventral hernia repair. However, it has been demonstrated that incisional hernia repair is associated with more complications since lysis of adhesions is more likely [2]. This increases the possibility of bowel injury either as single or multiple serosal tears, or as full thickness defects with perforation. Therefore, bowel injury can occur during enterolysis or adhesiolysis during incisional hernia repair or manipulation of instruments during ventral hernia repair. If recognized, the bowel should be immediately repaired either via the robotic approach, or with conversion to an open procedure if not feasible. Most likely, however, a robotic repair of any enterotomy or serosal tear can be appropriate due to the multiple benefits offered by the robotic technology and with adequate surgical skills.

Changes in plans regarding the approach to repair the hernia and with respect to mesh selection may occur after an inadvertent bowel injury. These changes must be carefully considered to prevent long-term issues like chronic mesh contamination or infection.

Postoperative complications are more common than intra operative complications. Wound issues, though less likely after robotic or minimally invasive surgery, can occur. Wound disruption can be seen due to pressure necrosis of the skin from the trocar during surgery. This can be avoided by creating the correct size incision to match the trocar size. After surgery, these issues are quite self-limiting and can be dealt with using simple wound care.

A trocar site wound infection can occur, especially in an obese patient where wound healing is not optimized due to excessive subcutaneous fat with poor blood supply. This will be recognized 5–10 days post operatively. Management is similar to all surgical wound infections, beginning with opening the wound and instituting antibiotic therapy, if indicated. These wounds are of low risk, since they are typically remote to the location of the hernia and mesh placement. Therefore, significant concern for mesh infection is not warranted.

Hematomas and seromas at the trocar site can also occur without an associated infection. These can be observed with patience and will spontaneously resolve.

Seromas at the area of the hernia repair are more common, despite the introduction of robotic surgery and techniques for fascial closure. A 2017 study by the Americas Hernia Society Quality Collaborative Analysis demonstrated higher rates of surgical site occurrence (SSO) in the laparoscopic intraperitoneal onlay mesh (IPOM) repair arm compared to the robotic arm, 14% vs 5%, respectively [3].

Gonzalez et al (not published) have educated many surgeons on the prevention of seromas with a post-operative dressing that included Kerlix rolls over the hernia repair with an abdominal binder. This applies pressure to the hernia sac, if the sac is left in situ, or over the subcutaneous space, if the sac is resected, and diminishes the formation of a seroma or hematoma at that location. Others have popularized the incorporation of the hernia sac in the defect primary closure to diminish the formation of a seroma.

If seromas develop in the immediate postoperative period, application of the above Gonzalez Hernia Binder technique can eliminate all that fluid from the subcutaneous space through the still semipermeable mesh. If more than 2 weeks have expired since surgery, it is unlikely that this binder would help. Management of the seroma would depend on whether it is symptomatic. If asymptomatic, no treatment is needed. If the patient is symptomatic from the seroma, aspiration in the office setting and application of the pressure binder is feasible. This may be repeated if needed. For recurrent, symptomatic seromas involving a significant granulation tissue cavity, surgical drainage of the fluid and excision of the seroma cavity may be needed. Drain placement after excision should be strongly considered.

Bleeding intraoperatively should be dealt with using basic surgical techniques as described above. Postoperative hematomas can be subcutaneous in the area of the hernia sac, especially if the sac was resected, or intraabdominal in location. Subcutaneous hematomas can be observed, since needle aspiration increases the risk of infection, as blood is a good milieu for bacterial growth. If they fail to resolve in 3–6 months and continue to be symptomatic, operative drainage and excision can be performed similarly to seromas. Intraabdominal hematomas are more likely to resolve and rarely require treatment. If super-infection of the hematoma occurs, percutaneous drainage using interventional radiology techniques is possible.

If an intraabdominal hematoma becomes infected, contamination of the mesh is possible. If the mesh becomes contaminated, treatment with long-term antibiotics is the initial step. Many lightweight meshes available today will resist infection and continue to incorporate themselves into the surrounding tissues [4]. If the infection causes a systemic inflammatory response and sepsis, or if it becomes chronic in nature, the management would change to operative exploration and explantation of the mesh. This can be attempted via laparoscopic or robotic approaches, but most likely would have to be dealt with via an open procedure since the presence of inflammation and infection usually precludes a minimally invasive approach.

If exploration of the surgical site via an open approach is performed, the unincorporated mesh is explanted, while the peritoneal cavity (or the portion of it exposed by the wound) and the abdominal wall are thoroughly lavaged. The hernia is repaired via an open approach with monofilament absorbable suture. Use of biological mesh can be used to reinforce the repair and decrease the chance of recurrence of the hernia [5].

Intra-abdominal adhesions can occur after any operation but have been proven to occur less frequently with minimally invasive surgery. After robotic ventral hernia repair, the likelihood of intraabdominal adhesions and resulting small bowel obstruction depends on where the mesh has been implanted. It has been postulated that the intraperitoneal onlay mesh (IPOM) technique has a higher likelihood of intraabdominal adhesions due to mesh placement within the peritoneal cavity [6]. Despite the adhesive barrier provided on the mesh, the inflammatory response by the mesh itself will propagate adhesions [7].

When the mesh is placed in the extraperitoneal location the occurrence of intraabdominal adhesions is less common [8]. When a small bowel obstruction occurs, management is similar to all initial medical management of bowel obstruction with nasogastric tube placement and intravenous fluids for resuscitation in the setting of third-space volume losses. When these occur in the early post-operative period, resolution is more likely [9]. If the bowel obstruction fails to resolve with medical management, operative exploration via laparoscopy or laparotomy is indicated.

Pain after robotic ventral hernia repair is common. Studies have demonstrated decreased pain with the robotic approach likely due to the elimination of tacks and suture fixation of the mesh [10]. This immediate postoperative pain is dealt with via a multimodal pain approach as recommended by multiple societies [11]. Scheduled acetaminophen and NSAIDS are used as a foundation for pain control, with judicious use of opiates as needed. The addition of an intraoperative nerve block, particularly in the preperitoneal plane with bupivacaine, may reduce the need for opiates in the immediate post-operative period [12].

Long term pain for more than a few weeks or a month would be categorized as chronic pain. This is less likely with the robotic approach, since transfacial sutures are not used. The use of transfacial sutures is associated with more chronic pain because nerve entrapment can occur with this technique [13]. Since the recommendation for mesh fixation is implantation with a monofilament absorbable suture, as the suture absorbs in 6–9 months, most pain associated with the fixation of the mesh should resolve. If chronic pain continues, attempts at nerve block in the office setting and nerve "destruction" can be managed by a pain specialist.

Hernia recurrence has been described as an important complication, which may occur in the early postoperative period as well as a chronic adverse event months to years later. As is expected, the patient's habitus and body mass index (BMI) play a crucial role, in addition to activity level and other factors such as diabetes mellitus type 2, chronic steroid use, smoking, connective tissue diseases and overall immune status, to name a few. Other factors include age, simultaneous bowel surgery, hernia defect size, and method of hernia repair [14]. Regarding the hernia size and BMI, Oviedo *et al* described the use of the robotic platform to repair large hernia defects with intracorporeal suturing for primary closure and mesh implantation with the IPOM technique, combined with an external oblique endoscopic component separation to decrease tension, with low recurrence rates in patients with BMI > 30 kg/m^2. Such a technique can be safely implemented in a community hospital setting with proper team training [15, 16]. Moreover, Gonzalez et al have demonstrated the benefit of the robotic approach to decrease hernia recurrence rates when repairing ventral hernias. Primary closure of the defect with intracorporeal suturing is facilitated by the robotic instruments, which empower the surgeon's dexterity when suturing. This is followed by meticulous mesh implantation [17, 18].

With respect to the incidence of venous thromboembolism or deep venous thrombosis (DVT) in addition to pulmonary embolism (PE), these possible complications are intricately related to the patient's overall condition and risk factors such as obesity, sedentary habits, propensity for venous stasis, among other well-known factors that do not necessarily have to do with the presence of a hernia. Therefore, specifically for the field of abdominal wall reconstruction and simple to complex hernia repair, with or without minimally invasive techniques such as robotics, DVT prophylaxis prior to surgery is not indicated unless the patient has a history of prior DVT and/or PE. Otherwise, normal measures for DVT prophylaxis in the post-operative period while recovering in the hospital are taken, including pharmacologic prophylaxis with subcutaneous Heparin or low-molecular weight Heparin (Lovenox), along with mechanical prophylaxis with sequential compression devices and frequent ambulation. If the surgery is planned to be ambulatory, then post-operative pharmacologic DVT prophylaxis is not indicated unless, again, if the patient has a prior history of DVT and/or PE [18]. In fact, large studies have already demonstrated that robotic ventral hernia repair is associated with shorter length of stay and complication rates, where DVT and PE do not play a significant role [19].

Hospital-acquired pneumonia (HAP) has also been studied as a possible adverse event following minimally invasive ventral or incisional hernia repair, including the robotic approach. The literature results vary, but a recent study showed higher rates of pneumonia in patients who underwent robotic ventral hernia repair compared to those who had the procedure with laparoscopic techniques. However, after controlling for confounding variables, there was no significant difference [20]. Part of the reason may be that the patients who are selected to undergo a robotic repair tend to be of more advanced age and with a higher American Society of Anesthesiologists (ASA) classification, which puts them at a higher risk for pneumonia. Aspiration precautions in this patient population are essential. On the other hand, the use of incentive spirometry on robotic ventral or incisional hernia repair patients is part of the fundamental principles of postoperative recovery, both in the hospital and at home, to counteract the effects of atelectasis and prevent pneumonia.

Finally, the discussion of adverse events during or after robotic ventral or incisional hernia repair cannot be complete without an analysis of system malfunction. This topic has been a very important one for the Food and Drug Administration (FDA) for several years since the robotic platform was approved in the United States. At least in the urology international literature, possible malfunction mechanisms during urologic robotic procedures have included the arm system, the optical system, the power system with the connector, endoscopic instruments, and the software itself [21]. The most important lesson is the proper training of the surgical team to manage the malfunction in a timely fashion and, if not possible, to convert to a traditional laparoscopic approach if possible before considering conversion to open. In either case, patient safety is at the forefront of any action taken in the operating room.

In the American literature, a very large retrospective series of 14 years of data has revealed some important lessons, as well, specifically pertaining to the surgical specialties that utilize the robot more often. These specialties, including gynecology, urology, and general surgery, exhibit lower rates of mortality, injuries, and conversions to open compared to those specialties where the robotic platform is not frequently used, such as cardiothoracic surgery and otolaryngology. System malfunction was also studied in terms of adverse events dealing with the components of the platform, including burnt or broken pieces of instruments falling into the patient, electrical arcing, unintended operation of instruments, system errors, and problems with the visual system. The procedure was interrupted to restart the system sometimes, while other times the procedure was rescheduled when critical portions were not performed. Education is of paramount importance, both for the surgical team and for the industry, so that adverse events are reported properly and dealt with as soon as they occur [22].

To summarize, robotic ventral and incisional hernia repair has become one of the most frequently performed minimally invasive procedures for general surgeons in the last few years, with the development of advanced techniques for abdominal wall reconstruction that go beyond a traditional laparoscopic intraperitoneal onlay mesh (IPOM) repair. These advanced techniques expand to the realm of intracorporeal primary closure of the hernia, preperitoneal or extraperitoneal mesh implantation, with or without posterior component separation via the transversus abdominis release (TAR) approach. Patients who were traditionally not considered for minimal access surgery are being offered a robotic repair, with successful outcomes and low rates of complications, including recurrence. Adverse events do and will continue to occur, but their incidence can be lowered with the use of meticulous technique especially during adhesiolysis and enterolysis, the primary repair of the defect, the implantation of the mesh in the selected plane, and the adherence to sound surgical principles just as it is done during open surgery. Constant awareness and knowledge of possible system malfunction scenarios and potential injuries to the patient must always be mastered by the entire team to achieve the highest standards of quality and patient safety.

References

1. Warren JA, Love M. Incisional hernia repair – minimally invasive approaches. Surg Clin N Am. 2018;98:537–59. https://doi.org/10.1016/j.suc.2018.01008
2. Bensley RP, et al. Risk of late-onset adhesions and incisional hernia repairs after surgery. J Am Coll Surg. 2013;216(6):1159–116812. https://doi.org/10.1016/j.jamcollsurg.2013.01.060.
3. Prabhu AS, et al. Laparoscopic vs robotic Intraperitoneal mesh repair for incisional hernia: an Americas hernia society quality collaborative analysis. J Am Coll Surg. 2017;225(2):285–93.
4. Li J, Ji Z, Zhang W, Li L. The comparison of lightweight mesh and standard mesh in incisional hernia repair with the open sublay technique: the results of a meta-analysis. Surg Laparosc Endosc Percutan Tech. 2015;25:238–44.
5. Darehzereshki A, et al. Biologic versus nonbiologic mesh in ventral hernia repair: a systematic review and meta-analysis. World J Surg. 2014;38:40–50. https://doi.org/10.1007/s00268-013-2232-1.
6. Kennedy M, et al. Robotic TAPP ventral hernia repair: early lessons learned at an inner city safety net hospital. JSLS. 2018;22(1):e2017.00070. https://doi.org/10.4293/JSLS.2017.00070.
7. Sharma A, Chowbey P, Kantharla NS, Baijal M, Soni V, Khullar R. Previously implanted intraperitoneal mesh increases morbidity during re-laparoscopy: a retrospective, case-matched cohort study. Hernia. 2018;22:343–51. https://doi.org/10.1007/s10029-017-1686-8
8. Haitian Z, et al. Totally extraperitoneal laparoscopic hernioplasty – the optimal surgical approach. Surg Laparosc Endosc Percutan Tech. 2009;19(6):501–5.
9. Williams SB, Greenspon J, Young HA, Orkin BA. Small bowel obstruction: conservative vs surgical management. Dis Colon Rectum. 2005;48:1140–6. https://doi.org/10.1007/s10350-004-0882-7.
10. Carbonell AM, et al. Reducing length of stay using a robotic-assisted approach for retromuscular ventral hernia repair. Ann Surg. 2018;267(2):210–7. https://doi.org/10.1097/SLA.0000000000002244.

11. Chou R, et al. Guidelines on the management of postoperative pain: a clinical practice perspective from the American pain society, the American Society of Regional Anesthesia and Pain Medicine, and the American Society of Anesthesiologists' Committee on Regional Anesthesia, Executive Committee, and Administrative Council. J Pain. 2016;17(2):131–57.
12. Boerboom SL, et al. Preperitoneal bupivacaine infiltration reduces postoperative opioid consumption, acute pain, and chronic postsurgical pain after bariatric surgery: a randomized controlled trial. Obes Surg. 2018;28(10):3102–10.
13. Tayar C, Karoui M, Cherqui D, Fagniez PL. Robot-assisted laparoscopic mesh repair of incisional hernias with exclusive intracorporeal suturing: a pilot study. Surg Endosc. 2007;21:1786–9. https://doi.org/10.1007/s00464-007-9247-3.
14. Lindmark M, Strigard K, Lowenmark T, Dahlstrand U, Gunnarsson U. Risk factors for surgical complications in ventral hernia repair. World J Surg. 2018;42(11):3528–36.
15. Oviedo RJ, Robertson JC, Desai AS. Robotic ventral hernia repair and endoscopic component separation: outcomes. JSLS. 2017;21(3):e2017.00055.
16. Oviedo RJ, Brownstein NC, Smith SL, Robertson JC, Nair-Collins S. First 200 robotic general surgery cases in a community hospital: a retrospective cohort study. World J Surg Surgical Res. 2018;1:1034.
17. Gonzalez AM, Romero RJ, Seetharamaiah R, Gallas M, Lamoureux J, Rabaza JR. Laparoscopic ventral hernia repair with primary closure versus no primary closure of the defect: potential benefits of the robotic technology. Int J Med Robot. 2015;11:120–5. https://doi.org/10.1002/rcs.1605.
18. Gonzalez A, et al. Robotic-assisted ventral hernia repair: a multicenter evaluation of clinical outcomes. Surg Endosc. 2017;31:1342–9. https://doi.org/10.1007/s00464-016-5118-0.
19. Beekman R, Crowther M, Farrokhyar F, Birch DW. Practice patterns for deep vein thrombosis prophylaxis in minimal-access surgery. Can J Surg. 2006;49(3):197–202.
20. Altieri MS, Yang J, Xu J, Talamini M, Pryor A, Telem DA. Outcomes after robotic ventral hernia repair: a study of 21,565 patients in the state of New York. Am Surg. 2018;84(6):902–8.
21. Coakley KM, et al. A nationwide evaluation of robotic ventral hernia surgery. Am J Surg. 2017;214:1158–63. https://doi.org/10.1016/j.amjsurg.2017.08.022.
22. Chen CC, et al. Malfunction of the da Vinci robotic system in urology. Int J Urol. 2012;19:736–40. https://doi.org/10.1111/j.1442-2042.2012.03010.x.

Incisional Hernia in Oncologic Surgery

27

John M. Lyons III

The past 50 years has seen major changes in the field of cancer surgery. Where previously, radical surgery was thought to be a prerequisite for cure, modern cancer surgeons understand that radicality can be superfluous; and bigger procedures do not always lead to better cancer outcomes. Today, preoperative surgical evaluation considers technology, multimodal therapy, and minimally invasive techniques. While great advances in multimodal cancer treatment have been realized, surgery remains the mainstay of treatment for most solid organ intra-abdominal malignancies. Rather than replacing surgery as a treatment modality, systemic therapy has, in many cases, enabled surgeons to expand their services to patients previously considered unresectable.

A good example is colorectal liver metastasis. Previously, very conservative criteria limited resectability only to those with unilobar, small volume, liver-only disease in whom a very wide margin could be achieved. However, liver surgery has become safer in the past 30 years [1]. This fact as well as advances in portal vein embolization, ablation techniques, and multi stage hepatectomy has led to an increase in the number of complex resections [2]. Moreover, pre-operative chemotherapy has the ability convert select patients with advanced disease to a resectable status [3]. Preoperative "conversion therapy" is now discussed regularly in patients with locally advanced pancreas cancer, gastric cancer, and several other solid organ malignancies [4, 5]. A similar trend has been seen in the management of primary and secondary peritoneal malignancies. Once thought to be a futile endeavor, now select patients with good functional status and low volume peritoneal disease are offered large cytoreductive surgeries with concomitant administration of intraoperative chemotherapy routinely.

J. M. Lyons III (✉)
Our Lady of the Lake Physician Group, Baton Rouge, LA, USA

Louisiana State University Health Sciences Center, New Orleans, LA, USA
e-mail: John.lyons@fmolhs.org

K. A. LeBlanc (ed.), *Robotic Assisted Hernia Repair*,
https://doi.org/10.1007/978-3-030-23025-8_27

While our ability to support these patients through complex oncologic resections has improved greatly, postoperative incisional hernia (IH) remains a source of major morbidity. About 1/3 of patients with postoperative IH will have symptoms of pain/discomfort, obstruction, or limitations of activity which can translate into worse physical and social functioning, general health perception, and overall lower body image [6, 7]. An estimated 17% of these patients present with incarceration or strangulation necessitating an urgent or emergent operation [8]. Moreover, the incidence of these defects appears to be rising as does the cost of repairs with a recent estimate of over $3 billion per year [9, 10].

Several technical and patient-related factors have been identified as predictive of postoperative IH. These include obesity, poor glycemic control, smoking, loss of domain, surgical site infection [11]. This chapter reviews several risk factors associated with the development of postoperative IH, focusing on those which have unique significance or prevalence in the cancer patient.

27.1 Size of the Incision

The choice of incision in abdominal surgery depends on adequacy of exposure, previous abdominal incisions, body habitus, the anticipated pathology, and surgeon preference. Traditional (open) approaches to cancer surgery include midline, paramedian, transverse, and oblique incisions.

The midline incision is the most commonly used in abdominal surgery as it is the simplest and provides adequate exposure to practically all four quadrants [12]. It is rapid to open and close; it is usually bloodless; and no muscle fibers are divided. However, IH is a major problem following midline incision with rates ranging up to 20% [13].

The paramedian incision may be an alternative to the midline incision. It is usually made by incising the skin down to the anterior rectus sheath over its the middle third. The rectus muscle is dissected free from its anterior and medial attachments and mobilized laterally to expose the posterior sheath, which is then incised longitudinally. The rectus muscle is not divided and its blood supply and innervation is maintained so that it bolsters the closure of the posterior and anterior sheaths at the conclusion of the case [14]. One of the challenges in evaluating this incision is that not all paramedian incisions are the same. Some groups using a medial paramedian (closer to the midline) have shown rates of IH very similar to those of a midline laparotomy [15, 16]. However, other groups using the lateral paramedian incision have seen virtually no incisional hernias [17]. Cahalane et al. combined prospective data from several series using the lateral paramedian incision and observed hernias in only four of 1203 (0.33%) cases at 1 year, without a single dehiscence [17]. Thus, the closer the fascial incision is to the midline, the less effective the paramedian incision is in the prevention of IH. In addition, the paramedian incision tends to be more limiting and more time-consuming than the midline incision.

Transverse and/or oblique incisions are associated with fewer IH, and some have suggested less respiratory compromise, less overall morbidity than midline incisions [18, 19]. However, similar exposure constraints limit the utility of these approaches to cases with a very narrow focus.

The field of minimally invasive surgery has grown considerably since the report of the first laparoscopic appendectomy by Dr. Kurt Semm in the early 1980s [20]. Since that time, it has been applied to several types of oncologic resection; however the most comprehensive and thorough analysis of minimally invasive oncologic resection has been in the arena of colorectal surgery. The first laparoscopic colectomies were performed in the early 1990s [21]. While these early cases demonstrated technical feasibility, concerns regarding adequacy of lymph node staging, the effect of abdominal insufflation on tumor dissemination, and the risk of trocar site implants made the oncologic merits of laparoscopy less certain. To address these oncologic concerns, several randomized controlled trials were conducted comparing laparoscopic to open colon resections [22–25]. In general, laparoscopy was found to have lower blood loss, less need for narcotics, quicker return of bowel function. Moreover, they all demonstrated oncologic equivalency with regard to survival and recurrence in long-term follow-up. The range of laparoscopic procedures has now expanded to include resection for gastric cancer, esophageal cancer, gynecologic cancer, as well as prostate and bladder cancer [26–29]. Minimally invasive pancreatic and liver resection surgery is also being evaluated [30, 31].

Incisional hernia rates following laparoscopic and open surgery have been compared by many. A retrospective analysis of 1057 colectomies (289 laparoscopic, 768 open) performed in a single British training center focused exclusively on patients with colorectal cancer [32]. The primary outcome was incidence of IH relative to surgical approach. They found the overall incidence of IH was 14.8% and noted no significant difference between the open and laparoscopic technique (14.4% vs. 15.9%, $p = 0.566$). These findings were corroborated by a larger British registry study looking at IH incidence in colorectal cancer patients [33]. However, this is contrary to data obtained from the Danish Colorectal Cancer Group and the Dutch National Patient Registry which did show a difference in IH incidence favoring laparoscopy (5.3% vs. 7.3%, $p < 0.001$) [34]. In general, the published rates of IH after laparoscopy vary greatly in non-randomized studies likely reflecting different methods of IH detection (some using radiology, other using only clinical examination) and varying length of follow up. Two of the randomized multicenter trials designed to assess oncological outcome did not detect a decrease in IH after laparoscopic access, although a trend in favor of laparoscopy was seen in follow-up of the CLASICC trial [35, 36]. Kossler-Ebs et al., performed a meta-analysis on 24 randomized controlled trials comparing IH rates after laparoscopic versus open surgery for all indications [37]. This included analysis of 3490 patients. The authors found that IH was significantly reduced among patients whose surgery was completely laparoscopic (4.3% vs. 10.1%, $p = 0.0002$). However, this difference was not observed in the subgroup of patients having "laparoscopic assisted" surgery with the hernia incidence at the extraction site comparable to that of open surgical approaches (5.5% vs. 7.8%, $p = 0.31$).

Proponents of robotic-assisted surgery have suggested that the rate of IH is lower than that of typical laparoscopy because the robotic technique enables the use of smaller port incision sites and wristed instruments which promote less direct tissue trauma [38]. To date, there are few series reporting IH rates following robotic abdominal surgery; and most of these reports are small, single institutional series. However, data that do exist suggest that the reduction in IH following robotic surgery is negligible. One single-institution retrospective review of 259 patients undergoing a robotic colorectal surgery from 2009 to 2014 found the overall IH rate to be 5.8% [39]—a rate similar to that reported by several laparoscopic series [40, 41]. A relatively recent study from the Memorial Sloan Kettering Cancer Center compared IH rates among patients who had undergone laparoscopic versus robotic right colectomy for colon cancer [42]. The clinical and demographic characteristics between the two groups were similar except that patients in the laparoscopic group had more advanced stage on average. Overall complication rates between the two groups were similar as was the incidence of IH. The rate of IH development was 22% and 17% ($p = 0.39$) for the laparoscopic and robotic groups, respectively.

27.2 Obesity

Obesity is a critical world health problem. A 2005 pooled analysis indicated that 937 million adults are overweight, and 396 million are obese. Taken together this means that approximately 1/3 of the world population is considered either overweight or obese; and if that trend continues, the incidence of overweight and obese people worldwide is projected to reach approximately 58% by 2030 [43]. The physiologic relationship between obesity and oncogenesis is complex, but the biological mechanisms that have received most attention include insulin, insulin-like growth factors, sex hormones, and adipokines. Briefly, in the obese patient, insulin resistance develops as a metabolic adaptation to increased levels of circulating free fatty acids released from intra-abdominal adipose tissue. This is compensated by increased pancreatic insulin secretion. This chronic hyperinsulinemia has been linked to oncogenesis in several types of cancers [44].

The link between obesity and cancer has been demonstrated in numerous clinical studies as well [45]. In 2002, the International Agency for Research on Cancer (IARC) concluded that there is adequate evidence of an association between obesity and several cancers including colon, postmenopausal breast, endometrial, kidney, and esophageal [46]. In 2009, a collaborative analysis of 57 prospective studies was reported evaluating the relationship between body mass index (BMI) and cause specific mortality evaluating over 900,000 patients [47]. These authors found that for every increase in BMI by 5 kg/m^2, all cancer mortality increased by 10%.

Obesity is also a major risk factor for the development of incisional hernias. This is likely because of the increased abdominal wall tension observed in obese patients. According to Laplace's law, abdominal wall tension is directly related to the radius of the abdomen and intra-abdominal pressure, and studies have confirmed a direct correlation between obesity and increased intra-abdominal pressure [48, 49]. In consideration of these pathophysiological mechanisms, central obesity plays a very strong role in IH development. Some have contended that rather than central obesity or BMI, the degree of visceral adiposity is a better predictor of IH in cancer patients.

Using pre-operative CT scans, Aquina at el. assessed several radiographic measurements of abdominal fat volume in a series of patients undergoing surgery for colorectal cancer. With very good interobserver reliability, they found that visceral fat volume determined by preoperative imaging was more predictive of IH than BMI alone (HR 2.04, 95% CI 1.07–3.91) [50]. In addition, visceral fat is metabolically active and is likely to alter the normal immune function [51]. This alteration has been linked to an increased risk of surgical site infection after colon resection; another independent risk factor for incisional hernia development [52].

27.3 Malnutrition

In order to promote healing, the surgical wound mediates the release of amino acids from muscles, gluconeogenesis, and other metabolic responses through afferent nerve fibers that perceive pain, inflammation, and changes in pH [53]. Successful healing also requires vitamins C, A, and B6 for collagen synthesis and cross-linking and essential fatty acids for cell synthesis. It is an anabolic process that occurs during a state of postoperative catabolism. Without these substances, wound healing is impaired. Naturally, patients with inadequate nutrition possess a limited supply of nutritional building blocks and not unexpectedly experience poor wound healing. This association between poor nutritional parameters and IH development has been demonstrated by many studies [54, 55]. One of the largest series to demonstrate this comes from the National Surgery Quality Improvement Program (NSQIP). Data from NSQIP (a large, multicenter, risk-adjusted, database) have consistently shown low serum albumin to be a risk factor for IH formation [55].

While malnutrition is not a feature exclusive to cancer patients, cancer has a profound impact on patient metabolism [56]. Advanced cancer patients can experience accelerated proteolysis, lipolysis, and diminished muscle protein synthesis [57]. Altered carbohydrate metabolism leads to increased hepatic glucose production and decreased insulin sensitivity. These alterations cause increased energy expenditure, loss of lean body mass, and generalized wasting [58]. The link between cancer-related malnutrition and IH has been noted in clinical studies as well. Researchers from the University of Wisconsin studied 265 patients following cytoreductive surgery for gynecologic malignancy [59]. At 1-year follow up, they found that poor nutritional status (preoperative albumin 3 g/dL or less) was an independent risk factor for early onset IH development. These nutritional considerations deserve special attention in cancer patients who are undergoing surgery; and taken together, it may explain why several authors have found that just harboring a cancer diagnosis is a risk factor for incisional hernia.

27.4 Immunosuppression

When cancer cells are encountered in vivo, the immune system recognizes tumor specific antigens on the surface of cancer cells in a manner similar to the recognition of non-self-pathogens [60]. Innate immune cells, such as NK cells, recognize the lack of MHC-I surface molecules on cancer cells, engage in active killing of these cells, and then recruit other inflammatory cells through their cytokine production. Recruited monocytes phagocytose tumor cells and then present tumor-associated antigens on their surface which activates a specific cytolytic T cell response that is directed against the tumor. Then, like a pathogen induced immune response, these specific effector T cells clonally expand and travel to the tumor to eradicate it from the body. Over time, selective cancer cells develop the ability to evade the immune system by decreasing their immunogenicity while at the same time promoting a highly immunosuppressive microenvironment that continues to support their own nutrition, angiogenesis and matrix remodeling.

Data from transplant recipients indicate that the immunosuppression is an important and potentially modifiable risk factor for IH formation. Several studies have found variable results but seem to implicate high dose steroids and sirolimus with higher rates of hernia formation [61, 62]. One study from 2002 compared mycophenolate mofetil and sirolimus directly and found significantly more wound complications with sirolimus, a finding supported by a similar study in heart transplant patients [63, 64]. Conversely, another study noted that failure to initiate immunosuppression therapy following transplantation was associated with a higher risk of hernia formation [65]. However, the decision to withhold immunosuppression following transplantation is likely representative of other clinical factors (i.e. delayed graft failure or presence of postoperative infections) that could also likely be risk factors for IH development.

Cytotoxic chemotherapy has long been known to affect the immune system. Most cytotoxic agents work by indiscriminant interference with the proliferation of rapidly dividing cells. This causes a major suppressive effect on the cellular mediators of both humoral and cell-mediated immunity during treatment. In addition, some have demonstrated diminished levels of immune parameters persisting for up to 12 months following cessation of treatment suggesting a more extended immunological effect than has previously been considered [66]. The relationship between chemotherapy and IH has been discussed in the literature. While some authors have found postoperative chemotherapy to be a risk for IH formation, Nilson et al., and others observed that preoperative, but not postoperative chemotherapy, was associated with IH [67–69]. They also noted that longer duration (>6 cycles) of preoperative chemotherapy was predictive of IH formation, and that the greatest risk factor observed was the administration of bevacizumab. This anti-VEGF agent has long been associated with impaired healing and has been implicated by others in the formation of postoperative IH [67].

27.5 Age

The median age of a new cancer diagnosis is in the United States is 66, and over 75% of patients with cancer are older than 55 [70]. Between 1982 and 2003, the population older than 65 doubled, and the population older than 85 quadrupled [71]. As a result, seniors with cancer are more frequently referred to surgeons for consideration of resection. Aging is associated with decline in functional reserve as well as physiologic changes in major organs that may affect the ability to heal from surgical procedures. Several authors have demonstrated age to be a significant risk for the development of postoperative IH [13, 72]. Itatsu et al., studied this in a prospective observation of over 4000 patients who underwent abdominal surgery from November 2009 to February 2011 [69]. They noted an estimated incidence of IH to be 10.3% at 2 years. Moreover, in multivariable analysis, increasing age by 10 year interval (HR-1.3, 1.6 to 1.45) was found to be an independent risk factor for the development of IH.

27.6 Special Considerations: Cytoreductive Surgery

Surgical cytoreduction with hyperthermic intraperitoneal chemotherapy (HIPEC) is a strategy used to treat primary and secondary peritoneal malignancies. The first descriptions of cytoreductive surgery were in the 1930s when Dr. JV Meigs described tumor debulking surgery for ovarian cancer theorizing that reducing macroscopic disease would improve symptoms [73]. Phase 1 trials were eventually conducted in the 1980s [74]; and through work conducted by Sugarbaker and others, guidelines regarding patient selection, technical feasibility, in adequacy of cytoreduction have been assembled [75].

Current indications exist for gynecologic, colorectal, appendiceal, and primary peritoneal neoplasms. The technique involves stripping disease from the peritoneum and visceral organs and leaving minimal residual tumor volume within the abdomen. Following surgery, a heated chemotherapy perfusate is administered intraoperatively into the abdomen to cover all peritoneal surfaces. Intraperitoneal chemotherapy allows a high local concentration of cytotoxic drugs to target any microscopic residual tumor volume [76]. Patients undergoing these procedures can experience significant morbidity and mortality, up to 52% and 5.8% in some series [76]. More common sources of morbidity include fistula formation, abscess, anastomotic leakage, and significant abdominal wall complications as well. Valle et al. reported an increased risk of abdominal wall infection in patients with colorectal surgery undergoing HIPEC [77]. This was attributed to longer operative time, intraoperative contamination during enteric resections, and treatment-related immunosuppression. In 2017, Struller et al., described the abdominal wall morbidity of 271 patients undergoing HIPEC at a single European comprehensive cancer center [78]. They noted an abdominal wall rupture rate of 4% which they acknowledged as elevated, but they also noted an IH incidence of only 7%. They felt that this rate was low secondary to shorter follow up. Risk factors for these complications included age, cardiopulmonary comorbidities, and certain histiotypes including pseudomyxoma and mesothelioma.

Several reconstructive strategies have been undertaken to mitigate the degree of abdominal wall morbidity that is experienced postoperatively. Scholer et al. described their experience using a combination of biologic mesh, component separation, and rectus abdominis myocutaneous flap to reconstruct HIPEC patients undergoing abdominal wall resection [79]. They compared outcomes of patients with abdominal wall resection and subsequent reconstruction to those of patients who did not require abdominal wall resection and just had primary closure. They observed similar IH rates among both groups. Additionally, they determined that abdominal wall reconstruction did not impact overall survival, R0 resection rate, postoperative morbidity or mortality.

27.7 Future Thoughts

Recognizing the significant morbidity of postoperative IH, several authors have investigated the placement of prophylactic mesh at the time of initial operation. This has been studied in benign, as well as malignant settings [80–82]. In addition, there have been several randomized controlled trials which have evaluated the role of intraoperative prophylactic mesh placement as a means to reduce postoperative IH. Recently, Borab et al., conducted a meta-analysis and review of all these trials [83]. They analyzed 14 studies representing 2114 patients comparing prophylactic mesh placement to primary suture closure in elective, midline laparotomy at index abdominal closure. The primary outcome of the analysis was IH. The authors found that prophylactic mesh placement significantly reduced the risk of postoperative IH (10% v 25%, RR 0.23; $p < .0001$). This reduction was noted regardless of mesh composition or location (ie whether onlay, retrorectus, or preperitoneal).

Additional analysis is required to further delineate optimal indications, patient selection, and cost effectiveness before universal application can be supported. In addition, patient-centered outcomes including quality of life should be further analyzed to identify patient populations that are most apt to benefit from prophylactic mesh placement. Prophylactic mesh placement does appear to hold promise in select patients, and it may be effective at reducing the incidence of this very debilitating problem in patients with both benign and malignant disease.

References

1. Carpizo DR, Are C, Jarnagin W, DeMatteo R, Fong Y, Gonen M, et al. Analysis of the extent of resection for adenocarcinoma of the gallbladder. Ann Surg Oncol. 2009;16:2138–46.
2. Lyratzopoulos G, Tyrrell C, Smith P, Yelloly J. Recent trends in liver resection surgery activity and population utilization rates in English regions. HPB (Oxford). 2007;9(4):277–80.
3. Basso M, Dadduzio V, Ardito F, Lombardi P, Strippoli A, Vellone M, et al. Conversion chemotherapy for technically unresectable colorectal liver metastases. Medicine (Baltimore). 2016;95(20):e3722.
4. Heinemann V, Haas M, Boeck S. Neoadjuvant treatment of borderline resectable and nonresectable pancreatic cancer. Ann Oncol. 2013;24(10):2484–92.
5. Kim SW. The result of conversion surgery in gastric cancer patients with peritoneal seeding. J Gastric Cancer. 2014;14(4):266–70.
6. Mudge M, Hughes LE. Incisional hernia: a 10 year prospective study of incidence and attitudes. Br J Surg. 1985;72:70–1.

7. van Ramshorst GH, Eker HH, et al. Impact of incisional hernia on health related quality of life and body image: a prospective cohort study. Am J Surg. 2012;204:144–50.
8. Reed RC, Yoder G. Recent trends in the management of incisional herniation. Arch Surg. 1989;124:485–8.
9. Trujillo CN, Fowler A, Al-Temimi MH, Ali A, Johna S, Tessier D. Complex ventral hernias: a review of past to present. Perm J. 2018;22:17-015.
10. Poulose BK, Shelton J, Phillips S, Moore D, Nealon W, Penson D, Beck W, Holzman MD. Epidemiology and cost of ventral hernia repair: making the case for hernia research. Hernia. 2012;16(2):179–83.
11. Malcher F, Cavazzola LT, Kingsnorth A. Open repair. In: Leblanc KA, Kingsnorth A, Sanders DL, editors. Management of abdominal hernias. 5th ed. New York: Springer; 2018. p. 365–79.
12. Ellis H. Midline abdominal incisions. Br J Obstet Gynaecol. 1984;91(1):1–2.
13. Höer J, Lawong G, Klinge U, Schumpelick V. Factors influencing the development of incisional hernia. A retrospective study of 2,983 laparotomy patients over a period of 10 years. Chirurg. 2002;73(5):474–80.
14. Hughes K, Selim NM. The lateral paramedian: revisiting a forgotten incision. Am Surg. 2009;75(4):321–3.
15. Brennan JM, Jones NA, et al. Lateral paramedian incision. Br J Surg. 1987;74:736–7.
16. Donaldson DR, Hegarty JH, Brennan TG, Guillou PJ, Finan PJ, Hall TJ. The lateral paramedian incision--experience with 850 cases. Br J Surg. 1982;69(10):630–2.
17. Cahalane MJ, Shapiro ME, Silen W. Abdominal incision: decision or indecision? Lancet. 1989;1(8630):146–8.
18. Greenall MJ, Evans M, Pollock AV. Midline or transverse laparotomy? A random controlled clinical trial. Part I: influence on healing. Br J Surg. 1980;67(3):188–90.
19. Greenall MJ, Evans M, Pollock AV. Midline or transverse laparotomy? A random controlled clinical trial. Part II: influence on postoperative pulmonary complications. Br J Surg. 1980;67(3):191–4.
20. Bhattacharya K. Kurt Semm: a laparoscopic crusader. J Minim Access Surg. 2007;3(1):35–6.
21. Jacobs M, Verdeja JC. Goldstein HS minimally invasive colon resection (laparoscopic colectomy). Surg Laparosc Endosc. 1991;1(3):144–50.
22. Lacy AM, Garcia-Valdecasas JC, Delgado S, et al. Laparoscopy-assisted colectomy versus open colectomy for treatment of non-metastatic colon cancer: a randomised trial. Lancet. 2002;359(9325):2224–9.
23. Clinical Outcomes of Surgical Therapy Study Group. A comparison of laparoscopically assisted and open colectomy for colon cancer. N Engl J Med. 2004;350(20):2050–9.
24. Jayne DG, Guillou PJ, Thorpe H, et al. Randomized trial of laparoscopic-assisted resection of colorectal carcinoma: 3-year results of the UK MRC CLASICC Trial Group. J Clin Oncol. 2007;25(21):3061–8.
25. Buunen M, Veldkamp R, Hop WC, et al. Survival after laparoscopic surgery versus open surgery for colon cancer: long-term outcome of a randomized clinical trial. Lancet Oncol. 2009;10(1):44–52.
26. Lee WJ, Wang W, Chen TC, Chen JC, Ser KH. Totally laparoscopic radical BII gastrectomy for the treatment of gastric cancer: a comparison with open surgery. Surg Laparosc Endosc Percutan Tech. 2008;18(4):369–74.
27. Francescutti V, Choy I, Biertho L, Goldsmith CH, Anvari M. Gastrectomy and esophagogastrectomy for proximal and distal gastric lesions: a comparison of open and laparoscopic procedures. Surg Innov. 2009;16(2):134–9.
28. Moran PS, O'Neill M, Teljeur C, Flattery M, Murphy LA, Smyth G, et al. Robot-assisted radical prostatectomy compared with open and laparoscopic approaches: a systematic review and meta-analysis. Int J Urol. 2013;20(3):312–21.
29. Woods ME, Wiklund P, Castle EP. Robot-assisted radical cystectomy: recent advances and review of the literature. Curr Opin Urol. 2010;20(2):125–9.
30. Fisher SB, Kooby DA. Laparoscopic pancreatectomy for malignancy. J Surg Oncol. 2013;107(1):39–50.

31. Gkegkes ID, Iavazzo C. Single incision laparoscopic hepatectomy: a systematic review. J Minim Access Surg. 2014;10(3):107–12.
32. Mishra A, Keeler BD, Maxwell-Armstrong C, Simpson JA, Acheson AG. The influence of laparoscopy on incisional hernia rates: a retrospective analysis of 1057 colorectal cancer resections. Color Dis. 2014;16(10):815–21.
33. Burns EM, Currie A, Bottle A, Aylin P, Darzi A, Faiz O. Minimal-access colorectal surgery is associated with fewer adhesion-related admissions than open surgery. Br J Surg. 2013;100(1):152–9.
34. Jensen KK, Krarup PM, Scheike T, Jorgensen LN, Mynster T. Incisional hernias after open versus laparoscopic surgery for colonic cancer: a nationwide cohort study. Surg Endosc. 2016;30(10):4469–79.
35. Leung KL, Kwok SP, Lam SC, Lee JF, Yiu RY, Ng SS, et al. Laparoscopic resection of rectosigmoid carcinoma: prospective randomised trial. Lancet. 2004;363(9416):1187–92.
36. Green BL, Marshall HC, Collinson F, Quirke P, Guillou P, Jayne DG, et al. Long-term follow-up of the Medical Research Council CLASICC trial of conventional versus laparoscopically assisted resection in colorectal cancer. Br J Surg. 2013;100(1):75–82.
37. Kössler-Ebs JB, Grummich K, Jensen K, Hüttner FJ, Müller-Stich B, Seiler CM, et al. Incisional hernia rates after laparoscopic or open abdominal surgery-a systematic review and meta-analysis. World J Surg. 2016;40(10):2319–30.
38. Huck MB, Powell M, McNatt S, Westcott C, Fernandez A. Incisional hernias after robotic assisted surgery. SAGES abstracts [Internet]. Available from: https://www.sages.org/meetings/annual-meeting/abstracts-archive/incisional-hernias-after-robotic-assisted-surgery.
39. Harr JN, Juo YY, Luka S, Agarwal S, Brody F, Obias V. Incisional and port-site hernias following robotic colorectal surgery. Surg Endosc. 2016;30(8):3505–10.
40. Lee L, Abou-Khalil M, Liberman S, Boutros M, Fried GM, Feldman LS. Incidence of incisional hernia in the specimen extraction site for laparoscopic colorectal surgery: systematic review and meta-analysis. Surg Endosc. 2017;31(12):5083–93.
41. Buckley FP, Vassaur HE, Jupiter DC, Crosby JH, Wheeless CJ, Vassaur JL. Influencing factors for port-site hernias after single-incision laparoscopy. Hernia. 2016;20(5):729–33.
42. Widmar M, Keskin M, Beltran P, Nash GM, Guillem JG, Temple LK, et al. Incisional hernia is after laparoscopic and robotic right colectomy. Hernia. 2016;20(5):723–8.
43. Kelly T, Yang W, Chen CS, Reynolds K, He J. Global burden of obesity in 2005 and projections to 2030. Int J Obes. 2008;32(9):1431–7.
44. Calle EE, Kaaks R. Overweight, obesity and cancer: epidemiological evidence and proposed mechanisms. Nat Rev Cancer. 2004;4(8):579–91.
45. Calle EE, Rodriguez C, Walker-Thurmond K, Thun MJ. Overweight, obesity, and mortality from cancer in a prospectively studied cohort of U.S. adults. N Engl J Med. 2003;348(17):1625–38.
46. Vainio H, Bianchini F. IARC handbooks of cancer prevent weight control and physical activity. Lyon: IARC press; 2002.
47. Prospective Studies Collaboration, Whitlock G, Lewington S, Sherliker P, Clarke R, Emberson J, et al. Body-mass index and cause-specific mortality in 900 000 adults: collaborative analyses of 57 prospective studies. Lancet. 2009;373(9669):1083–96.
48. Lau B, Kim H, Haigh PI, Tejirian T. Obesity increases the odds of acquiring and incarcerating noninguinal abdominal wall hernias. Am Surg. 2012;78(10):1118–21.
49. Lambert DM, Marceau S, Forse RA. Intra-abdominal pressure in the morbidly obese. Obes Surg. 2005;15(9):1225–32.
50. Aquina CT, Rickles AS, Probst CP, Kelly KN, Deeb AP, Monson JR, et al. Visceral obesity, not elevated BMI, is strongly associated with incisional hernia after colorectal surgery. Dis Colon Rectum. 2015;58(2):220–7.
51. Fontana L, Eagon JC, Trujillo ME, Scherer PE, Klein S. Visceral fat adipokine secretion is associated with systemic inflammation in obese humans. Diabetes. 2007;56(4):1010–3.
52. Tsujinaka S, Konishi F, Kawamura YJ, Saito M, Tajima N, Tanaka O, et al. Visceral obesity predicts surgical outcomes after laparoscopic colectomy for sigmoid colon cancer. Dis Colon Rectum. 2008;51(12):1757–65.

53. Kavalukas SL, Barbul A. Nutrition and wound healing: an update. Plast Reconstr Surg. 2011;127(Suppl 1):38S–43S.
54. Heimann TM, Swaminathan S, Greenstein AJ, Steinhagen RM. Incidence and factors correlating with incisional hernia following open bowel resection in patients with inflammatory bowel disease: a review of 1000 patients. Ann Surg. 2018;267(3):532–6.
55. Best WR, Khuri SF, Phelan M, Hur K, Henderson WG, Demakis JG, et al. Identifying patient preoperative risk factors and postoperative adverse events in administrative databases: results from the Department of Veterans Affairs National Surgical Quality Improvement Program. J Am Coll Surg. 2002;194(3):257–66.
56. Franz MG. The biology of hernia formation. Surg Clin North Am. 2008;88(1):1–15.
57. Delano MJ, Moldawer LL. The origins of cachexia in acute and chronic inflammatory diseases. Nutr Clin Pract. 2006;21(1):68–81.
58. Bosaeus I, Daneryd P, Svanberg E, Lundholm K. Dietary intake and resting energy expenditure in relation to weight loss in unselected cancer patients. Int J Cancer. 2001;93(3):380–3.
59. Spencer RJ, Hayes KD, Rose S, Zhao Q, Rathouz PJ, Rice LW, et al. Risk factors for early-occurring and late-occurring incisional hernias after primary laparotomy for ovarian cancer. Obstet Gynecol. 2015;125(2):407–13.
60. Markman JL, Shiao SL. Impact of the immune system and immunotherapy in colorectal cancer. J Gastrointest Oncol. 2015;6(2):208–23.
61. Knight RJ, Villa M, Laskey R, Benavides C, Schoenberg L, Welsh M, et al. Risk factors for impaired wound healing in sirolimus-treated renal transplant recipients. Clin Transpl. 2007;21:460–5.
62. Janßen H, Lange R, Erhard J, Malagó M, Eigler FW, Broelsch CE. Causative factors, surgical treatment and outcome of incisional hernia after liver transplantation. Br J Surg. 2002;89:1049–54.
63. Valente JF, Hricik D, Weigel K, Seaman D, Knauss T, Siegel CT, et al. Comparison of Sirolimus vs. Mycophenolate Mofetil on surgical complications and wound healing in adult kidney transplantation. Am J Transplant. 2003;3:1128–34.
64. Kuppahally S, Al-Khaldi A, Weisshaar D, Valantine HA, Oyer P, Robbins RC, et al. Wound healing complications with de novo sirolimus versus mycophenolate mofetil-based regimen in cardiac transplant recipients. Am J Transplant. 2006;6:986–92.
65. Smith CT, Katz MG, Foley D, Welch B, Leverson GE, Funk LM, et al. Incidence and risk factors of incisional hernia formation following abdominal organ transplantation. Surg Endosc. 2015;29(2):398–404.
66. Kang DH, Weaver MT, Park NJ, Smith B, McArdle T, et al. Significant impairment in immune recovery after cancer treatment. Nurs Res. 2009;58(2):105–14.
67. Rettenmaier MA, Abaid LN, Brown JV, Micha JP, Goldstein BH. Chemotherapy and patient co-morbidity in ventral site hernia development. J Gynecol Oncol. 2009;20(4):246–50.
68. Nilsson JH, Strandberg Holka P, Sturesson C. Incisional hernia after open resections for colorectal liver metastases - incidence and risk factors. HPB (Oxford). 2016;18(5):436–41.
69. Itatsu K, Yokoyama Y, Sugawara G, Kubota H, Tojima Y, Kurumiya Y, et al. Incidence of and risk factors for incisional hernia after abdominal surgery. Br J Surg. 2014;101(11):1439–47.
70. NCI's surveillance, epidemiology, and end results program [Internet]. 2015. Available from: https://www.cancer.gov/about-cancer/causes-prevention/risk/age.
71. Korc-Grodzicki B, Downey RJ, Shahrokni A, Kingham TP, Patel SG, Audisio RA. Surgical considerations in older adults with cancer. J Clin Oncol. 2014;32(24):2647–53.
72. Caglià P, Tracia A, Borzì L, Amodeo L, Tracia L, Veroux M, et al. Incisional hernia in the elderly: risk factors and clinical considerations. Int J Surg. 2014;12(Suppl 2):S164–9.
73. Meigs JV. Tumors of the female pelvic organs. New York: The MacMillan Company; 1934.
74. Zimm S, Cleary SM, Lucas WE, Weiss RJ, Markman M, Andrews PA, et al. Phase I/pharmacokinetic study of intraperitoneal cisplatin and etoposide. Cancer Res. 1987;47(6):1712–6.
75. Sugarbaker PH. Surgical management of peritoneal carcinosis: diagnosis, prevention and treatment. Langenbecks Arch Chir. 1988;373:189–96.

76. Chua TC, Yan TD, Saxena A, Morris DL. Should the treatment of peritoneal carcinoma ptosis by cytoreductive surgery and hyperthermic intraperitoneal chemotherapy still be regarded as a highly morbid procedure? Ann Surg. 2009;249(6):900–7.
77. Valle M, Federici O, Carboni F, Toma L, Gallo MT, Prignano G, et al. Postoperative infections after cytoreductive surgery and HIPEC for peritoneal carcinomatosis: proposal and results from a prospective protocol study of prevention, surveillance and treatment. Eur J Surg Oncol. 2014;40(8):950–6.
78. Struller F, Koenigsrainer I, Horvath P, Koenigsrainer A, Beckert S. Abdominal wall morbidity following cytoreductive surgery and hyperthermic intraperitoneal chemotherapy. Scand J Surg. 2017;106(4):294–8.
79. Scholer AJ, Oliver JB, Rosado J, Patel JS, Lynch LJ, Spiegler KM, et al. Abdominal wall reconstruction after cytoreduction surgery-hyperthermic intraperitoneal chemotherapy. J Surg Res. 2018;221:266–74.
80. Bevis PM, Windhaber RA, Lear PA, Poskitt KR, Earnshaw JJ, Mitchell DC. Randomized clinical trial of mesh versus sutured wound closure after open abdominal aortic aneurysm surgery. Br J Surg. 2010;97(10):1497–502.
81. El-Khadrawy OH, Moussa G, Mansour O, Hashish MS. Prophylactic prosthetic reinforcement of midline abdominal incisions in high-risk patients. Hernia. 2009;13(3):267–74.
82. Ventham NT, Brady RR, Stewart RG, Ward BM, Graham C, Yalamarthi S, et al. Prophylactic mesh placement of permanent stomas at index operation for colorectal cancer. Ann R Coll Surg Engl. 2012;94(8):569–73.
83. Borab ZM, Shakir S, Lanni MA, Tecce MG, MacDonald J, Hope WW, et al. Does prophylactic mesh placement in elective, midline laparotomy reduce the incidence of incisional hernia? A systematic review and meta-analysis. Surgery. 2017;161(4):1149–63.

Part IV

Diaphragmatic Hernia

28 Operating Room Set Up in the Repair of Diaphragmatic Hernia

Elizabeth Colsen

The diaphragm is a thin muscle used for respiration in the upper abdomen [1]. There are two main types of congenital diaphragmatic hernias that occur through the diaphragm complex and their description is based on the location of the diaphragmatic defect. The Morgagni hernia is in the anteromedial subcostosternal diaphragmatic space and constitutes 2–4% of congenital diaphragmatic hernias [2]. The Bochdalek hernia is in the lumbocostal trigone or diaphragmatic dome. This is a more common type of hernia with a prevalence of one per 2200 live births. Both hernias can remain asymptomatic until adulthood; however, the exact prevalence as an adult is still unknown as these are uncommon hernias. A third type of diaphragmatic hernia is the traumatic hernia, and its location can be anywhere on the diaphragm depending if the mechanism is blunt or penetrating trauma [3].

In the adult patient, these hernias often present with abdominal pain or incarceration [4]. Advanced imaging like a CT scan allows for better visualization of hernia contents and the defect location. Adequate pre-operative imaging also permits for an improved operative plan.

All diaphragmatic hernias pose a challenge to repair due to the location of the diaphragm high in the abdomen, and the likelihood of intraabdominal contents herniating into the chest. This makes the laparoscopic approach appealing given the relative ease of visualization and accessibility to the upper abdominal contents. The da Vinci® surgical robot (Intuitive Surgical, Inc., Sunnyvale, CA) affords the surgeon advanced laparoscopic capacity with 3D visualization and wristed instruments.

This chapter will describe each of the hernia types and the operating room set up for the Si and Xi da Vinci® robotic platforms.

E. Colsen (✉)
Minneapolis VA Medical Center, Minneapolis, MN, USA
e-mail: ziemb027@umn.edu

K. A. LeBlanc (ed.), *Robotic Assisted Hernia Repair*,
https://doi.org/10.1007/978-3-030-23025-8_28

28.1 Morgagni Hernia

The Morgagni hernia is in the anteromedial subcostosternal diaphragmatic space. Patients usually present with symptoms related to the compressive effect of the intraabdominal organs into the chest or even incarceration/strangulation of abdominal contents [4]. For the subacute presentation, pre-operative imaging should include a CT scan of the chest/abdomen and pelvis to characterize the location, size, and contents of the hernia. Using this, the surgeon can formulate the operative approach.

Typically, the patient is placed supine on the operating room table with arms tucked and a foot board in place to allow for safety while in reverse Trendelenburg position. Port placement is based on location of the hernia, with care taken to not place ports too close to the defect.

28.1.1 Si

The Si robot is docked over the shoulder with ports placed subcostally. It is important to place the ports far enough away from the hernia defect to allow for either the creation of a pre-peritoneal flap or for intraperitoneal onlay mesh (IPOM) placement. Also, consideration should be made for how high the hernia reaches into the thoracic cavity. Ports can be advanced into the abdomen or placed higher if needed to reduce contents of the hernia (for very large hernias) (Fig. 28.1).

An important consideration is placing the patient in reverse Trendelenburg positioning to help reduce the hernia contents and keep the operative view clear. This should be done before docking the da Vinci® robot. Once docked, the operative table cannot be moved.

28.1.2 Xi

The Xi robot is side docked at either side of the patient. The robot boom is then centered over the patient. Port placement is similar to the Si, with the ports triangulated toward the hernia defect. If your robotic system has robotic table motion (TruSystem® 7000dV Table, Trumpf Medical, Chicago, IL) then you will be able to move the bed while docked; however, without this operative table, the patient should be placed in to reverse Trendelenburg position before docking (Fig. 28.2).

28.2 Bochdalek Hernia

The Bochdalek hernia is in the lumbocostal region which is more posterior in location on the diaphragm [4]. They can be on either the left or right side; however, 85% of the time are on the left [4]. Because of the lateral and posterior location, positioning the patient in a lateral position may be needed. Pre-operative imaging will facilitate

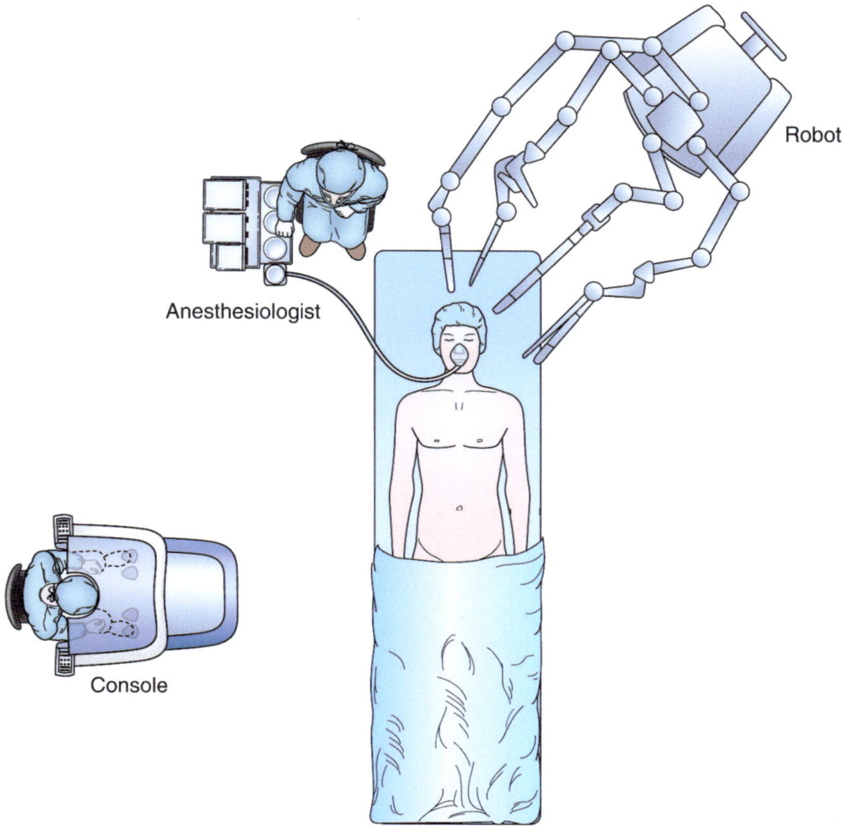

Fig. 28.1 Room set up for Robotic diaphragmatic hernia repair with da Vinci® Si system

adequate characterization of the exact location of the hernia. If on the left, the patient may need to be in left lateral decubitus position utilizing a bean bag for positioning.

28.2.1 Si

The Si robot is docked over the shoulder with ports placed in a subcostal fashion. The port placement depends on the location of the hernia. If located in the most common location left posterior, the patient should be in left lateral decubitus position with ports placed subcostally. Additionally, these hernias can be approached from the chest thoracoscopically [4] if repair from the abdomen is unable to be achieved. Again, slight reverse Trendelenburg positioning for either robot may help to reduce hernia contents and operative field of view. This will need to be done before docking the robot.

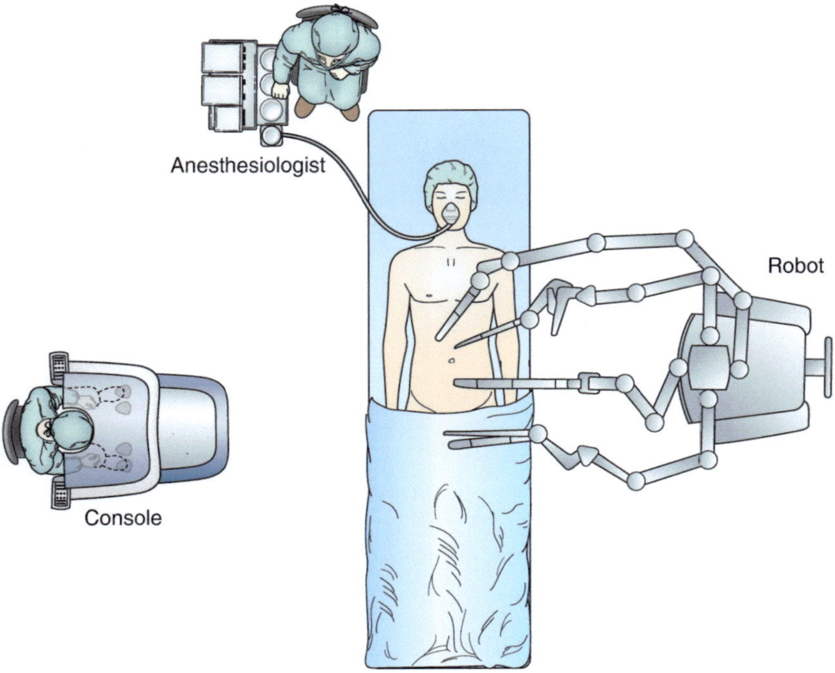

Fig. 28.2 Room Set up for Robotic diaphragmatic hernia repair with the da Vinci® Xi system

28.2.2 Xi

The Xi robot is side docked with the arms centered over the working area. Ports are placed similarly to the Si positioning. As noted earlier, if your robotic system has the TruSystem® 7000dV table then the bed will be able to move while docked; however, without this table, the patient should be placed in to reverse Trendelenburg position before docking. Generally, the appropriate position is achieved prior to docking even with the TruSystem®.

28.3 Traumatic Diaphragmatic Hernia

The location of the traumatic diaphragmatic hernia can be any location on the diaphragm; however, the liver does appear to have some protective effect as they are more common on the left [5]. If the nature of the trauma is blunt, the defect may be quite large and contain multiple viscera [3]. These hernias are repaired in a similar fashion to the congenital variety depending on size and location. The placement of the trocars and robot in the room would like that of the congenital hernias.

28.4 Summary

In summary, diaphragmatic hernias are easily approached laparoscopically utilizing the da Vinci® robotic platform. The port and robot positioning depend on the location of the hernia defect. Adequate pre-operative imaging can serve as a road map to how the room should look. Optimally, the placement of ports and final positioning of the robot should be made after initial laparoscopic visualization of the hernia. The repair technique depends on surgeon preference and is discussed in Chap. 30.

References

1. Sanford Z, Weltz AS, Brown J, Shockcor N, Wu N, Park AE. Morgagni hernia repair: a review. Hernia. 2018;22(4):697–705. https://doi.org/10.1007/s10029-018-1760-x.
2. Dapri G, Himpens J, Hainau B, Roman A, Stevens E, Capelluto E, Germay O, Cadière G. Surgical technique and complications during laparoscopic repair of diaphragmatic hernias. Hernia. 2007;11:179–83. https://doi.org/10.1007/s10029-006-0161-8.
3. Thiam O, Konate I, Gueye M, Toure A, Seck M, Cisse M, Diop B, Dirie E. Traumatic diaphragmatic injuries: epidemiological, diagnostic and therapeutic aspects. Springerplus. 2016;5:1614. https://doi.org/10.1186/s40064-016-3291-1.
4. Lima M, Di Salvo N, Ugolini S, Libri M, Ruggeri G. Robot-assisted thoracoscopic repair of a late-onset Bochdalek hernia: a case report. Pediatr Med Chir. 2018;40:173.
5. Magagi I, Habou O, Adamou H, Adakal O, Ali Ada M, Moustapha H, Abarchi H. Isolated right-sided posttraumatic diaphragmatic hernia. Case Rep Surg. 2018;1:1–3. https://doi.org/10.1155/2018/8758021.

Robotic Assisted Morgagni Hernia Repair

29

Francesco M. Bianco, Yevhen Pavelko, and Antonio Gangemi

29.1 Introduction

Morgagni hernias (MH) are rare congenital defects of the antero-medial portion of the diaphragm. Discovered and named after the Italian anatomist Giovanni Battista Morgagni in 1769, the hernia originates from an area of weakness of the anterior diaphragm, between the sternal and costal origin of the diaphragm muscles at the level of the xiphoid process and the central tendon [1]. This space is traversed by the internal mammary artery, which continues to form the superior epigastric artery in the abdomen [1, 2]. The most common localization of the defect is on the right side (91%) of the diaphragm because the left side (5%) is protected by the pericardium. A bilateral defect is even more rare and is present in 4% of cases (Fig. 29.1) [3].

MH accounts for <3% of all diaphragmatic hernias. As a congenital defect, it can be associated with atrial septal defects, ventricular septal defects, Down syndrome and Cantrell's Pentalogy [4–7]. The hernia is generally quite small and, in 30–40% of the cases, will be discovered incidentally [3, 4, 8] in adulthood and will not be associated with any other congenital anomaly [9, 10].

When MH is diagnosed, elective surgical repair is indicated, due to the risk of viscus incarceration or strangulation [11]. In the past, thoracotomy (49%), followed by laparotomy (30%) were the most common surgical approaches to treat MH [3]. In 1992 Kuster was the first to report a laparoscopic repair of the defect [12]. Since then, minimally invasive surgical (MIS) approach has gained popularity. More than 154 cases are reported in the literature, including laparoscopic, robotic assisted and thoracoscopic surgery [5, 10, 13–27].

Laparoscopy is proven to be a safe and feasible technique, but has several limitations that include a greater difficulty in the excision of the sac that is successfully

F. M. Bianco · Y. Pavelko (✉) · A. Gangemi
Division of General, Minimally Invasive and Robotic Surgery, University of Illinois, Chicago, IL, USA
e-mail: ypavelko@uic.edu

K. A. LeBlanc (ed.), *Robotic Assisted Hernia Repair*,
https://doi.org/10.1007/978-3-030-23025-8_29

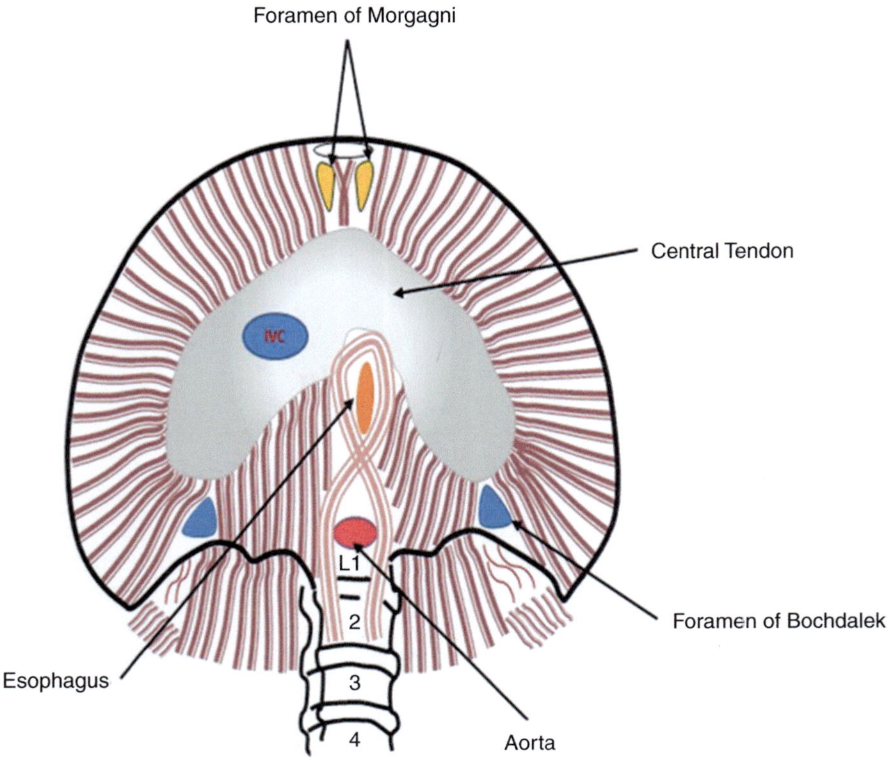

Fig. 29.1 Anatomical location of the Morgagni foramen

accomplished in only 31% of the cases and in placing the mesh for the definitive repair of the defect [28]. It is worth noting that hernia sac excision, primary tissue repair, and mesh implantation are considered critical steps of the MH repair [29].

Whether or not to excise the hernia sac during MH repair is still a controversial topic [30]. Many authors report that the excision of the hernia sac has proven to reduce the recurrence rate for paraesophageal hernias, as well as seroma formation, and the same concept can potentially be extended to the Morgagni hernias [3, 13, 29, 31–33]. On the other end, several studies, have showed that when severe adhesions between the hernia sac and mediastinum are present, attempts to excise the sac can cause damage of the superior epigastric vessels, pneumomediastinum, or even fatal pneumopericardium [3, 12, 29, 34].

In these cases, it is advised to leave the sac behind. There are several reports that support the evidence that seroma formation is not very high and there is evidence as well that at 30 days post-op the sac might not be detectable on ultrasound and/or CT scan [34, 35].

The ideal laparoscopic approach for primary closure of the defect and for mesh fixation is still debated as indicated by the several techniques proposed by various authors and centers. The robotic platform and approach may lessen the technical challenges associated with the three aforementioned critical steps [19, 29].

However, the limited surgical experience associated with the low incidence of this type of hernia does not allow one to draw any definitive conclusions on which approach and/or treatment would be the gold standard for this technically challenging repair.

The only area where a wide consensus seems to have been reached is in regard to the thoracic approach for those patients who have developed giant hernias and severe adhesions between the hernia sac and parietal pleura [25, 27].

29.2 Preoperative Evaluation

The hernia bulging into the thoracic cavity can cause compression on various organs and anatomical structures including the herniated abdominal viscus and/or tissue. The severity of the respiratory and gastrointestinal symptoms associated with this occurrence varies depending on the size and the content of the defect [8].

Symptoms can include cough, dyspnea, paroxysmal nocturnal dyspnea, recurrent pulmonary infections, cardiac arrhythmias, chest discomfort, substernal pain, wheezing, or can involve the GI tract with dysphagia, epigastric pain, bloating, periodic regurgitation of solids and liquids and bowel obstruction [3, 20, 28, 29, 36].

The hernia content may consist of transverse colon, omentum, extraperitoneal fat, stomach, small bowel and (rarely) a portion of the liver [3, 28]. Obesity, pregnancy, chronic constipation and cough tend to increase intra-abdominal pressure, which in turn increases hernia size and risk of further herniation through the defect. As a consequence of this process, the risk of incarceration and subsequent strangulation is increased [29].

The diagnostic workup should start with a thorough history and physical examination followed by radiographic studies [3]. Chest X-ray is the first-line imaging and usually shows a mediastinal mass with air-fluid levels, suggestive of viscus herniation [8]. When no air-fluid levels are seen in the mediastinum, the hernia can be confused with the cardiophrenic fat pad, or other conditions such as intrathoracic and abdominal wall tumors, pericardial cysts, thymoma, lymphoma, atelectasis, pneumonia and localized anterior segmental eventration of the diaphragm or diaphragmatic rupture [5, 34, 37–39].

Computed tomography (CT) is used to confirm the diagnosis and for better characterization of the anatomy of the defect and its content/s, which will help to plan the appropriate surgical approach [11]. Similarly, magnetic resonance imaging (MRI) may help to differentiate the diagnosis of MH from other pathologic conditions and to characterize the hernia sac [3, 40]. For patients who present with non-specific gastrointestinal symptoms, barium swallow study may be an appropriate initial approach in the diagnostic work up [37]. Sonography (US) can also be useful in differentiating MH vs right sided partial diaphragmatic eventration involving a portion of the liver without exposing the patient to the radiation and/or high costs associated with CT scan and/or MRI [41].

Pre-operative assessment for elective repair will include routine blood work, ECG and anesthesiologist evaluation. Based on patient history and medical conditions, further testing might be indicated for optimal risk stratification prior to surgical intervention [42].

29.3 Patient Selection

There are no absolute contraindications to a robotic approach. Ideally the extent of the learning curve and experience of the surgeon and his/her team with the robotic system should dictated by the complexity of the case.

A relative contraindication can be represented by very large defects with anticipated adhesions to the pleura or recurrent herniation where a transthoracic approach might be better suited. Nonetheless, an initial evaluation can be done from the abdominal side and the decision to convert could be made intra-operatively if a safe reduction of the hernia content/s and resection of its adhesions are not feasible transabdominally. In those cases, a double lumen endotracheal tube should be used in order to exclude one lung as needed. The minimally invasive approach for incarcerated hernias or strangulated hernias should be evaluated on a case by case basis.

29.4 Operating Room Setup, Cart Positioning and Robot Docking

The operating room setup is crucial for a smooth flow of the procedure. It is important to invest time and effort in standardization of all of the details of docking and robotic cable set up. This will reduce docking time and unexpected issues that can slow down the procedure creating frustration among the surgical team members.

For the Intuitive Si system, the robotic cart is placed in the corner of the operating room that will be closer to the left shoulder of the patient. The cart placement is done before the patient enters the room. This will facilitate the docking, as once ready, the patient table can be rotated to have the patient head pointing at the cart. With the Intuitive Xi platform the robotic cart can be docked from any direction so there is no need to move it before the patient enters the room.

In our setup, the robotic vision tower and accessories boom are positioned by the patient's right foot. In this way, the camera cables, the energy cables and all other connecting cables reach the surgical field by running over the drape on top of the patient's leg. The cables are grouped together and clipped to the drape at the level of the leg. The first assistant is positioned in between the patient's legs, the scrub tech is standing at the left side of the patient. Laparoscopic screens will be positioned to the left and right shoulder of the patient.

The anesthesia machine is generally kept at the head of the patient, slightly moved to the right side. An intravenous line extension is used in order to move the IV posts away from the field as far as possible and to reduce the need to access them under the drapes and under the robotic arms. The console is always placed in a position that facilitates communication with the rest of the team and direct vision of the surgical field by the console surgeon (Fig. 29.2).

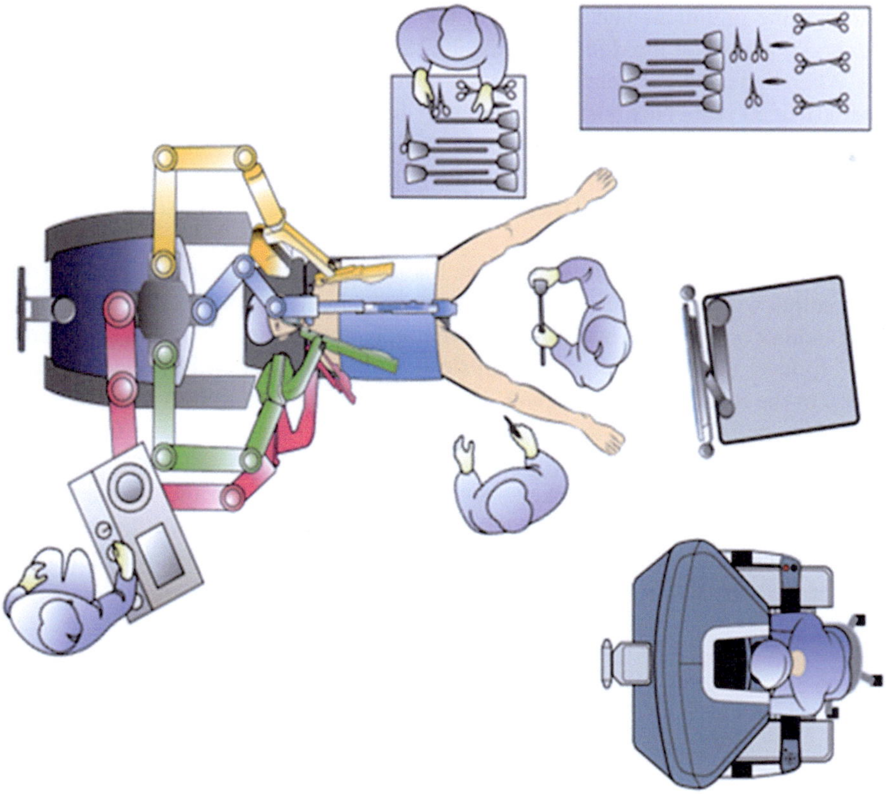

Fig. 29.2 OR setup

29.5 Patient Positioning and Port Placement

The patient is positioned supine on the operative table with split legs and on a “bean bag” for adequate support during reverse Trendelenburg position. This position allows the assistant to sit comfortably in between patient’s legs and facilitate triangulation of the instruments.

In non-obese patients, the first trocar is placed in the umbilicus via an open access technique. This requires the use of an 8 mm port for the Xi or a 12 mm disposable port for the Si platform. In obese patients, where the umbilicus is not a reliable landmark due to the caudal stretching of the abdominal pannus, a Veress needle is placed at the Palmer’s point and a 5 mm disposable port is placed under direct visualization approximately 20 cm from the xiphoid process.

Based on the hernia size and herniated contents, three or four ports are used. The standard triangulation calls for two operative ports, one on each flank, roughly along the transverse umbilical line for the Xi platform. For the Si platform the two operative trocars are placed a little closer to the hernia site along a concave line passing through the umbilicus and pointing at the defect. The fourth arm, when used, is generally placed on the right side (Fig. 29.2).

When indicated, a 12 mm assistant port can be placed in between the camera and the left sided port. This port will eventually be used to introduce the mesh and the sutures for the reinforcement of the repair. For the three port technique without an assistant, the camera port has to be 12 mm to allow easy introduction of the mesh inside the peritoneal cavity. The sutures can be introduced through the 8 mm operative ports.

The operative trocars must be placed sufficiently lateral and cephalad on the abdominal wall so that the robotic arms can move freely and without colliding with one another or with the patient's legs. Eventually, the surgical table can be flexed at the hip level to alleviate possible collisions. This maneuver will provide a greater reach to the robotic arms when working in the "ceiling" position. Another possible trick is to pull the robotic arms up (burp up) as much as possible after the docking has been completed.

The patient is placed in steep reverse Trendelenburg and the robotic cart is docked over the patient's head if the Si platform is being used for the repair. As mentioned earlier, the more versatile Xi platform can be docked from virtually any side of the patient (Fig. 29.3).

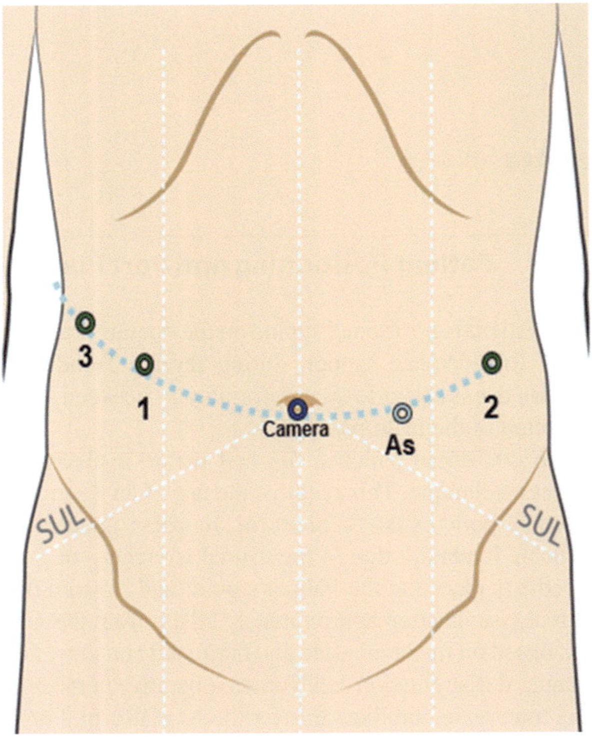

Fig. 29.3 Trocar placement (As = assistant port)

29.6 Intraoperative Considerations

After docking has been completed, the robotic 30° scope is connected and set to the up position. The procedure starts with reduction of contents of the hernia. The content of small defects usually reduce back into the abdomen by gravity. In case of incarceration, the hernia content will have to be reduced using Pro-grasp forceps and/or the Cadiere grasper. In our experience, the use of two large graspers during this step allows for gentler manipulation and reduction in the risk of injuries to the herniated content. It is particularly important to carefully weigh the tension applied on the anatomical structures based on the deformation of the tissue. This sort of visual compensation for the lack of tactile feedback is something that is usually acquired by the robotic surgeon after relatively few procedures. In some cases, and for the less experienced surgeon, this step can be safely performed with laparoscopic instruments. Once the larger part of the hernia content is reduced, the few attachments left can be dissected with a combination of blunt traction and sharp dissection using the Prograsp and monopolar hook. We prefer the monopolar hook to the scissors because of its combination of curved and rectilinear shape and a blunt tip which allow for (in our opinion) an easier and safer dissection of anatomical planes while reducing the costs as they are less expensive than the robotic scissors.

For large hernias with bulky herniated content, the fourth arm or the assistant trocar instrument can help to pull the hernia content back into the abdominal cavity while the console surgeon keeps the area of dissection under constant tension. During the dissection of the hernia sac, the assistant can also use a suction cannula to provide tissue retraction and at the same time keep the surgical field clean by suctioning out smoke or blood.

Hemostasis should be meticulous and timely as soon as small bleeders are encountered. This will contribute to keeping the surgical field clean which in turns improves visualization as blood absorbs light. Once the hernia contents are safely reduced into the abdominal cavity and inspected for serosal tears, the falciform ligament is transected to facilitate the hernia dissection and the mesh placement. Any serosal tears must be repaired immediately when recognized since it may be difficult to recognize any of the occurrences later in the procedure.

The next step will be the excision of the hernia sac. This is achieved with a combination of blunt traction and sharp dissection with the Prograsp forceps and the monopolar hook. It is important to resect the hernia sac completely while assuring the integrity of the pleura. The robot can offer a potential advantage over conventional laparoscopy during this step of the procedure as the third robotic arm generally facilitates exposure of the tissues while the assistant is using the suction cannula to keep the field clean.

As previously discussed, complete excision of the hernia sac has proven to reduce the recurrence rate for paraesophageal hernias. Various authors advocate for the same strategy with the MH repairs as potentially reducing the rate of recurrence [13, 31, 32]. However, occasionally the dissection of the medial aspect of the sac can be challenging due to its proximity to the pericardium. In this situation, it is acceptable to leave some of the medial aspect of the sac behind to avoid the risk of potentially disastrous pericardial injuries.

Once the hernia sac is excised, the primary closure of the defect follows. This allows for a more physiological repair and tends to reestablish the normal anatomical dynamics of the diaphragm. Primary closure is achieved with a 0 permanent, barbed suture. Based on the size of the defect, multiple sutures might be needed. The suture is used only for half of its length and then run backwards to lock itself without tying knots. It is important to make sure that the suture is deep enough on the abdominal wall side in order to include sturdy fascia. In some cases it is advisable to perform some dissection of the pre-peritoneal fat in order to expose the posterior rectus fascial plane.

When the diaphragm is particularly thin, the use of Teflon pledgets, along with multiple interrupted stiches of braided or monofilament sutures has been described. This is a potentially good solution to reduce the stress on the muscle in order to avoid the risk of cutting through it due to the tension on the closure [20].

Before completion of the primary closure of the defect, the anesthesiologist should give a few Valsalva maneuvers in order to expel the CO_2 from the space previously occupied by the hernia. After primary closure, small defects can be just covered again with the falciform ligament that is generally tucked in place with a Vicryl 3/0 suture. This is seldom used as this is a less reliable repair in most cases.

Larger defects are repaired using mesh. There are multiple reports in the literature suggesting the use of almost any possible type of prosthetic material currently available, from permanent to biologic. We will not discuss the details of mesh choice as these are described in a different chapter of this book. The mesh should follow the general and widely accepted rules for the overlap of the defect.

The mesh should be marked on the anti-adherent side (double-layer meshes) before deploying. The longer side has longer markings and the shorter side is marked with N for North (anterior) and S for South (posterior). These marks serve to more easily orient the mesh inside the abdominal cavity (Fig. 29.4.)

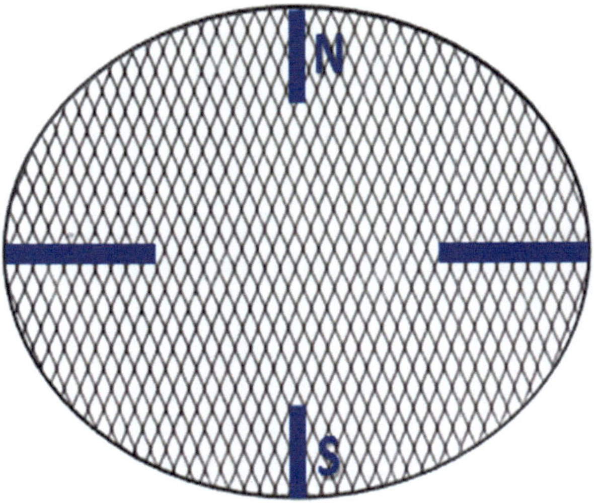

Fig. 29.4 Mesh fixation

Once deployed, the North and South edges are sutured in place using a 2/0 Prolene suture approximately 20–25 cm long. The sutures are placed to assure that the two marks are aligned with and parallel to the midline of the abdomen. This can be confirmed on the abdominal side by pushing below the xiphoid and on the diaphragm by following the line of the falciform ligament. In this phase the mesh is held in place by the third robotic arm or by the assistant.

After the midline edges are sutured, the two lateral edges are sutured with the same technique. Once good overlap is confirmed, the four sutures are run clockwise to complete the mesh fixation. Special attention must be paid to the placement of those sutures. Ideally the sutures should not be too tight (to prevent ischemia of the thin diaphragm tissue) nor too deep (to avoid damage of the underlying pericardium).

The suturing is performed with a Large or Mega Suture Cut Needle Driver™ if there is no assistant as this latter instrument enables the console surgeon to stitch and cut the sutures without using the robotic or laparoscopic scissors.

29.7 Recommended Instruments

In order to reduce costs, it is important to plan in advance which instrument will be used. The surgeon should be familiar with the cost per use of each device as well as the advantages and drawbacks of each instrument. This is a surgery with limited financial margins and in order to make it cost-effective the surgeon must judiciously select the right instruments and supplies while achieving good outcomes. This has been shown to be easily accomplished across many procedures and specialities.

The table below describes the instruments for different steps of the procedure with the main features and costs to keep in mind when making these decisions (Table 29.1).

Table 29.1 Instrument comparison based on cost and effectiveness

Graspers	Cost	Strength
Prograsp	++	+++
Cadiere	++	++
Fenestrated Bipolar Forceps™	+++	++
Maryland Bipolar Forceps™	+++	+
Energy	**Cost**	**Blunt dissection**
Hot Shears Monopolar Curved Scissors™	+++	++
Permanent Cautery Hook™	++	+++
Vessel Sealer™	++++	+
Harmonic ACE Curved Shears™[a]	++	+++
Suturing	**Cost**	**No assistant**
Large Suture Cut Needle Driver™	++	+
Mega Suture Cut Needle Driver™	++	+
Large Needle Driver™	++	–
Mega Needle Driver™	++	–

[a]Not endowristed

29.8 Postoperative Care

Patients are generally extubated immediately after surgery. In some instances it is advisable to keep the patient intubated longer especially if a large defect and/or pleural damage with CO2 reabsorption have been encountered.

Patients with small hernias are admitted overnight and if fulfilling criteria for discharge, can be sent home on post-op day 1. A clear liquid diet is generally started on the day of surgery and advanced as tolerated. There is no evidence that identifies a benefit from the continuation of the antibiotic prophylaxis during the post-op period. The use of deep venous thrombotic prophylaxis is to be implemented based upon standard guidelines. Routine post-op imaging is not required. A postoperative chest x-ray should be obtained selectively and based on the complexity and extent of the dissection and/or the onset of symptoms indicating a possible complication.

Patients usually report immediate improvement of their pre-operative symptoms following the surgery and should be seen for routine follow-up in the surgical office 2 weeks after the procedure.

Imaging and/or further diagnostic work up in the office setting should be implemented only if patient is reporting symptoms suspicious for possible complications and/or recurrence.

29.9 Conclusion

The repair of the rate Morgagni hernia can be complex depending on the status of the patient and the size of the hernia and its contents. The robotic repair facilitates this repair. Proper workup, operative technique and management of postoperative care will effect excellent outcomes.

References

1. Morgagni G. The seats and causes of diseases investigated by anatomy; in five books, containing A Great Variety of Dissections, with Remarks. To Which are Added Very Accurate and Copious Indexes of the Principal Things and Names therein contained. Translated from the Latin of John Baptist Morgagni, Chief Professor of Anatomy, and President of the University at Padua, by Benjamin Alexander, M. D. in Three Volumes. London: printed for A. Millar; and T. Cadell, his Successor, in the Strand; and Johnson and Payne, in Pater-Noster Row; MDCCLXIX. [1769].
2. Minneci PC, Deans KJ, Kim P, Mathisen DJ. Foramen of Morgagni hernia: changes in diagnosis and treatment. Ann Thorac Surg. 2004;77(6):1956–9.
3. Horton JD, Hofmann LJ, Hetz SP. Presentation and management of Morgagni hernias in adults: a review of 298 cases. Surg Endosc. 2008;22(6):1413–20.
4. Escarcega P, Riquelme MA, Lopez S, Gonzalez AD, Leon VY, Garcia LR, et al. Multi-institution case series of pediatric patients with laparoscopic repair of Morgagni hernia. J Laparoendosc Adv Surg Tech A. 2018;28(8):1019–22.
5. Tarcoveanu E, Georgescu S, Vasilescu A, Andronic D, Danila N, Lupascu C, et al. Laparoscopic management in Morgagni hernia - short series and review of literature. Chirurgia (Bucur). 2018;113(4):551–7.

6. Al-Salem AH, Zamakhshary M, Al Mohaidly M, Al-Qahtani A, Abdulla MR, Naga MI. Congenital Morgagni's hernia: a national multicenter study. J Pediatr Surg. 2014;49(4):503–7.
7. Pokorny WJ, McGill CW, Harberg FJ. Morgagni hernias during infancy: presentation and associated anomalies. J Pediatr Surg. 1984;19(4):394–7.
8. Abraham V, Myla Y, Verghese S, Chandran BS. Morgagni-larrey hernia- a review of 20 cases. Indian J Surg. 2012;74(5):391–5.
9. Kaida T, Ikeda A, Shimoda H, Sako H, Uchida H, Wada M, et al. Laparoscopic mesh repair of a Morgagni hernia using the double-crown technique: a case study. Asian J Endosc Surg. 2014;7(4):323–6.
10. El-Sharkawy A, Higashi Y, Lobo D. Education and imaging. Gastrointestinal: foramen of Morgagni hernia in an adult. J Gastroenterol Hepatol. 2012;27(3):616.
11. Aghajanzadeh M, Khadem S, Khajeh Jahromi S, Gorabi HE, Ebrahimi H, Maafi AA. Clinical presentation and operative repair of Morgagni hernia. Interact Cardiovasc Thorac Surg. 2012;15(4):608–11.
12. Kuster GG, Kline LE, Garzo G. Diaphragmatic hernia through the foramen of Morgagni: laparoscopic repair case report. J Laparoendosc Surg. 1992;2(2):93–100.
13. Ryan JM, Rogers AC, Hannan EJ, Mastrosimone A, Arumugasamy M. Technical description of laparoscopic Morgagni hernia repair with primary closure and onlay composite mesh placement. Hernia. 2018;22(4):697–705.
14. Fu SS, Carton MM, Ghaderi I, Galvani CA. Robotic-assisted simultaneous repair of paraesophageal hernia and Morgagni hernia: technical report. J Laparoendosc Adv Surg Tech A. 2018;28(6):745–50.
15. Kawasaki H, Ueki T, Tetsuo T, Terada R, Miyashita K, Okabe N, et al. A case of combined Morgagni and esophageal hiatal hernias successfully repaired by endoscopy and laparoscopy. Nihon Shokakibyo Gakkai Zasshi. 2017;114(10):1836–44.
16. Ozawa H, Shinozaki H, Kimata M, Ozawa S. Case of giant paraesophageal hiatal hernia associated with Morgagni hernia. Asian J Endosc Surg. 2018;11(1):43–6.
17. Sahsamanis G, Terzoglou A, Theodoridis C, Kiakou M, Mitsopoulos G, Deverakis T, et al. Laparoscopic repair of an excessive Morgagni hernia in an adult presenting as upside-down stomach. Int J Surg Case Rep. 2017;41:443–5.
18. Pironi D, Palazzini G, Arcieri S, Candioli S, Manigrasso A, Panarese A, et al. Laparoscopic diagnosis and treatment of diaphragmatic Morgagni hernia. Case report and review of the literature. Ann Ital Chir. 2008;79(1):29–36.
19. Arevalo G, Harris K, Sadiq A, Calin ML, Nasri B, Singh K. Repair of Morgagni hernia in adults with primary closure and mesh placement: first robotic experience. J Laparoendosc Adv Surg Tech A. 2017;27(5):529–32.
20. Wei B, Pittman BC Jr. Robotic Morgagni hernia repair: an emerging approach to a congenital defect. J Robot Surg. 2019;13(2):309–13.
21. Janssens W, Schoneveld M, Allaeys M, De Backer A. Robotic repair of large Morgagni hernia in an adolescent girl. J Pediatr Surg Case Rep. 2019;41:51–3.
22. Yavuz N, Yigitbasi R, Sunamak O, As A, Oral C, Erguney S. Laparoscopic repair of Morgagni hernia. Surg Laparosc Endosc Percutan Tech. 2006;16(3):173–6.
23. Agalar C, Atila K, Arslan NC, Derici ZS, Bora S. Adult morgagni hernia: a single-center experience of five cases and a review of literature. Turk J Surg. 2018:1–4. https://doi.org/10.5152/turkjsurg.2018.3929.
24. Arikan S, Dogan MB, Kocakusak A, Ersoz F, Sari S, Duzkoylu Y, et al. Morgagni's hernia: analysis of 21 patients with our clinical experience in diagnosis and treatment. Indian J Surg. 2018;80(3):239–44.
25. Nakashima S, Watanabe A, Hashimoto M, Mishina T, Obama T, Higami T. Advantages of video-assisted thoracoscopic surgery for adult congenital hernia with severe adhesion: report of two cases. Ann Thorac Cardiovasc Surg. 2011;17(2):185–9.
26. Amore D, Bergaminelli C, Di Natale D, Casazza D, Scaramuzzi R, Curcio C. Morgagni hernia repair in adult obese patient by hybrid robotic thoracic surgery. J Thorac Dis. 2018;10(7):E555–E9.

27. Ambrogi V, Forcella D, Gatti A, Vanni G, Mineo TC. Transthoracic repair of Morgagni's hernia: a 20-year experience from open to video-assisted approach. Surg Endosc. 2007;21(4):587–91.
28. Gedik E, Tuncer MC, Onat S, Avci A, Tacyildiz I, Bac B. A review of Morgagni and Bochdalek hernias in adults. Folia Morphol (Warsz). 2011;70(1):5–12.
29. Sanford Z, Weltz AS, Brown J, Shockcor N, Wu N, Park AE. Morgagni hernia repair: a review. Surg Innov. 2018;25(4):389–99.
30. Arraez-Aybar LA, Gonzalez-Gomez CC, Torres-Garcia AJ. Morgagni-Larrey parasternal diaphragmatic hernia in the adult. Rev Esp Enferm Dig. 2009;101(5):357–66.
31. Edye M, Salky B, Posner A, Fierer A. Sac excision is essential to adequate laparoscopic repair of paraesophageal hernia. Surg Endosc. 1998;12(10):1259–63.
32. Dallemagne B, Quero G, Lapergola A, Guerriero L, Fiorillo C, Perretta S. Treatment of giant paraesophageal hernia: pro laparoscopic approach. Hernia. 2018;22(6):909–19.
33. Watson DI, Davies N, Devitt PG, Jamieson GG. Importance of dissection of the hernial sac in laparoscopic surgery for large hiatal hernias. Arch Surg. 1999;134(10):1069–73.
34. Palanivelu C, Rangarajan M, Rajapandian S, Amar V, Parthasarathi R. Laparoscopic repair of adult diaphragmatic hernias and eventration with primary sutured closure and prosthetic reinforcement: a retrospective study. Surg Endosc. 2009;23(5):978–85.
35. Mullins ME, Saini S. Imaging of incidental Bochdalek hernia. Semin Ultrasound CT MR. 2005;26(1):28–36.
36. Yap KH, Jones M. Late presentation of congenital diaphragmatic hernia after a diagnostic laparoscopic surgery (a case report). J Cardiothorac Surg. 2013;8:8.
37. Catalona WJ, Crowder WL, Chretien PB. Occurrence of hernia of Morgagni with filial cervical lung hernia: a hereditary defect of the cervical mesenchyme? Chest. 1972;62(3):340–2.
38. Pillai SA, Chinnappan S. Congenital right Morgagni hernia presenting in an adult-a case report. Indian J Surg. 2016;78(3):238–40.
39. Kamiya N, Yokoi K, Miyazawa N, Hishinuma S, Ogata Y, Katayama N. Morgagni hernia diagnosed by MRI. Surg Today. 1996;26(6):446–8.
40. Collie DA, Turnbull CM, Shaw TR, Price WH. Case report: MRI appearances of left sided Morgagni hernia containing liver. Br J Radiol. 1996;69(819):278–80.
41. Yeh HC, Halton KP, Gray CE. Anatomic variations and abnormalities in the diaphragm seen with US. Radiographics. 1990;10(6):1019–30.
42. McAneny D. Preoperative preparation. In: Doherty GM, editor. CURRENT diagnosis & treatment: surgery, 14e. New York: McGraw-Hill Education; 2015.

Robotic Paraesophageal Hernia Repair 30

Robert F. Cubas, Joslin N. Cheverie, and Santiago Horgan

30.1 Introduction

Paraesophageal hernias present a clinical and anatomical entity that must be fully appreciated for safe and effective management. They are an uncommon form of hiatal hernia that tend to present clinically in the population of patients over 65 years of age. The most common symptomatic presentations of a paraesophageal hernia (PEH) include dysphagia, regurgitation, gastroesophageal reflux, dyspnea, chest or epigastric pain or pressure, and anemia. Weight loss in this patient population may be common and dramatic. Acute presentations may demonstrate signs and symptoms of bleeding (due to friction ulcer) or obstruction (due to gastric volvulus). The risk of hemorrhage and ischemia in the acute setting are a particular subset of PEH presentation.

There are four types of hiatal hernias as depicted below (Fig. 30.1). Type 1 hernias account for 90% of all hiatal hernias and are often asymptomatic or present with predominantly reflux symptoms. Type 2, type 3, and type 4 reflect the paraesophageal component and involve movement of the gastric fundus through the hiatus into the thorax. Type 3 or "mixed" hernias are the most common representing 90% of all PEH. Giant PEH are defined as type 2, 3, or 4, but with over 50% of the stomach in an intrathoracic position [1, 2].

Symptomatic hernias should be repaired unless there are clinical parameters precluding safe and effective surgical intervention. The timing and preoperative evaluation varies depending on the patient and disease factors and will be discussed below. Elective repair in the symptomatic patient has been associated with an increase in patient quality of life with satisfaction rates in the literature ranging between 85 and 96%. Revisional surgery is known for its technical difficulty, higher complication rate, and decreased patient satisfaction. Clinical assessment and

R. F. Cubas · J. N. Cheverie (✉) · S. Horgan
Division of Minimally Invasive Surgery, Department of Surgery, UC San Diego Medical Center, San Diego, CA, USA
e-mail: jcheverie@ucsd.edu

K. A. LeBlanc (ed.), *Robotic Assisted Hernia Repair*,
https://doi.org/10.1007/978-3-030-23025-8_30

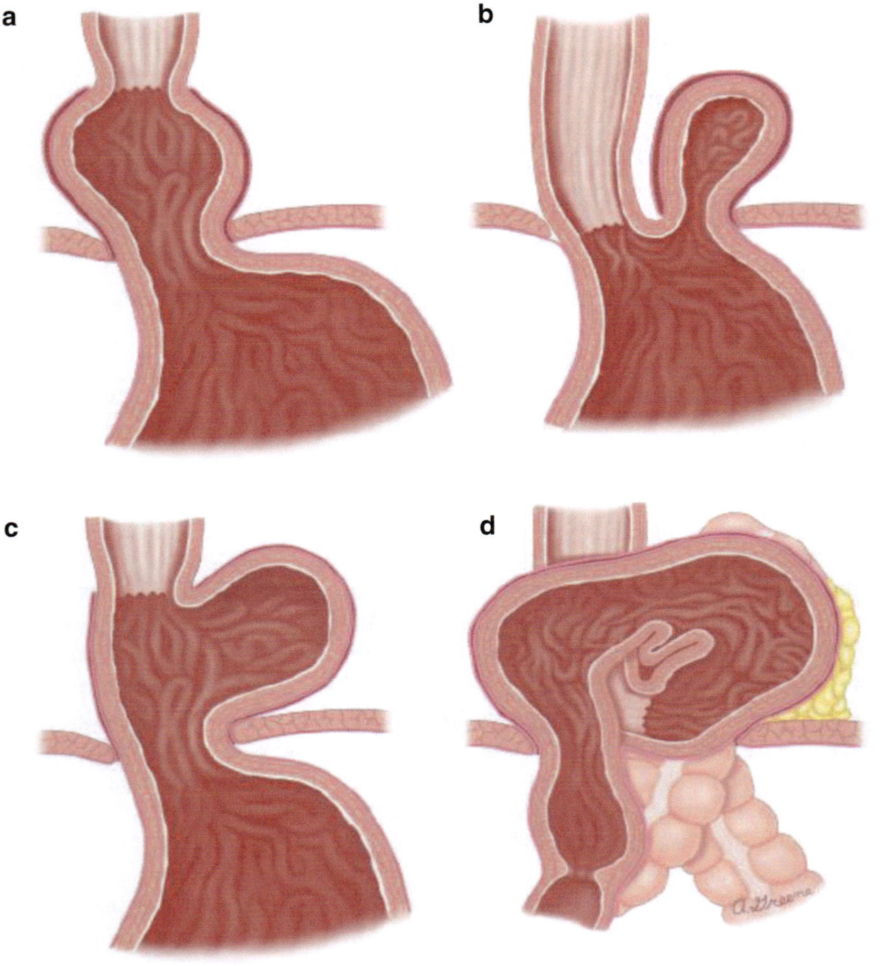

Fig. 30.1 Types of hiatal hernias. (**a**) Type I—Sliding hernia. (**b**) Type-II—"True" paraesophageal hernia. (**c**) Type-III—"Mixed" paraesophageal hernia. (**d**) Type-IV—"Giant" paraesophageal hernia

perioperative considerations are imperative in this group in order to properly stratify surgical candidates and optimize outcomes [3, 4].

Robotic repair of a paraesophageal hernia is an efficient and ergonomic approach to this challenging anatomical problem. Added precision and extended accessibility and visualization of the thorax from an abdominal approach makes the robotic repair a preferred surgical method. In addition to the mentioned clinical manifestations, this chapter will review the preoperative workup required. Surgical technique will then focus on the robotic approach in a step-wise fashion. Evidentiary review of outcomes will highlight this approach as a feasible if not superior approach [5, 6].

Special considerations for emergent and prophylactic repair, esophageal lengthening, crural closure with regards to mesh and relaxing incisions will be addressed. In addition, a brief comparative cost analysis with robotic and laparoscopic approach will be highlighted.

30.2 Preoperative Evaluation

As with all foregut surgery, preoperative preparation is critical. A carefully documented history of current symptoms, previous treatment modalities and outcomes, as well as comorbid cardiac and pulmonary processes must be completed. This may alter the pathway to surgery with involvement of other respective specialists to investigate further any underlying cardiac, pulmonary or systemic disease processes. In addition to symptomatology, patient characteristics and comorbidities may help alter or adjust operative approach.

The proposed workup in our institution consists of esophagogastroduodenoscopy, pH testing (only performed if patients had disabling reflux symptoms), upper GI series and high-resolution manometry. Variations to this may be reasonable depending on the patient symptoms, the surgical approach, as well with acute presentations. In the case of acute volvulus CT scan of the chest and abdomen may suffice but would lack more specific functional information which may preclude knowledge of underlying motility disorders.

30.2.1 Upper Endoscopy

Endoscopy is performed for every patient to assess the anatomy with regards to esophageal length, size of hernia, esophagitis, presence of Cameron's erosions at the level of the diaphragm, and assessment of gastric volvulus. Retroflexion views as well as assessment of the gastroesophageal junction (GEJ) are crucial.

30.2.2 Barium Swallow

This contrast study demonstrates the size, location, orientation, and reducibility of the paraesophageal component. It also provides functional information with regards to dysphagia and regurgitation. Esophageal length is also assessed.

30.2.3 High Resolution Esophageal Manometry

Esophageal manometry is indicated in the assessment of dysphagia or non-cardiac chest pain in patients without evidence of mechanical obstruction, ulceration, or inflammation. It is imperative for surgical planning when an anti-reflux procedure is indicated.

The fundamental difference between conventional manometry and high-resolution manometry (HRM) is the number of pressure sensors used and the spacing between them. In contrast to conventional manometry where sensors are spaced at 3–5 cm intervals, in HRM sensors are typically spaced 1 cm apart along the length of the manometric assembly. Catheters with up to 36 sensors distributed longitudinally and radially in the esophagus allow for simultaneous pressure readings spanning both sphincters and the interposed esophagus [7].

30.2.4 pH Monitoring

Ambulatory pH monitoring is performed by placing a wireless pH capsule, (Bravo System, Medtronic, Inc., Minneapolis, MN), 6 cm above the upper border of the LES. At the time of endoscopic insertion, the Bravo delivery catheter is introduced through the mouth, and the capsule is attached to the esophageal mucosa. The patient wears a Bravo pH receiver around the waist. Data is transmitted to a receiver worn by the patient, and data recording is carried out for 48 h. A standard DeMeester scoring system is compiled for objective assessment [8].

30.3 Operative Technique

Paraesophageal hernia repair can be performed via a trans-thoracic or trans-abdominal approach. Open, laparoscopic, and robotic techniques may be applied.

We prefer the robotic system for trans-abdominal paraesophageal hernia repair in our institution for both elective and emergency settings provided a suitable clinical scheme. The operation is performed using the Da Vinci Surgical System (Intuitive Surgical, Sunnyvale, CA), which combines robotics and computer imaging to enable microsurgery in a laparoscopic environment. The most notable benefit of the robot with this approach is the 7 degrees of freedom provided by the instrument arms. Tip articulation mimics the up/down and side-to-side flexibility of the human wrist. These articulations extend the surgeon's minimally invasive abilities within the confines of the intracorporeal space [9].

30.3.1 Operating Room (OR) Setup

The room size of the OR must accommodate the robotic system consisting of three to four integrated components. Before the patient is brought into the room it should be confirmed that all appropriate equipment is present, turned on, and functioning properly including all three components of the da Vinci® Robotic System, for this matter an experienced OR and robotic support staff is crucial [10].

The patient cart is sterilely draped and is advanced towards the patient over the head (Si system) or from the side (Xi system). This cart is physically docked with the patient through robotic arms and adapting robotic trocars. A variety of robotic instruments exist which are manually connected and inserted at the patient cart. A vision cart, which include the system processors, sits at side of the patient and allows for a camera and energy interface between the patient cart and the surgical console.

The endoscope is calibrated through the vision cart accordingly. The surgical console may be single or dual (training) depending on the requirements of the institution. The integration of visual cues allows for precise activation and control of the robotic arms within the surgical field. All of the unit components must be appropriately positioned with spatial allowance to accommodate regular intraoperative conduct.

30.3.2 Patient Positioning

The patient is initially placed in the supine position over a bean bag. Pneumatic compression stockings are routinely placed on the lower extremities. All pressure points should be comfortably padded. After satisfactory induction of general endotracheal anesthesia, the legs are placed in split leg attachments, and the arms out to the side on padded arm boards (Fig. 30.2). Preoperative antibiotics are given, and the abdomen is prepped from the nipples down to the pubic symphysis and as far lateral as possibly, especially on the left side.

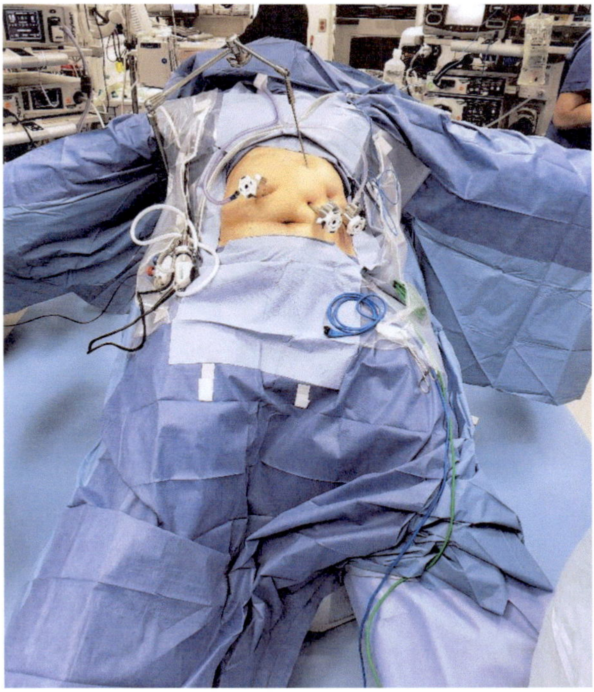

Fig. 30.2 Patient in supine position with outstretched arms to 80° and split legs in steep reverse Trendelenburg

30.3.3 Trocar Placement

A 12-mm, 8.5 mm or 8 mm trocar (depending on the system being used; Si vs Xi) is initially placed, under direct vision using an optical trocar system. This is the preferred location for the camera and is in the left mid abdomen two fingerbreadths lateral to the umbilicus and one palm-width inferior to the left costal margin. Two additional robotic 8-mm trocars are then placed: one on the left subcostal midclavicular line, one on the right subcostal midclavicular line. A 5 mm assistant trocar is positioned in the left flank and is used during the case for retraction. It may be upsized to a 12 mm trocar to accommodate sutures or mesh as desired. The patient is positioned in steep reverse Trendelenburg. A small sub-xiphoid incision is used for the placement of the Nathanson liver retractor (Fig. 30.3).

30.3.4 Docking

At this point, the robotic surgical cart is brought into position and the arms are attached to the three specific trocars. The position of the patient cart will depend on the system used; the Si will have to come in from the patient's left shoulder or head, whereas the Xi can approach the patient perpendicularly from the left or right side and the boom will have to rotate 90° counter clock or clockwise respectively (Fig. 30.4). A Cadiere Forceps or Force bipolar instrumentation is placed in the surgeon's left hand, and in the right hand, the articulated robotic vessel sealer device is introduced. The assistant at the bedside usually performs the setup of the robot. The assistant surgeon is positioned on the patients' left side. During the case, the assistant is in charge of switching the robotic instruments and introducing and extracting the sutures, Penrose or mesh (if used) for the operating surgeon. For this reason, basic training in laparoscopic surgery and robotics is essential for the assistant surgeon.

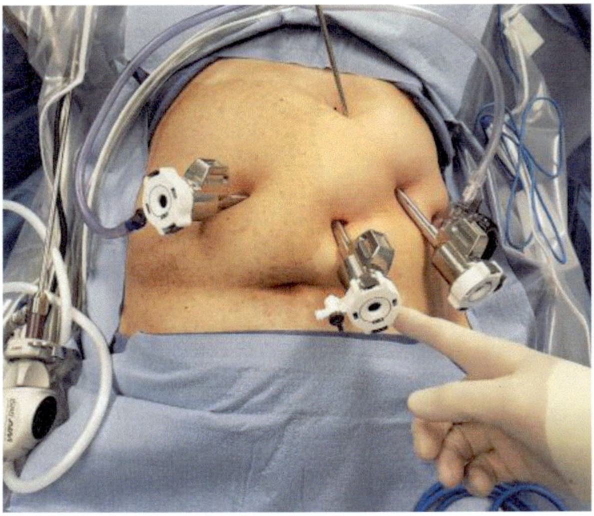

Fig. 30.3 Assistant's finger pointing at the camera port. Insufflation cannula connected to the 12 mm assistant port and smoke evacuator cannula connected to the right 8 mm port

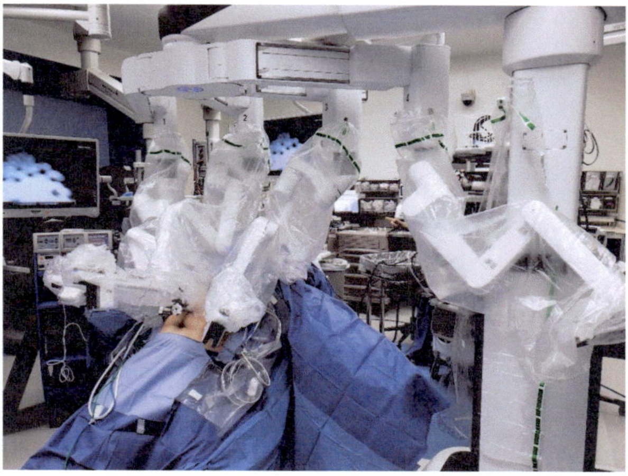

Fig. 30.4 Da Vinci Xi; patient cart approaching perpendicularly from the left side, with the boom rotated 90° counterclockwise

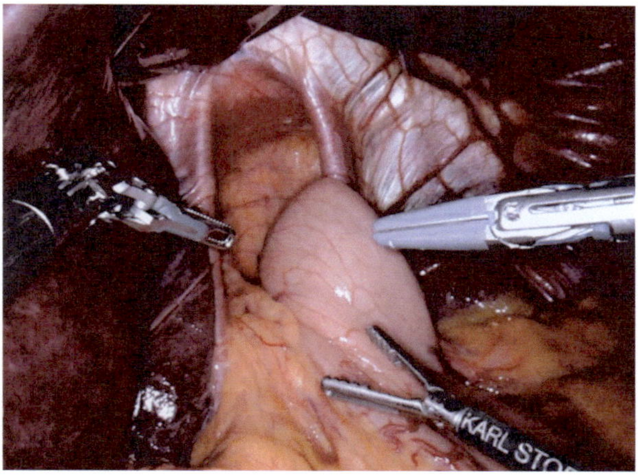

Fig. 30.5 Exposure of the hiatus with a large paraesophageal hernia

30.3.5 Visualization

The left mid-abdominal port is used for the 30° robotic camera selecting the downward view. After the left lobe of the liver is retracted anteriorly using the Nathanson retractor, the hiatus is exposed. At this point, the hernia is visualized (Fig. 30.5). Often, with positioning, herniated contents will reduce spontaneously at this point.

30.3.6 Reduction of Hernia

The herniated contents are reduced manually, as required, and the robotic vessel sealer may be used (along with the Forced bipolar) in a hand-over-hand manner. An additional formal grasper, such as the Cadiere, may be required. The left crus approach is preferred (Fig. 30.6) beginning with division of the short gastric vessels using the robotic vessel sealer from the level of the inferior pole of the spleen

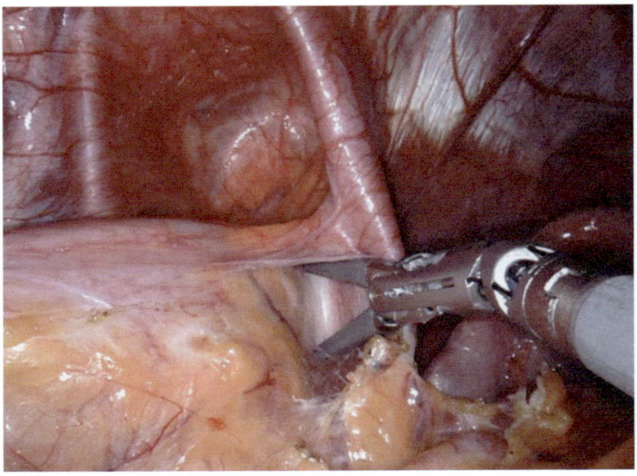

Fig. 30.6 Left crus approach

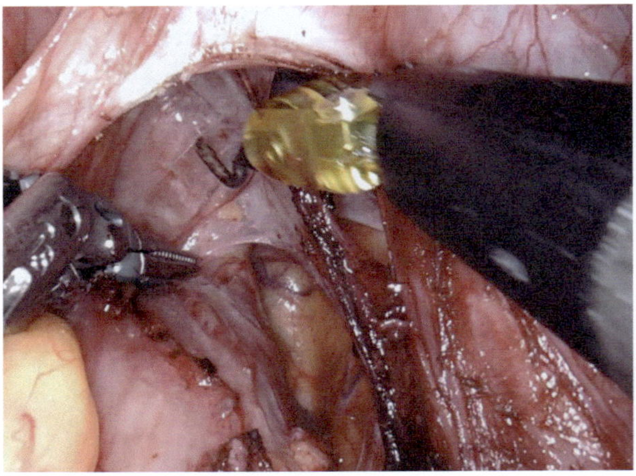

Fig. 30.7 Hernia sac dissected off the mediastinum

allowing for left crural exposure. In the event of massive herniation, the surgical approach may have to be modified with initial dissection commencing at the interface of the hernia sac and the left crura avoiding excessive short gastric vessel division. Incision of the hernia sac is started at its junction with the left crus and continued around the rim of the hiatus in a circumferential fashion. Entry into the correct plane will ease the dissection and minimize bleeding and disorientation. Reduction of the sac is performed as much as possible from this position whilst avoiding injury to the anterior vagus nerve. Once the left crus is exposed, the dissection is then focused on the right side of the esophagus. The pars flaccida is opened, and the right crus is mobilized with a combination of blunt dissection, hook dissection, and robotic vessel sealer, reducing further the intrathoracic component of the hernia and sac. A retroesophageal window is created and a Penrose drain passed and secured with an 0-PDS endoloop which is used for further manipulation and retraction by the assistant as the dissection continues into the mediastinum.

Next, the hernia sac is dissected off its mediastinal attachments (Fig. 30.7). This can be a tedious process requiring technical precision and a circumferential approach.

Care must be taken to identify the pleural attachments that are often intimate with the hernia sac. Any violation of the pleura should be addressed by means of immediate closure with suture or clip placement. Subsequent desufflation of the abdomen and 1 min of bag-ventilation per anesthesia will obviate any clinical implication.

The aorta is identified posteriorly and the esophageal attachments divided allowing for circumferential mobilization. The anterior and posterior vagal nerves are identified and are kept with the esophagus. Once the position of a tension-free intraabdominal esophagus has been achieved the hernia dissection is complete [11].

30.3.7 Esophageal Lengthening

If a 3 cm intra-abdominal esophageal length cannot be obtained with esophageal mobilization alone, a Collis gastroplasty may be performed to obtain additional esophageal length. Failure to lengthen a shortened esophagus can lead to recurrence as it produces strain on the repair. The Collis procedure entails the creation of a gastric tube by vertically stapling the proximal stomach from the angle of His, parallel to a large bougie placed alongside the gastric lesser curvature. This neoesophagus permits that the new esophagogastric junction be located intra-abdominally. Collis gastroplasty is not without its complications. The neoesophagus created by the gastroplasty does not display the normal peristaltic activity of the esophagus and can lead to dysphagia. Persistent parietal cells can also lead to recurrent heartburn and esophagitis. In addition, the presence of a staple line can lead to leak rates of 1–3% even in high volume, experienced centers [12]. We prefer a modality of lengthening that involves retraction of the fundus so that level of the angle of His is pulled into the jaws of the blue load stapling device in a parallel fashion necessitating a single staple line.

30.3.8 Crural Closure

The esophagus is retracted anteriorly and to the left. Closure of the diaphragmatic defect is started at the junction of the right and left crus to decrease tension on every stitch, and is carried cephalad. The closure is performed using a running 0 non-absorbable barbed suture (Fig. 30.8). A 52 Fr bougie is passed down the esophagus during the repair to tailor the closure and to avoid undue angulation as the esophagus passes through the hiatus. We also ensure visualization and of the aorta and keep this structure away from the approximating suture. Furthermore, a C-shaped GORE® Bio-A hiatal mesh is used routinely to reinforce the closure of the diaphragmatic defect. The mesh is secured in place to the antero- and retro-esophageal diaphragm using fibrin sealant. Additional anchoring sutures may be required. In the event that the diaphragmatic crura cannot be approximated primarily without tension, a relaxing incision may be necessary [13].

30.3.9 Relaxing Incisions

Relaxing incisions are typically performed on the right side unless excessive scarring or close proximity to the inferior vena cava (IVC) is prohibitive in which case

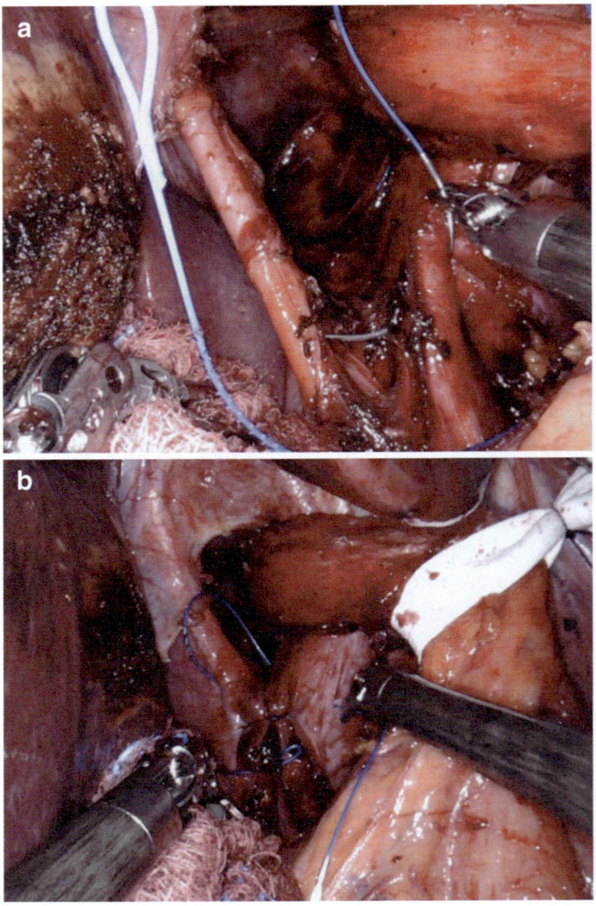

Fig. 30.8 (**a**, **b**) Posterior crural closure using a running non absorbable barbed suture

a left-sided incision is performed. A right-sided relaxing incision is made by incising the diaphragm 2 cm lateral to the crus, between the right crus and IVC, and carrying this full thickness without violating the pleural space. Caution must be taken to avoid the anterior crural vein and the thoracic duct near the aortic hiatus. A left-sided incision is performed in a similar fashion between the left crus and the left seventh rib taking care not to injure the left-sided phrenic nerve. In cases where a unilateral relaxing incision is not sufficient, bilateral relaxing incisions can be performed. The crural closure and relaxing incisions should be reinforced and covered with a mesh [14].

30.3.10 Fundoplication

The creation of a floppy tension-free 360° fundoplication is calibrated over a 52 F bougie. If the fundus is not completely free of hiatal or posterior attachments then additional dissection is performed. The fundus is then placed up on the left crus and is grasped from the posterior retroesophageal window. The shoeshine maneuver is

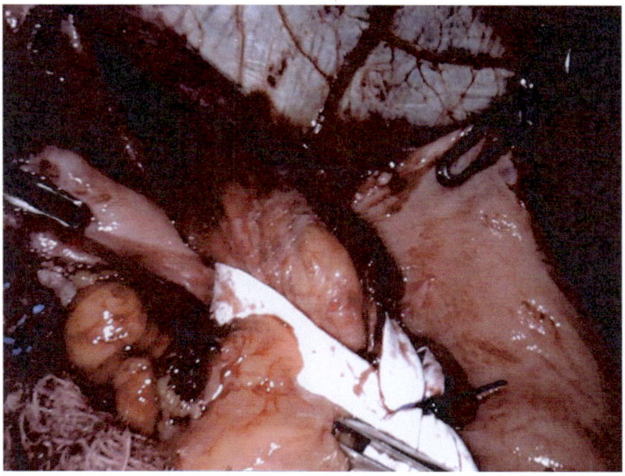

Fig. 30.9 Shoeshine maneuver

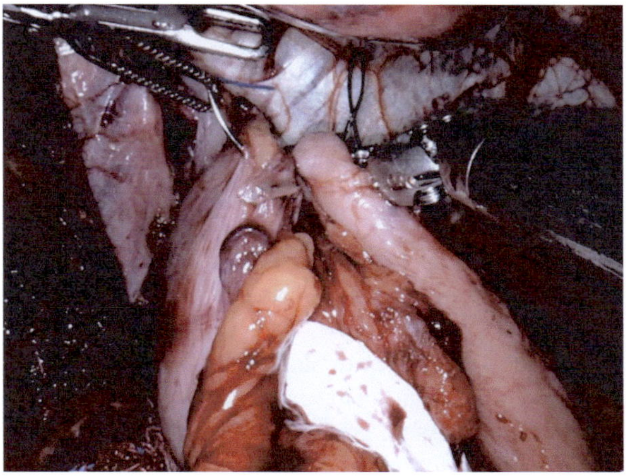

Fig. 30.10 Floppy Nissen fundoplication

fundamental to ensure the proper orientation of the wrap demonstrating a "short-gastric to short-gastric" association (Fig. 30.9). This confirms proper fundal placement of the wrap which serves to prevent wrap herniation. It also avoids undue twisting of the fundus as it comes around the esophagus. Once this maneuver is satisfied, an initial 2-0 silk suture attaches stomach to stomach using the divided short gastric vessels as landmarks for approximation (Fig. 30.10). The Penrose drain is removed at this point. A second 2-0 silk suture then encompasses stomach, esophagus and stomach to truly anchor the wrap in a proper location. A final suture incorporating only the stomach may be placed. We prefer to anchor the wrap posteriorly to the midline crura. Other techniques of fixation such as lateral crural suture fixation may be used with caution not to alter the orientation of the wrap. Upper endoscopy is performed at the completion of the case to check the integrity of the mucosa of the esophagus, stomach, and to verify the adequacy, orientation, and patency of the fundoplication. In the presence of impaired or unknown esophageal motility, a partial (270°) Toupet fundoplication is preferred.

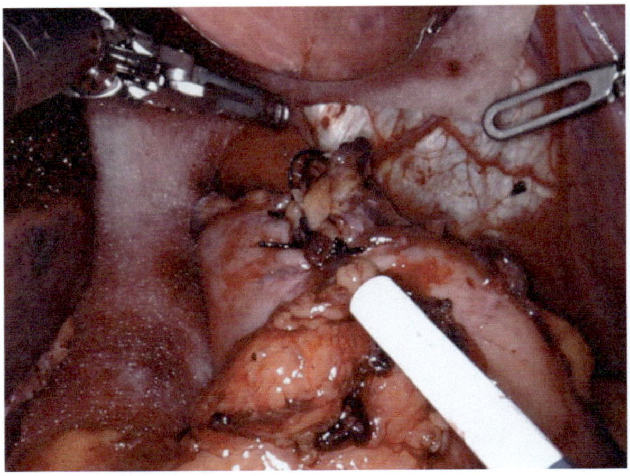

Fig. 30.11 Bio-A mesh (Gore®) placed in a C-shape to reinforce the anterior and posterior hiatus

30.3.11 Mesh Reinforcement

Both permanent and biologic meshes have been shown to be effective in reducing early recurrences in separate randomized trials. In a 2016 meta-analysis of four randomized trials including 406 patients, compared with suture closure alone, mesh reinforcement of the crural closure reduced the rate of reoperation but not recurrence or complication rates. On the other hand, no comparative large studies have been performed on the use of bio-absorbable mesh (Fig. 30.11), however these short studies demonstrated its safety and effectiveness [15, 16].

The ideal hernia repair should result in a permanent retention of the stomach in the abdominal cavity. However, the recurrence rate following PEH repair is high because of a pressure gradient resulting from the positive intra-abdominal pressure and negative intrathoracic pressure. While not routinely applied at our institution, such fixation techniques are described below and may be useful in acute presentations or in giant hernias for which the reduced and enlarged stomach seems functionally impaired [11].

30.3.12 Anterior Gastropexy with Sutures

Gastropexy with sutures to the anterior abdominal wall may be performed at the end of a PEH repair.

30.3.13 Posterior Gastropexy with Sutures (Hill Repair)

Sutures placed from the lower esophageal sphincter to the arcuate ligament, performed less often due to its technical difficultness and poor results. An anterior gastropexy is preferred [17].

30.3.14 Anterior Gastropexy with PEG Tubes

An endoscopic hernia reduction with or without laparoscopic assistance, followed by anterior gastropexy with two PEG tubes may be performed for patients who are too frail to undertake a formal PEH repair or for patients in an emergency setting. The placement of two PEG tubes reduces the potential risk of stomach volvulus around a single PEG tube. This procedure relieves symptoms from a paraesophageal hernia, prevents the occurrence of gastric volvulus, and does not preclude a formal hernia repair at a later time [18].

30.4 Peri-Operative Complications

30.4.1 Pneumothorax

Violation of the pleural is a common complication of the challenging dissection of the hernia sac in the mediastinum. This usually has minimal clinical consequences, but immediate communication with anesthesia is imperative. Primary closure with suture or clips is appropriate. This sometimes requires further dissection to remove tension of the scarred hernia sac off of the pleura. Abdominal de-sufflation and hand-bag mask ventilation can alleviate any notable capnothorax. Of course, one must be prepared for more aggressive intervention such as thoracostomy tube if clinically warranted. However, it is important in the perioperative setting to remember the mechanism of pneumothoraces in this surgical patient population.

30.4.2 Vagal Injury

Inadvertent injury to the anterior or posterior vagal nerves are possible at multiple points of the procedure. Both traction and sharp/thermal injuries are possible. Careful dissection and early as well as continued identification are key to avoid inadvertent injury.

There is a concern for gastroparesis and gastric outlet obstruction after vagal injury. However, Oelschlager et al performed a review of 30 patients undergoing a vagotomy during the course of an esophageal lengthening procedure; 20 anterior, six posterior, and four bilateral and compared the results with 72 patients that did not have a vagotomy. The primary presenting symptoms were improved in both groups. Similarly, there was no difference in the severity of abdominal pain, bloating, diarrhea, or early satiety between the Vagotomy and No Vagotomy groups at follow-up (median of 19 months). No patient required a subsequent operation for gastric outlet obstruction [19].

30.4.3 Esophageal Perforation

Although rare, esophageal perforation can be a catastrophic complication leading to mediastinitis and death if not recognized and managed appropriately. They are frequently associated to Collis gastroplasty (88%) and its overall occurrence and presentation as a post-operative leak is 2.5%. Our preference would be complete exposure including endoscopic evaluation followed by primary full thickness repair [4].

30.4.4 Gastric Perforation

This is a very rare event (0.3%) and should be managed as above with full exposure and primary repair. The location will often be optimally incorporated in the fundoplication [4].

30.4.5 Bleeding

A most common source of bleeding may be from the short gastric vessels following transection with thermal energy. It is often due to bleeding at the angle of division and subsequent temporary retraction.

A more concerning intrathoracic bleeding event may occur from small arterial vessels branching from the aorta during the posterior dissection. Larger vessel bleeding may occur. Inflammation of the sac can lead to diffuse oozing during the mediastinal dissection. Regardless of location, general principles of surgery including pressure, communication, exposure and control are necessary. The robotic platform adds 3-D visualization and ergonomic ease of access in confined spaces. We prefer initial control with pressure by insertion of Ray-tec® gauze. Adjuncts such as 10 mm suction devices may be useful. Assessment and definitive control through application of thermal energy device or clips may then ensue. Communication with anesthesia is crucial.

30.4.6 Dysphagia

As with any hiatal surgery, dysphagia may ensue and has multiple possible etiologies. Thorough evaluation by means of UGI, EGD, and manometry are often required. Common causes can be undue angulation of the esophagus as it enters the abdomen due to the crural closure. A wrap may be functionally too tight. Both of these may be alleviated by serial endoscopic dilatation. Slippage of the fundoplication may necessitate revisional surgery.

30.4.7 Reflux

According to a prospective study of 111 patients performed at Johns Hopkins University where a validated gastroesophageal reflux disease-specific quality of life (QOL) tool was administered to patients before and at 2, 12, and 36 months after the procedure, (higher QOL scores represented greater severity of symptoms). Overall, patients experienced significant symptom improvement at postoperative months 2 (mean QOL score, 10.18 [7.39]), 12 (mean QOL score, 9.74 [8.69]), and 36 (mean QOL score, 10.58 [9.14]) compared with baseline (mean QOL score, 28.50 [11.13])

($P < 0.001$) [20]. This would indicate the benefits of the procedure as a disease treatment.

30.5 Outcomes

PEH is a potentially devastating condition frequently manifesting in patients of advanced age with other substantial medical problems.

The pressure gradient across the abdominal and thoracic cavities predisposes the patient to a recurrence after a PEH repair. A meta-analysis of 13 studies, including 965 patients reported an overall recurrence of 10.2% and a "true" recurrence rate of 25.5% when a follow up barium esophagogram was used [21].

Most patients with a radiographic recurrence after PEH repair are asymptomatic, and patients with a clinical recurrence often have reflux symptoms that can be controlled with proton pump inhibitors. Only a small fraction of patients will require a reoperation for complications or intractable symptoms.

Robotic assisted paraesophageal hernia repair is a safe procedure that has a learning curve of about 36 cases. Upon review of the literature, this approach seems to have the same benefits as those of the laparoscopic approach in terms of, total surgical time, complication rate, length of hospital stay and quality of life; in addition, the robotic platform may be associated with a lower recurrence rate than the laparoscopic approach according to small retrospective series [22].

30.6 Reoperative Considerations

Reoperation for a symptomatic paraesophageal hernia should be performed by highly experienced surgeons, as these procedures present a significant technical challenge, especially if permanent mesh has been placed at the time of the index operation. In this setting, the robotic platform presents an invaluable approach, as it contributes to a decrease in the rate of conversion to an open procedure, especially in the presence of perforation, ischemia, or significant blood loss, intraoperative complications that can still be fixed while sitting in the console.

In more complex reoperative cases (patients who failed numerous transabdominal repairs), a transthoracic approach can offer a virgin territory for repair.

30.7 Emergent Repair: Timing and Indication

Over 40 years ago, life-threatening complications such as gastric ischemia, perforation, or severe hemorrhage were thought to occur in up to 30% of patients diagnosed with PEH. As a result, operative repair of any PEH was sought, irrespective of symptoms. Recent literature and modern operative techniques challenge these historical estimates. Stylopoulos used a Markov Monte Carlo model to predict clinical outcomes related to elective laparoscopic hernia repair and watchful waiting. He found an annual probability of developing acute complications requiring emergent surgery of 1.1% in the watchful waiting group and a mortality rate of 1.4 and 5.4% for laparoscopic elective surgery and emergency surgery, respectively.

Giant paraesophageal hernias may present acutely with Borchard's triad: severe epigastric pain, retching, and inability to pass a nasogastric tube. The best timing for an operative repair after an acute presentation is a subject of ongoing debate. Although any clinical or radiological suspicion of acute ischemia or perforation requires immediate surgical management, most acute presentations can be initially managed conservatively providing the opportunity for semi-elective repair [23].

30.8 Cost analysis of Laparoscopic Vs Robotic Fundoplication

Robotic assisted compared to purely laparoscopic Nissen fundoplication and hiatal hernia repair has been demonstrated to be associated with increased costs in previously published studies. Müller-Stich et al. conducted a randomized controlled trial comparing laparoscopic to robotic fundoplication. They identified a shorter operative time for robotic fundoplication at 88 min, compared to 102 min for laparoscopic ($p = 0.033$). Costs were higher for the robotic procedure compared to laparoscopic procedures (€3244 vs. €2743, respectively; $p = 0.003$). A study on robotic fundoplication costs using the United Health System Consortium database included 12,079 patients who underwent robotic, laparoscopic, or open fundoplication. When laparoscopic was compared to robotic fundoplication, there was no significant difference in morbidity, mortality, or length of stay. Robotic fundoplication was associated with an increased 30-day readmission rate compared to a laparoscopic approach (3.6 vs. 1.8%; $p < 0.05$). Costs were also higher in robotic procedures in this study ($10,644 robotic vs. $7968 laparoscopic; $p < 0.05$). Another large database study, this time using the Nationwide Inpatient Sample, evaluated 297,335 patients undergoing robotic compared to laparoscopic gastrointestinal surgery, including both fundoplication and gastroenterostomy without gastrectomy. In the fundoplication cohort, there was no difference in the length of stay or complications. Costs were significantly higher with robotic fundoplication ($37,638 vs. $32,947; $p < 0.0001$).

According to Higgins et al., after retrospectively evaluating 22 robotic and 115 laparoscopic fundoplication procedures, robotic cases were associated with a statistically significant increase in operative time and overall supply cost. The mean and median number of robotic instruments used for fundoplication was 4.9 and 4.0, respectively. The mean total cost of robotic instruments, excluding outliers, was $1320.70, and $2925.20 including outliers. Among the 22 robotic fundoplications performed, 13 outlier instruments were used (individual case cost of >$1000). These instruments included primarily bowel graspers and cautery spatulas. To account for the amortized upfront cost of the robotic instruments, an additional analysis of standardizing the cost of each robotic instrument as $200 per case was performed. From this, it was determined that there was no difference in total supply cost between robotic and laparoscopic fundoplications [24].

30.9 Conclusion

Robot-assisted laparoscopic hiatal hernia repair has demonstrated low short-term clinical recurrence rates with morbidity and quality of life comparable to the literature for laparoscopic repair, even in older patients and those with high operative risks. With increasing numbers of robotic trained general surgeons in the community, a wider application of the robotic platform for the repair of paraesophageal hernia, even in complex cases, is expected which will bring shorter operative times. It will also allow wider application of minimally invasive technique although surgeon experience and knowledge of anatomy may not be substituted. The ergonomic and visual advantages of the robotic platform add surgical precision and potentially lower recurrence rates.

Financial Disclosure Statement Dr. Horgan- Gore (Grant) having received honoraria from W. L. Gore & Associates to provide educational training of their products. Additionally, W. L. Gore & Associates provides financial support for the Minimally Invasive Surgery Fellowship that Drs. Horgan and Cheverie are instructors. One of the products made by W. L. Gore & Associates was reviewed in this invited article. Dr. Cubas has no financial interest in any of the products, devices, or drugs mentioned in this manuscript.

References

1. Geha AS, Massad MG, Snow NJ, Baue AE. A 32-year experience in 100 patients with giant paraesophageal hernia: the case for abdominal approach and selective antireflux repair. Surgery. 2000;128(4):623–30. https://doi.org/10.1067/msy.2000.108425.
2. Seetharamaiah R, Romero RJ, Kosanovic R, Gallas M, Verdeja JC, Rabaza J, Gonzalez AM. Robotic repair of giant paraesophageal hernias. JSLS. 2013;17(4):570–7. https://doi.org/10.4293/108680813X13654754534594.
3. Hall T, Warnes N, Kuchta K, Novak S, Hedberg H, Linn JG, Haggerty S, Denham W, Joehl RJ, Ujiki M. Patient-centered outcomes after laparoscopic paraesophageal hernia repair. J Am Coll Surg. 2018;227(1):106–14. https://doi.org/10.1016/j.jamcollsurg.2017.12.054.
4. Luketich JD, Nason KS, Christie NA, Pennathur A, Jobe BA, Landreneau RJ, Schuchert MJ. Outcomes after a decade of laparoscopic giant paraesophageal hernia repair. J Thorac Cardiovasc Surg. 2010;139(2):395–404.e1. https://doi.org/10.1016/j.jtcvs.2009.10.005.
5. Vasudevan V, Reusche R, Nelson E, Kaza S. Robotic paraesophageal hernia repair: a single-center experience and systematic review. J Robot Surg. 2018;12(1):81–6. https://doi.org/10.1007/s11701-017-0697-x.
6. Dunnican WJ, Singh TP, Guptill GG, Doorly MG, Ata A. Early robotic experience with paraesophageal hernia repair and Nissen fundoplication: short-term outcomes. J Robot Surg. 2008;2(1):41–4. https://doi.org/10.1007/s11701-008-0079-5.
7. Wirsching A, Zhang Q, McCormick SE, Hubka M, Low DE. Abnormal high-resolution manometry findings and outcomes after paraesophageal hernia repair. J Am Coll Surg. 2018;227(2):181–8 e2. https://doi.org/10.1016/j.jamcollsurg.2018.03.033.
8. Pohl D, Tutuian R. Reflux monitoring: pH-metry, Bilitec and oesophageal impedance measurements. Best Pract Res Clin Gastroenterol. 2009;23(3):299–311. https://doi.org/10.1016/j.bpg.2009.04.003.

9. Diez Del Val I, Martinez Blazquez C, Loureiro Gonzalez C, Vitores Lopez JM, Sierra Esteban V, Barrenetxea Asua J, Del Hoyo Aretxabala I, Perez de Villarreal P, Bilbao Axpe JE, Mendez Martin JJ. Robot-assisted gastroesophageal surgery: usefulness and limitations. J Robot Surg. 2014;8(2):111–8. https://doi.org/10.1007/s11701-013-0435-y.
10. DeUgarte DA, Hirschl RB, Geiger JD. Robotic repair of congenital paraesophageal hiatal hernia. J Laparoendosc Adv Surg Tech A. 2009;19(Suppl 1):S187–9. https://doi.org/10.1089/lap.2008.0185.
11. Galvani CA, Loebl H, Osuchukwu O, Samame J, Apel ME, Ghaderi I. Robotic-assisted paraesophageal hernia repair: initial experience at a single institution. J Laparoendosc Adv Surg Tech A. 2016;26(4):290–5. https://doi.org/10.1089/lap.2016.0096.
12. Zaman JA, Lidor AO. The optimal approach to symptomatic paraesophageal hernia repair: important technical considerations. Curr Gastroenterol Rep. 2016;18(10):53. https://doi.org/10.1007/s11894-016-0529-6.
13. Asti E, Sironi A, Bonitta G, Lovece A, Milito P, Bonavina L. Crura augmentation with Bio-A((R)) mesh for laparoscopic repair of hiatal hernia: single-institution experience with 100 consecutive patients. Hernia. 2017;21(4):623–8. https://doi.org/10.1007/s10029-017-1603-1.
14. Crespin OM, Yates RB, Martin AV, Pellegrini CA, Oelschlager BK. The use of crural relaxing incisions with biologic mesh reinforcement during laparoscopic repair of complex hiatal hernias. Surg Endosc. 2016;30(6):2179–85. https://doi.org/10.1007/s00464-015-4522-1.
15. Memon MA, Memon B, Yunus RM, Khan S. Suture cruroplasty versus prosthetic hiatal herniorrhaphy for large hiatal hernia: a meta-analysis and systematic review of randomized controlled trials. Ann Surg. 2016;263(2):258–66. https://doi.org/10.1097/SLA.0000000000001267.
16. Tam V, Winger DG, Nason KS. A systematic review and meta-analysis of mesh vs suture cruroplasty in laparoscopic large hiatal hernia repair. Am J Surg. 2016;211(1):226–38. https://doi.org/10.1016/j.amjsurg.2015.07.007.
17. Park Y, Aye RW, Watkins JR, Farivar AS, Louie BE. Laparoscopic hill repair: 25-year follow-up. Surg Endosc. 2018;32(10):4111–5. https://doi.org/10.1007/s00464-018-6150-z.
18. Kercher KWMB, Ponsky JL, Goldstein SL, Yavorski RT, Sing RF, Heniford BT. Minimally invasive management of paraesophageal herniation in the high-risk surgical patient. Am J Surg. 2001;182(5):510–4.
19. Oelschlager BK, Yamamoto K, Woltman T, Pellegrini C. Vagotomy during hiatal hernia repair: a benign esophageal lengthening procedure. J Gastrointest Surg. 2008;12(7):1155. https://doi.org/10.1007/s11605-008-0520-0.
20. Lidor AO, Steele KE, Stem M, Fleming RM, Schweitzer MA, Marohn MR. Long-term quality of life and risk factors for recurrence after laparoscopic repair of paraesophageal hernia. JAMA Surg. 2015;150(5):424–31. https://doi.org/10.1001/jamasurg.2015.25.
21. Rathore MA, Andrabi SI, Bhatti MI, Najfi SM, McMurray A. Metaanalysis of recurrence after laparoscopic repair of paraesophageal hernia. JSLS. 2007;11(4):456–60.
22. Brenkman HJ, Parry K, van Hillegersberg R, Ruurda JP. Robot-assisted laparoscopic hiatal hernia repair: promising anatomical and functional results. J Laparoendosc Adv Surg Tech A. 2016;26(6):465–9. https://doi.org/10.1089/lap.2016.0065.
23. Wirsching A, El Lakis MA, Mohiuddin K, Pozzi A, Hubka M, Low DE. Acute vs. elective paraesophageal hernia repair: endoscopic gastric decompression allows semi-elective surgery in a majority of acute patients. J Gastrointest Surg. 2018;22(2):194–202. https://doi.org/10.1007/s11605-017-3495-x.
24. Higgins RM, Frelich MJ, Bosler ME, Gould JC. Cost analysis of robotic versus laparoscopic general surgery procedures. Surg Endosc. 2017;31(1):185–92. https://doi.org/10.1007/s00464-016-4954-2.

Magnetic Sphincter Augmentation for Management of Gastroesophageal Reflux Disease

31

Mark G. Hausmann and Karl A. LeBlanc

31.1 Introduction

Gastroesophageal reflux disease (GERD) occurs when gastric contents flow retrograde from the stomach to the esophagus. The most common anatomic issue that can allow this to occur is diminished function of the lower esophageal sphincter. Medical therapies reduce the acidity of the refluxate, but do not address the mechanism of the reflux. Antireflux surgeries are intended to recreate the anatomic valve-like barrier that prevents reflux at the gastroesophageal (GE) junction.

The surgical management of GERD has had many modifications over the years. Rudolph Nissen performed the first fundoplication in 1955. Multiple other iterations of the fundoplication have evolved over the years including procedures such as the Belsey Mark IV (1952), Collis gastroplasty (1957), the Dor (1962), Toupet (1963), and Hill (1967) fundoplications among the more better-known modifications [1]. During this path of operative innovations, the Angelchik device (introduced in 1979) was developed. This was a C-shaped ring of silicon that was placed around the gastroesophageal junction. While its introduction was seen as a significant advance, it soon fell out of favor due to complications of dysphagia, migration and erosion. Through these years of development of these methods, the surgical approach to GERD management and hiatal hernia repair has been modified from laparotomy or thoracotomy to laparoscopy, and now most recently to robotic approaches (Table 31.1)

Magnetic sphincter augmentation (LINX®, Torax Medical, Inc., Shoreview, MN) has been shown to be an effective alternative to fundoplication, with a favorable side effect profile. This device is composed of a ring of individually interconnected

M. G. Hausmann (✉) · K. A. LeBlanc
Our Lady of the Lake Physician Group, Baton Rouge, LA, USA
e-mail: mark.hausmann@fmolhs.org

K. A. LeBlanc (ed.), *Robotic Assisted Hernia Repair*,
https://doi.org/10.1007/978-3-030-23025-8_31

Table 31.1 Chronology of hiatal hernia surgery

Year	Surgical approach/proponent
1919	Transabdominal repair/Soresi
1950	Transthoracic repair/Sweet
1951	Association of incompetent LES and reflux esophagitis (crural sling)/Allison
1952	Transthoracic approach for extensive esophageal mobilization/Belsey (Mark IV)
1954	Importance of the restoration of the cardiophrenic angle/Barrett
1955	Transabdominal approach to restore the angle (full wrap)/Nissen
1962	Partial anterior wrap/Dor
1963	Partial posterior wrap/Toupet
1965	Gastric patch for esophageal stricture/Thal
1967	Anchoring of phrenoesophageal bundles to median arcuate ligament/Hill
1977	"Floppy" Nissen and division of short gastric vessels/Donahue
1986	Two cm wrap to reduce bloat and dysphagia/Johnson and DeMeester
2008	Initial animal implantations of LINX® device
2012	FDA approval of the LINX® device

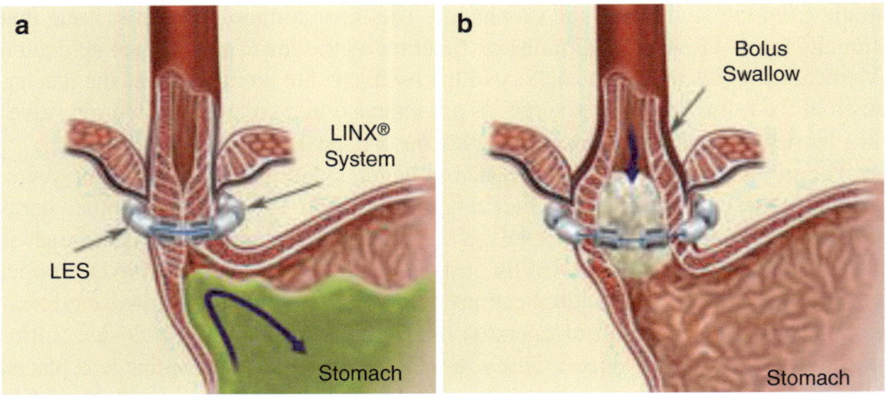

Fig. 31.1 (**a**) Prevention of acid reflux with closed LINX® device in place. (**b**) Opening of the LINX® device to allow food bolus to pass

titanium beads with magnetic cores that augment the lower esophageal sphincter without disruption of the normal gastric anatomy. These beads will separate upon the passage of a food bolus thereby allowing the introduction of food into the stomach (Figs. 31.1 and 31.2) [2].

Initial animal studies were completed in 2008 [3], followed by human feasibility studies [4], which led to FDA approval in March 2012. The magnetic sphincter augmentation was initially described via a laparoscopic approach with minimal dissection for small hiatal hernias, leaving the phrenoesophageal membrane intact. This significantly limited the introduction of this technology but with further experience the technique has evolved to include larger hiatal hernias along with full dissection of the hiatus. While the initial introduction of the LINX® was with the

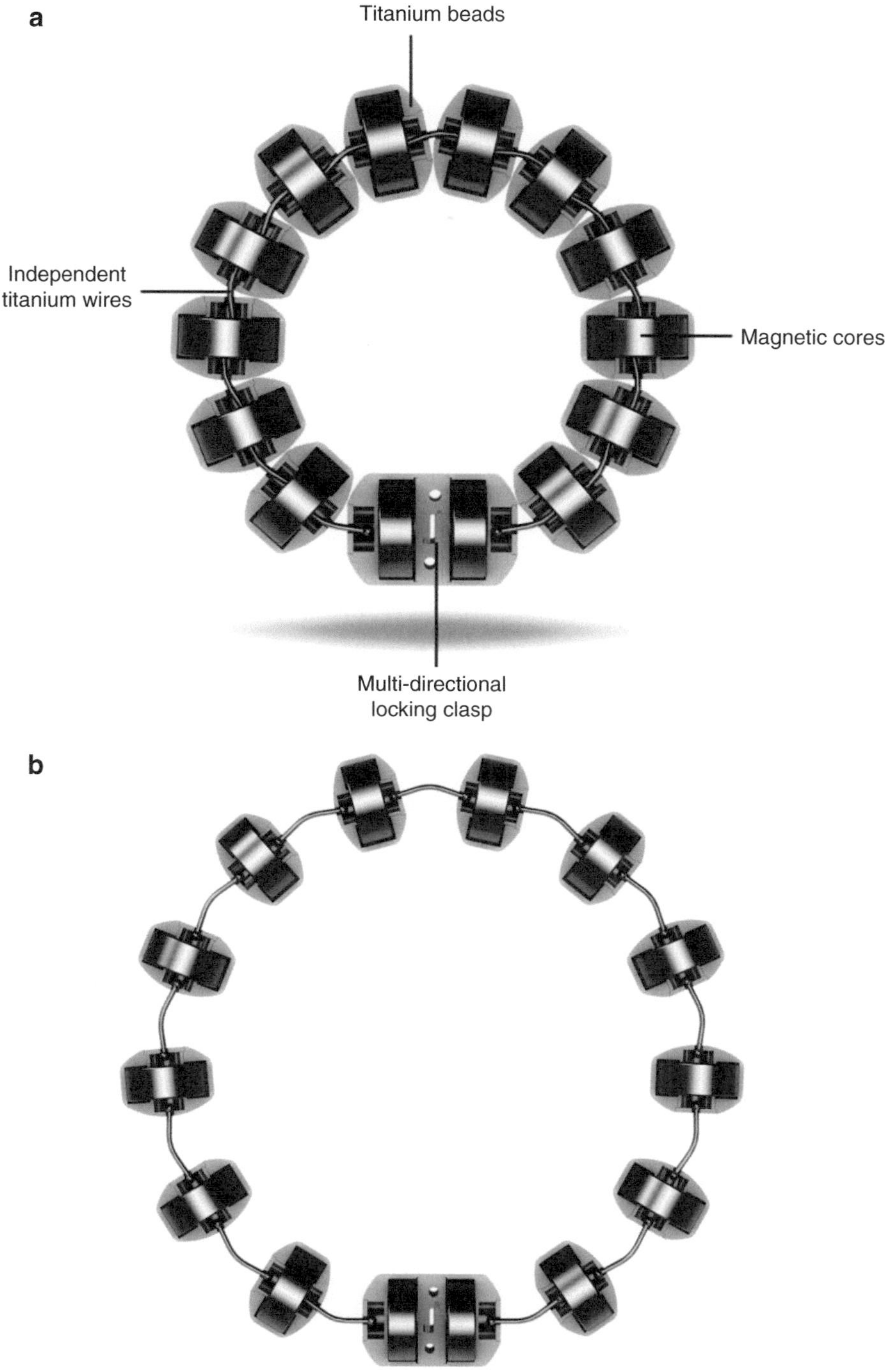

Fig. 31.2 (**a**) Cutaway image of LINX device closed—provided by J&J/Ethicon. (**b**) Cutaway image of LINX device open—provided by J&J/Ethicon

laparoscopic insertion, as the robot technology has evolved and expanded, many surgeons have found benefit in the use of the robot for the performance of the hiatal dissection, closure of the hernia and insertion of the LINX® device.

One common concern that is noted is that the magnets within the LINX® device may preclude magnetic resonance imaging (MRI) studies. However, the current LINX® device is approved for magnetic resonance imaging (MRI) systems up to 1.5 T. As over 80% for MRI machines in the U.S. are 1.5 T or lower, this has not proven to be a significant issue [5]. The potential effect of the use of one of the other MRI machines is the de-magnetization of the magnets of the LINX® device. This would render the device ineffective thereby allowing the recurrence of GERD. If needed, the LINX® could be removed and replaced. This is a very rare occurrence to date.

31.2 Surgical Indications

Surgical management of GERD should be considered in individuals that have inadequate or incomplete symptom control with medical management or those with complications of GERD (Table 31.2). The indications for the LINX® device are no different than the traditional surgical treatment of GERD.

The initial trials using the LINX® Reflux Management System included patients with heartburn, abnormal esophageal acid exposure, and normal esophageal peristalsis. Anatomic exclusion criteria included a hiatal hernia size ≥3 cm (as determined by endoscopy), Los Angeles grade B, C or D erosive esophagitis (Table 31.3), and body mass index >35 [6] so as to limit treatment and patient variability and by exclusion of reflux patients with complicated reflux disease [7–9].

Table 31.2 Surgical indications of GERD

Inadequate symptom control with medical management
Regurgitation
Nocturnal recumbent reflux and/or aspiration
Atypical symptoms (chest pain, sore throat, hoarseness, dental decay)
Patient desire to eliminate medical therapy
Barrett's esophagus/dysplastic mucosal changes
Cameron's ulcerations
Esophageal stricture

Table 31.3 Los Angeles classification

Grade	Mucosal breaks
A	One or more <5 mm in maximal length
B	One or more >5 mm in maximal length without continuity across mucosal folds
C	Continuous between >2 mucosal folds involving <75% of the esophageal circumference
D	Involves >75% of the esophageal circumference

Rona et al., studied hiatal hernia repair in conjunction with magnetic sphincter augmentation in patients with more advanced reflux disease including hiatal hernia as large as 7 cm. They found the frequency of improvement or resolution of symptoms as well as the percentage of patients requiring intervention for dysphagia was similar to patients with less complex reflux disease and smaller hernias [10]. Buckley et al. studied 200 patients with hiatal hernias greater than 3 cm and demonstrated similar results as those reported from studies of hiatal hernias ≤3 cm [11]. Research such as these have resulted in the expansion of the use of the LINX® beyond the limited indications when this device was initially introduced.

There are reports regarding the use of LINX® in patients as an option for patients who have severe reflux symptoms following sleeve gastrectomy surgery and with reflux following Roux-en-Y gastric bypass [12, 13]. The results from these studies as well as ample anecdotal experience has provided patients with these difficult situations and limited options with a new surgical option. This is especially beneficial when these individuals have failed medical therapy. While most studies describe magnetic sphincter augmentation via a laparoscopic approach, many surgeons using robotic technology for the hiatal dissection are very likely to place the LINX® device robotically as well. It is anticipated that the results utilizing robotic methods will be published in the near future.

31.3 Preoperative Evaluation

The evaluation of the foregut is paramount in the surgical treatment of GERD. This requires both radiologic and functional testing. The initial evaluation includes radiographic contrast evaluation of the esophageal and upper gastrointestinal tract. While necessary, these tests do not provide the mucosal evaluation of these tissues that upper GI endoscopy provides. It is preferred, when feasible, that the operating surgeon performs the endoscopic evaluation to better appreciate the anatomy that is to be treated. Additional functional tests will be needed and will depend upon the experience and requirements of the surgeon and may include esophageal manometry, the Bravo™ (Medtronic, Minneapolis, MN) pH study or the impedance pH probe study. Nuclear medicine gastric emptying evaluation may be considered in selected patients (i.e. when this issue may be the source of reflux). It should be assumed that these studies are complementary rather than exclusive [14]. Especially for the consideration of the LINX® device, more information rather than less is preferred.

The esophagram provides a radiographic assessment of the foregut anatomy. Videoesophagography provides a radiographic image of the foregut and some surgeons have applied a modification to assess motility radiographically. This protocol assesses the food bolus transit with the patient prone in 15° Trendelenburg position. Adequate esophageal clearance is considered to be the allowance of passage of the food bolus within 2 esophageal peristaltic strips [15]. This evaluation may not be familiar to many radiologists but in our practice, this has proven to be a viable option to those patients that are unable or unwilling to undergo the traditional functional studies.

Due to the innate function of the LINX® device, esophageal motility is one of the most important considerations in the selection of this option in these patients. Magnetic sphincter augmentation can be considered in hiatal hernia and reflux patients with adequate motility. While all of the important considerations of esophageal motility are beyond the scope of this chapter, the general parameters regarding esophageal motility (in which this device can be an option) would require a distal esophageal amplitude of ≥35 mmHg, distal contractile integral ≥500 by Chicago classification, and ≥70% peristaltic propagation. This can be evaluated effectively by high resolution manometry [16, 17].

Physiologic confirmation of acid reflux may be obtained via a Bravo™ pH study. There is a plethora of patients that exhibit a varied presentation of acid reflux complaints. Many of these have some other source of symptomology and not reflux. It is critical to differentiate these individuals to ascertain the best course of clinical treatment. If nonacid reflux is a consideration, impedance pH may be the test of choice. This method of study is quite important but must be critically interpreted to determine the results [18].

If there is suspicion of delayed gastric emptying, (excessive nausea, vomiting or bloating) the addition of a nuclear medicine gastric emptying study should be considered. As is well known, this entity can cause GERD symptoms and the anti-reflux procedures will not alleviate these problems and, in fact, could make them worse.

31.4 Surgical Technique

The procedure is performed under general anesthesia, with the patient in the supine position. The initial entry in the abdomen is via an 8 mm robotic trocar with transparent obturator superior to the umbilicus, about 15 cm below the xyphoid, just to the left of midline (2–3 cm) so that the camera trocar is to the left of the falciform ligament. Another form of entry is the use of a 5 mm laparoscopic optical trocar at this location. If this is selected, this trocar will be exchanged for an 8 mm robotic trocar after insertion of additional trocars. After laparoscopic exploration of the abdomen, the patient is then placed in 10–20° of reverse Trendelenburg position. This will vary slightly based upon the habitus of the patient. The technique described below is for the Da Vinci Xi system by Intuitive Surgical but can be modified for other systems such as the Da Vinci Si or X platform. The pneumoperitoneum is established at a pressure of 15 mmHg. Two additional robotic ports are then placed parallel to the camera port in the left anterior axillary line just above the reflection of the left colon (arm 4). The next port (arm 3) is placed midway between trocars 2 and 4 in order to maximize the robotic arm position which results in a location approximately in the left mid-clavicular line. Because the fourth port on the right side of the abdomen (arm 1) will be used to measure the circumference of the esophagus at the lower esophageal sphincter, it is placed higher than the initial 3 trocars (Fig. 31.3). It is positioned in the mid-clavicular line or more lateral just below the costal margin. This location is necessitated so that the approach to the GE junction of the esophagus by the LINX® sizing device is perpendicular to the that anatomy.

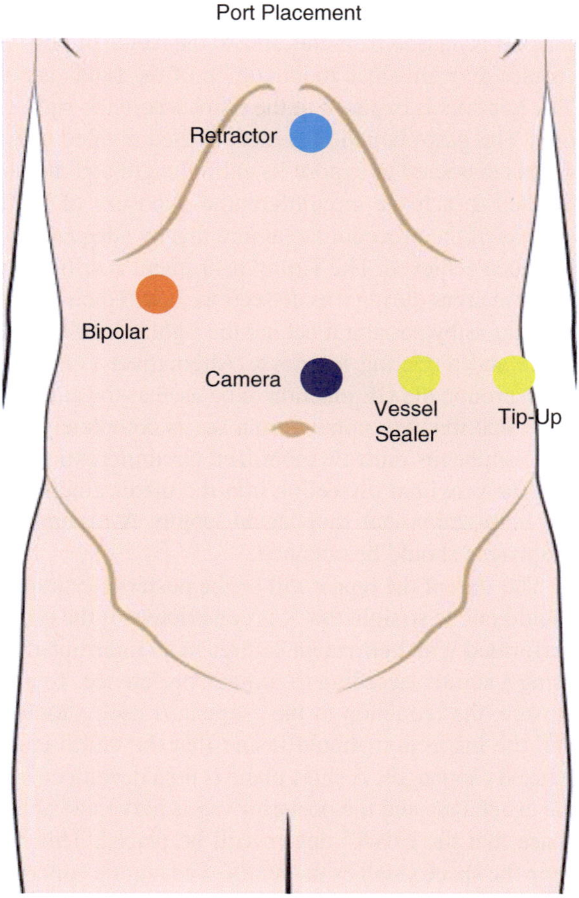

Fig. 31.3 Port placement

Alternatively, this robotic port can be placed in line with the initial 3 ports and an accessory port can be positioned in the immediate subcostal position and used as access for the measurement of the lower esophageal sphincter circumference.

We prefer to use the Nathanson liver retractor that is placed in the subxiphoid region to retract the left lobe of the liver anteriorly to expose the hiatus. It is preferred to place the Nathanson at this point so that the liver position is established prior to introduction of the right sided trocar through which sizing of the esophagus will take place. The smallest sized Nathanson retractor that accommodates the left lobe is preferred, so as to limit the profile and avoid interference with the robotic arms.

A Fenestrated Bipolar Grasper is placed in arm 1, the Vessel Sealer or the newer Vessel Sealer Extend in arm 3 and Tip-up Fenestrated Grasper in arm 4. Some surgeons may prefer to use the Harmonic ACE® Curved Shears in arm 3, but the benefit of articulation of the Vessel Sealer is sacrificed.

The dissection is initiated at the superior pole of the spleen whereupon the peritoneum is incised from this area to the Angle of His. The short gastric vessels do not require division since mobilization of the funds is not required for fundoplication. The left crus is exposed to the point where the right crus can be visualized posteriorly. The gastrohepatic ligament is then divided exposing the right crus. The right crus is dissected to expose its entire length and the phrenoesophageal membrane is divided to achieve circumferential exposure of the hiatus. These are the critical aspects of the procedure to assure that an adequate mobilization of the GE junction has been achieved. The Tip-up instrument is critical to provide the needed exposure of these areas during this dissection. It will then be used to provide retraction of the esophagus by passing it behind the right side of the GE junction, flexing it at a right angle and retracting inferiorly. Alternatively, one might prefer to place a Penrose drain around the GE junction to be used as the aid for retraction of the esophagus. It is critical that any noted hernia sac is completely reduced from the mediastinum. The esophagus must be mobilized circumferentially to the extent needed to assure that the proximal dissection into the mediastinum allows for maximal increase of the intra-abdominal esophageal length. A minimum of 2 cm of intra-abdominal esophagus should be obtained.

The start of the repair will be the posterior cruraplasty. The crural approximation should not be so tight that it is constrictive of the esophagus. The cruraplasty can be performed with permanent sutures in an interrupted fashion or in a running fashion using a suture according to surgeon preference. To assess the adequacy of the crural closure, the retraction of the esophagus itself should be relaxed. After this maneuver, the inspection should insure that the crural closure is not constrictive on the relaxed esophagus. A short plane is then developed between the posterior surface of the esophagus and the posterior vagus nerve just above the GE junction. This is the space that the LINX® device will be placed. This dissection should be limited to keep the space small as the retained adventitia superiorly and inferiorly are intended to limit the migration of the device until it is encapsulated by scar tissue. A silicone-based Penrose drain can be placed to maintain this tunnel location for the measurement of the esophageal circumference and the placement of the LINX® device. The circumference of the esophagus is measured at this site from the right subcostal trocar (arm 1). The LINX® sizing device has a stiff shaft with the actual sizing mechanism at the end consisting of a flexible tube with a magnet on its end. The flexible portion is passed around the circumference of the GE junction and will connect with another magnet on the end of the sizing instrument shaft. The sizing device should be tightened until the tubing is close to the esophageal circumference, but not constrictive in any fashion (Fig. 31.4). The measurement on the sizing device coincides with the numbers on the proximal portion of the shaft which correlate with the number of beads of the LINX® device (from 13 beads to 17 beads) to be selected. We recommend that this sizing should be done in at least triplicate fashion to assure appropriate selection. The sizer should be tightened slowly as it is manipulated to assess the space between it and the esophagus and the ability to move it around the esophagus. As it is tightened, it will be appreciated that its movement becomes restricted and ultimately, the magnets of the sizing device will separate.

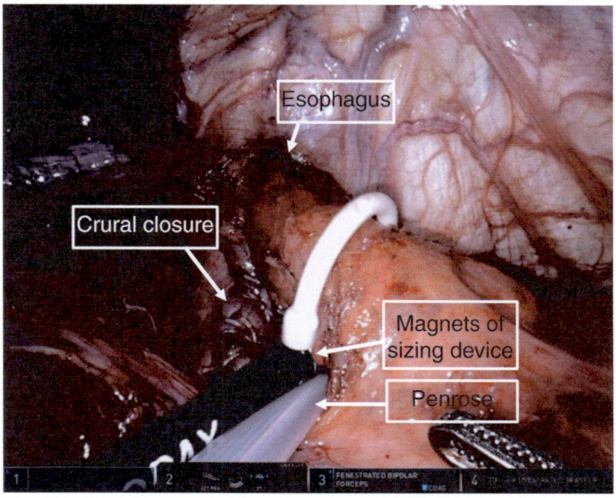

Fig. 31.4 Sizing the LINX device

The appropriately sized device should allow movement of the sizer. This will differ from patient to patient and represents the most critical portion of the procedure. This cannot be overstated. If it is too large, reflux will be poorly controlled; if too tight, dysphagia can result. If any question, we recommend to "size up" the selected device. In other words, if needed one should select one size larger than that noted by the sizing device if the exact size to be selected is not perfectly assured.

The LINX® device is introduced through the 8 mm metal robotic trocar to the right of the patient, the robotic arm should be undocked, and the cap removed from the trocar. The magnetic beads will adhere to the proximal well of the metal trocar, so the beads must be directed into the cannula portion of the trocar. The cap can then be replaced and the LINX® pushed down the cannula with a 5 mm laparoscopic instrument. (If introducing through an accessory laparoscopic port, the LINX® device requires an 8mm Medtronic (Minneapolis, MN) or Ethicon (Sommerville, NJ) trocar, but will fit down a 5 mm trocar by Applied Medical (Rancho San Margarita, CA)

The appropriately sized LINX® device is then passed through the tunnel between the Penrose and the esophagus and buckled (Fig. 31.5a, b). Using an instrument via the right subcostal trocar (arm 1) the path over the Penrose drain (and posterior to the esophagus) is followed and one of the sutures at the end of the LINX® device is grasped and pulled gently through the tunnel, stopping when 2 beads are visible on the right side of the esophagus. This will allow the buckling to occur on the right anterolateral aspect of the esophagus. If the beads are pulled too far through the tunnel, the beads making up the clasp will be positioned on the left side of the esophagus, making visualization more difficult. When buckling the clasp, hold the suture of one of the clasping beads still and bring the other clasping bead near and allow them to mate magnetically. In order to seat the clasp, the sutures should be pulled perpendicular to the orientation of the beads and 180° from each other. Then the clasping beads are finessed until the clasp is buckled securely. Full engagement of

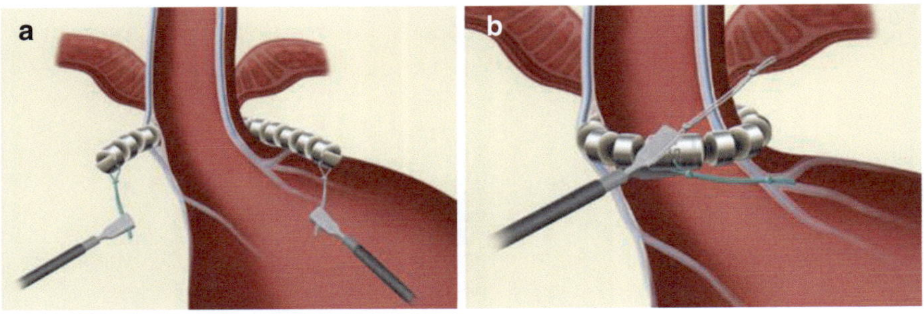

Fig. 31.5 (**a**) LINX placed at GE junction. (**b**) LINX ends fully engaged

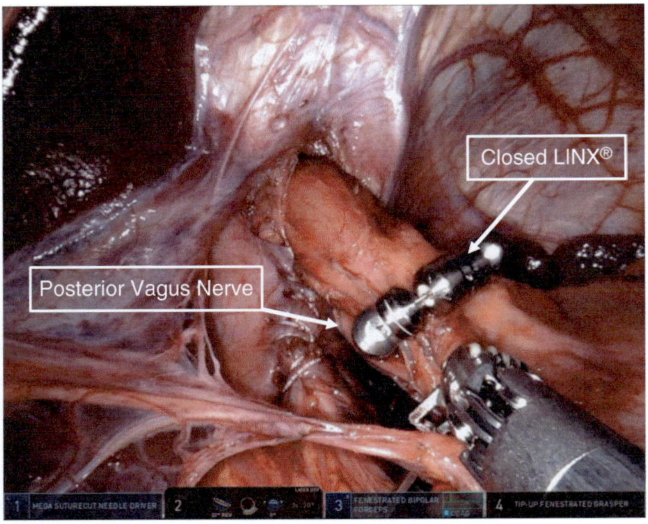

Fig. 31.6 LINX® at completion of procedure

the clasp is indicated by the presence of a single window in the clasp. Security of the clasp can be confirmed by gently pulling the clasp sutures opposite each other, perpendicular to the LINX®. The clasp should not separate easily. The positioning sutures are then excised. There is a bit of a challenge in learning the best method to link the ends of the device. As these are magnets, the device will attach itself to the instruments used in the operation. With experience, this is easily overcome. The robot does offer an advantage to achieving the connection of the ends of the device (Fig. 31.6).

If there is a need to add some type of reinforcement to the crural closure such as with a mesh material we prefer to place this material prior to the sizing and placement of the LINX® device. The manipulation of the mesh will be hampered due to the magnetic attraction of the device to the surgical instruments. One can either glue or suture the mesh in place. After this has been completed, the method to place the LINX® will then be performed.

Table 31.4 Postoperative diet

First 24 h—soft food
After 24 h—regular diet
Continuous—small bit of soft or solid food every 2–3 h between meals for 6–8 weeks

After all of the above has been completed, the Nathanson retractor is removed. The robotic instruments are removed, and the robot is undocked. Generally, we elect to close the skin incisions with absorbable sutures. For the most part, these procedures are performed as an "outpatient" and the patients are thus sent home shortly after surgery.

31.5 Postoperative Care

Patients are instructed to eat a bit of soft or solid food every two hours for the initial six weeks following the procedure in order to regularly activate the device and avoid contracture of the scar tissue around the device (Table 31.4). We refer to this activity as "physical therapy" for the magnets and to prevent scarring that will inhibit or restrict the movement of the magnets. Patients comprehend this analogy fairly well.

As this is a foreign body, the magnetic ring will become encapsulated with scar tissue postoperatively. This scarring process will cause most patients to experience dysphagia at approximately 2–4 weeks following the procedure. Dysphagia is expected and peaks 2–4 weeks postoperatively. If dysphagia is severe, to the point that small bites of soft or solid food is not tolerated, a course of steroids should be trialed to abate the inflammatory reaction. If a methylprednisolone dose pack is insufficient, a short course of higher dose steroid can be tried (i.e. 10 mg/kg for 5 days). If possible, dilation should be delayed as much as 3 months postoperatively. If necessary, balloon dilation should be performed under fluoroscopy using contrast in the balloon so as to allow visualization of the filling of the balloon. The goal is the separation of one third of the magnets of the device to assure adequate enlargement of the opening of the device. It is not necessary that all bead spaces separate.

If all interventions fail, device removal should be considered as a last resort. The individual beads of the device do become encapsulated. Removal requires identification of the device within the capsule followed by dissection of each bead from its encapsulation. The LINX® beads are individually interconnected and are not threaded onto a single wire; therefore, only one of the inter-bead wires needs to be divided. The beads will not "spill" off of the wire. The need to remove the device is very uncommon.

31.6 Outcomes

Magnetic sphincter augmentation appears to be a safe and effective intervention for the management of hiatal hernia and reflux. Available 5-year data have shown a 90% patient satisfaction with symptom resolution. There is also a significant reduction in the GERD-Heath Related Quality of Life score and normalization of esophageal pH exposure occurred in 70%. Compete discontinuation of PPIs was obtained in 87.8% [19]. The most common side effect is dysphagia, which can occur in as many as 70% in the early postoperative period, but only 10% report dysphagia at 1 year. Endoscopic dilation is required in 6–12% of patients. Explanation has been required for 3–6% of patients. Erosion is a rare event occurring in 0.1% of patients. Erosion can be treated with device removal without significant long-term sequelae. There have been no reports of either migration of the device or device related mortality [20].

Studies comparing laparoscopic fundoplication with magnetic sphincter augmentation suggest that GERD control is similar, but there is reduced side effect profile with the magnetic augmentation of the sphincter with documentation of a lower incidence of gas bloat and flatulence with maintenance of the ability to belch [21].

31.7 Conclusion

The use of magnetic sphincter augmentation in the treatment of GERD has added an alternative to the management of this disease process. The use of the robot appears to offer improved ergonomics to the operation and allows improved movement of the linking of the device. Longer term outcomes in the future will allow the surgeon do select the best method of surgical intervention for the patients with GERD.

References

1. Stylopoulos N, Rattner DW. The history of hiatal hernia surgery: from Bowditch to laparoscopy. Ann Surg. 2005;241(1):185–93.
2. Torax Medical. The LINX Reflux management system: stop reflux at its source. 2018. Available at http://www.toraxmedical.com/linx/. Accessed 22 Dec 2018.
3. Ganz RA, Gostout CJ, Grudem J, Swanson W, Berg T, DeMeester TR. Use of a magnetic sphincter for the treatment of GERD: a feasibility study. Gastrointest Endosc. 2008;67(2):287–94.
4. Bonavina L, Saino GI, Bona D, Lipham J, Ganz RA, Dunn D, DeMeester T. Magnetic augmentation of the lower esophageal sphincter: results of a feasibility clinical trial. J Gastrointest Surg. 2008;12(12):2133–40.
5. LINX. Diagnostic imaging with LINX. 2018. Available at http://www.linxforlife.com/mri-info. Accessed 22 Dec 2018.
6. Lipham JC, DeMeester TR, Ganz RA, Bonavina L, Saint G, Dunn DH, Fockens P, Bemelman W. The LINX® reflux management system: confirmed safety and efficacy now at 4 years. Surg Endosc. 2012;26:2944–9.
7. Armstrong D, Bennett JR, Blum AL, Dent J, De Dombal FT, Galmiche JP, Lundell L, Margulies M, Richter JE, Spechler SJ, Tytgat GN, Wallin L. The endoscopic assessment of esophagitis: a progress report on observer agreement. Gastroenterology. 1996;111:85–92.
8. Lundell LR, Dent J, Bennett JR, et al. Endoscopic assessment of oesophagitis: clinical and functional correlates and further validation of the Los Angeles classification. Gut. 1999;45:172–80.
9. Kasyap AK, Sah SK, Chaudhary S. Clinical spectrum and risk factors associated with asymptomatic erosive esophagitis as determined by Los Angeles classification: a cross-sectional study. PLoS ONE. 2018;13(2):e0192739. https://doi.org/10.1371/journal.pone.0192739.

10. Rona KA, Reynolds J, Schwameis K, Zehetner J, Samakar K, Oh P, Vong D, Sandhu K, Datkhouda N, Bildzudewicz N, Lipham JC. Efficacy of magnetic sphincter augmentation in patients with large hiatal hernias. Surg Endosc. 2017;31:2096–102.
11. Buckley FP, Bell RCW, Freeman K, Doggett S, Heidrick R. Favorable results from a prospective evaluation of 200 patients with large hiatal hernias undergoing LINX magnetic sphincter augmentation. Surg Endosc. 2018;32(4):1762–8.
12. Munoz-Largacha JA, Hess DT, Litle VR, Fernando HC. Lower esophgeal sphincter augmentation for persistent reflux after roux-en-y gastric bypass. Obes Surg. 2016;26:464–6.
13. Crawford C, Gibbens K, Lomelin D, Krause C, Simorov A, Oleynikov D. Sleeve gastrostomy and anti-reflux procedures. Surg Endosc. 2017;31:1012–21.
14. Hewson EG, Ott DJ, Dalton CB, Chen YM, Wu WC, Richter JE. Manometry and radiology. Complementary studies in the assessment of esophageal motility disorders. Gastroenterology. 1990;98(3):626–32.
15. D'Alessio MJ, Rakita S, Bloomston M, Chambers CM, Zervos EE, Goldin SB, Poklepovic J, Boyce HW, Rosemurgy AS. Esophagography predicts favorable outcomes after laparoscopic Nissen fundoplication for patients with esophageal. Dysmotility. 2005;201:3335–42.
16. Bredenoord AJ, Fox M, Kahrilas PJ, Pandolfino JE, Schwizer W, Smout AJ. Chicago classification criteria of esophageal motility disorders defined in high resolution esophageal pressure topography. Neurogastroenterol Motil. 2012;24(Suppl 1):57–65.
17. Rohof WOA, Bredenoord AJ. Chicago classification of esophageal motility disorders: lessons learned. Curr Gastroenterol Rep. 2017;19:37.
18. Namasivayam V, Murray JA. Discounting the duration of bolus exposure in impedance testing underestimates acid reflux. BMC Gastroenterol. 2016;16:60. https://doi.org/10.1186/s12876-016-0471-y.
19. Saino G, Bonavina L, Lipham JC, Dunn D, Ganz RA. Magnetic sphincter augmentation for gastroesophageal reflux at 5 years: final results of a pilot study show long-term acid reduction and symptom improvement. J Laparoendosc Adv Surg Tech A. 2015;25(10):787–92.
20. Telem DA, Wright AS, Shah PC, Hytter MM. SAGES technology and value assessment committee (TAVAC) safety and effectiveness analysis: LINX® reflux management system. Surg Endosc. 2017;31:3811–26.
21. Louie BE, Farivar AS, Shultz D, Brennan C, Vallieres E, Aye RW. Short-term outcomes using magnetic sphincter augmentation versus Nissen fundoplication for medically resistant gastroesophageal reflux disease. Ann Thorac Surg. 2014;98(2):498–504.

Adverse Events in Robotic Assisted Hiatal Hernia Repair

32

Alexander C. Mertens and Ivo A. M. J. Broeders

32.1 Adverse Events in Hiatal Hernia Repair

Surgery for benign conditions, such as hiatal hernias, should have a low complication risk since in the vast majority of cases the goal of the procedure relates to quality of life while the health risk of conservative treatment is limited.

Antireflux surgery and procedures for hiatal hernia have been associated with high risk of morbidity and mortality and moderate subjective outcomes. The majority of information still leans on the evidence from the era of open surgery where these types of procedures where performed by many general surgeons, usually in low volume. Currently, laparotomy has been replaced by minimally invasive surgery and postoperative care has improved drastically. Surgeons have become aware of the importance of excellent knowledge of hiatal anatomy and the essential concepts of hiatal closure and anti-reflux procedures. An increase in referrals seems to parallel the concentration of surgical care. Nonetheless, surgery for large hiatal hernias and reoperative procedures can be very challenging making the awareness of potential risks essential.

In this chapter we will describe the possible adverse events in hiatal hernia surgery. We will try to explore why these events occur and the possible treatment options for when they do. We will divide this chapter in intraoperative, postoperative/in-hospital and late adverse events.

A. C. Mertens · Ivo A. M. J. Broeders (✉)
Department of Surgery, Meander Medical Centre Amersfoort, Amersfoort, The Netherlands

Robotics and Mechatronics, University of Twente, Enschede, The Netherlands
e-mail: iamj.broeders@meandermc.nl

K. A. LeBlanc (ed.), *Robotic Assisted Hernia Repair*,
https://doi.org/10.1007/978-3-030-23025-8_32

32.2 Intraoperative Adverse Events in Hiatal Hernia Surgery

Intraoperative complications may relate to bleeding, organ perforation and damage to vagal nerves or intrathoracic structures. We will not discuss the complications related to pneumoperitoneum as these have to be considered in any laparoscopic and robot assisted procedure.

32.3 Bleeding

The most common bleeding in laparotomy is caused by traction on the spleno-gastric ligament, resulting in splenic capsule tears or bleeding from the short gastric vessels. Splenectomy in hiatal hernia repair was not uncommon in the past and contributed to the unfavourable reputation to of these procedures. Today, the open approach to hiatal hernia surgery and fundoplication is outdated and should be strongly discouraged. Splenectomy has become rare due to the growing experience with laparoscopic techniques and the available equipment.

In the case of 270° and 360° fundoplication, avoidance of traction on the gastric fundus prevents injury to the short gastric vessels. It is most advisable to use a "high-tech" sealing and cutting device, such as an ultrasonic dissector, advanced bipolar sealing device or the robotic vessel sealer. In the case of bleeding originating from the short gastric vessels, damage can be controlled with these devices. A suction device should be on the table, or at the very least be quickly accessible at all times. Bleeding from small splenic capsule tears should be treated by gauze compression; these gauzes should be left for several minutes to allow for natural clotting to occur. If there is persistent bleeding, a resorbable gauze of surgeon preference can be applied on the splenic surface and left in situ.

Bothersome hemorrhage may also arise during dissection of the hernia sac and esophagus. Surgery usually starts with the incision of the gastro-hepatic ligament. This ligament often harbours a large aberrant artery supplying the left lobe of the liver. If possible, this artery should be spared, but this may be troublesome in big hiatal hernias. Alternatively, it can be ligated, but advanced sealing or clips such as Hem-o-lock® (Weck® Morrisville, NC) should be used in all instances to avoid serious bleeding. In large hiatal hernias special care is required for the left gastric artery or vein as these may project onto the operation field due to migration of the stomach towards the mediastinum.

Usually, the vena cava is out of the way, but one should always check its position before dissection or suturing of the crus. It can easily be visualized by lifting the caudate lobe of the liver. The vena cava can get close to the hiatal hernia in reoperative surgery due to scarring, and/or due to the need to apply traction on the hiatal pillars when approximating the crus. In the case of a small puncture, bleeding may be limited. Quick and careful suturing with a permanent polypropylene suture is possible. While preparing for suturing, a gauze should be applied at the site of injury to prepare for repair and avoid the occurrence of a massive pulmonary embolism with the insufflated CO_2. Surgeons attempting vena cava repair should possess excellent laparoscopic suturing skills.

In case of large tears and massive bleeding, immediate gauze compression should be applied. This is usually sufficient for controlling the bleeding due to the low pressure in the venous system. The patient can then be prepared for laparotomy and surgical support by a vascular surgeon can be arranged.

Other vascular structures that require awareness are the left and right diaphragmatic arteries and the inferior phrenic vein, which are always visible approximately one centimeter above the upper margin of the hiatal opening. Phrenic arteries can be damaged during dissection of the gastro-phrenic ligament or during crural reapproximation. Control is gained by sealing, or simply with tying the approximating sutures in hiatal repair.

In esophageal dissection, one may encounter small aorto-esophageal branches. Cutdown by sealing or diathermy is advised, while maintaining a safe distance from the esophagus and vagal nerve branches. If there is hemorrhage, a no touch approach or gauze compression is advisable to avoid thermal damage to essential structures. This type of bleeding is usually low volume and self-limited.

Special attention is required for the aorta when suturing the diaphragmatic crus. Especially in large type 3 and 4 hiatal hernias, the left crus can be stretched over the distal end of the thoracic aorta. The first two to three sutures below the esophagus should be positioned with great care and subtle needle handling to avoid puncturing of the aorta. One may lift the left crus or push it to the patients left with the left-hand needle driver to create space between the limb and the aorta. In case of injury to the aorta with subsequent bleeding, the surgeon should carefully remove the needle by pulling on the suture and maintain direct compression of the crus on the aorta with a needle driver followed by gauze compression. Puncture holes will stop bleeding within minutes and a *just compress* approach is highly advisable. In case the aorta is punctured, do not continue suturing and knot tying, because the needle path through the aorta is unknown and knot tying may result in an aortic tear with consequent massive bleeding.

32.4 Organ Perforation

Perforation of the small intestine and large bowel should be avoided by utilizing correct laparoscopic techniques. In robot assisted surgery, special care is required when exchanging instruments because the intestine could potentially move into a position in front of the ends of the trocar, resulting in a risk of injury when exchanging instruments blindly. Likewise, great care should be taken when moving robotic instruments outside the field of view. Recognized intestinal perforations or serosal tears should be sutured immediately to avoid real or potential contamination with intestinal content.

Gastric perforation may result from excessive traction with robotic instruments. The exerted forces can be high and increase when the size of the instrument tip diminishes. This risk is enhanced due to the absence of haptic feedback. The bigger the hernia, the larger the risk. Extreme reverse Trendelenburg position is very helpful in repositioning the hernia contents, because gravity will assist the spontaneous repositioning of an intrathoracic stomach.

Serosal tears of the stomach surface or superficial muscular tears need no repair. Transmural or deep tears should be closed immediately to avoid unnecessary spillage of content. A barbed suture is very helpful in closing these lacerations. At the end of the procedure the sutured area should be inspected again because extensive manipulation of the stomach may cause suture line dehiscence.

Small or microscopic gastric perforations may also result from fundoplication "takedown" during reoperative surgery, especially when removing previously placed sutures. If this occurs, an effort should be made when possible to cover this dissected area with the newly created fundoplication to protect this vulnerable surface.

Esophageal perforation is one of the most disastrous complications. It should be avoided at all times by careful dissection of the esophagus. Excessive traction is undesirable and dissection of the hernia sac from the gastro-oesophageal junction should be avoided because the anatomy can be unclear, putting both the distal esophagus and vagal nerves at risk. One can simply leave the hernia sac in the abdomen attached to the gastro-esophageal junction after the hiatal hernia repair and fundoplication. Most of it will atrophy in due time.

Special care is needed for gastric and esophageal dissection in reoperative surgery. The exact anatomy may be difficult to ascertain during dissection and adhesions can be very dense; especially at the dorsal side of the esophagus and stomach. Prior use of mesh for crural reinforcement may greatly increase the difficulty of dissection. In the worst case scenario, the procedure should be aborted but this is an infrequent occurrence. Conversion to laparotomy can be considered when the surgeon believes that manual or hand assisted release of adhesions may result in a better outcome.

Any recognized esophageal perforation should be closed and covered with the gastric wall in the subsequent fundoplication. If this occurs, we recommend the performance of an esophageal contrast swallow X-ray or a CT scan with oral contrast that day or the next day to rule out any leakage of intestinal content.

32.5 Damage to Vagal Nerves and Intrathoracic Structures

The pleura usually needs to be dissected from the hernia sac in big hiatal hernias. This may result in pleural tears which are usually easily noticed. The pleurae are especially at risk in reoperative surgery, and damage may be unavoidable. The pulmonary parenchyma will hardly ever incur injury and one should not attempt to close pleural defects. The anesthesiologist should be asked to check end-expiratory pressure and induce a post expiration end pressure (PEEP) exceeding the intra-abdominal pressure induced by the CO_2 pneumoperitoneum if the pleural tear results in significant physiologic changes. The surgeon may lower CO_2 pressure, in combination with adequate muscle relaxation. PEEP should be maintained until the surgeon uses suction to remove as much CO_2 as possible when removing the trocars [1]. A clinically significant pneumothorax will rarely result, but a chest X-ray is advisable in the recovery room. A small-bore pleural drain may be introduced in the case of pulmonary collapse such as a tension pneumothorax, although this is rarely necessary.

Pericardial and pulmonary veins can be differentiated when removing the hernia sac and dissecting the esophagus to create sufficient intra-abdominal length. Damage can be avoided at all times with careful and mostly gentle blunt dissection. Hernia sac dissection should be performed initially at the outer surface of the sac. This will facilitate blunt dissection for effective extraction of the sac from the mediastinum and avoid damage to mediastinal structures while minimizing blood loss.

Pericardial or myocardial injury could result from hiatal closure in giant hernias or from gastropexy to the diaphragm [2–4]. One should be aware of this if the patient should develop a cardiac arrhythmia or a sudden drop in cardiac output. The pericardium may be opened through the hiatal opening, or through a small cutdown of the diaphragm adjacent to the pericardium. One should avoid the use of tackers for mesh fixation at all times in the vicinity of aorta, vena cava or pericardium. The surgeon should be aware of the position of these structures which are often (partly) covered by the diaphragm.

Vagal nerve injury with subsequent delayed gastric emptying is a feared complication of anti-reflux surgery and hiatal hernia repair. In primary surgery the anterior and posterior vagal nerves can generally be easily identified and spared. Damage to these nerves can lead to delayed gastric emptying, further aggravating the recovery of normal intake in patients undergoing a fundoplication with some patients experiencing a lack of improvement over time resulting in permanent intestinal difficulties. The reported incidence of accidental vagal nerve injury in the available literature is around 2%, although these numbers mainly describe the incidence in open surgery [5–7]. The actual percentage is potentially much higher.

Damage can be avoided by dissection of the esophagus at a distance from the crural opening, preferably with gentle blunt techniques. The use of energy devices should be limited to a safe distance from the esophagus. The posterior vagal nerve branch is especially at risk during dissection of the posterior portion of the hernia sac. We recommend lifting the vagal nerve together with the esophagus with an atraumatic instrument or with a flat soft drainage tube. The posterior vagal nerve branch is adjacent to the posterior surface of the esophagus but may be found at a further distance in the mediastinum in giant hernias during sac dissection. It sometimes curves toward the area of the dissection at the level of the gastro-esophageal junction. Rarely, it can have more than one branch, making these especially vulnerable to injury.

The anterior vagal nerve branch is at risk when opening the mediastinum at the anterior side of the esophagus, especially in reoperative surgery. It may also be damaged during dissection of the hernia sac from the anterior surface of the esophagus.

The mediastinum should be opened as high as possible in the hiatus, and sac dissection should be attempted in a blunt fashion. When sharp dissection is necessary, it is recommended to initiate this dissection somewhat distally on the sac, away from the gastro-esophageal junction. Although initially this might require sharp dissection of the first layer, further dissection can be performed bluntly.

32.6 Postoperative In-hospital Complications

Robotic assisted hiatal hernia repair generally is a fairly sterile and safe operation [8–13]. Aside from the risk of surgical site infection present in any surgery, there is a small risk of gastro-intestinal organ perforation with accompanying infection. The most common sources of perforation are torn fundoplication sutures, laceration by a surgical instrument, trocar perforation or ischemic perforation. These sources of infection should be recognized and treated intraoperatively as described above. Thermal damage, both to the esophagus or stomach should be avoided by dissection at distance from the organ wall. Short gastric vessel division should be performed at least 0.5 cm away from the gastric border. In case of obvious thermal damage to the stomach wall, one can consider plication or resection with a linear endoscopic stapler.

As in any surgery, postoperative elevation of C-reactive protein or leukocyte count can be expected but a postoperative ileus is abnormal in hiatal hernia surgery. Severe gastric dilatation due to emptying disorders may occur and should be treated with a nasogastric tube perhaps combined with a jejunal feeding tube. Although most of these resolve in just a few days to weeks, some problems may not resolve.

When an intra-abdominal infection is suspected, we advise CT imaging as the primary diagnostic method due to its high specificity for the diagnosis of any free fluid. Perforation of the esophagus and/or stomach can be diagnosed using an orally administered contrast agent prior to scanning after performance a non-contrasted scan for reference.

Suspected gastric perforation should be treated by re-laparoscopy, perforation closure or partial gastric resection and drainage. When a perforation of the esophagus is diagnosed, endoscopic stenting can be used to close the defect as well as possible. Concomitant mediastinal collections and pleural empyema require immediate drainage. When possible, this can be performed by radiologic intervention but a thoracoscopic procedure or lateral thoracotomy may be required for adequate drainage. This procedure often needs to be repeated several times in case of serious mediastinitis. Esophageal perforation can be treated with low mortality by continuous close and aggressive, often repetitive, invasive intervention. The hospital stay often takes numerous weeks and the time to full recovery is frequently over one year.

The development of an abscess may also occur without identification of an overt perforation. These abscesses are usually located in the mediastinum or just below the diaphragm on the left side. In the event that imaging studies do not reveal evidence of a perforation, percutaneous or laparoscopic drainage should be performed.

Moderate dysphagia is common after fundoplication and these complaints should diminish over time. As long as sufficient nutritional intake of any kind is assured, it is advisable to delay intervention for 6–8 weeks as these will commonly resolve without treatment. When intake is impossible or highly painful, early intervention should be considered. The most common reasons for dysphagia during the in-hospital period are an overly tight repair and/or recurrent hiatal hernia. Several diagnostic options are available under those circumstances. If complaints are sufficient to consider a recurrent hiatal hernia, CT scanning should be considered using both oral and intravenous contrast. If the suspicion instead is a fundoplication that is too tight, a barium swallow is the preferred diagnostic tool.

In-hospital hernia recurrence or complete blockage of food and fluids should be treated within days. The area is well accessible in the first two weeks after surgery, and reoperative surgery can usually be performed laparoscopically, preferably with robotic assistance.

32.7 Late Complications

Fundoplications are designed to provide a one-way valve to prevent the reflux of gastric contents at the gastro-esophageal junction. Many side effects of this treatment are directly related to the function of this newly created valve function, one of which is the prevention of belching. In some patients this can be debilitating due to air trapping, with aerophagia or ingestion of carbonated drinks that will aggravate these symptoms. This side effect is usually called gas bloat and is accompanied with increased flatulence.Postoperative treatment consists of efforts to prevent the entrance of air into the stomach. This is most easily managed by limiting the intake of carbonated drinks. In the case of true aerophagia, treatment is more involved due to the variety of etiologies of the problem, ranging from chewing gum to unconscious behavioral traits or psychiatric problems. The most effective method to prevent gas bloating is operatively tailoring the fundoplication to the patient. Numerous high quality studies have proven the superiority of a partial fundoplication over a 360 Nissen fundoplication [14–17], with equal long term reflux control and less gas bloating. Preoperative manometric testing will greatly aid in the preoperative decision-making process for each patient regarding whether a partial or full fundoplication is most appropriate.

In the instance of a para-esophageal hernia, the anatomical defect is most likely the cause of problems, and an anterior fundoplication after hiatal hernia repair can be sufficient to avoid reflux. This fundoplication is closest to the normal anatomy and will usually result in physiologic reflux without bloating due to air trapping. Many studies have been published on this subject that report excellent long-term results.

Recurrent reflux after fundoplication is often a symptom of recurrent hiatal hernia, and should be considered when a prior successful repair has now failed to relieve reflux symptoms. Studies [9, 16, 18–20] have identified that some form of radiologic recurrence is identified in 40%, symptomatic recurrence in 20% and reoperative surgery is necessary in 10% of patients. The use of mesh seems to result in less recurrence at the short term but has equivalent long-term results.

Patients may also complain of symptoms comparable to the preoperative situation, even in the absence of pathologic reflux. This often leads to the resumption of the use of antacid medication. In order to ascertain the correct etiology for the symptomatology there are several diagnostic tools available to identify the source of the situation including CT scanning, barium swallow and 24-h esophageal pH-measurement. CT imaging is most valuable to confirm the development of a recurrent hiatal hernia and it will often have sufficient resolution to confirm a failed fundoplication. A barium swallow series can be useful for confirming gastro-esophageal reflux and can also indicate a significant hiatal hernia but, like CT scanning, does not reveal reflux over time. A 24-h esophageal pH measurement provides the best evidence for recurrent reflux and is the investigational method of choice should there be a lack of demonstration of a failed prior repair as demonstrated by imaging techniques.

If a recurrent hiatal hernia or failed fundoplication is proven, the choice of treatment is up to the surgeon and more importantly, the patient. In some cases, reinstitution of acid suppression therapy will be sufficient, while in more severe cases another hiatal hernia repair with fundoplication will be required. It is important to note that patient satisfaction after reoperation decreases from 85–90% to 70% [20–23]. Reoperative surgery can be very challenging and should only be performed by surgeons with a high-volume reflux and hiatal hernia repair practice. The ability to perform primary antireflux surgery does not mean that one has to be able to treat recurrence; referral to centers specialized in reoperative surgery is worthy of consideration.

The effects and complications of the use of mesh in hiatoplasty is a major source of controversy in the literature [9, 24]. There are many types and shapes of mesh, which can be categorized as follows; pledgets (small patches), strips, horseshoe or V shaped, and circular mesh or reverse “C” shaped. Many types of materials have been used, mostly polypropylene, ePTFE and biologic or absorbable synthetic materials.

Over time, mesh contracts. In circumferential mesh shapes this can cause dysphagia or even erosion into the esophagus. Because of these risks, circular meshes should be avoided at all times.

Mesh erosion into the esophagus is the most feared complication after using mesh. This may result from contraction in circular meshes, but usually results from friction over the edge of a mesh that is not covered by diaphragmatic muscle. Mesh should therefore never be used to bridge a gap in the hiatus. The sole role for mesh is to support and strengthen a hiatal repair. In case of high tension on the repair, left or right collateral diaphragmatic incisions need to be made instead of bridging a gap with artificial material. A lateral incision can be covered with an asymmetric mesh with V shape to cover both hiatal repair and diaphragm incision.

Mesh erosion may initially be suspected due to the development of dysphagia. Usually the area is scarred, and low-grade infection is limited to the direct location of the mesh.

Parts of the mesh can occasionally be removed by endoscopic techniques. Mesh removal by laparoscopy or laparotomy is very difficult and will always result in an esophageal defect that needs to be closed. Oftentimes the damage is tremendous and partial esophageal resection is required. Mesh erosion with limited symptoms should perhaps be accepted without intervention in a clinically stable patient.

As previously described in the paragraph on intraoperative complications, vagal nerve injury is a known complication of hiatal hernia surgery and anti-reflux surgery.

The most common symptoms are dyspeptic complaints, delayed gastric emptying with troublesome intake and/or diarrhea. Any of these complaints are often recognized after the repair of huge hernias because of extensive dissection to create enough esophageal length.

The risk of vagal nerve damage is higher in reoperative hernia repair because it is more difficult to recognize the branches in the often very scarred tissue. The majority of symptoms resolve over time. Meanwhile, conservative treatment should include drugs with prokinetic effects; such as erythromycin, cisapride, metoclopramide or domperidon in combination with professional advice on intake. Improvement of symptoms can be expected up to two years after surgery.

In case of persistent and very severe symptoms of gastroparesis, laparoscopic (robot-assisted) pyloromyotomy or pyloroplasty [25, 26] may be considered, but results are only moderately successful. Serious delayed gastric emptying has to be proven before consideration of this intervention.

Persistent pain after hiatal hernia repair and fundoplication is relatively rare and difficult to treat. Most patients complain of shoulder pain immediately after surgery. This referred pain usually subsides after a few days but may persist sometimes in combination with pain in any abdominal compartment. If the anatomic repair is proven to be intact and reflux is absent, this pain is very difficult to treat. Revision of the repair is not advisable and pain medication in combination with paramedical treatment is the approach of choice.

Two sources of pain are worth mentioning. Dysphagia is often reported as abdominal pain; further in-depth questioning allows for easy distinction. The most important characteristic of dysphagia over other abdominal causes of pain is that the pain always occurs shortly after swallowing.

A second cause of abdominal pain is splenic infarction. The literature is lacking in evidence on the incidence of splenic infarction after fundoplication but is estimated at 1% [27–29].

The probable cause of these infarctions is ligation of the short gastric vessels during the creation of a fundoplication. The short gastric vessels are responsible for part of the arterial blood supply of the superior pole of the spleen. Generally speaking, the splenic artery will soon take over the blood supply and symptoms subside, however in some cases the ischemia leads to a splenic abscess with possible chronic pain.

32.8 Conclusion

As with all surgical procedures, adverse events can and will occur. The surgeon should be vigilant to identify these during and after the operation. Those specific to the hiatal hernia repair are discussed above and will aid the surgeon to identify and treat these potential problems.

References

1. Joris JL, Chiche JD, Lamy ML. Pneumothorax during laparoscopic fundoplication: diagnosis and treatment with positive end-expiratory pressure. Anesth Analg. 1995;81:993–1000.
2. Farlo J, Thawgathurai D, Mikhail M, et al. Cardiac tamponade during laparoscopic Nissen fundoplication. Eur J Anaesthesiol. 1998;15:246–7.
3. Swide CE, Nyberg PF. Cardiac trauma: an unusual cause of dysrhythmias and electrocardiographic changes during laparoscopic Nissen fundoplication. Anesthesiology. 1996;85:209–11.
4. Kemppainen E, Kiviluoto TEK. Fatal cardiac tamponade after emergency tension-free repair of a large paraesophageal hernia. Surg Endosc. 2000;14:593. https://doi.org/10.1007/s004640000138.
5. Watson I, de Beaux AC. Surgical endoscopy complications of laparoscopic antireflux surgery. Surg Endosc. 2001;15:131. https://doi.org/10.1007/s004640000346.
6. Lindeboom MYA, Ringers J, van Rijn PJJ, et al. Gastric emptying and vagus nerve function after laparoscopic partial fundoplication. Ann Surg. 2004;240:785–90. https://doi.org/10.1097/01.SLA.0000143124.30911.0F.
7. Low DE, Mercer CD, James EC, Hill LD. Post Nissen syndrome. Surg Gynecol Obstet. 1988;167:1–5.
8. Mertens AC, Tolboom RC, Zavrtanik H, et al. Morbidity and mortality in complex robot-assisted hiatal hernia surgery: 7-year experience in a high-volume center. Surg Endosc. 2018;1:3. https://doi.org/10.1007/s00464-018-6494-4.
9. Zhang C, Liu D, Li F, et al. Systematic review and meta-analysis of laparoscopic mesh versus suture repair of hiatus hernia: objective and subjective outcomes. Surg Endosc. 2017;31:4913–22. https://doi.org/10.1007/s00464-017-5586-x.
10. Gehrig T, Mehrabi A, Fischer L, et al. Robotic-assisted paraesophageal hernia repair—a case–control study. Langenbeck's Arch Surg. 2013;398:691–6. https://doi.org/10.1007/s00423-012-0982-0.
11. Tolboom R, Broeders I, Draaisma W. Robot-assisted laparoscopic hiatal hernia and antireflux surgery. J Surg Oncol. 2015;112:266–70. https://doi.org/10.1002/jso.23912.
12. Brenkman HJF, Parry K, Van Hillegersberg R, Ruurda JP. Robot-assisted laparoscopic hiatal hernia repair: promising anatomical and functional results. J Laparoendosc Adv Surg Tech A. 2016;26(6):465–9. https://doi.org/10.1089/lap.2016.0065.
13. Müller-Stich BP, Reiter MA, Mehrabi A, et al. No relevant difference in quality of life and functional outcome at 12 months' follow-up-a randomised controlled trial comparing robot-assisted versus conventional laparoscopic Nissen fundoplication. Langenbeck's Arch Surg. 2009;394:441–6. https://doi.org/10.1007/s00423-008-0446-8.
14. Broeders JAJL, Mauritz FA, Ahmed Ali U, et al. Systematic review and meta-analysis of laparoscopic Nissen (posterior total) versus Toupet (posterior partial) fundoplication for gastro-oesophageal reflux disease. Br J Surg. 2010;97:1318–30. https://doi.org/10.1002/bjs.7174.
15. Du X, Wu J-M, Hu Z-W, et al. Laparoscopic Nissen (total) versus anterior 180° fundoplication for gastro-esophageal reflux disease: a meta-analysis and systematic review. Medicine (Baltimore). 2017;96:e8085. https://doi.org/10.1097/MD.0000000000008085.

16. Roks DJ, Broeders JA, Baigrie RJ. Long-term symptom control of gastro-oesophageal reflux disease 12 years after laparoscopic Nissen or 180° anterior partial fundoplication in a randomized clinical trial. Br J Surg. 2017;104:852–6. https://doi.org/10.1002/bjs.10473.
17. Broeders JA, Roks DJ, Ahmed Ali U, et al. Laparoscopic anterior 180-degree versus nissen fundoplication for gastroesophageal reflux disease: systematic review and meta-analysis of randomized clinical trials. Ann Surg. 2013;257:850–9. https://doi.org/10.1097/SLA.0b013e31828604dd.
18. Oelschlager BK, Pellegrini CA, Hunter JG, et al. Biologic prosthesis to prevent recurrence after laparoscopic paraesophageal hernia repair: long-term follow-up from a multicenter, prospective, randomized trial. ACS. 2011;213:461–8. https://doi.org/10.1016/j.jamcollsurg.2011.05.017.
19. Granderath FA, Schweiger UM, Kamolz T, et al. Laparoscopic Nissen fundoplication with prosthetic hiatal closure reduces postoperative intrathoracic wrap herniation: preliminary results of a prospective randomized functional and clinical study. Arch Surg. 2005;140:40–8. https://doi.org/10.1001/archsurg.140.1.40.
20. Furnée EJB, Draaisma WA, Simmermacher RK, et al. Long-term symptomatic outcome and radiologic assessment of laparoscopic hiatal hernia repair. Am J Surg. 2010;199:695–701. https://doi.org/10.1016/j.amjsurg.2009.03.008.
21. Furnée EJB, Draaisma WA, Broeders IAMJ, Gooszen HG. Surgical reintervention after failed antireflux surgery: a systematic review of the literature. J Gastrointest Surg. 2009;13:1539–49. https://doi.org/10.1007/s11605-009-0873-z.
22. Gee DW, Andreoli MT, Rattner DW. Measuring the effectiveness of laparoscopic antireflux surgery. Arch Surg. 2008;143:482. https://doi.org/10.1001/archsurg.143.5.482.
23. Terry M, Smith CD, Branum GD, et al. Outcomes of laparoscopic fundoplication for gastroesophageal reflux disease and paraesophageal hernia. Surg Endosc. 2001;15:691–9. https://doi.org/10.1007/s004640080144.
24. Tam V, Winger DG, Nason KS. A systematic review and meta-analysis of mesh vs suture cruroplasty in laparoscopic large hiatal hernia repair. Am J Surg. 2016;211:226–38. https://doi.org/10.1016/j.amjsurg.2015.07.007.
25. Toro JP, Lytle NW, Patel AD, et al. Efficacy of laparoscopic pyloroplasty for the treatment of gastroparesis. J Am Coll Surg. 2014;218:652–60. https://doi.org/10.1016/j.jamcollsurg.2013.12.024.
26. Shada AL, Dunst CM, Pescarus R, et al. Laparoscopic pyloroplasty is a safe and effective first-line surgical therapy for refractory gastroparesis. Surg Endosc. 2016;30:1326–32. https://doi.org/10.1007/s00464-015-4385-5.
27. Wilkinson NW, Edwards K, Adams ED. Splenic infarction following laparoscopic nissen fundoplication: management strategies. JSLS. 2003;7(4):359–65.
28. Ipek T, Eyuboglu E, Ozben V. Partial splenic infarction as a complication of laparoscopic floppy Nissen fundoplication. J Laparoendosc Adv Surg Tech A. 2010;20:333–7. https://doi.org/10.1089/lap.2009.0409.
29. Martínez DG, Sánchez AW, García AP. Splenic abscess after laparoscopic Nissen fundoplication: a consequence of short gastric vessel division. Surg Laparosc Endosc Percutan Tech. 2008;18:82–5. https://doi.org/10.1097/SLE.0b013e318159e837.

Reoperation After Robotic Diaphragmatic Hernia Repair

33

Jordan A. Bilezikian, Robert G. Johnson, W. Borden Hooks III, and William W. Hope

33.1 Introduction

Laparoscopic fundoplication is the gold standard for surgical treatment of gastroesophageal reflux disease (GERD) [1] (Fig. 33.1). However, robotic surgery is increasing in many institutions due to the benefits of the robotic approach compared with traditional laparoscopy. These benefits include better visualization for the operator, better dexterity of hand motions translated through instruments, and better ergonomics [2]. Many studies have compared robotic diaphragmatic hernia repair with laparoscopic diaphragmatic hernia repair and have reported similar in-hospital

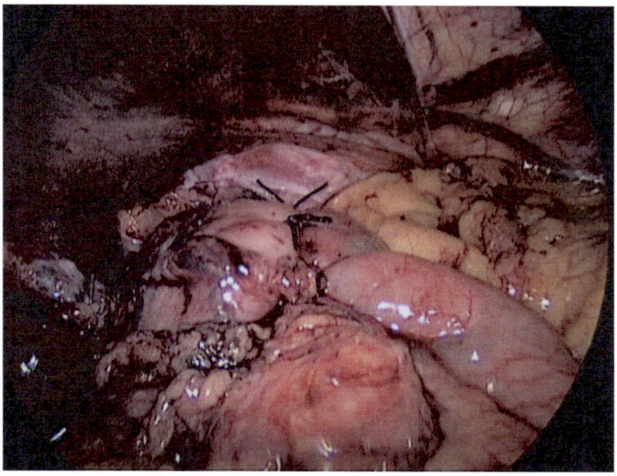

Fig. 33.1 Laparoscopic Nissen (360°) fundoplication performed for medically refractory GERD

J. A. Bilezikian (✉) · R. G. Johnson · W. Borden Hooks III · W. W. Hope
New Hanover Regional Medical Center, Wilmington, NC, USA
e-mail: Jordan.Bilezikian@nhrmc.org; Bobby.Johnson@nhrmc.org; Borden.Hooks@nhrmc.org; William.Hope@nhrmc.org

K. A. LeBlanc (ed.), *Robotic Assisted Hernia Repair*,
https://doi.org/10.1007/978-3-030-23025-8_33

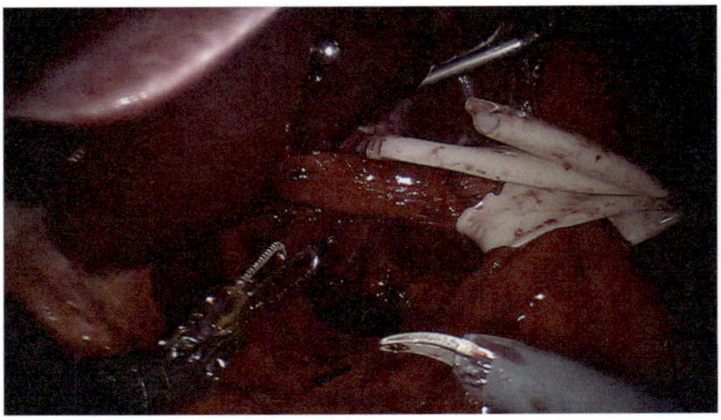

Fig. 33.2 Robotic Nissen (360°) fundoplication showing the esophageal mobilization and the good visualization possible with the robotic surgical approach

outcomes, postoperative quality of life, and functional outcomes [3–8]. Robotic reoperation after index operation failure is increasing as surgeons report that there is better visualization and easier dissection of anatomic planes [8]. Prospective studies with long term follow-up data are needed to guide surgical treatment during these difficult reoperations.

33.2 Rationale for Robotic Diaphragmatic Hernia Repair

Robotic diaphragmatic hernia repair is based on principles similar to laparoscopic repair and is described elsewhere in this book. Similar to other operations that have both laparoscopic and robotic approaches, the potential benefits of the robotic approach include better visualization, dexterity, and ergonomics [2] (Fig. 33.2). Benefits specific to diaphragmatic hernia repair include better visualization of relevant anatomy and easier dissection of difficult planes with potentially less risk of intraoperative complications [8]. Since many minimally invasive surgeons are increasing their robotic operative volumes, robotic surgery has become their default approach for selected operations.

33.3 Indications for Reoperative Diaphragmatic Hernia Repair

As with most hernia operations, the most common reason for reoperation is hernia recurrence (Fig. 33.3). However, unlike other types of recurrent hernias requiring reoperation, diaphragmatic hernia recurrences can be treated with conservative management in select patients. Conservative treatment can be justified in patients with mild to moderate symptoms. Severe dysphagia or recurrent reflux usually requires a reoperation. In a retrospective cohort study of 103 patients undergoing an antireflux operation at a single institution during a two-year period, the reasons for reoperation were dependent on the type of fundic wrap chosen in the index operation [9]. In patients undergoing a Nissen fundoplication, the most common reason was dysphagia, and in patients undergoing a Toupet, it was recurrent reflux [9].

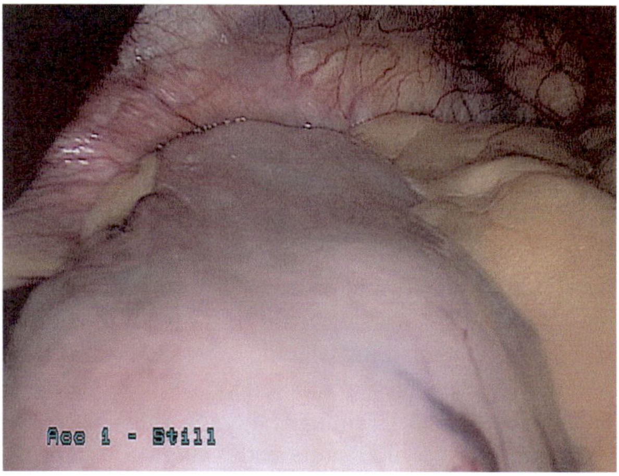

Fig. 33.3 Recurrent hiatal/paraesophageal hernia following robotic repair. The stomach is seen going through hiatal defect and into chest

33.4 Mechanism of Failures of Robotic Diaphragmatic Hernia Repair

Although no studies have analyzed robotic antireflux surgery failures, a consecutive series by Stein et al. of 105 patients delineated the causes of laparoscopic antireflux surgery failures [10]. In this study, technical factors and inappropriate patient selection were the most common reasons for failures of antireflux laparoscopic surgery [10]. More specifically, the reasons for failure were disruption of the initial antireflux procedure (46%), a displaced repair (23%), too-tight or too-long fundoplication (10%), an unrecognized motor disorder (9%), paraesophageal or axial herniation (6%), or gastric denervation (6%) [10]. Seventy-one of 105 patients required surgical revision, and the remaining 34 patients were treated with a conservative approach [10]. An intraoperative assessment of patients who required reoperation showed technical errors responsible for failure of the initial operation in 40 of 71 patients [10].

Other studies describe the failures and reoperation rates of laparoscopic antireflux surgery. Awais et al. retrospectively reviewed 275 patients undergoing redo surgery by thoracic surgeons for failed fundoplication and demonstrated that transmediastinal migration-recurrent hernia was the most common pattern of failure in 64% of patients [11]. Of note, the thoracic surgeons completing these complex redo esophageal antireflux operations had significant laparoscopic and open esophageal surgical experience [11].

Robotic antireflux surgery has mechanisms of failure similar to those listed above, which include disruption or displacement of original repair and improper fundoplication. Surgeons should analyze trends in their patients' technical failures that require reoperation and consider modifications to prevent future failures.

33.5 Treatment Options for Recurrent Diaphragmatic Hernia Following Robotic Repair: Overview of Strategies

As discussed, recurrent diaphragmatic hernias can be treated with reoperation or conservative therapy depending on symptom severity and other patient-specific factors. Reoperative repair presents unique challenges due to varying degrees of adhesions, inflammatory changes, and anatomic distortion (Fig. 33.4).

Reoperative diaphragmatic hernia repair applies principles similar to those described elsewhere in this book. The surgeon should obtain and review the previous operative notes. One should be aware of the original surgical approach, type of repair, aberrant anatomy, and intraoperative complications that occurred.

The surgeon's previous experience with reoperative approaches plays an important role in surgical planning and preoperative decision making. After consideration of all patient-specific factors and a surgical approach is chosen, three criteria are essential for a successful reoperation. These are: a complete takedown of the previous repair with identification of the normal anatomy, recognition of a short esophagus, and proper placement of the new fundoplication [11].

33.6 Open Repair

Open diaphragmatic hernia repair is increasingly rare as a primary fundoplication operation. However, it is still the most common approach for reoperations for recurrent diaphragmatic hernias. Although many general surgeons trained using open approaches, there is currently more use of the laparoscopic and robotic technique. Thoracic surgeons may have more experience with open diaphragmatic hernia repairs depending on their established practice. In some cases, thoracic approaches may be preferred in reoperative settings. When surgeons are not comfortable using these approaches, consultation with a thoracic surgeon may be warranted.

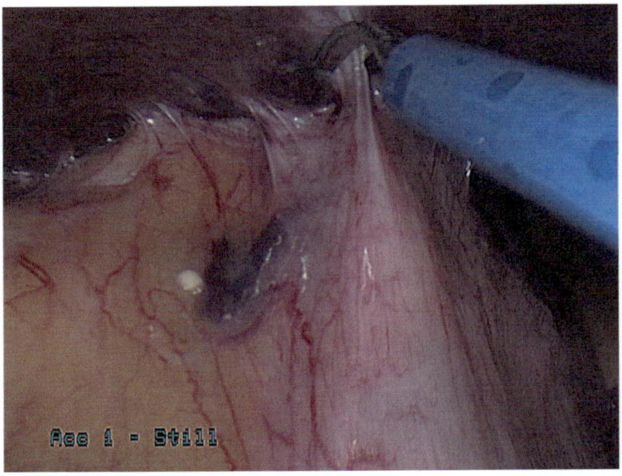

Fig. 33.4 Reoperative hiatal hernia repair with severe adhesions of stomach to liver requiring meticulous sharp dissection

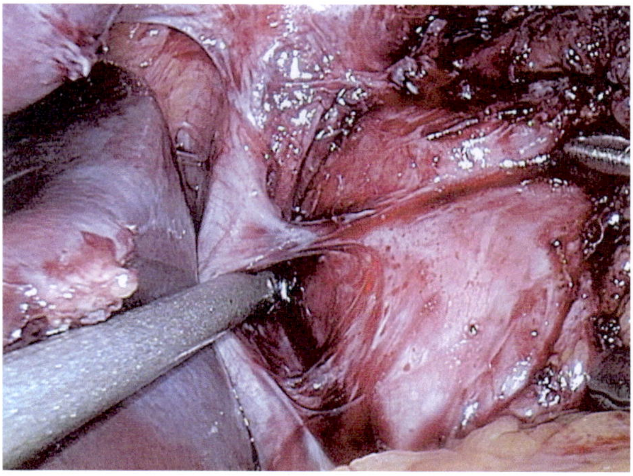

Fig. 33.5 Dissection of right crus. Previously done wrap has slipped/migrated above the crus and must be reduced. Tissue planes can often be difficult in reoperative foregut surgery, and careful delineation of the anatomy is crucial for a successful outcome

The patient's risk factors for undergoing an open repair must be considered, as should the risk/benefits of undergoing an invasive operation with increased risk of morbidity and increased hospital length of stay. Open repair is a fairly common reoperative approach, unless the surgeon is more experienced with reoperations using a laparoscopic/minimally invasive modality.

33.7 Laparoscopic Repair

Laparoscopic repair appears to be declining in usage for recurrent diaphragmatic hernias due to the advent of robotic technology in many institutions. Reoperative laparoscopic fundoplications have a significantly higher morbidity than primary laparoscopic fundoplications [12]. This is due to the complex nature of this procedure, the difficulty to clearly delineate tissue planes, and distorted anatomy due to the initial operation and resultant adhesions (Fig. 33.5). However, the surgeon may decide that the original repair failure is more easily repaired using a laparoscopic approach. The laparoscopic approach may be selected when a surgeon is well trained in this approach for reoperations and does not anticipate benefits in overall morbidity by using an open approach.

33.8 Robotic Repair

Robotic repair for recurrent diaphragmatic hernia is a reasonable surgical approach. Although some studies have demonstrated higher costs and longer operative times for robotic surgery, in general [13–15], there are potential benefits with robotic surgery for reoperations in these complex cases [13]. As previously stated, reoperative laparoscopic diaphragmatic hernia repair has higher morbidity than primary laparoscopic repair. It is assumed that robotic surgery is similar. Interestingly, in a recent

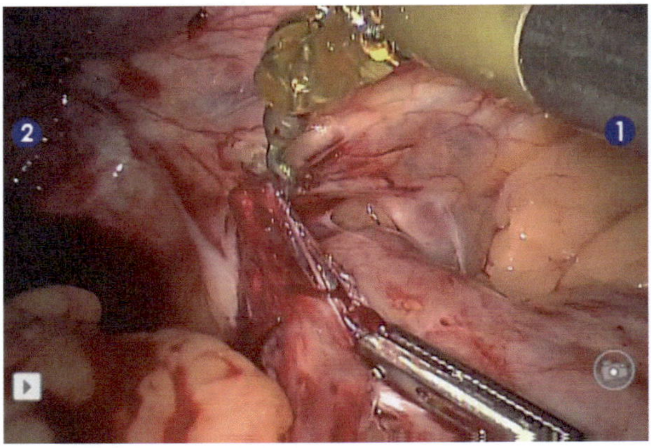

Fig. 33.6 Robotic repair of recurrent hiatal hernia following previous robotic repair. Improved visibility and dexterity are beneficial with complex foregut reoperations

5-year retrospective review of 200 patients undergoing primary or reoperative robotic antireflux surgery, the robotic approach showed minimal morbidity [12].

Open repair is usually selected as the approach of choice in these reoperations due to better exposure of the operative field compared with laparoscopic repair. Better visualization using the robotic approach may obviate this as a benefit of open surgery. A recent study by Tolboom et al. included 75 patients at a single institution undergoing redo surgery for recurrent GERD-related symptoms or dysphagia [16]. Thirty patients underwent a standard laparoscopic redo operation, and the remaining 45 patients underwent a robot-assisted operation [16]. The robotic group had more patients who had undergone an open index procedure [16]. This study demonstrated that early postoperative complication rates were similar and that conversion to open surgery occurred more often when using laparoscopic approaches compared with robotic approaches. [16] Robotic repair for reoperation of antireflux surgery has several benefits to the surgeon experienced in minimally invasive/robotic techniques (Fig. 33.6).

33.9 Conclusions

As surgeons strive to optimize surgical technique and patient outcomes, reoperations for recurrent diaphragmatic hernias are inevitable. Repairs fail due to technical failure factors and risk factors inherent in improper patient selection. The decision whether to reoperate depends on the patient's severity of symptoms and patient-related risk factors. Although the optimal approach has not been categorically demonstrated, most surgeons use an open approach while some choose laparoscopic or robotic approaches. Ultimately, this selection is based on surgeon experience with the different approaches and patient-specific factors such as complexity of the original operation and type of wrap performed. While there is some evidence suggesting that robotic repair of recurrent diaphragmatic hernia has some benefits, large, prospective, randomized studies are needed to identify long term outcomes.

References

1. Stefanidis D, Hope WW, Kohn GP, Reardon PR, Richardson WS, Fanelli RD, et al. Guidelines for surgical treatment of gastroesophageal reflux disease. Surg Endosc. 2010;24:2647–69. https://doi.org/10.1007/s00464-010-1267-8.
2. Lanfranco AR, Castellanos AE, Desai JP, Meyers WC. Robotic surgery: a current perspective. Ann Surg. 2004;239:14–21. https://doi.org/10.1097/01.sla.0000103020.19595.7d.
3. Draaisma WA, Buskens E, Bais JE, Simmermacher RK, Rijnhart-de Jong HG, Broeders IA, et al. Randomized clinical trial and follow-up study of cost-effectiveness of laparoscopic versus conventional Nissen fundoplication. Br J Surg. 2006;93:690–7. https://doi.org/10.1002/bjs.5354.
4. Markar SR, Karthikesalingam AP, Hagen ME, Talamini M, Horgan S, Wagner OJ. Robotic vs. laparoscopic Nissen fundoplication for gastro-oesophageal reflux disease: systematic review and meta-analysis. Int J Med Robot. 2010;6:125–31. https://doi.org/10.1002/rcs.309.
5. Morino M, Pellegrino L, Giaccone C, Garrone C, Rebecchi F. Randomized clinical trial of robot-assisted versus laparoscopic Nissen fundoplication. Br J Surg. 2006;93:553–8. https://doi.org/10.1002/bjs.5325.
6. Muller-Stich BP, Reiter MA, Wente MN, Bintintan VV, Koninger J, Buchler MW, et al. Robot-assisted versus conventional laparoscopic fundoplication: short-term outcome of a pilot randomized controlled trial. Surg Endosc. 2007;21:1800–5. https://doi.org/10.1007/s00464-007-9268-y.
7. Muller-Stich BP, Reiter MA, Mehrabi A, Wente MN, Fischer L, Koninger J, et al. No relevant difference in quality of life and functional outcome at 12 months' follow-up-a randomised controlled trial comparing robot-assisted versus conventional laparoscopic Nissen fundoplication. Langenbeck's Arch Surg. 2009;394:441–6. https://doi.org/10.1007/s00423-008-0446-8.
8. Rebecchi F, Allaix ME, Morino M. Robotic technological aids in esophageal surgery. J Visc Surg. 2017;3:7. https://doi.org/10.21037/jovs.2017.01.09.
9. Jensen JS, Antonsen HK, Durup J. Two years of experience with robot-assisted anti-reflux surgery: a retrospective cohort study. Int J Surg. 2017;39:260–6. https://doi.org/10.1016/j.ijsu.2017.02.014.
10. Stein HJ, Feussner H, Siewert JR. Failure of antireflux surgery: causes and management strategies. Am J Surg. 1996;171:36–9. https://doi.org/10.1016/S0002-9610(99)80070-1.
11. Awais O, Luketich JD, Schuchert MJ, Morse CR, Wilson J, Gooding WE, et al. Reoperative antireflux surgery for failed fundoplication: an analysis of outcomes in 275 patients. Ann Thorac Surg. 2011;92:1083–9. https://doi.org/10.1016/j.athoracsur.2011.02.088.
12. Elmously A, Gray KD, Ullmann TM, Fahey TJ, Afaneh C, Zarnegar R. Robotic reoperative anti-reflux surgery: low perioperative morbidity and high symptom resolution. World J Surg. 2018;42(12):4014–21. https://doi.org/10.1007/s00268-018-4708-5.
13. Ceccarelli G, Patriti A, Biancafarina A, Spaziani A, Bartoli A, Bellochi R, et al. Intraoperative and postoperative outcome of robot-assisted and traditional laparoscopic Nissen fundoplication. Eur Surg Res. 2009;43:198–203. https://doi.org/10.1159/000223751.
14. Heemskerk J, van Gemert WG, Greve JW, Bouvy ND. Robot-assisted versus conventional laparoscopic Nissen fundoplication: a comparative retrospective study on costs and time consumption. Surg Laparosc Endosc Percutan Tech. 2007;17:1–4. https://doi.org/10.1097/01.sle.0000213756.76761.b7.
15. Nakadi IE, Melot C, Closset J, DeMoor V, Betroune K, Feron P, et al. Evaluation of da Vinci Nissen fundoplication clinical results and cost minimization. World J Surg. 2006;30:1050–4. https://doi.org/10.1007/s00268-005-7950-6.
16. Tolboom RC, Draaisma WA, Broeders IA. Evaluation of conventional laparoscopic versus robot-assisted laparoscopic redo hiatal hernia and antireflux surgery: a cohort study. J Robot Surg. 2016;10:33–9. https://doi.org/10.1007/s11701-016-0558-z.

Index

K. A. LeBlanc (ed.), *Robotic Assisted Hernia Repair*,
https://doi.org/10.1007/978-3-030-23025-8

J

L

MIX
Papier aus verantwortungsvollen Quellen
Paper from responsible sources
FSC® C105338
FSC
www.fsc.org

If you have any concerns about our products,
you can contact us on
ProductSafety@springernature.com

In case Publisher is established outside the EU,
the EU authorized representative is:
Springer Nature Customer Service Center GmbH
Europaplatz 3, 69115 Heidelberg, Germany

Printed by Libri Plureos GmbH
in Hamburg, Germany